Fundamental Orthopedic
Management for the
Physical Therapist Assistant

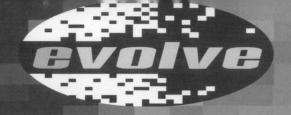

The Latest *Evolution* in Learning.

Evolve provides online access to free learning resources and activities designed specifically for the textbook you are using in your class. The resources will provide you with information that enhances the material covered in the book and much more.

Visit the Web address listed below to start your learning evolution today!

▶▶ **LOGIN:** *http://evolve.elsevier.com/Shankman/orthopedic/*

Evolve Instuctor Learning Resources for Shankman: *Fundamental Orthopedic Management for the Physical Therapist Assistant* offers the following features:

- **Electronic Image Collection**
  Search, view, and download the selection of hundreds of images from the textbook. Instructors can print out the majority of images from the book or transform them into PowerPoint slides for use in class.

- **Dissection and Cadaver Image Collection**
  View and download this selection of 28 images from Jacob S: Anatomy: A Dissection Manual and Atlas. Churchill Livingstone, 1996.

- **WebLinks**
  An exciting resource that lets you link to hundreds of websites carefully chosen to supplement the content of the textbook. The WebLinks are regularly updated, with new ones added as they develop.

- **Suggestion Box**
  An opportunity to submit your suggested improvements to the text to the author for possible inclusion in the next edition.

NOTE: Instructors should check with their sales representative for turther information.

Evolve Student Learning Resources for Shankman: *Fundamental Orthopedic Management for the Physical Therapist Assistant* offers the following features:

- **WebLinks**
  An exciting resource that lets you link to hundreds of websites carefully chosen to supplement the content of the textbook. The WebLinks are regularly updated, with new ones added as they develop.

- **Suggestion Box**
  An opportunity to submit your suggested improvements to the text to the author for possible inclusion in the next edition.

Think outside the book... evolve.

Fundamental Orthopedic Management for the Physical Therapist Assistant

GARY A. SHANKMAN, PTA
Floyd Medical Center
Rome, Georgia
Floyd Outpatient Rehabilitation Center
Rome, Georgia

SECOND EDITION

*with **454** illustrations*

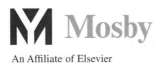

Mosby

An Affiliate of Elsevier

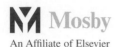
An Affiliate of Elsevier

11830 Westline Industrial Drive
St. Louis, Missouri 63146

FUNDAMENTAL ORTHOPEDIC MANAGEMENT FOR THE
PHYSICAL THERAPIST ASSISTANT, SECOND EDITION

ISBN 0-323-02002-X

NOTICE

Physical therapy is an ever-changing field. Standard safety precautions must be followed, but as
new research and clinical experience broaden our knowledge, changes in treatment and drug
therapy may become necessary or appropriate. Readers are advised to check the most current
product information provided by the manufacturer of each drug to be administered to verify the
recommended dose, the method and duration of administration, and contraindications. It is the
responsibility of the licensed prescriber, relying on experience and knowledge of the patient, to
determine dosages and the best treatment for each individual patient. Neither the publisher nor the
author assumes any liability for any injury and/or damage to persons or property arising from this
publication.

Previous edition copyrighted 1997

Library of Congress Cataloging-in-Publication Data

Shankman, Gary A.
    Fundamental orthopedic management for the physical therapist assistant / Gary A.
Shankman.— 2nd ed.
        p. ; cm.
    Includes bibliographical references and index.
    ISBN 0-323-02002-X (alk. paper)
     1. Orthopedics. 2. Physical therapy. 3. Physical therapy assistants. I. Title.
    [DNLM: 1. Orthopedic Procedures. 2. Allied Health Personnel. 3. Physical Therapy
Techniques. WE 168 S527f 2004]
    RD731.S5513 2004
    616.7—dc22

                                                                                        2003070637

Acquisitions Editor: Marion Waldman
Developmental Editor: Marjory Fraser
Publishing Services Manager: Patricia Tannian
Project Manager: Sharon Corell
Design Manager: Gail Morey Hudson

Printed in China

Last digit is the print number: 9 8 7 6 5 4 3 2 1

Contributors

MITCHELL A. COLLINS, EdD, FACSM
Professor
Department of Health, Physical Education, and Sport Science
Kennesaw State University
Kennesaw, Georgia

SANDRA ESKEW CAPPS, PT
Instructional Designer
Medical College of Georgia
Augusta, Georgia

GARY A. SHANKMAN, PTA
Floyd Medical Center
Rome, Georgia
Floyd Outpatient Rehabilitation Center
Rome, Georgia

In loving memory of my parents
Arthur and **Yvonne Shankman**

To my sons
Kyle, Tyler, and **Jordan**

To my grandson
Trevor

To my extended family
Clark, Mandy, and **Payne**

To my wife
Pebbles
my heart and soul, my best friend,
my purpose, and my teacher

Foreword to the First Edition

In the past, the duties and activities that surrounded the orthopedic management of a patient have existed solely within the purview of the physical therapist. The physical therapist assistant had little or no contribution to the process of evaluating a patient's functional status and usually was expected to follow the directions of the attending physical therapist with little room for modification. Tradition dictated that the physical therapist assume responsibility for the majority of a patient's treatment, with the delegation of only minor tasks to the physical therapist assistant. In the past, the physical therapist assistant did not really need to be concerned with the processes for the appropriate orthopedic management of a patient as such matters were handled exclusively by the physical therapist. The present, however, requires a different mode of operation and a different set of expectations for the physical therapist assistant.

The contemporary scheme of orthopedic management has evolved from the traditional system to a newer system of managed care. The physical therapist is still directly responsible for the disposition of a patient's treatment, but delegates as many clinical management duties as are possible to the physical therapist assistant. The current real world expectation for orthopedic management is this "evaluate and delegate" model for physical therapist and physical therapist assistant practice. Although this new model certainly expands the scope of practice for the physical therapist assistant, it also requires much more clinical responsibility in the management of patients who have orthopedic disorders. Such new responsibility requires knowledge, which is the purpose of this book.

Fundamental Orthopedic Management for the Physical Therapist Assistant is the first text that consolidates the orthopedic knowledge expected of the physical therapist assistant under the new "evaluate and delegate" model of clinical physical therapy care. The author, Gary A. Shankman, PTA, is very well experienced and qualified as an expert in the arena of orthopedic management and does an excellent job of presenting the important information contained in this book in a clear and comprehensive manner. Mastery of the knowledge presented in this text will help to ensure that physical therapist assistants meet, if not exceed, the expectations for their clinical role in the modern system of orthopedic health care.

Kent E. Timm, PhD, PT, SCS, OCS, ATC, FACSM
St. Luke's Healthcare Association
Saginaw, Michigan

Foreword to the Second Edition

Fundamental Orthopedic Management for the Physical Therapist Assistant, second edition, establishes a standard of excellence for physical therapist assistant (PTA) texts. Gary Shankman is a PTA with a passion for educating and writing and an understanding of what knowledge PTAs need to successfully treat orthopedic conditions. This book establishes a foundation on which to build the orthopedic knowledge and skills of the student and expands the knowledge and skills of the practicing PTA clinician. The Appendixes alone contain a wealth of reference information that can be used on a daily basis in the clinic.

Between the publication of the first edition of this text and the second edition, the profession of physical therapy experienced a small earthquake. This earthquake came in the form of the American Physical Therapy Association's (APTA) *Guide to Physical Therapist Practice*. While many in our profession have not begun to appreciate the far-reaching effects of the *Guide*, Gary Shankman incorporates the *Guide to Physical Therapist Practice* in his text. He strives to use the *Guide* to assist PTAs in identifying common elements of examination, evaluation, and assessment within the scope of practice for the PTA. In helping the PTA apply the language of the *Guide* to physical assessment procedures, Gary Shankman acknowledges that it is essential that the physical therapist and PTA speak the same language to provide successful physical therapy treatment.

The inclusion of Orthopedic Pharmacology adds to the value of this text. Understanding basic pharmacologic concepts is important for the delivery of safe and effective physical therapy interventions. With the addition of chapters on physical agents, connective tissue, neurovascular healing, and biomechanics, Gary Shankman has written in a clear and concise manner a text that should be on every clinic reference shelf.

Lola Sicard Rosenbaum, PT, MHS, OCS
Cantrell Center for Physical Therapy and Sports Medicine
Warner Robins, Georgia

Preface to the First Edition

Within the discipline of physical therapy, "orthopedics has emerged as the largest specialty group,"[1] requiring that the physical therapist assistant play a key role in the care of patients suffering from injury or disease of the musculoskeletal system. An introduction to basic concepts and applied principles of orthopedics is necessary for the physical therapist assistant (PTA), who needs a source for learning the key elements consistent with responsible, appropriate rehabilitation team management of patient care. Yet there have been very few texts written specifically for the PTA student and the practicing PTA clinician. This text responds to the absence of appropriate textbooks, intending to fill this long-neglected void in PTA education, and will serve as a primary resource, supplemental guide, and valuable reference.

Current popular orthopedic texts used in both physical therapy and physical therapist assistant education focus on comprehensive, objective evaluation procedures, differential diagnosis, and the development of treatment plans related to anatomy, biomechanics, and pathophysiology of injury. Care has been taken throughout this text to focus instead on fundamental, basic scientific principles, as well as on clinical applications of physical therapy interventions related to the scope and use of the physical therapist assistant. It is the intent and design of this text that the reader immediately recognize this focus on the application of fundamental orthopedic physical therapy principles.[1,2,4,5]

Additionally, this text seeks to show the student and the clinician that individual differences exist between patients experiencing the same general pathology. A consistent effort is made to clearly identify the interrelationship between soft tissue and bone healing time constraints, severity of injury, methods of immobilization or bone fixation, as well as the outgoing evaluation and reassessment procedures used to design a precise, individualized treatment plan. This element necessitates the introduction of individual criteria-based rehabilitation programs applying tissue healing mechanisms and the patient's individual tolerance (or intolerance) to advance in physical therapy interventions.[6] Yet a specific presentation of a clearly defined treatment protocol does not expose the PTA to the many complex variables the physical therapist takes into account when designing an appropriate plan of care for each patient. For this reason specific protocols have been omitted throughout this text. In the presence of so many conflicting opinions about how to manage the same injury or disease, it becomes necessary to define the intent of specific protocols rather than the protocols themselves.

Those familiar with physical therapy departments or outpatient clinics recognize that many different protocols exist for the same pathology, each influenced by the training and practical experiences of the physicians and physical therapists involved. In order to minimize conflicts of opinion on this subject, I decided to focus on aiding the physical therapist assistant in understanding the fact that many complex factors dictate patient care following injury, surgery, or disease of the musculoskeletal system. Most important for the PTA is the ability to first recognize the patient's individual response to treatment and then, after consultation with the physical therapist, to modify, add, or delete the treatment procedures of the physical therapy plan of care.

To achieve this result, the text strives to actively involve the reader in the concept of *teamwork* in the care of all patients. An often overused term and under-applied concept, *teamwork*, is necessary to successful patient care. In each chapter the need for immediate, open, accurate, and purposeful communication between the physical therapist assistant, physical therapist, patient, and others in made clear to highlight the interdependance of all team members in patient care. In all, the PTA must realize that the elements of effective and responsible patient supervision, understanding the mechanisms affecting musculoskeletal tissue healing, and communication with other rehab team members all play a critical role in developing individual treatment plans. This text gives the instructor, student, and clinician greater freedom to investigate and critically analyze rationale for treatment progression.

The body of the text is organized into eighteen chapters, each evolving to include more complex and practical applications. Chapter one, "Patient Supervision and Observation During Treatment," introduces a concept vital to the assistant's scope of practice: patient care is a *shared responsibility*, and the physical therapist assistant must assume a proactive role in that responsibility. Chapters two through five move on to develop rudimentary concepts of flexibility, strength, endurance, balance, and coordination, with specific references to applying these basic scientific principles to orthopedic physical therapy.

Because it is clinically relevant for the assistant to appreciate the magnitude of the events and factors that influence healing and, ultimately, the course of physical therapy treatment, chapters six through nine introduce appropriate concepts of injury and repair of musculoskeletal tissue. The relationships of injury, disease, surgery, and immobilization to restoration of motion, strength, and function are consistently emphasized. Chapter eleven outlines and describes fundamentals of peripheral joint mobilization. The appropriate use of specific joint mobilization techniques are quite useful for pain reduction and for enhancing joint motion, and in clinical practice the physical therapist may elect to have the assistant perform patient set-up and provide select techniques to peripheral joints. Clinical instructors, students, and practicing clinicians may effectively use the fundamental principles found in this chapters to enhance specific goals of treatment.

The foundation of this text appears in chapters twelve through eighteen. In these chapters the foot and ankle, knee, hip, spine and pelvis, shoulder, elbow, and the wrist and hand are reviewed in sequence. The chapters introduce the reader to the common soft tissue injuries, fractures, and diseases of each area. Although examples of surgery for specific injuries are included, the emphasis is on rehabilitation treatment options used to reduce pain and swelling, increase motion and strength, enhance balance and proprioception, and ultimately, to restore purposeful function.

As important as it is to discuss what this text is, it is equally important to identify what it is not. Although this text provides essential, practical information related to afflictions of the musculoskeletal system appropriate to the scope of the physical therapist assistant, it does not substantially cover anatomy, physiology, kinesiology, or include a comprehensive review of all musculoskeletal injuries. It is imperative, therefore, that the student or practicing clinician thoroughly study and review these essential subjects prior to and throughout the study of this text.[1-5] Those who have already acquired, or are in the process of acquiring, familiarity with these fundamental areas will find this text's focus on the application of fundamental orthopedic physical principles a great compliment to the pursuit of increased information, awareness, and knowledge. This textbook was written solely for the physical therapist assistant using the experience, education, and clinical perspective of a practicing physical therapist assistant, and I hope this book will be judged by instructors and readers to be the solution to the problem of finding appropriate textbooks for PTA curricula.

Gary A. Shankman

SUGGESTED READINGS

1. Donatelli R, Wooden MJ: Orthopaedic Physical Therapy. New York, Churchill Livingstone, 1989.
2. Kisner C, Colby LA: Therapeutic Exercise: Foundations and Techniques, 2nd ed. Philadelphia, FA Davis, 1990.
3. Lippert L: Clinical Kinesiology for Physical Therapist Assistants, 2nd ed. Philadelphia, FA Davis, 1994.
4. Norkin C, Levangie P: Joint Structure and Function: A Comprehensive Analysis, 2nd ed. Philadelphia, FA Davis, 1992.
5. Richardson JK, Iglarsh ZA: Clinical Orthopaedic Physical Therapy. Philadelphia, WB Saunders, 1994.
6. Timm KE: Knee. In Richardson JK, Iglarsh ZA (eds): Clinical Orthopaedic Physical Therapy. Philadelphia, WB Saunders, 1994.

Preface to the Second Edition

The second edition of *Fundamental Orthopedic Management for the Physical Therapist Assistant* has been expanded from 18 chapters to 24 chapters.

Within Part I, two new essential chapters have been added as key components of efficient and effective physical therapy intervention. The first new chapter—The Role of the Physical Therapist Assistant in Physical Assessment—incorporates and applies language consistent with the *Guide to Physical Therapist Practice*. The chapter strives to identify common elements of examination, evaluation, and assessment within the scope of practice of the physical therapist assistant.

In addition, this new chapter provides practice patterns and techniques of systems review and a systems approach to physical assessment. Key components of data collection, documentation, and modification of the plan of care are presented. Other texts may mention or suggest concepts related to physical assessment and evaluation, but generally they lack the central theme of essential, practical, and purposeful information consistent with the clinical practice and expectations of the physical therapist assistant.

The other new chapter addition to Part I is Physical Agents Used in the Treatment of Common Musculoskeletal Conditions. The therapeutic application of various physical agents constitutes core knowledge in all clinical settings for the physical therapist assistant. Basic physiology and physics related to thermal and electrotherapeutic agents are covered along with supporting physical and physiologic theory and evidence. Selection of appropriate physical agents according to their response characteristics and clinical applications in treating various musculoskeletal conditions represent a key feature of this chapter, as well as spanning the gap between basic science and clinical utility.

Within Part I, chapters on flexibility, strength, endurance, balance, and coordination remain. However, in response to suggestions regarding the first edition, a section on Strength Training for Younger Populations with subsections on physiologic adaptations, injury risk, and relevant clinical applications has been added.

Part II has been enhanced with the addition of a new chapter—Composition and Function of Connective Tissue. The general cellular response to injury is addressed. Cell structure, repair, and regeneration are introduced, as well as cell signaling molecules, cytokines, and growth factors and their involvement in inflammation, fibroplasia, coagulation, remodeling, and tissue maturation. Part II has been further expanded to include a new chapter—Neurovascular Healing and Thromboembolic Disease.

The highly complex and sophisticated interrelationship between bone and soft tissue healing would not be complete without a discussion of neurovascular anatomy, vascular supply to peripheral nerve tissue, the mechanical behavior of nerves; the structure and composition of vascular tissue; as well as the signs, symptoms, and pathophysiology of thromboembolic disease.

Substantial updated and relevant material has been added to chapters on ligament healing, bone healing, cartilage healing, and muscle and tendon healing. I believe that Part II is of significant importance to all students, educators, and practicing clinicians. An effort has been made therefore to unite the basic science of bone and soft tissue injury and repair with the application of specific therapeutic interventions that parallel time healing constraints as well as criteria-based rehabilitation programs. Whereas some popular texts focus on technical delivery of "protocols," I strongly believe that an understanding of healing characteristics of musculoskeletal tissues greatly enhances the delivery of physical therapy services by broadening the scope of awareness of the intricate and complex relationship between injury, repair, healing, and rehabilitation.

Perhaps a deviation from traditional texts, a brief, cursory, albeit important introduction to pharmacology is presented in a new chapter—Concepts of Orthopedic Pharmacology. General terms and concepts are introduced to students and practicing clinicians regarding pharmacokinetics, antibiotics, infections, bacterial adherence to orthopedic implants, corticosteroids, and nonsteroidal antiinflammatory drugs.

Two key topics discussed are infections and antiinflammatory medications. The clinical importance and awareness of the delivery of various medications used in orthopedic infectious and inflammatory conditions cannot be overstated. I feel that it is important for students, educators, and practicing physical therapist assistants not to lose focus of the significant role that therapeutic medications play in orthopedics. The very foundation of acute and chronic pain management and infection control is based on the appropriate and judicious use of medications.

In concert with understanding the physics and physiology of physical agents to control pain and inflammation, it is imperative to appreciate terms and definitions and be exposed to various rudimentary concepts related to orthopedic infection and antiinflammatory medications. Although this chapter is not designed by any means to be a comprehensive review of all medications used in orthopedics, it is meant to establish an awareness of how drugs are delivered; how different antiinfective drugs exert their actions against specific organisms; how organisms adhere to implants; and how and why steroids are used versus nonsteroidal antiinflammatory drugs to control pain and inflammation. Once again, the rationale for presenting this information is not only to expand the student's awareness but also more importantly to involve the application of basic science with the student's abilities to provide various physical therapy interventions.

A new section—Biomechanical Basis for Movement—has been added to substantially enhance the students' understanding of the complexities of fundamental orthopedic sciences. This new addition provides students, educators, and clinicians with foundations governing the principles of human movement. As an introductory chapter, Biomechanics will build on previous sections regarding basic science and will "set the stage" for the body of the text, which involves application of therapeutic interventions for various orthopedic afflictions.

Each chapter in this new edition includes multiple choice, labeling, short answer, essay, fill-in, and true/false questions and pertinent critical thinking applications with case study development, role playing activities, and application of therapeutic interventions consistent with the body of the text.

The design method used in developing the review questions lends itself to concept exploration, independent thinking, and student collaboration through critical thinking questions that foster interaction and stimulate comprehension of fundamental principles.

An Appendix has been added to include listings of common medications, laboratory reference ranges for commonly used tests, lab values with explanation of results, units of measurement and terminology in exercise science, as well as common fracture eponyms.

This text is further enhanced with the addition of the Evolve website, which includes the unique features of human cadaver dissection slides and an electronic image collection of reference figures found in the text. Also included are a number of generic physical therapy Web-Links, which instructors and students will find highly useful. The Evolve website is a regularly updated developmental tool that will further serve as an essential adjunct to the text for instructors, students, and clinicians. Updated relevant orthopedic science information, case studies, and therapeutic applications will be added over time.

I think that this second edition will serve to stimulate students to more fully appreciate the complexity of and relationships among all disciplines of orthopedic medicine. Although the second edition is certainly not a comprehensive text, I am confident that the new additions will greatly enhance and broaden the scope of understanding of students and clinicians involved in orthopedic physical therapy.

Gary A. Shankman

Acknowledgments

This edition would not be possible without the professional wisdom, creativity, and talents from everyone at Elsevier.

Without question, Marjory I. Fraser, Senior Developmental Editor for Health Professions at Elsevier in Philadelphia, has personally directed each and every step in the creation of this work. Her leadership, organization, timely suggestions, and attention to detail are truly noteworthy of praise and respect.

A very special and sincere thank you to Sharon Corell and her co-workers at Elsevier in St. Louis for their attention to detail, diligence, and profound patience during many weeks of hard work putting this project together.

Carol DiBerardino is an extraordinary talent. She was able to decipher my unintelligible ramblings and compile them into a structured, organized, and formal document. Always on time, professional beyond reproach, eager to offer suggestions (all of which were appropriate, clear, concise, and useful); I could not have written this text without her.

Sandra Eskew Capps is a true friend. Without any reservation or hesitation whatsoever, she eagerly agreed to contribute two new chapters. Her knowledge, keen insight, skills, talents, and experience as a physical therapist and educator have added immeasurably to the substance and quality of this text. She agreed to complete this work while moving to a new city to begin a new chapter in her life as an instructional designer for the physical therapy program at the Medical College of Georgia. At the same time, she was caring for her children on her own because her husband was out of the country. I am indeed grateful and fortunate to call Sandy my friend and colleague.

Dr. Mitchell Collins' new chapter entitled "Biomechanical Basis for Movement" has greatly enhanced the core knowledge of this text. A widely respected educator in exercise science and sought-after speaker, Dr. Collins agreed to undertake this task while lecturing in Brazil. Such unselfish sharing of his valuable time and expansive knowledge of the subject is exceeded only by his kindness, friendship, and passionate enthusiasm.

Many people have strongly influenced my professional and personal life. Few have had such a profound affect on my life as the late Fred L. Allman, Jr., MD. Dr. Allman taught me patience, perseverance, the importance of listening carefully to my patients, and most important, how to be a better person.

I thank every physical therapist, physician, educator, and scientist who has personally molded my views and has given me the knowledge and motivation to share with others, Tab Blackburn, Dr. Mike Voight, Dr. Steve Tippett, George Davies, Carolyn Wadsworth, Dr. Don Chu, Dr. William Kraemer, Dr. Mike Stone, Al Jones, Gary Sutton, Dr. Rick Hammesfahr, and many others for shaping my understanding of physical therapy and for enriching my life.

I wish to personally recognize and thank my close friends, administrators, and supporters of the National Strength and Conditioning Association (NSCA) for many years of valued education, and to my friends with the American Society of Orthopedic Physician Assistants (ASOPA), who openly share my commitment for a greater understanding and appreciation of orthopedic basic science. Thanks to the membership and leaders of the Orthopedic Section and Education Committee of the American Physical Therapy Association for their continued support of specific physical therapist assistant education and for their enthusiasm and vision in encouraging greater physical therapist assistant involvement within the orthopedic section and the physical therapy profession. Special thanks go to Lola Rosenbaum, who has supported the orthopedic education of physical therapist assistants and who has graciously offered to author the Foreword of this text.

I wish to publicly thank two very special friends, Trudy Golstein and Jeff Konin, who have demonstrated continued friendship and strong personal commitment to enhance the orthopedic continuing education of physical therapist assistants.

A project of any magnitude demands organization and time. My family has stood by my efforts and has shown support during my long hours away from home. My dear wife Pebbles had to endure my efforts on many fronts. Her loving support held my head up every step of the way. Her love and encouragement inspires me. The family is held together by Jim and Fannie Clark, Nan Payne and her late husband Don, who to this day provides comfort and love that literally allowed this project to take shape.

Finally, I thank every patient in whose care I have ever had the pleasure and opportunity to participate for their confidence that has allowed me to better understand their needs and for the faith they have shown in me, which continue to humble me.

Gary A. Shankman, PTA

SUGGESTED READINGS

American Physical Therapy Association: Guide to Physical Therapist Practice. *Physical Therapy* 1997;77:1163-1650.

American Physical Therapy Association: Physical Therapist Assistant Clinical Performance Instrument. Alexandria, VA, APTA, 1998.

Browner BD, Jupiter JB, Levine AM, Trafton PG (eds): Skeletal Trauma: Fractures, Dislocations, Ligamentous Injuries. Philadelphia, WB Saunders, 1998.

Buckwalter JA, Einhorn TA, Simon SR: Orthopedic Basic Science: Biology and Biomechanics of the Musculoskeletal System, 2nd ed. AAOS, 2000

Donatelli R, Wooden MJ: Orthopaedic Physical Therapy. New York, Churchill Livingstone, 1989.

Goodman CC, Fuller KS, Boissonnault WG: Pathology: Implications for the Physical Therapist. Philadelphia, WB Saunders, 2003.

Kisner C, Colby LA: Therapeutic Exercise: Foundations and Techniques, 2nd ed. Philadelphia, FA Davis, 1990.

Konin JG, Wiksten DL, Isear JA: Special Tests for Orthopedic Examination. Thorofare, NJ, Slack, Inc., 1997.

Lesh SG: Clinical Orthopedics for the Physical Therapist Assistant. Philadelphia, FA Davis, 2000.

Lippert L: Clinical Kinesiology for Physical Therapist Assistants, 2nd ed. Philadelphia, FA Davis, 1994.

Norkin C, Levangie P: Joint Structure and Function: A Comprehensive Analysis, 2nd ed. Philadelphia, FA Davis, 1992.

Richardson JK, Iglarsh ZA (eds): Clinical Orthopaedic Physical Therapy. Philadelphia, WB Saunders, 1994.

Timm KE: Knee. In Richardson JK, Iglarsh ZA (eds): Clinical Orthoapedic Physical Therapy. Philadelphia, WB Saunders, 1994.

Contents

PART **I**
BASIC CONCEPTS OF ORTHOPEDIC MANAGEMENT

1 Patient Supervision and Observation During Treatment, 3

2 The Role of the Physical Therapist Assistant in Physical Assessment, 13
SANDRA ESKEW CAPPS

3 Physical Agents Used in the Treatment of Common Musculoskeletal Conditions, 37
SANDRA ESKEW CAPPS

4 Flexibility, 57

5 Strength, 75

6 Endurance, 99

7 Balance and Coordination, 107

PART **II**
REVIEW OF TISSUE HEALING

8 Composition and Function of Connective Tissue, 123

9 Ligament Healing, 137

10 Bone Healing, 147

11 Cartilage Healing, 162

12 Muscle and Tendon Healing, 175

13 Neurovascular Healing and Thromboembolic Disease, 193

PART **III**
COMMON MEDICATIONS IN ORTHOPEDICS

14 Concepts of Orthopedic Pharmacology, 207

PART **IV**
GAIT AND JOINT MOBILIZATION

15 Fundamentals of Gait, 219

16 Concepts of Joint Mobilization, 229

xxiii

PART V
BIOMECHANICAL BASIS FOR MOVEMENT

17 Biomechanical Basis for Movement, 239
MITCHELL A. COLLINS

PART VI
MANAGEMENT OF ORTHOPEDIC CONDITIONS

18 Orthopedic Management of the Ankle, Foot, and Toes, 259

19 Orthopedic Management of the Knee, 289

20 Orthopedic Management of the Hip and Pelvis, 334

21 Orthopedic Management of the Lumbar, Thoracic, and Cervical Spine, 359

22 Orthopedic Management of the Shoulder, 392

23 Orthopedic Management of the Elbow, 421

24 Orthopedic Management of the Wrist and Hand, 437

ANSWERS TO REVIEW QUESTIONS, 455

APPENDIX

A Commonly Used Medications in Musculoskeletal Medicine, 467

B Reference Ranges for Commonly Used Tests, 474

C Laboratory Values as Clues, 476

D Units of Measurement and Terminology for the Description of Exercise and Sport Performance, 488

E Fracture Eponyms, 490

F Major Movements of the Body and the Muscles Acting at the Joints Causing the Movement, 492

GLOSSARY, 501

Fundamental Orthopedic Management for the Physical Therapist Assistant

PART I

BASIC CONCEPTS OF ORTHOPEDIC MANAGEMENT

The foundations for the appropriate application of skills and therapeutic techniques related to orthopedic physical therapy are based on the interdependence of basic science principles and the relationships between patient and therapist. The physical therapist assistant, although responsible for proper patient supervision and clinical observation during treatment, is frequently guided and directed to modify or adjust therapeutic interventions in consultation with the physical therapist based on specific physiologic responses from the patient. Keen observation skills and properly directed patient supervision techniques, and a thorough understanding of physiologic and therapeutic adaptations to exercise techniques, serve the physical therapist assistant to effectively and skillfully apply rudimentary, as well as advanced, rehabilitation techniques.

Therefore this section introduces basic orthopedic physical therapy components of patient supervision; the role of the physical therapist assistant in physical assessment with specific reference to the *Guide to Physical Therapist Practice* and related key elements of systems review and a systems approach to physical assessment; physical agents used in treatment of musculoskeletal conditions, flexibility and soft tissue management, and muscular strength, power, and plyometrics; unique characteristics of strength and adaptation in young and elderly patients; and closed kinetic chain exercise; neuromuscular fatigue; and balance, coordination, and the enhancement of the afferent neural input system related to orthopedic physical therapy management.

The focus and specific intent of this section is to provide a sound, practical, and purposeful introduction to the principles of basic orthopedic management, as well as the therapeutic application of these critical components related to specific tissue healing constraints, immobilization, and postsurgical recovery after orthopedic surgery.

1 Patient Supervision and Observation During Treatment

LEARNING OBJECTIVES

1. Identify and discuss the rationale for clear and concise communication among all members of the rehabilitation team.
2. Discuss the skills necessary to provide patient supervision.
3. Define objective scales of measurements used to communicate changes in a patient's status to the physical therapist.
4. Apply proactive listening skills and objective scales of measurement to provide appropriate, accountable, and responsible observation and supervision of the patient during treatment.
5. Define open-ended and closed-ended questioning.
6. Define the quadrants of the basic dimensional model.
7. Discuss the four categories of behavior of the physical therapist assistant: dominance, submission, hostility, and warmth.
8. Describe the differences between "prompting" and "cueing."

KEY TERMS

Responsibility
Communication
Listening
Accountability
Proactive

Probing questions
Open-ended questions
Closed-ended questions
Dominance
Submission

Hostility
Warmth
Basic dimensional model
Recognition

CHAPTER OUTLINE

Supervising the Patient During Treatment
    Components of Patient Supervision
    Patient Supervision by the Rehabilitation Team
    Basic Patient Supervision Skills
Modifications During Treatment
Understanding Different Philosophies of Therapists

SUPERVISING THE PATIENT DURING TREATMENT

Among the many challenges for the physical therapist assistant (PTA) are the supervision of the patient during treatment and the making of appropriate decisions. The assistant must recognize that interpersonal communication skills, patient supervision methods, and responsive clinical decision making must be learned, practiced, and demonstrated to function efficiently and effectively.

Initial contact with a patient establishes a framework of rapport and sets the stage for all future interactions with that individual. The assistant has the opportunity to convey confidence, capability, and sensitivity during the initial introductions by the physical therapist. This leads the patient to trust the assistant and minimizes fear and anxiety in the patient.

The physical therapist assistant is responsible for carrying out prescribed treatments in patient supervision and appropriate clinical decision making. For proper care to be given, the physical therapist assistant must monitor the patient's response to therapeutic interventions and accurately and swiftly report changes to the supervising therapist. This involves constant patient interaction, observation, palpation, reassessment of initial data, and responsive action to clarify and enhance the effectiveness of prescribed treatments. Changes in the patient's status, both positive and negative, can occur throughout the treatment program, whether during a single visit or over the span of multiple treatments. Some of these changes are subtle and require keen awareness of the initial objective data and acute sensitivity to the patient's subjective reports. Other changes are profound and sudden. In either situation, the physical therapist assistant observes a patient's range of motion, strength, pain, balance, coordination, swelling, endurance, or gait deviations. When reported to the supervising therapist, these changes dictate and significantly affect the course of treatment.

Components of Patient Supervision

Clinical patient supervision can be viewed as a process with the following purposes:
■ To gather relevant information
■ To establish and enhance rapport, trust, and confidence
■ To facilitate understanding of the physical therapist assistant's concept of the patient's problem as outlined, described, and initially determined by the physical therapist
■ To assist in the management of the patient
■ To provide a conduit or therapeutic outlet for the patient to voice concerns about his or her problem

Clearly gathering information from the patient and interpreting those data during the initial evaluation are functions primarily done by the physical therapist. However, the physical therapist assistant must help the patient understand the problem throughout the course of rehabilitation. The assistant must recognize how difficult it is for patients to grasp all the components of the situation well enough to fully appreciate the rationale for the prescribed treatment. Therefore the physical therapist assistant's role is to help the patient understand the disorder being treated and reassure him or her concerning the appropriateness of care.[3] In so doing the assistant must be keenly aware of and sensitive to subtle or overt signs of patient apprehension, fear, and anxiety.

Although direct patient supervision is frequently the task of one individual, **responsibility** for the patient's care is shared by the entire rehabilitation team. In addition, the patient must be actively involved in the treatment and accept shared responsibility for his or her own care.

During treatment the assistant makes observations of the patient and develops an objective assessment using appropriate scales of measurement (Box 1-1). Using applicable questioning techniques ensures that the patient is actively involved. This interactive approach to supervision, as well as the skills of the physical therapist assistant to seek, understand, and accurately relay information related to the patient's status distinguishes the assistant from a physical therapist aide.[4]

Patient Supervision by the Rehabilitation Team

The assistant must be aware of the key members of the rehabilitation team. The physical therapist and rehabilitation aide are involved with direct patient care on a daily basis. The occupational therapist and occupational therapy assistant, along with the speech language pathologist, audiologist, rehabilitation counselor, nurse, respiratory therapist, psychologist, and dietitian, play significant roles in daily patient care. These rehabilitation specialists seek to maximize recovery for each patient and always must be regarded as resources to meet specific patient needs as they are identified by any member of the team. Thus the assistant charged with direct patient care and supervision is only one vital member of the team, and he or she can take comfort in knowing that every member of the team is prepared to provide appropriate skills so that the patient can achieve the highest functional gains in recovery. Developing a team mindset helps the physical therapist assistant to be responsible and accountable to the other members of the team for his or her own contribution and to reach out to others when their expertise is needed.[5]

Effective **communication** is the hallmark of a great team and should be maximized. To effectively supervise and provide the greatest care for the patient, the assistant must learn to communicate openly and freely, with honesty and respect, and in a professional manner with every member of the team.[5] He or she must differentiate

---

BOX 1-1

General Scales of Measurements

STRENGTH: MANUAL MUSCLE TESTING

−5/5 *Normal:* Full resistance against gravity

−4/5 *Good:* Some resistance against gravity

−3/5 *Fair:* No resistance against gravity

−2/5 *Poor:* No movement against gravity

−1/5 *Trace:* Slight contraction, no movement

−0/5 *Zero:* No contraction

PAIN: ANALOG SCALE

Graded from 0 to 10 (0 absent, 10 severe)

SWELLING: GENERALLY MEASURED BY

Circumferential measurement

Water displacement

Blood pressure: 120/80 normal, use sphygmomanometer and stethoscope

Pulse: Average 72 BPM. Pulse can be lower (e.g., 55) for trained athletes

Respirations: Average 12 to 16/min

COORDINATION

Tapping foot or hand

Finger to nose

Heel on shin

Coordination activities are tested first with eyes open, then with eyes closed. All events are described as degrees of rhythmic, symmetric, even, and consistent.

STRETCH REFLEX (DTR) *[handwritten: Deep tendon Reflex]*

0 = Areflexia

+ = Hyperreflexia   *[handwritten: 2 = Normal]*

1 to 3 = Average

3 + to 4 = Hyperreflexia

RANGE OF MOTION: STANDARD GONIOMETRY

Shoulder

Flexion 0 to 180°

Extension 0 to 60°

Abduction 0 to 180°

Internal rotation 0 to 70°

External rotation 0 to 90°

Hip

Flexion 0 to 120°

Extension 0 to 30°

Abduction 0 to 45°

Abduction 0 to 30°

External rotation 0 to 45°

Internal rotation 0 to 45°

Ankle

Dorsiflexion 0 to 20°

Plantar flexion 0 to 50°

Inversion 0 to 35°

Eversion 0 to 15°

Knee

Flexion 0 to 135°

Elbow

Flexion 0 to 150°

---

between the language used for communicating among peers and that used to define and explain injury, disease, and physical therapy procedures to a patient. The assistant must employ appropriate and professional medical language to outline and describe an orthopedic problem to a physical therapist and must be able to use familiar terms to describe the same pathologic condition to a patient or family member. If the assistant uses medical jargon inappropriately, the patient or family member might perceive the therapist as insensitive, aloof, and impersonal. Generally use of language appropriate to the patient's comprehension conveys understanding, sensitivity, warmth, and reassurance and removes uncomfortable and unnecessary barriers to communication.[3]

The physical therapist assistant also must be aware that **listening** is an effective communication tool. Listening demonstrates interest and provides the opportunity for a better understanding of the patient's concept of the problem. By active listening, the assistant is better able to integrate verbal and nonverbal messages that the patient may have received.[3] In addition, patients may be more comfortable and trusting with a good listener, more at ease, and more willing to provide information.

Supervision of patients by the physical therapist assistant must be done systematically and reliably with an emphasis on **accountability.** Appropriate and responsible investigative questioning of the patient during treatment helps the assistant focus on the areas to probe, findings to quantify, and objective changes to assess. The assistant is responsible for reporting all findings to the physical therapist so that modifications can be made in accordance with changes in patient status.*

Basic Patient Supervision Skills

Communication Skills

The physical therapist assistant can be most effective if he or she develops an understanding of human behavior and adopts a **proactive** role in supervising patients. In a proactive role the assistant does not wait to be placed in a reactive position. Use of appropriate **probing questions** is a proactive method to use during patient supervision. Questioning patients during treatment can be insightful, rewarding, and helpful for both the physical therapist and the assistant. The format of asking probing questions is critical and strongly influences the responses received (Fig. 1-1). Using **open-ended questions** invites the patient to share feelings, thoughts, and opinions. Examples are as follows:

"Tell me about your pain."

"How does that feel?"

"What do you think about this exercise?"

These types of questions are generally not answered by "yes" or "no." They open discussions and prompt the patient to express a wide range of views and opinions.

Open-ended questions for patients have been described as "a good medium for facilitating rapport and, as such, are particularly useful. . . ."[3] Using open-ended questions promotes personal interactions between the therapist and patient, may allow the patient to give a more in-depth explanation of the problem, and may lead to discussions of what the patient identifies as important. Although this type of questioning does not enable the patient to give precise, clear answers, it is appropriate in situations that require compassion and empathy from the assistant and shared feelings between the assistant and patient.

Closed-ended questions are directed toward finding facts, obtaining specific responses, and filling in details. By asking the patient questions such as, "Where is your pain?" "When does your knee feel unstable?" or "Does your back hurt when you bend forward?" the assistant proactively directs the discussion and sequence of questions instead of sifting out pertinent information from among all the data gathered in open-ended questioning.

Summary-type statements check understanding, help the patient clarify thinking, and provide direction for the therapist. Examples include the following: "So your back hurts only at night?" and "Then your knee doesn't hurt with this exercise." Using precise closed-ended questions with summary statements elicits information that can lead to an objective assessment of the patient. The approach the assistant takes influences the balance of questioning between open-ended and closed-ended questions.

Behavior

The behavior of the physical therapist assistant during supervision can either reassure the patient and demonstrate appropriate responsive professional care or create a sense of indifference. Four broad categories of behavior are: dominance, submission, hostility, and warmth.[1] Buzzotta and Lefton[1] define these four categories as follows:

Dominance

Dominance can be defined as exercising control or influence. People who show dominant behavior are forceful, dynamic, and assertive. They push their ideas forward or try to sway the way other people think or behave. They take charge, guide, lead, and move other people to action.

Submission

Submission can be defined as being passive. People who show submissive behavior are willing to take a back seat. They are ready to comply, quick to give in, and reluctant to try to exert influence.

Hostility

Hostility can be defined as being unresponsive or insensitive to others and their needs. People showing hostile behavior tend to care only about themselves; they lack regard for other people's feelings and ideas. Although anger is a form of hostility, people can be hostile while showing no open anger.

Warmth

Warmth can be defined as being responsive and sensitive to others and their needs. People who show warm behavior are open and caring and have a high regard for other people's ideas and feelings. This does not mean they automatically gush with affection. A person can be warm without being openly affectionate.

These four categories of behavior are used to describe the extremes of the **basic dimensional model** (Fig. 1-2). Quadrants (Q) are formed (Fig. 1-3) and certain patterns of behavior exist when two dimensions are combined, as described in the following:

Q1 Dominant hostile

Q2 Submissive hostile

Q3 Submissive warm

Q4 Dominant warm

Four patterns, or types, of human behavior come from this (Fig. 1-4).

---

*From Guide for Conduct of the Affiliate Member. American Physical Therapy Association, Alexandria, Virginia.

Probe	Definition	Objectives	Characteristics	Examples
Open-ended questions	A question or statement that invites a wide-ranging response, often asks for ideas, opinions, or views.	• Open up discussion • Invite broad response • Give other freedom to talk • Gets involvement	• Can't be answered "yes" or "no" • Gets at feelings, opinions, thoughts	• "What do you think about. . . ?" • "Tell me about. . . " • "Why do you feel. . .?" • "What's your opinion?"
Pause	An intentional, purposeful period of silence.	• Give other a chance to think and respond • Slow down pace • Draw out other	• Usually follows open-ended question • Deliberate	• "Why do you say that?" (silence) • "Tell me more." (silence)
Reflective	A statement that describes and reflects a feeling or emotion (without implying agreement or disagreement).	• Identify emotions • Show you understand • Vent interfering emotions	• Names a feeling or emotion • Usually uses the word "you" or "you're" • May state cause of the emotion	• "You're pretty mad about it." • "You seem reluctant to talk about it." • "Sounds like you're excited."
Neutral phrase or question	A question or statement that encourages other to elaborate.	• Get other to tell more about a subject	• Few words • About subject under discussion	• "Tell me more." • "Please elaborate." • "Explain that." • "Amplify on that."
Brief assertion	A short statement, sound, or gesture, which shows involvement.	• Encourage other to continue • Increase receptivity	• Elicits additional information • Occurs automatically	• "Oh, okay." • "Yes, sure." • "I see." • Nodding your head.
Summary statements	A brief statement, in your own words, of the content of what was said.	• Check understanding • Prove you're listening • Give structure and direction • Help other clarify thinking • Invite other to comment or expand	• Summarizes content, not feelings • Restatement of essential ideas • In own words	• "So you disagree about. . . ." • "The way you see it is. . . ." • "You prefer working overtime. . . ." • "Let me summarize how I. . . ."
Close-ended questions	A question that limits the answer by requesting specific facts, or a "yes" or "no" answer.	• Find out details, specifics • Check understanding • Direct the discussion • Get other to take a stand	• Often starts with "Who," "Which," "When," "Where," "How many," etc. • Can sometimes be answered with a simple "yes" or "no"	• "Who is. . . ?" • "Which order. . . ?" • "When will you. . . ?" • "Do you think. . . ?"
Leading questions	A question that implies only one answer, or a rhetorical question—no answer is needed.	• Pin down positions or agreements • Can verify assumptions • Can be threatening	• The question gives the answer • No answer is required	• "Shouldn't we discuss. . . ?" • "This is the best way to go, isn't it?"

Fig. 1-1 Probes and probing questions: The use of questions, statements, and pauses to elicit information, thoughts, and opinions. The type of questions used elicits a characteristic response. (From Buzzotta VR, Lefton RE: Dimensional Management Training. St. Louis, Psychological Associates, 1989.)

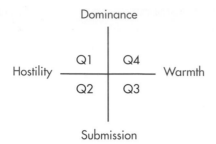

Dominance—Active behavior: leading, controlling, making things happen

Submission—Passive behavior: following, letting things happen, reacting

Hostility—A lack of concern or regard, and unresponsiveness for other people and their position/ideas

Warmth—Concern, regard, and responsiveness for other people and their position/ideas

Fig. 1-2 The dimensional model: A tool to size up behavior. The model applies to subordinates, peers, and superiors. General behavior characteristics are dominance, submission, hostility, and warmth. (From Buzzotta VR, Lefton RE: Dimensional Management Training. St. Louis, Psychological Associates, 1989.)

Applying this model when asking open-ended and closed-ended questions shows such questions to be equally balanced within Quadrant 4 (Q4). The goal of the physical therapist assistant during supervision of the patient is to consistently demonstrate those qualities found in Q4; for example, being appropriately friendly, attentive, responsive, involved, exploring, analytical, and task oriented.

While supervising patients according to the Q4 model, the assistant must understand the differences between prompting and cueing a patient to perform a specific task. Prompting a patient to perform a task can be viewed as the presentation of a question. For example, when instructing a patient to ambulate with a standard walker, the assistant should prompt the patient by asking, "After you move the walker, what foot do you move next?" Prompting allows patients to decipher information, solve problems, and provide solutions to activities they must overcome during recovery. Cueing can be viewed as a direction. An example is, "After you move the walker, move your injured leg." Although the solution is provided for the patient, he or she must still demonstrate appropriate follow-through and proper understanding of the command.

MODIFICATIONS DURING TREATMENT

Using attentive Q4 behavior with balanced open-ended and closed-ended questioning of the patient helps the physical therapist assistant identify and quantify

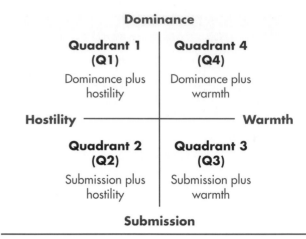

Fig. 1-3 Quadrants are formed among dominance, submission, hostility, and warmth that create certain patterns of behavior. (From Buzzotta VR, Lefton RE: Dimensional Management Training. St. Louis, Psychological Associates, 1989.)

changes in the patient's condition. After consulting the physical therapist and receiving direction, the assistant can effectively modify a specific treatment procedure in accordance with changes in patient status.*

The following example helps to clarify the scope of treatment modifications during postoperative rehabilitation after anterior cruciate ligament (ACL) reconstruction.

Swelling (joint effusion) after knee surgery is common and occurs in about 12% of cases after ACL reconstruction.[6] Usually the effusion is a hemarthrosis (blood within the joint). As little as 60 ml of fluid within a joint can cause a 30% to 50% inhibition of voluntary muscle contraction. In such a case the physical therapist provides baseline evaluation data about the degree of swelling present by making comparative circumferential measurements at midpatella, 2 inches superior to the midpatella, and 2 inches inferior to the midpatella. The physical therapist assistant maintains daily records of the three comparative circumferential measurements. Because reeducation and strengthening of muscle is influenced negatively by postoperative swelling, any increase or decrease in swelling necessitates a modification in the initial program outlined by the physical therapist. Thus the degree of swelling documented influences the adjustment made in the exercise prescription.

As the physical therapist assistant identifies objective changes in the patient's status each day, the concept of visual, nonresponsive, and noninteractive supervision is altered to one of appropriate, responsive, and accountable supervision.

---

*From Guide for Conduct of the Affiliate Member. American Physical Therapy Association, Alexandria, Virginia.

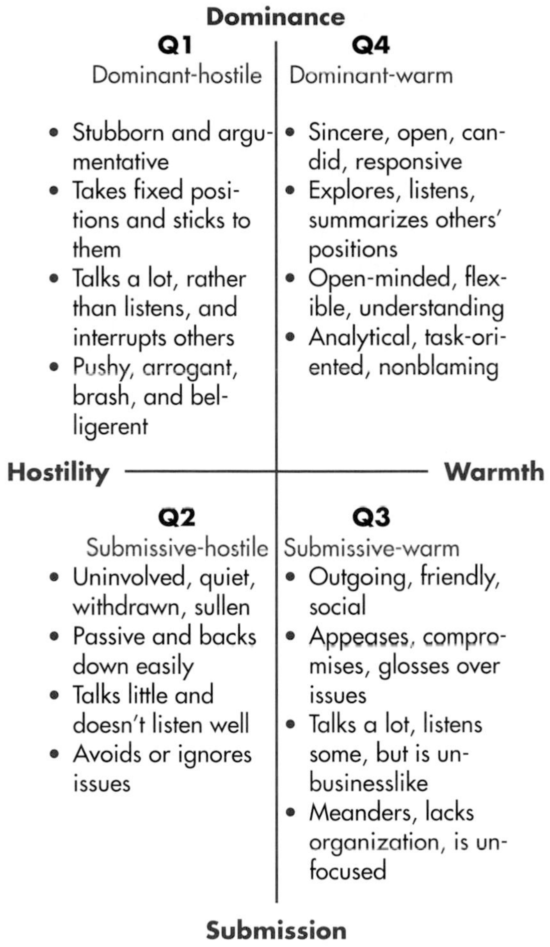

Dominance

Q1	**Q4**
Dominant-hostile	Dominant-warm
• Stubborn and argumentative	• Sincere, open, candid, responsive
• Takes fixed positions and sticks to them	• Explores, listens, summarizes others' positions
• Talks a lot, rather than listens, and interrupts others	• Open-minded, flexible, understanding
• Pushy, arrogant, brash, and belligerent	• Analytical, task-oriented, nonblaming

Hostility ——————————— **Warmth**

Q2	**Q3**
Submissive-hostile	Submissive-warm
• Uninvolved, quiet, withdrawn, sullen	• Outgoing, friendly, social
• Passive and backs down easily	• Appeases, compromises, glosses over issues
• Talks little and doesn't listen well	• Talks a lot, listens some, but is unbusinesslike
• Avoids or ignores issues	• Meanders, lacks organization, is unfocused

Submission

Fig. 1-4 Four distinct patterns and characteristics are formed between the four quadrants: Q1, dominant-hostile; Q2, submissive-hostile; Q3, submissive-warm; and Q4, dominant-warm. (From Buzzotta VR, Lefton RE: Dimensional Management Training. St. Louis, Psychological Associates, 1989.)

Isometric exercises generally are used early in the rehabilitation of acute postoperative knee injuries. Concentric and eccentric exercises are introduced as rehabilitation proceeds. Concentric and eccentric exercises are defined as dynamic, producing work, and creating changes in joint angles and muscle length.[2] The progression from isometric to dynamic exercise produces an increase in force generated, increases muscle soreness, and causes greater articular stresses.[7] If swelling and pain increase as the patient progresses from isometric to concentric and eccentric contractions, the physical therapist assistant, with direction and input from the physical therapist, can adjust or modify the program back to isometrics or reduce the amount of resistance, joint angle of exercise, volume of exercise, or velocity of movement. The specific sequence or combination of these modifications depends on the patient's specific needs, the surgical procedure, and the patient's toler-

---

BOX 1-2

Knee Extension: Isotonic Exercise Modifications

If pain and swelling develop during full range of motion isotonic knee extension:

- Adjust the resistance. Reduce the amount of weight being used.
- Adjust the range of motion to limit full knee flexion. Example: Begin knee extension exercises from 45° of flexion or less instead of 90° or greater. *Note:* Some acute, chronic, and post-surgical conditions prohibit terminal knee extension (0°). In this case, limit full extension to −10° or greater.
- Adjust the speed or velocity of the performance of the exercise. Closely observe the speed of the exercise. Perform slow, controlled, nonballistic exercise.
- Adjust the volume of exercise.
  a. Reduce the number of repetitions being performed.
  b. Reduce the number of sets being performed.
  c. Reduce the number of days per week performing the exercise.
- Change the performance of exercise.
  a. Perform only isometric holds followed by eccentric loads. No concentric lifting.

---

ance to exercise. Usually it is prudent to begin with the least drastic change in exercise prescription and then progress (Box 1-2).

The clinical decision-making process used by the physical therapist assistant involves recognizing that a problem exists, then taking orderly and specific steps to notify the therapist and adjust the program accordingly. Thus the assistant takes an active, participatory role while supervising patients, using his or her training and skills to the fullest extent.

Note that the **recognition** of changes in patient status does not imply interpretation of objective, measurable data by the assistant. The assistant's task is to provide information to the physical therapist on a daily basis, keep the therapist informed concerning patient status, and provide insightful and meaningful suggestions for modifications.

The objective data supplied to the therapist by the assistant include goniometric measurements, circumferential measurements, manual muscle testing, endurance grading, heart rate, blood pressure, respirations, dynamic balance, and coordination measurements, according to the scope of the assistant's training.

UNDERSTANDING DIFFERENT PHILOSOPHIES OF THERAPISTS

Fundamental differences exist among therapists concerning the methods, protocols, and directives they use to treat patients. In addition, just as the physical therapist assistant is directed by the therapist, the physical therapist is often directed by the physician. Within a hospital physical therapy department, the assistant may have contact with many therapists and physicians, each with different backgrounds, experiences, and education. The assistant sees therapists and physicians use various protocols to manage the same pathologic condition. It is not the task of the assistant to change or modify treatment plans or protocols without the therapist's direction. Opinions and controversies exist concerning how best to manage various orthopedic pathologic conditions. Changes in surgery and physical therapy occur because of advanced technology and rigorous research in rehabilitation medicine and orthopedic surgery. New procedures in arthroscopic ACL surgery allow a more rapid return to function, motion, and strength than ever before. Although ideally we presume all surgical procedures and rehabilitation techniques to be universally accepted, in fact the specialties of orthopedics and physical therapy are both art and science; therefore diversity is accepted.

The physical therapist assistant can be placed in frustrating and confusing situations when dealing with therapists with different backgrounds and opinions concerning the management of patients. To minimize the confusing array of treatment protocols, the assistant must communicate with the supervising therapist to clarify differences in patient care, always remembering that the responsibility for patient care is a shared one. The assistant does not divest interest in the care of any patient because of a disagreement in strategy with the therapist. The assistant's task requires a broader perspective and understanding that there are many ways to effectively manage the same pathology.

Having strong opinions on how to care for orthopedic patients is appropriate and shows passion, interest, and confidence in a certain method or protocol that has demonstrated good results. However, particular experience with the successful management of patients by one therapist may in fact conflict with the course of treatment prescribed by another. On the surface this situation may seem particularly frustrating and stressful. To better understand this difference the assistant must identify the key elements of disagreement and seek an appropriate explanation from the therapist. This gives each therapist the opportunity to teach and explain the rationale for the particular treatment and exposes the assistant to new information. The assistant then can observe and learn new methods that may actually prove equally or more successful than the previous plan of care.

Fully understanding the rationale and purpose of each treatment allows for improved delivery of service to the patient. During direct patient supervision the assistant can reinforce any procedure the therapist directs him or her to perform so long as the safety and welfare of the patient are not compromised.

The well-adapted assistant views any apparent roadblocks as learning opportunities. The assistant is advised to take advantage of the broad knowledge and experience of many therapists, constantly inquire about the rationale and scientific basis for a particular program, and establish himself or herself as an eager learning participant who is open to innovative ways of managing various pathologic conditions.

❖ ADDITIONAL FEATURES

Accountability: Systematic, reliable, and appropriate investigative questioning, listening, and active participation at all levels of patient care.

Behaviors: *Dominance*—exercising control or influence. *Submission*—passive and quick to comply. *Hostility*—unresponsive and insensitive. *Warmth*—responsive and sensitive.

Closed-ended Questions: Technique that requires a "yes" or "no" answer. This method effectively directs specific responses aimed at details of the patient's condition.

Listening: An effective communication tool. Demonstrates interest and concern for the patient and his or her individual needs.

Open-ended Questions: Allows patients the opportunity to provide substantial information concerning their care. A technique to facilitate rapport and lets the patient see that the PTA is effectively listening.

Proactive Supervision: By using probing questions and appropriate communications skills, accountability, listening, and responsibility, the patient avoids being placed in a reactive position.

Probing Questions: Techniques of questioning patients leading to insightful, rewarding, and responsive care.

Purpose of Communication: To gather information relevant to the patient's problem; to establish rapport and to provide confidence. To facilitate understanding of the patient's problem to assist in comprehensive patient management.

Responsibility: A component of active involvement of all areas of patient care.

Summary-Type Statements: Techniques that validate understanding of the patient's needs. Helps to clarify and specify patient's awareness and places emphasis on listening and responding appropriately.

REFERENCES

1. Buzzotta VR, Lefton RE: Dimensional Management Training. St. Louis, Psychological Associates, 1989.
2. Jokl PJ: Muscle. In Albright JA, Brand RA, eds. The Scientific Bases of Orthopaedics, 2nd ed, Norwalk, CT, Appleton & Lange, 1987.
3. Lombardo P, Stolberg S: Interviewing and communication skills. In Ballweg R, Stolberg S, Sullivan EM, eds. Physician Assistant: A Guide to Clinical Practice. Philadelphia, WB Saunders, 1994.
4. Lupi-Williams FA: The PTA, role and function. An analysis in three parts. I. Education, Clinical Management 3;3.

5. Mallory C: Team Building. Leadership Series. National Press Publications, 1991.
6. Sacks RA, et al: Complications of knee ligament surgery. In Daniel D, Akeson W, O'Connor J, eds. Knee Ligaments Structure: Function, Surgery and Repair. New York, Raven Press, 1990.
7. Sapaga AA: Muscle performance evaluation in orthopaedic practice. *J Bone & Joint Surg* 1990;72A:1562–1574.

REVIEW QUESTIONS

Multiple Choice

1. Throughout patient supervision and observation, the physical therapist assistant does which of the following?
   A. Observes the patient and notes any and all changes in objective clinical data
   B. Provides intermittent supervision throughout treatment
   C. Assesses changes noted in initial clinical data obtained by the physical therapist and immediately alters the treatment program before consultation with the physical therapist
   D. Constantly interacts, observes, and supervises each patient, comparing initial clinical evaluation data with any changes noted in the patient's condition, then reporting these changes to the supervising therapist before altering the treatment program
   E. A, B, and C
   F. A and D

Short Answer

2. List five components of patient supervision.

3. Identify six members of the rehabilitation team who also may be involved with patient supervision.

4. Effective _____ is the hallmark of a great team and should be maximized.

5. Appropriate medical language used with the patient and his or her family helps to convey _____ , _____ , _____ , and _____ .

6. The physical therapist assistant also must be aware that _____ is an effective communication tool.

7. Which type of probing questions invites the patient to share feelings, thoughts, and opinions?

8. Which type of probing questions is directed toward finding facts, obtaining specific responses, and filling in details?

9. Give three examples of open-ended probing questions that may be appropriate during the course of patient observation and interactive supervision.

10. Give three examples of closed-ended probing questions that may be appropriate during the course of patient observation and interactive supervision.

11. Which type of statement checks understanding, helps patients clarify thinking, and provides direction for the clinician?

12. Give two examples of summary-type statements.

13. Identify four categories of human behavior as described by Buzzotta and Lefton.

14. In the following figure, label and identify the components of the dimensional model and the quadrants formed by combining two dimensions.

15. Applying the dimensional model to the use of open-ended and closed-ended probing questions, which quadrant represents the behavioral goal of the physical therapist assistant during patient supervision?

16. List seven qualities that are found in Q4 behavior.

17. Give an example of "prompting" a patient to attempt a specific task.

18. Give an example of "cueing" a patient to attempt a specific task.

19. Give nine examples of objective, measurable data that can help guide the assistant and supervising physical therapist to make appropriate modifications in a patient's treatment.

Essay Questions

Answer on a separate sheet of paper.
20. Identify and discuss the rationale for clear and concise communication among all members of the rehabilitation team.
21. Discuss the skills required to provide patient supervision.
22. Define objective scales of measurements used to communicate changes in a patient's status to the physical therapist.

23. Apply proactive listening skills and objective scales of measurement to provide appropriate, accountable, and responsible observation and supervision of the patient during treatment.
24. Define open-ended and closed-ended questioning.
25. Define the quadrants of the basic dimensional model.
26. Discuss the four categories of behavior: dominance, submission, hostility, and warmth.
27. Describe the differences between "prompting" and "cueing."

Critical Thinking Application

As a role-playing activity, one student acts the part of a patient, and another student plays the role of a practicing PTA. Using the dimensional model as a guide, the PTA should demonstrate proactive, participatory supervision skills, using appropriate probing questions and behavior consistent with the Q4 quadrant. Guide the patient in developing open-ended questions, closed-ended questions, and summary statements to convey compassion, understanding, interest, focus, and task-specific actions to clarify and enhance the effectiveness of treatment. The students switch roles and the student now playing the PTA uses behaviors consistent with Q1, Q2, and Q3 quadrants of the dimensional model. Compare the effectiveness of using Q4 behavior with patient supervision with that of Q1, Q2, and Q3. If you were a patient, how would you prefer to be treated? Which supervisory skills convey trust? Which behavior would you, as a patient, expect from the PTA?

2

The Role of the Physical Therapist Assistant in Physical Assessment

SANDRA ESKEW CAPPS

LEARNING OBJECTIVES

1. Apply the language of the *Guide to Physical Therapist Practice* to physical assessment procedures.
2. Identify the common elements of examination, evaluation, and assessment.
3. Describe the role of the physical therapist assistant in the performance of physical assessment based on the physical therapy plan of care.
4. Discuss the role of the physical therapist assistant in data collection.
5. Explain methods of modifying the physical therapy plan of care or actions to be taken in response to physical assessment of the patient.
6. Identify critical elements to include with documentation of physical assessment.
7. Relate physical assessment to goals and outcomes of a physical therapy plan of care.

KEY TERMS

Assessment	Volumetrics	Orthostatic hypotension
Examination	Brawny edema	Pulse oximetry
Evaluation	Pitting edema	Rate of perceived exertion
Clinical Performance	Peripheralization	(RPE)
Instrument (CPI)	Centralization	End-feel
Judgment	Intermittent claudication	Tone
Data collection skills	Referred pain	Accessory joint motions
Granulomatosis	Visceral pain	Crepitus
Induration	Trigger points	
Pallor	Valsalva maneuver	

CHAPTER OUTLINE

American Physical Therapy Association Guiding Documents
   The Guide to Physical Therapist Practice
   The Clinical Performance Instrument
   The Normative Model of Physical Therapist Assistant Education
Inflammation
   What Is Inflammation?
General Contraindications and Precautions with Inflammation
   Acute versus Chronic
Temperature
   Fever and Infection Control
   Fever and Exercise
   Fever and Lymph Nodes
Redness and Skin Color Changes
Edema

Continued

CHAPTER OUTLINE—cont'd

Pain
    "Red Flag" Pain Symptoms
    Intermittent Claudication
    Referred Pain
    Visceral Pain
    Trigger Points
    Pain: A Final Note
Vital Signs
    Pulse (Heart Rate)
    Respiration
    Blood Pressure
    Pulse Oximetry
    Vital Signs and Exercise
Fatigue
Assessment of Musculoskeletal Structures
    End-Feel
    Contractile Tissue
    Strength Testing
    Stretching and Palpation
    Flexibility
    Overuse
Bones
Joints and Ligaments
    Accessory Joint Motions
    Distraction and Compression
    Ligamentous Integrity
    Gait
    Balance
Documentation
Conclusion

As any prospective or current student in the field of physical therapy (PT) is aware, changes in the profession are emerging rapidly. In an effort to bring physical therapy professionals to the "health care table" for discussion of legislative, regulatory, and reimbursement issues, the leaders of our profession are striving for standardization of terminology and recognition and application of evidence-based practice.[3] Needless to say, controversy or at least animated debate occurs among interested parties any time such an in-depth self-scrutiny of a profession takes place. One significant element of this debate in physical therapy revolves around the physical therapist assistant's role in the profession, including how the physical therapist assistant (PTA) participates in the administration of the physical therapy plan of care, including assessment and interventions and the terminology associated with the PTA's role. The purpose of this chapter is to summarize available standards and guidelines associated with the PTA's role in physical assessment and to discuss techniques and implications of specific assessment procedures for the patient with a musculoskeletal condition.

AMERICAN PHYSICAL THERAPY ASSOCIATION GUIDING DOCUMENTS
The Guide to Physical Therapist Practice

The *Guide to Physical Therapist Practice* (the *Guide*) is a tool that was developed by the American Physical Therapy Association[3] in part to ". . . describe physical therapist practice in general; . . . standardize terminology used in and related to physical therapist practice; . . . delineate preferred practice patterns that will help physical therapists . . . promote appropriate utilization of health care services; [and] increase efficiency and reduce unwarranted variation in the provision of services . . . ."[3] The stated purpose of the *Guide* reads, in part, that it is: ". . . a resource not only for physical therapist clinicians, educators, researchers, and students, but [also] health care policy makers, administrators, managed care providers, third-party payers, and other professionals." According to the *Guide*, the definition of the PTA is: "a technically educated health care provider who assists in the provision of physical therapy interventions."[3] **Assessment** is defined as "the measurement or quantification of a variable or the placement of a value on something."[3] Further, the *Guide* states, "Assessment should not be confused with examination or evaluation." **Examination** involves preliminary gathering of data and performing various screens, tests, and measures to obtain a comprehensive base from which to make decisions about physical therapy needs for each individual patient. **Evaluation** is the specific process reserved solely for the physical therapist in our profession, in which clinical judgments are made from this base of data (obtained from examination), including the possibility of referral to another health care provider.

The Clinical Performance Instrument

The **Clinical Performance Instrument** (CPI), a uniform clinical education grading tool developed by the American Physical Therapy Association,[4] includes the following criteria related to the PTA's role in assessing the patient:

■ Participates in patient status **judgments*** within the clinical environment based on the plan of care established by the physical therapist (criterion #9)

---

*The following definition for the term **judgments** is offered in the *Glossary* of the *CPI:* "decisions made within the clinical environment that are based on the established physical therapy plan of care. . . ." Furthermore, included as a part of this definition, the designers of the instrument refer to the process of "problem-solving," taken into account with consideration toward safety and including, ". . . decision rules (e.g., codes, protocols), thinking, data collection, and interpretation."[4]

- Obtains accurate information by performing selected data collection[†] consistent with the plan of care established by the physical therapist (criterion #10)
- Discusses the need for modifications to the plan of care established by the physical therapist (criterion #11)

The Normative Model of Physical Therapist Assistant Education

The *Normative Model of Physical Therapist Assistant Education* (the *Model*) is a consensus-based document developed by the American Physical Therapy Association. Briefly, the *Model* was designed to provide a representation of all of the elements that provide the foundation for the development and evaluation of approved educational programs preparing physical therapist assistants.[5] According to the *Model*, PTAs ". . . assist with data collection; . . . make appropriate judgments; (and) *modify interventions* within the PT's established plan of care. . . ."[5]

Interestingly, the *Model* includes objectives specifically related to the content of "chain of communication" and "role theory" to ensure that PTAs have a clear understanding of what their professional role is, including the objective of explaining it others.[5]

The content areas (referred to as "Performance Expectation Themes") that most closely relate to the role of the PTA and assessment include "Clinical Problem Solving and Judgments," "Data Collection," "Plan of Care," and "Outcomes Measurement and Evaluation." Each theme includes a description of the content, examples of behavioral objectives, and examples of instructional objectives.

Frequently, the response to the question about the "difference between PTs and PTAs" is simply, "PTAs don't do evaluations." Considering the elements of judgment and decision-making involved with evaluation and from the preceding discussion, does this imply that the PTA does not exercise judgment or make decisions? Of course not. However, the judgments and subsequent decisions of the PTA are made within the context of the existing physical therapy plan of care, established by the physical therapist through the examination and evaluation process. This process occurs on an ongoing basis.[20] Without effective data collection and reporting by the PTA, the PT would lack key information on which this "data management" process relies.[20]

It may be helpful to consider the functions of data collection and management as integral parts of manag-ing a patient's physical therapy case, which is a dynamic process. According to Bella J. May, EdD, PT and Jancis Dennis, PhD, PT, "Clinical decision making is really a feedback loop system that requires ongoing determination of whether the outcomes are desired."[20] A visual model to represent the respective roles of the PT and PTA functioning as a team to meet the physical therapy needs of a patient is presented in Figure 2-1.

This discussion of specific assessment techniques and issues begins with two conditions frequently encountered among patients with musculoskeletal involvement: inflammation and pain.

INFLAMMATION
What Is Inflammation?

Inflammation is a living organism's first response to injury or disruption of normal processes. It is a normal response, and actually can be considered the body's immediate trigger for healing. Inflammation involves the responses of several body constituents, including vascular components, fluid and semifluid (humoral) substances, and neurologic and cellular reactions. Inflammation that does not resolve within expected time frames may develop into a chronic state (as a result of either abnormality in the individual's immune or inflammatory response or as a result of prolonged, continuous, or repeated exposure to the injurious agent). Chronic inflammation (considered a pathologic condition) may result in secondary complications or permanent changes in the makeup of the involved tissue, including scarring or **granulomatosis.** Two important factors must be kept in mind: that inflammation is a normal and necessary response to trigger tissue healing; and that unresolved (chronic) inflammation may lead to permanent and undesired tissue changes. Therefore it is imperative for the PTA to monitor changes in the inflammatory response of the area being treated. In addition, extreme changes in the appearance of inflammation may signal the onset of serious complications, necessitating further evaluation by the PT or, in some cases, referral to the physician for immediate medical evaluation.

As discussed elsewhere in this book, certain physical agents are employed to control (but not eliminate) the acute inflammatory response or accelerate it, thus moving the healing process along. Depending on the degree of inflammation present, certain physical agents may be contraindicated; these are discussed in the chapter on physical agents. So how does the PTA differentiate between "normal" inflammation and an inflammatory reaction indicating the potential for contraindicated procedures or serious complications?

The commonly accepted and normal ("cardinal") signs and symptoms of inflammation are localized heat,

---

[†]**Data collection skills** are defined as, "those processes/procedures used to gather information through observation, measurement, subjective, objective, and functional findings; progression toward goals; and interpretive processes/procedures applied to formulate a judgment/decision within the plan of care established by the physical therapist." The definition also states that [data collection skills] "must be integrated to achieve the most effective interventions and optimal outcomes."[4]

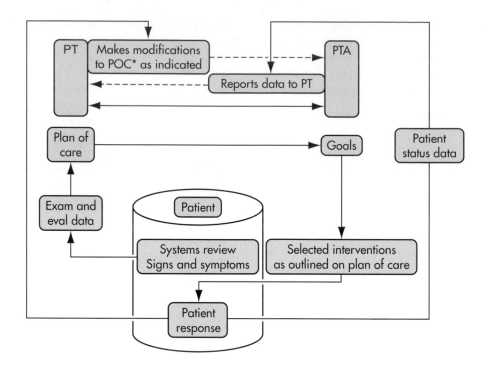

Representation of PT: PTA relationship, examining interaction of basic elements of patient physical therapy experience. The model is intended to illustrate and emphasize the importance of the interactive relationship, which serves to enhance outcomes for the patient.
*POC = Plan of care

Fig. 2-1 Representation of the physical therapist–physical therapist assistant relationship, examining interaction of basic elements of patient physical therapy experience. The model is intended to illustrate and emphasize the importance of the interactive relationship, which serves to enhance outcomes for the patient. (POC, plan of care.)

redness, swelling, and pain with a resultant loss of range of motion in the injured area. Temperature and redness are discussed here in relation to the PTA's role in collecting data and communicating concerns appropriately to the PT. The discussion of the assessment of edema and pain are discussed in separate sections.

GENERAL CONTRAINDICATIONS AND PRECAUTIONS WITH INFLAMMATION

In general remember that inflammation is a reaction to tissue trauma or injury; the increased inflammatory reactions after exercise or other interventions may indicate that the intervention is too aggressive or contraindicated, resulting in "new" trauma or injury to healing tissues. Furthermore, responses to interventions between visits also must be assessed; a patient may report signs of increased inflammation up to 24 hours after an intervention, particularly after administration of exercise or manual stretching techniques.

Acute versus Chronic

Under normal circumstances, signs of acute inflammation persist for 4 to 6 days, assuming the precipitating condition, agent, or event is removed. In the initial 48 hours after tissue injury, the observable signs of inflammation are associated with the normal inflammatory vascular response to trauma. An important distinction to make is the definition of *acute* versus *chronic* in relation to the actual cause of injury or trauma. It is common for sources to refer to these tissue states in terms of time frames only, with the acute phase defined as the first 24 to 48 hours after injury and the chronic phase defined as longer than 48 or 72 hours after injury. A more useful way to consider inflammation incorporates the concept of whether there is real or impending tissue damage present. The significance of this designation relates to the PTA's role in determining whether, based on the stage of inflammation present, certain interventions may be implemented or contraindicated. If an intervention normally results in an inflammatory reaction, it is contraindicated when the tissue is in an acute inflammatory state that indicates ongoing tissue damage. For example, in the presence of acute inflammation (indicating an active state of injury, tissue damage, or early tissue healing), dynamic resistance exercises are contraindicated.[16] However, the PTA also may proceed with interventions included in the plan of care that accelerate the inflammatory process if it has been determined that the original causal agent or condition no longer results in ongoing tissue damage. Contraindications related to specific diagnoses or associated with the application of specific physical agents are discussed elsewhere in this book.

During interventions involving range of motion (ROM) activities, the PTA also may note that the patient reports pain before tissue resistance is felt (before "end" ROM); this is an indication of acute inflammation. Pain reported at the same time end ROM is reached is indicative of a subacute inflammatory state, and pain reported as a "stretching" sensation at the limit of ROM is a sign of inflammation in the chronic state.[16] If the PTA determines that the established plan of care includes interventions that are not appropriate for the apparent stage of inflammation, the PT must be consulted to adjust goals, time frames, or possibly the plan itself to ensure that the treatment does not contribute to a prolonged or abnormal state of inflammation.

TEMPERATURE

The PTA must be able to differentiate between expected temperature responses in a normal inflammatory response versus abnormal responses. A normal increase in temperature is local and initially mild to moderate (compared with the contralateral anatomic region) versus a more pervasive change, which may manifest as significant either as compared with the contralateral side or as a systemic increase in temperature (fever). In the former case joint effusion may be present; the latter may represent a systemic response to the injury (e.g., infection) or an unrelated condition, such as an acute disease process (e.g., flu). Either of these situations warrants action on the part of the PTA. In the presence of systemic infection, the patient's ability to participate in the physical therapy plan is affected. Because of the exclusive one-on-one time traditionally associated with physical therapy care, it is not uncommon for the PTA to be the member of the health care team who provides important "pieces to the puzzle" of the patient's total health or illness picture.

Both the degree of temperature elevation and duration of fever are relevant to diagnostic processes when elevated body temperature is evident. During the initial PT examination and evaluation, any abnormality in temperature, either locally or systemically, should be noted. The PTA's role is then to note deviations from the examination findings, determine the length of time the fever has been present (through patient interview) and note other possible related signs and symptoms: rash, cough, complaints of sore throat, and so on. Also it should be noted if the patient reports any pattern of temperature changes, because this may have diagnostic implications for the physical therapist or physician. Immediate implications include whether or not exercise or other interventions may be contraindicated and to what extent infection control issues must be addressed. Normal body temperature (oral measurement) ranges from 96.8° F to 99.5° F (36° C to 37.5° C). Temperature is affected by factors including age, time of day, immune system function, and drug use. Temperature responses to acute infectious diseases usually include fever not greater than 102° F and lasting up to 7 days. In the case of the presence of fever, the PTA must gather the related data, document it, and report it to the supervising PT. The data and report should include adequate information to enable the PT to respond appropriately, either in terms of immediate modification to the PT plan of care or consultation with the medical team.

Fever and Infection Control

As always, the PTA must attend to his or her responsibility of exercising appropriate precautions for both the patient and himself or herself. The importance of handwashing by the caregiver and patient cannot be overstated as an effective means of controlling the transmission of infectious agents. In addition, treatment areas should be properly cleaned and disinfected as a routine procedure, not only in the case of patients with obvious infectious conditions. (Detailed information and guidelines for handwashing in the health care setting are available through the web site of the Centers for Disease Control and Prevention, *www.cdc.gov/health*).

Fever and Exercise

In terms of exercise precautions, "discretionary caution" should be applied with any patient with a fever, because of stresses on the cardiopulmonary and immune systems and the possible further complications related to dehydration.[9] The PTA must be familiar with specific exercise techniques (e.g., aquatic exercise) contraindicated in the presence of diseases transmitted via water or air.

Fever and Lymph Nodes

Another condition that may become readily apparent to the PTA in the course of carrying out elements of the PT plan of care is tenderness or exquisite pain in particular

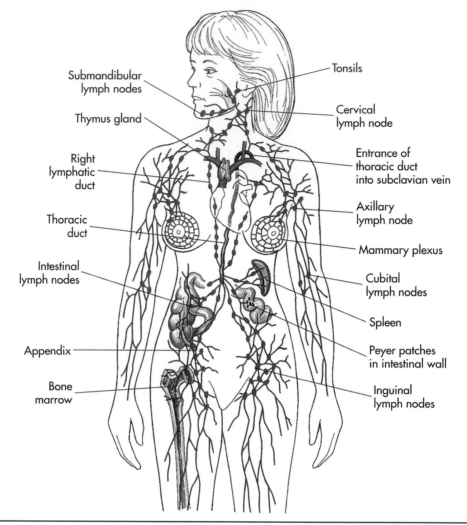

Fig. 2-2 Location of lymph vessels and nodes. Note clusters of nodes in axilla and groin areas. (Modified from Seeley RR, Stephens TD, Tate PT: Anatomy and Physiology, 3rd ed. St. Louis, CV Mosby, 1993.)

regions of the body. The presence of tender or enlarged lymph nodes is of particular concern to the PTA who is performing soft-tissue interventions on a patient with an elevated body temperature (or otherwise). Figure 2-2 provides a visual reference for the location of lymph nodes.[21] PTAs using hands-on techniques such as soft-tissue massage and manual stretching are incidentally afforded the opportunity during the course of treatment to assess for the presence of unusual conditions in areas of lymph node clusters (e.g., in the neck and axilla). Because these symptoms can signify the presence of potentially serious pathologic conditions, the presence of pain, tenderness or enlargement of lymph nodes are situations in which the PTA must consult with the supervising PT to pursue medical follow-up for definitive diagnosis. In addition, certain interventions are considered contraindicated if the patient has an underlying pathology related to changes in the lymph nodes.

REDNESS AND SKIN COLOR CHANGES

Redness *(erythema)* is a normal component of the inflammatory reaction. The PTA must be alert to abnormal or unexpected changes in skin color, which may indicate the presence of secondary complications or underlying pathologies. Redness may be considered normal when it is noted in the immediate area of injury and is associated with local temperature changes. Depending on the patient's pigmentation, color changes may appear in tones other than red.

Unexpected findings in terms of changes in skin color should be reported to the PT for further evaluation. These changes include rashes or redness that appears as a streak originating from the site of injury. Red streaks may indicate an acute inflammation caused by a bacterial infection (streptococci, staphylococci, or both), resulting in acute inflammation of the lymph vessels.[9] Redness along with superficial tenderness and "hardness"

Table 2-1	*Risk Factors for Deep Vein Thrombosis (DVT)*

IMMOBILITY (VENOUS STASIS)
Prolonged bed rest (e.g., burns, fracture)
Prolonged air travel
Neurologic disorder (e.g., spinal cord injury, stroke)
Cardiac failure
Absence of ankle muscle pump

TRAUMA (VENOUS DAMAGE)
Varicose veins
Surgery
Local trauma (e.g., direct injury)
Intravenous injections
Fracture or dislocation
Childbirth and delivery
Sclerosing agents

OTHER
Diabetes mellitus
Genetic
Obesity
Previous deep vein thrombosis (DVT)
Buerger disease
Age >60 yr
Idiopathic

LIFESTYLE
Hormonal status
Oral contraceptive use
Hormone replacement therapy
Hormonal medications (e.g., tamoxifen, doxorubicin [Adriamycin])
Pregnancy
In vitro fertilization (?)
Smoking

HYPERCOAGULATION
Hereditary thrombotic disorders
Neoplasm (especially viscera, ovary)
↑ Levels of coagulation factors (VIII, XI)
Prothrombin mutation
↓ Levels of homocysteine
Activated protein C syndrome

From Goodman CC, Fuller KS, Boissonnault WG: Pathology: Implications for the Physical Therapist, 2nd ed. Philadelphia, WB Saunders, 2001.

(**induration**) of the area is a sign of superficial thrombophlebitis; these findings should be reported to the supervising PT because this condition may be a precursor to more serious conditions. A loss of skin color (paleness or **pallor**) associated with temperature changes, edema, or pain may be indicative of an occlusion in a blood vessel and warrants immediate medical referral. A commonly used quick assessment technique to rule out the presence of a deep vein thrombosis (DVT) is Homans' sign, performed by gentle passive stretching of the ankle into full dorsiflexion and assessing for pain in the calf. Some clinicians also incorporate a gentle "squeezing" of calf musculature during the passive dorsiflexion to assess for tenderness. However, these tests are far from 100% reliable in confirming the presence of a DVT. Other structures that are stretched during this test include the calf muscles and the Achilles tendon; thus a positive Homans' sign may be noted in error if a patient has tightness or inflammation of these structures. According to Catherine C. Goodman, PT, in *Pathology: Implications for the Physical Therapist* (Saunders, 2003), ". . . this test is insensitive, non-specific, and present in fewer than 30% of documented cases of DVT . . . more than one-half of all people with a positive Homans' sign do not have evidence of venous thrombosis." Furthermore, a serious potential complication of a DVT is that a piece of the coagulated blood (the clot) may break free from the inside of the vessel wall as a result of the test (or otherwise) and travel through the bloodstream, lodging in a pulmonary artery, causing a life-threatening condition (pulmonary embolism). Therefore it is recommended that the PTA refrain from conducting the Homans' test and be alert to the other signs and risk factors associated with thrombophlebitis and DVT (Table 2-1),[9] and report these findings to the PT for further investigation and possible immediate medical referral.

Furthermore, the PTA should be aware of differences in superficial skin changes based on the patient's skin color. In other words, these findings in individuals with darkly pigmented skin may be less obvious and do not manifest as the same changes in skin tones as with light-skinned individuals. A critical element to be included in the lab practice and skill development of the PTA student is exposure to a number of "normal" subjects of different body types, skin tones, and so on (often represented within a classroom population of adult learners). By observing and "practicing" on different subjects, the PTA student develops an awareness of normal variations, which will subsequently enhance his or her ability to recognize differences or abnormalities in a patient population.

EDEMA

Because edema and its management have significant implications in the practice of physical therapy, the entry-level PTA is expected to possess the following skills related to the assessment of edema.[5]

- Describe factors (activities and posture) that affect edema.
- Recognize changes in edema (including classification levels).
- Measure edema (through techniques of girth, palpation, and **volumetrics,** when indicated, to measure changes in overall body fluids).

BOX 2-1

Sample Format for Documenting Edema

UE	Right	Left
Axilla	_____ inches	_____ inches
4" above elbow	_____ inches	_____ inches
2" above elbow	_____ inches	_____ inches
Elbow*	_____ inches	_____ inches
2" below elbow	_____ inches	_____ inches
4" below elbow	_____ inches	_____ inches
Wrist*	_____ inches	_____ inches

*A standard for "elbow" could be from the cubital fossa around the elbow, crossing the olecranon process; a standard for "wrist" could be just distal to the radial and ulnar styloid processes.

BOX 2-2

Technique for Figure-of-Eight Edema Measurement of Ankle

1. Position the patient so that the lower leg is supported and the ankle is in a neutral position of dorsiflexion or plantarflexion.
2. Place the (0) edge of the tape measure at the slight fossa located midway between the tibialis anterior tendon (superficially palpable just medial and anterior to the medial malleolus, on the dorsal surface of the ankle).
3. Wrap the tape medially across the bottom surface of the foot, just distal to the navicular tuberosity (palpable projection on the anteromedial aspect of the hindfoot).
4. Draw the tape straight across the sole of the foot, winding it back to the dorsum of the foot just proximal to the tuberosity (base) of the fifth metatarsal (palpable projection on the lateral aspect of the hindfoot).
5. Cross back over the tibialis anterior tendon, with the edge of the tape crossing just perpendicular to the starting edge.
6. Wrap the tape measure around the ankle, drawing it just distal to the tip of the medial malleolus, crossing the calcaneal ("Achilles") tendon and drawing the tape measure just distal to the lateral malleolus, back to the starting point.
7. For consistency, it is recommended that this process be repeated three times, with the average of the three measurements recorded.

Adapted from Magee DJ: Orthopedic Physical Assessment. Philadelphia, WB Saunders, 2002; Tatro-Adams D, McGann S, Carbone W: Reliability of the figure-of-eight method on subjects with ankle joint swelling. J Orthop Sports Phys Ther 1995;22(4):161–163. (With permission of the Orthopaedic and Sports Physical Therapy Sections of the American Physical Therapy Association.)

For purposes of this text, the focus is on localized edema, resulting from injury or trauma to musculoskeletal tissue or structures. Other terms and conditions are defined or discussed in relation to the PTA's responsibility in the event unrelated or unexpected conditions are discovered.

Edema refers to excessive pooling of fluid in the spaces between tissues (interstitial spaces). In relation to patients with orthopedic injuries or conditions, the main consideration for assessment by the PTA is measurement of the edematous part or extremity. Typically, the technique used to measure edema in an extremity is straightforward—use of a tape measure to obtain circumferential dimensions of the involved part. The data must be reliable and the measurement reproducible, regardless of who is conducting the assessment. To ensure this level of consistency, the PTA must use precisely the same landmarks as the evaluating physical therapist. Specifically, palpable bony landmarks must be used as the starting standard reference point; then circumferential measurements can be taken at determined distances from that point. For example, to measure the lower leg, circumference measured with the tape measure at the inferior pole of the patella may be used as a reference point, with measurements then taken every 2 inches distally and at the ankle. An example of a flow chart for recording circumferential measurements is provided in Box 2-1.

A figure-of-eight technique may be used at the ankle to ascertain a gross estimate of generalized ankle edema. Refer to Box 2-2 for the steps involved in this procedure.

Another technique used to obtain a quantitative measure of edema in a limb involves immersing the limb into a specially designed container of fluid (a volumeter) and measuring the amount of water displaced. A recent study established correlation between different techniques of "volumetric" measurement but also emphasized the importance of ensuring reliability of the data for a given patient, in terms of employing a consistent technique for edema measurement of the same patient. In other words, as stated, the PTA must use the method of measurement, employing the same technique chosen by the evaluating PT.[14]

In addition to a quantitative measurement of edema through circumferential measurement or volumetrics, data relating to the quality of edema should be collected and documented by the PTA. Characteristics of edema that may be observed are described as "**brawny**" or "**pitting.**" Brawny edema refers to edema that feels hard, tough, or thick and leathery. This indurated quality is frequently associated with chronic inflammation or systemic pathologies involving fluid shift abnormalities (e.g., congestive heart failure [CHF]). Pitting edema is characterized by the formation of a sustained indentation when the swollen area is compressed. Pitting edema may be further quantified according to the scale in Box 2-3.[17]

Unlike transient inflammatory reactions that may normally occur in response to certain PT interventions, a significant increase in edema should be regarded as abnormal and reported accordingly. Upon first noticing edema in the extremity being treated, the PTA must determine if the swelling is confined to the involved extremity or if the contralateral extremity is also involved. If the opposite extremity is also edematous, this finding could indicate a systemic pathologic condition. For example, bilateral pitting edema of the distal lower extremities is a common manifestation in CHF, a relatively common diagnosis encountered among individuals with cardiac disease and those more than 65 years old. Because this pathology is common among a significant population and it develops gradually, the PTA may play an important role in the diagnostic process via astute recognition of signs and symptoms associated with the onset of CHF. In addition to bilateral lower extremity pitting edema, the PTA also may note a decrease in tolerance to exercise (fatigue, shortness of breath, and muscle weakness). The presence of this clinical response necessitates prompt consultation with the supervising PT for medical diagnostic workup and possible subsequent modifications to the PT plan of care.

A potentially serious condition involving edema is *compartment syndrome*. This condition occurs in anatomic compartments (of the calf or, less frequently, the antebrachium) as a result of increased fluids in an area tightly bound by fascia. Because fascia does not "give" to allow more space to accommodate this fluid buildup, this edema can compress on nerves and blood vessels as they course through the compartment, leading to ischemia and possible nerve damage. Because the edema is contained within the compartment, the PTA should be alert to other associated signs and symptoms:

pain ("cramping") with activity that improves with rest; increased superficial temperature of the region; a tight, shiny appearance of the skin; and, in advanced cases, changes in the sensation in the area and distally. Immediate consultation with the supervising PT and possibly immediate medical referral are warranted if the signs and symptoms are noted.

PAIN

In the *Normative Model of Physical Therapist Assistant Education*,[5] entry-level PTA data collection skills related to pain include the following:

- Recognize pain behavior and reaction during specific movements.
- Recognize muscle soreness during specific movements.
- Describe pain and soreness with joint movement.
- Describe pain perception (e.g., phantom pain).

An important skill that novice clinicians must develop along the path to entry-level competence is to attend to the patient as a whole being, with the various elements being assessed working together to produce full function. It is crucial for the PTA to conduct an assessment of pain responses and behaviors throughout each patient interaction. A common behavior of a novice clinician performing basic assessment skills is for the clinician to focus on the involved body part and overlook the overall response of the patient to specific procedures. For example, a patient may exhibit strength of the quadriceps muscle group that measures 4+/5. However, if the student PTA performing the assessment of strength fails to observe that the patient is grimacing in pain during the resisted isometric test, he or she is overlooking an important determinant of true function of the muscle group. Likewise, other components of function, such as range of motion and flexibility, must include pain-free performance to be wholly functional. Ideally the PTA student will make the transition from focusing only on the involved body part during assessment procedures and interventions to performing assessments that include comprehensive observation of the patient's responses and behaviors.

Although pain is considered subjective, because there are multiple internal factors that determine a patient's perception of pain, complaints of pain always should be addressed as legitimate or "real." The PTA's role in assessing pain is to gather data that present a clear picture of the following:

- Changes in pain since last PT visit or examination
- Responses of the patient in terms of how interventions to date or at present affect pain
- Patterns of pain (e.g., physical or temporal)
- Modalities, types, or characteristics of pain (e.g., "sharp" or "burning")

Several standardized instruments are available to record findings of pain assessment. As with all assessment procedures, the PTA must use the same instrument or same technique for recording data related to a patient's pain complaints as was used by the evaluating PT during the initial examination. Two examples of simple and commonly used tools are a pain rating scale and a visual analog scale. Refer to Figures 2-3, 2-4, and 2-5 for examples.[19]

During the course of carrying out elements of the plan of care, the PTA may notice a change in the quality of a patient's pain from more acute to chronic pain. As described in the section on inflammation, a chronic state is one in which the symptoms (pain in this case) persist for a period of time longer than expected, based on physiologic principles of tissue healing. Chronic pain has been described as that which lasts more than 3 months.[10] Recall also that one descriptive feature of a chronic condition relates to the lack of real, ongoing, or pending tissue damage. In regard to pain, this circumstance also often coincides with complaints of pain that are nonspecific, diffuse, or indirectly proportional to the physical appearance or presentation of the patient.

McGill-Melzack
PAIN QUESTIONNAIRE

Patient's name ________ Age ________
File No. ________ Date ________
Clinical category (e.g., cardiac, neurological, etc.): ________

Diagnosis: ________

Analgesic (if already administered):
1. Type ________
2. Dosage ________
3. Time given in relation to this test ________

Patient's intelligence: circle number that represents best estimate
1 (low) 2 3 4 5 (high)

****

This questionnaire has been designed to tell us more about your pain. Four major questions we ask are:

1. Where is your pain?
2. What does it feel like?
3. How does it change with time?
4. How strong is it?

It is important that you tell us how your pain feels now. Please follow the instructions at the beginning of each part.

© R. Melzack, Oct. 1970

Part 1. Where Is Your Pain?

Please mark, on the drawings below, the areas where you feel pain. Put E if external, or I if internal, near the areas which you mark. Put EI if both external and internal.

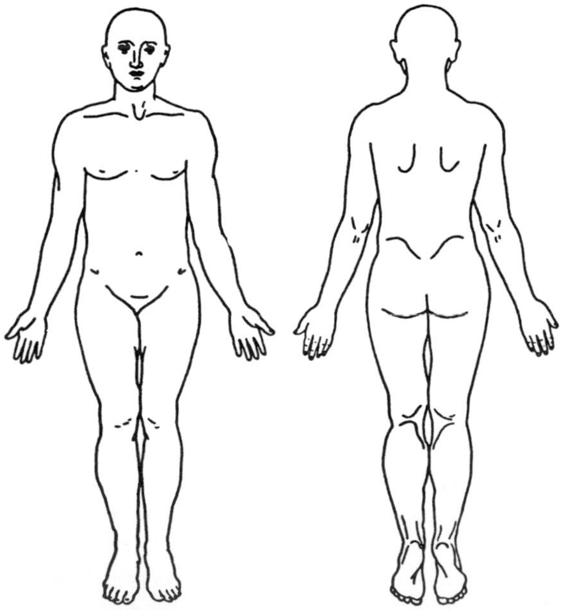

Part 2. What Does Your Pain Feel Like?

Some of the words below describe your present pain. Circle ONLY those words that best describe it. Leave out any category that is not suitable. Use only a single word in each appropriate category—the one that applies best.

1	2	3	4
Flickering Quivering Pulsing Throbbing Beating Pounding	Jumping Flashing Shooting	Pricking Boring Drilling Stabbing Lancinating	Sharp Cutting Lacerating
5	**6**	**7**	**8**
Pinching Pressing Gnawing Cramping Crushing	Tugging Pulling Wrenching	Hot Burning Scalding Searing	Tingling Itchy Smarting Stinging
9	**10**	**11**	**12**
Dull Sore Hurting Aching Heavy	Tender Taut Rasping Splitting	Tiring Exhausting	Sickening Suffocating
13	**14**	**15**	**16**
Fearful Frightful Terrifying	Punishing Gruelling Cruel Vicious Killing	Wretched Blinding	Annoying Troublesome Miserable Intense Unbearable
17	**18**	**19**	**20**
Spreading Radiating Penetrating Piercing	Tight Numb Drawing Squeezing Tearing	Cool Cold Freezing	Nagging Nauseating Agonizing Dreadful Torturing

Part 3. How Does Your Pain Change With Time?

1. Which word or words would you use to describe the pattern of your pain?

1	2	3
Continuous	Rhythmic	Brief
Steady	Periodic	Momentary
Constant	Intermittent	Transient

2. What kind of things relieve your pain?

3. What kind of things increase your pain?

Part 4. How Strong Is Your Pain?

People agree that the following 5 words represent pain of increasing intensity. They are:

1	2	3	4	5
Mild	Discomforting	Distressing	Horrible	Excruciating

To answer each question below, write the number of the most appropriate word in the space beside the question.

1. Which word describes your pain right now? ________
2. Which word describes it at its worst? ________
3. Which word describes it when it is least? ________
4. Which word describes the worst toothache you ever had? ________
5. Which word describes the worst headache you ever had? ________
6. Which word describes the worst stomach-ache you ever had? ________

Fig. 2-3 McGill-Melzack Pain Questionnaire. (From Melzack R: The McGill Pain Questionnaire. Major properties and scoring methods. *Pain* 1975;1:280–281.)

On the line provided, please mark where your "pain status" is today.

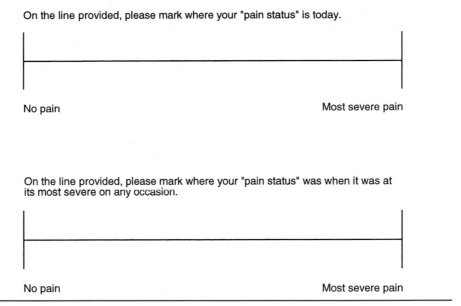

No pain   Most severe pain

On the line provided, please mark where your "pain status" was when it was at its most severe on any occasion.

No pain   Most severe pain

Fig. 2-4 Visual analog scales for pain. (From Magee DJ: Orthopedic Physical Assessment, 4th ed. Philadelphia, WB Saunders, 2002:7.)

Instructions:
Below is a thermometer with various grades of pain on it from "No pain at all" to "The pain is almost unbearable." Put an × by the words that describe your pain best. Mark how bad your pain is AT THIS MOMENT IN TIME.

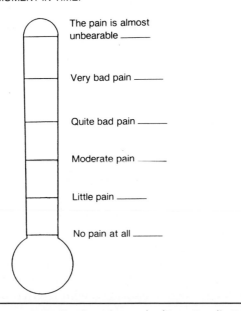

The pain is almost unbearable _____

Very bad pain _____

Quite bad pain _____

Moderate pain _____

Little pain _____

No pain at all _____

Fig. 2-5 "Thermometer" pain rating scale. (From Brodie DJ, Burnett JV, Walker JM, et al: Evaluation of low back pain by patient questionnaires and therapeutic assessment. *J Orthop Sports Phys Ther* 1990;11:528.)

In this case the PTA's documentation or other interaction with the supervising PT may include recommendations for changes in the goals and plan of care to address the pain by incorporating interventions that will attend to the more complex issues involved with chronic pain. Specifically, depression and a cycle involving decreased activity levels and associated decreased tolerance to activity often ensues with chronic pain. The PTA may recommend the inclusion of relaxation exercises and a comprehensive gradual conditioning program in this case. Furthermore, when the PTA notices that a patient is exhibiting signs and symptoms of chronic pain, further diagnostic workup may be indicated, because the presence of chronic pain may signal involvement of systems or factors other than musculoskeletal structures (e.g., depression).

Certain changes that occur in complaints of pain in response to therapeutic interventions are expected. **Peripheralization** (spreading to areas outside of or distant from the immediate area of involvement) may indicate a worsening or progressive condition. A typical example of this occurs with a progressively herniating spinal disk, indicating increasing compression of the associated nerve root. **Centralization** (increasing signs and symptoms in the immediate area of the lesion) of pain symptoms may indicate improvement of the condition, such as in the case of decreasing compression on a nerve root as a disk herniation is reduced.

The PTA must establish the location of pain when the patient reports changes in pain symptoms associated with certain positions or movements. For example, the patient with a primary diagnosis of low back pain

Table 2-2	*Red Flag Pain Symptoms*
Pathology or Body System	**Pain Complaint or Symptom**
Cardiovascular	Pain or feeling of heaviness in the chest
	Pulsating pain anywhere in the body
	Constant and severe pain in lower leg
Cancer	Persistent pain at night or pain that awakens patient
	Constant pain unrelieved by change in position or activity
Gastrointestinal	Frequent or severe abdominal pain
Neurologic	Frequent or severe headaches

Adapted from Magee DJ: Orthopedic Physical Assessment, Philadelphia, WB Saunders, 2002; Tatro-Adams D, McGann S, Carbone W: Reliability of the figure-of-eight method on subjects with ankle joint swelling. *J Orthop Sports Phys Ther* 1995;22(4):161–163. (With permission of the Orthopaedic and Sports Physical Therapy Sections of the American Physical Therapy Association.)

secondary to *HNP (herniated nucleus pulposus)* may complain of pain when lying prone. The PTA must not assume that the pain is in the area of the disk lesion, which is a positive indication of centralization and a desired response. If, on further questioning, it is determined that the pain is referred to the lower extremity along the neural distribution for the involved spinal segment, then this is a sign of peripheralization of the symptoms, indicating that the prone position is not appropriate at this time. Thus the importance of understanding neuromuscular anatomy and function cannot be overlooked. The PTA student must become familiar with these anatomic relationships to fully understand the implications of data collected during pain assessment.

"Red Flag" Pain Symptoms

The PTA also must be keenly aware of pain that sends a "red flag" signal. In this case, the PTA should not proceed with any interventions that are potentially contraindicated and should also report this condition to the supervising PT. Table 2-2[19, 25] presents a summary of "red flag" or potentially serious pain conditions and the possible associated pathology or body system.

In addition to the "red flag" symptoms described here, the PTA working with any clientele must be alert to signs and symptoms of myocardial infarction (MI, heart attack). Certain patterns of pain have been identified as early warning signs of a heart attack (Fig. 2-6).[10] The PTA working with a patient exhibiting any of these patterns of pain should consult with the supervising PT right away for possible immediate medical referral. Concurrent symptoms of MI may include nausea, pallor, and profuse perspiration. Myocardial infarction may occur over a period of time and may be experienced while the patient is undergoing exertion or even at rest.

Intermittent Claudication

Another distinct pattern or type of pain that may manifest coincidentally with musculoskeletal symptoms or conditions is that of **intermittent claudication,** which is the term used to describe activity-related discomfort associated with peripheral arterial disease (PAD). Intermittent claudication is typically described as "aching" or "cramping" that is localized in the region affected by the impaired circulation.[10] Because it involves a systemic condition, it typically manifests bilaterally and usually involves the calves, thighs, or buttocks, areas that are often symptomatic with musculoskeletal pathologies.[2, 10] Once the aggravating activity is discontinued, it is characteristic for the symptoms of claudication (pain or cramping) to improve rapidly.

The assessment for intermittent claudication consists of determining what is referred to as "claudication time." The basic protocols most commonly used consist of having the patient walk at a particular speed (2.0 mph) and incline grade (in 2.0% or 3.0% increment increases) and then measuring the time until onset of symptoms occurs and the time of maximal walking tolerance.[2] As with other standardized tests and measures, the technique employed by the PTA must be the same technique used by the evaluating PT.

It is also possible that the PTA may be the first clinician to recognize the symptoms associated with undiagnosed occlusive vascular disease, in terms of the nature, characteristics, and location of symptoms as described. Other signs and symptoms that are consistent with PAD include pallor, decrease in peripheral pulses, sensory changes, and weakness of the involved area (distal to the site of blocked circulation). Diabetes mellitus and nonhealing wounds on the feet also are frequently associated with PAD.[9] Obviously observation of the signs of undiagnosed PAD should be reported to the supervising PT immediately.

Referred Pain

The term **referred pain** describes pain related to patterns of innervation to organs or other anatomic structures. Referred pain is defined as pain that is "referred from deep somatic or visceral structures to a distant region within the same neural segment, with or without hyperalgesia and hyperesthesia, deep tenderness, muscle spasms, and autonomic disturbance."[11] True neurologic findings (muscle weakness and diminished deep tendon reflexes) are not associated with referred pain.[11]

Visceral Pain

The term **visceral pain** refers to pain that originates from a body organ. The primary concern for the PTA related to this type of pain is for the PTA to be aware of how

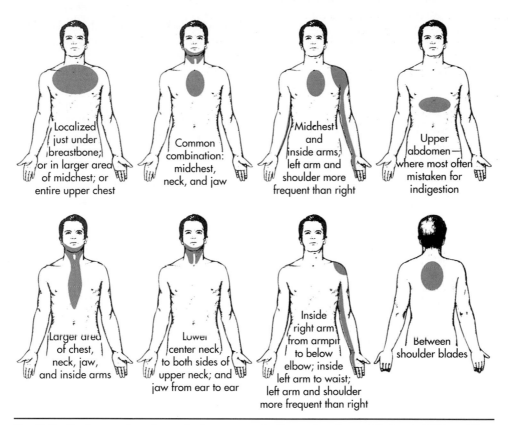

Fig. 2-6 Early warning signs of a heart attack. (From Goodman CC, Snyder TEK: Differential Diagnosis in Physical Therapy, 3rd ed. Philadelphia, WB Saunders, 2003:127.)

visceral pain may manifest and report suspicious pain symptoms to the supervising PT. Often disease processes involving specific or multiple organs reveal themselves through a variety of symptoms and not just pain. However, it is quite possible for a patient to have more than one pathologic condition at the same time. In other words a patient with a confirmed diagnosis of herniated disc in the lumbar spine also could have some type of developing abdominal pathology. Pain of a visceral origin may present as musculoskeletal symptoms because of the innervation pattern of the involved organ. Figure 2-7 provides a visual representation of innervation to major internal organs in terms of spinal levels of nerve supply.[10] Note that the organs are supplied via plexuses or ganglia, resulting in innervation from multiple segmental levels. For this reason organ pain may be diffuse and difficult for the patient to localize, appearing as nonspecific musculoskeletal discomfort. In the case of disease processes that develop over time, the PTA must be alert to changes in the patient's complaints of pain and reports from the patient of patterns that are not consistent with musculoskeletal conditions.

Trigger Points

"**Trigger points** are discrete, focal, hyperirritable spots located in a taut band of skeletal muscle."[1] Trigger points are associated with musculoskeletal conditions

such as temporomandibular joint dysfunction, cervical strain, fibromyalgia, and myofascial pain syndrome. The pain produced by trigger points is characterized by tenderness and a referred pattern of pain to palpation, usually in upper quarter or pelvic girdle muscles. According to a recent article in *American Family Physician*,[1] "Palpation of a hypersensitive bundle or nodule of muscle fiber of harder than normal consistency is the physical finding typically associated with a trigger point. Palpation of the trigger point will elicit pain directly over the affected area or cause radiation of pain toward a zone of reference and a local twitch response." If, during the process of applying hands-on soft-tissue interventions or passive exercises, the PTA notices signs and symptoms of possible trigger points that have not been previously documented, these findings should be reported to the evaluating PT to be included in the complete diagnostic picture of the patient.

Pain: A Final Note

On occasion the PTA may be faced with the circumstance that the patient's complaints of pain do not match observed behaviors of the patient. In this case, it is not the role of the PTA to judge the patient and conclude that the patient is malingering or "faking" the condition. Instead the PTA should report and record his or her observations objectively and include in the

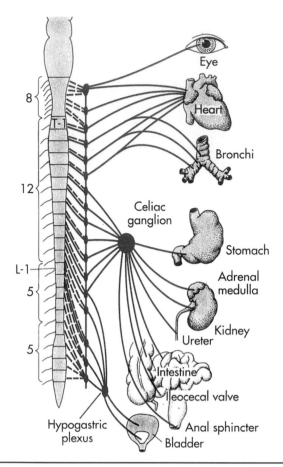

Fig. 2-7 Diagram of the autonomic nervous system. The visceral afferent fibers mediating pain travel with the sympathetic nerves, except for those from the pelvic organs, which follow the parasympathetics of the pelvic nerve. (From Guyton AC, Hall JE: Textbook of Medical Physiology, 9th ed. Philadelphia, WB Saunders, 1996.)

assessment his or her judgment that the observed behaviors are not consistent with the patient's reported pain symptoms or with the PT diagnosis.

VITAL SIGNS

An objective measure of physiologic status, particularly as related to cardiopulmonary function, can be obtained quickly through measurement and assessment of vital signs. Body temperature is discussed in the section on inflammation; heart rate, blood pressure, and respiration are discussed here. It may be observed that vital signs are not routinely assessed in the outpatient clinic that serves mainly patients with orthopedic diagnoses. However, as the profession of physical therapy strives toward achieving the status of a recognized point of entry for the health care consumer, we must shift our perception of "routine" procedures to

include a more thorough and comprehensive assessment of the patient's overall health status and responses to our treatments.

The student is encouraged to become proficient with effective assessment of vital signs through repeated practice on a variety of subjects and on subjects in different positions (supine versus sitting, versus standing), as well as subjects performing different activities (e.g., activities of daily living [ADLS] and exercise).

It is not within the scope of this text to discuss or review detailed physiology related to cardiopulmonary function or pathology. General guidelines for collecting vital sign data and determining when modification to planned interventions is warranted are discussed.

Pulse (Heart Rate)

Heart rate should be measured at the time of evaluation to establish a baseline rate and subsequently when beginning any exercise program or new activity. Accepted values for normal heart rate in adults range from 60 to 100 beats per minute (BPM). Factors that influence heart rate include age, gender, emotional state, and exercise or conditioning level.[24]

In addition to the quantitative measure, the quality of the pulse should be noted. Often in a setting where the PTA is working primarily with "healthy" clients (e.g., trained or conditioned athletes), it may be sufficient to perform a 6-second beat-count and multiply by 10 to quickly determine the cardiovascular response to an activity. However, if the PTA perceives any abnormal quality to the pulse, such as an irregular rhythm or a "thready" pulse (lacking distinct beats), the heart rate should be monitored for a full minute. In such a case, if the abnormality has not previously been noted, this finding should be reported to the supervising PT immediately. Otherwise, as in the case with other assessment procedures, the PTA should employ the same technique as the PT uses during the initial evaluation to enhance consistency and better determine any deviation from the baseline measure.

Several textbooks commonly used by PTA educational programs offer specific guidelines for setting exercise intensity using heart rate as a determinant.[7,16,24] A basic guideline to determine a safe exercise level is a return of the pulse to its resting rate within 5 minutes of discontinuing exercise and avoid exceeding resting heart rate by more than 20 BPM during exercise.[9]

Respiration

As with pulse, respirations should be assessed for both rate and quality. In the healthy adult, normal respiratory rate ranges from 10 to 20 breaths per minute. Variations in the range of "normal" respiration rate are expected among age groups. Other factors influencing respirations include age, body size, stature, exercise, and body position.[24]

At rest, respiration should be smooth and steady, with uniform chest movement. Observe for excessive use of accessory breathing muscles (anterior upper quarter, anterolateral shoulder, and cervical muscles), which may indicate ventilatory compromise (e.g., chronic obstructive pulmonary disease, asthma, chronic bronchitis caused by smoking, or other pathologic conditions). Also observe to ensure that chest expansion is symmetric bilaterally. Because respiration includes voluntary control, it is best to discreetly assess respiration in conjunction with heart rate to avoid the patient inadvertently altering breathing pattern or rate in response to feeling self-conscious if he or she is aware that the PTA is observing the rise and fall of the chest. Refer to the section of this chapter on fatigue for information relating specifically to the assessment of pulmonary response to exercise and activity.

Blood Pressure

Assessment of *blood pressure* provides an objective measurement of the amount of force blood is exerting against vessel walls at a given time. The pressure exerted by blood is influenced by various factors and conditions, including age and cardiac output, both of which are directly proportional to systolic blood pressure. Obviously, age is a nonmodifiable factor, so an increase in systolic blood pressure of elderly patients may not necessarily indicate an active pathologic process. As always, these findings should be noted in relation to the baseline measurement obtained by the PT during the initial examination.

The PTA working with patients who have musculoskeletal dysfunction or impairment is most concerned with noting responses in blood pressure as new therapeutic activities are introduced or advanced during the course of progression through the established plan of care. Most notably, blood pressure is affected by exercise and activity level in the following ways. Cardiac output increases proportionally to increased physical activity.[12] An even greater and potentially dangerous increase in blood pressure also may occur if the patient holds his or her breath during periods of exertion with exercise. Patients may do this subconsciously in an effort to increase the weight-bearing function of the abdominal cavity, which becomes more stable with an attempt at strong exhalation against a closed glottis, nose, and mouth. As noted in the discussion about pain, the PTA must be alert to the patient's total response to interventions. When the observant PTA notices that the patient is holding his or her breath during exertion, the patient should be educated in techniques to avoid this behavior. The PTA also may want to reassess blood pressure at this time, although the effect on blood pressure from this activity, known as the **Valsalva maneuver,** is transient. It is particularly critical that the Valsalva maneuver be avoided by patients with a known history of hypertension or cardiac disease.[12]

Another important blood pressure response that may occur during a physical therapy session is a sudden drop in blood pressure, called **orthostatic hypotension.** This rapid drop in blood pressure is associated with a sudden change in the patient's position. It is most frequently the result of the patient being immobile or recumbent for prolonged periods of time. Signs of orthostatic hypotension include lightheadedness, weakness, dizziness, or diaphoresis. If not addressed (by returning the patient to at least a semireclined position), the patient may lose consciousness. Because of the rapid change in blood pressure, the PTA must be prepared to assess the blood pressure immediately upon the change in position. The blood pressure response is critical to obtain, record, and report because the symptoms associated with orthostatic hypotension also could be caused by other serious medical conditions.

Three final points should be noted by the student PTA. First, the PTA should check to be sure of any precautions or contraindications for the assessment of blood pressure that may be present. If the patient has a history of circulatory or lymphatic drainage compromise in one upper extremity, blood pressure must be assessed in the contralateral upper extremity. Second, as mentioned in relation to assessment of other vital signs, the PTA student should practice taking and monitoring blood pressure on a variety of "healthy" individuals to reinforce a sense of values and ranges considered "normal." Finally, the psychomotor skill involved with applying and securing the blood pressure cuff and attached sphygmomanometer, applying and holding the stethoscope diaphragm, pumping air into the bulb, releasing pressure from the cuff, and reading the meter while listening for the blood pressure sounds (called *Korotkoff sounds*) does take coordination and skill. Although the process is basic and consistent, practice reinforces efficient application in actual patient care situations.

Pulse Oximetry

In addition to the measurement of vital signs described, **pulse oximetry** is a tool used to provide instant information about a subject's cardiopulmonary status. Specifically, the pulse oximeter is a noninvasive probe (in the form of a clip-on device placed on the ear, finger, foot, or nose) that provides a digital readout of oxyhemoglobin saturation. Most commonly, this device is employed in the acute and critical care settings or during exercise testing and training.[13] However, for the patient in the hospital setting who has coexisting cardiopulmonary and musculoskeletal involvement, pulse oximetry is a viable tool for establishing goals to address tolerance to progressive activities.

The standard "normal" value for oxygen saturation ranges from 95% to 98%; this value is not expected to change with activity or exercise in the healthy individual.[9,12] This level noticeably decreases in patients with chronic respiratory disease; the PTA must be aware of normal ranges for a given individual in this case. Activity should be halted if the value of oxygen saturation drops below 90% in the acutely ill patient or below 86% in the patient with chronic lung disease.[9] If the referring physician has indicated any other specific level of oxygen saturation to use as a guideline for a given patient, the PTA must be sure to be aware of this level, so that exercise tolerance will not be exceeded.[12]

Vital Signs and Exercise

As the profession of physical therapy evolves, with the pursuit of uniform direct access throughout the country, physical therapists will more often be the "point of entry" for the health care consumer. Along with this increased autonomy and recognition also come increased responsibilities of physical therapy providers, including PTAs, to assess and monitor the patient's general health status, making decisions and judgments accordingly. For the PTA working with orthopedically involved patients, this responsibility included being aware of normal and expected vital signs, values, and responses and monitoring for the unexpected.

Certain responses in vital signs are expected with exercise. In a "Scientific Statement" published by The American Heart Association,[8] detailed guidelines for exercise testing and training are provided, taking into consideration the cardiovascular health status of the patient. Abnormal blood pressure responses include the absence of an increase in systolic pressure or a drop in systolic pressure with exercise; a normal response is an increase that correlates to the rate and intensity of exercise initiation.[13] If the patient's systolic blood pressure elevates to >250 mmHg or if the diastolic pressure elevates to >110 mmHg during exercise, the activity should be discontinued.[9] Further, the systolic pressure should not rise >20 mmHg with minimal to moderate exercise or >40 to 50 mmHg with intensive exercise.[9] Diastolic blood pressure is not expected to increase or decrease more than 10 mmHg with exercise in the healthy adult.[9] Refer to Table 2-3 for a summary of abnormal responses of vital signs to exercise.[12]

FATIGUE

In general the PTA is expected to be competent with participating in making judgments about a patient's status to determine the need for adjusting or withholding intervention accordingly.[5] In relation to fatigue, this may translate as observing and reporting abnormal responses to activity and making modifications to the interventions within the context of the existing plan of care. Fatigue may be specific to an individual muscle or muscle group, or it may affect the entire body, mani-

Table 2-3	*Abnormal Responses to Exercise*
Heart rate increases more than 20 to 30 BPM above resting heart rate	
Heart rate decreases below resting heart rate	
Systolic blood pressure increases more than 20 to 30 mmHg above resting level	
Systolic blood pressure decreases more than 10 mmHg below resting level	
Oxygen saturation drops below prescribed level	
Patient becomes short of breath or respiratory rate increases to a level not tolerated by the patient	
Electrocardiogram changes	

From Hillegass EA, Sadows HS: Essentials of Cardiopulmonary Physical Therapy, 2nd ed. Philadelphia, WB Saunders, 2001.

festing as cardiopulmonary (also called *cardiorespiratory* or *general*) fatigue.[16]

A muscle in a state of fatigue is unable to generate a normal contraction, which may manifest by decreased force, range of motion, or quality of the contraction. The patient may complain of discomfort or cramping in the muscle being exercised.[16] When a muscle is fatigued, the patient may compensate by consciously or subconsciously substituting with another muscle or muscle group that performs the same or similar action. For this reason, it is very important for the PTA to be particularly familiar with muscle actions and potential substitutions and observe patients during exercise activities. In terms of quality of motion, fatigue may result in tremulous or "jerky" motions, instead of a smooth contraction through the range of motion.[16]

Generalized fatigue is apparent when the patient is experiencing *dyspnea* or inability to breathe normally with activity, indicating a decreased ability of the body to use oxygen efficiently.[13,16] One tool that has been determined to be a fairly good indicator of a patient's pulmonary tolerance to exercise is a standardized scale referred to as **Rate of Perceived Exertion** (RPE).[12] This instrument calls for the patient to place an objective grade on the amount of exertion he or she perceives with exertion, thus making a subjective report more measurable. Similar instruments for rating the level of shortness of breath, or dyspnea, also exist; these consist of a 5- or 10-point scale or a visual analog scale on which the patient rates the amount of dyspnea experienced with activity.[12] As with all standardized instruments, the PTA uses the form, instrument, or technique consistent with that of the evaluating PT when the initial examination occurred. If the PT chose to use a standardized instrument to document examination data related to the patient's tolerance to activity, it is likely that a goal addressing that impairment is included in the plan of care, with the outcome to be measured using the same instrument.

ASSESSMENT OF MUSCULOSKELETAL STRUCTURES

Detailed reviews of anatomy and function of specific structures are not covered here because the scope of this chapter is limited to the PTA's role in assessment. Rather, this section provides information relating to entry-level data collection and assessment procedures pertaining to structures involved with musculoskeletal diagnoses commonly encountered by the PTA.

End-Feel

End-feel is the term used to describe the quality of limitation (normal or pathologic) obtained by passively moving a body part to its extreme range of motion. Because different types of tissue have different characteristics and qualities to their constituency, there are associated normal and abnormal end-feels for each tissue. Normal end-feels are described simply as soft, firm, or hard. Other terms used to denote normal end-feels include "soft tissue approximation," such as occurs with full elbow flexion; "tissue stretch" or "leathery," such as occurs with ankle dorsiflexion; and "bony," "bone contacting bone," or "bone-to-bone," such as occurs with knee extension.[16,19,23] Obviously these terms are descriptive of the specific anatomic relationships of structures that normally limit the motion of each joint. The PTA student is encouraged to practice assessing the different normal end-feels on a variety of subjects, because the exact perception varies depending on the structure and build of each individual tested.

When one of the end-feels (described in the preceding) is noted in a joint that normally exhibits a different end-feel, it is considered to be abnormal or pathologic. A soft end-feel perceived in a joint that normally has a firm or hard end-feel may be described as "boggy" and could be indicative of soft-tissue edema or synovial inflammation.[23] A pathologic firm end-feel also has been described as "capsular" and may result from muscle guarding or inflammatory conditions.[11] A hard or bony end-feel ("bony block") that occurs unexpectedly in a joint or at a point in mid–range of motion could signify the presence of a loose body (bony fragment) in the joint, a fracture, or other pathologic skeletal condition.[11,23] As always, when the PTA recognizes these abnormal circumstances, these findings must be reported to the evaluating PT.

One additional pathologic end-feel is termed the *empty* end-feel. An empty end-feel is one in which the PTA is unable to determine the actual end range response, because of the presence of pain that prevents the patient from achieving full range. Obviously if this finding was not present at the time of initial examination, interventions must be halted and the supervising PT must be notified immediately.

Contractile Tissue

The term *contractile tissue* refers to soft tissues that have properties of contractility and irritability.[11] Contractility is the term used to describe the muscle's ability to contract and relax, by virtue of the actin–myosin filament cross-bridges; *irritability* refers to the tissue's response to electrical impulses that either stimulate or inhibit the muscle's action (contraction, relaxation, or other change in state of tone).

Strength Testing

It is beyond the scope of this text to provide detailed instruction in the performance of techniques used to measure strength of specific muscles. However, because specific strength increases are frequently included as physical therapy goals, the PTA must be competent with measuring strength, by use of both specific and gross testing techniques. Procedures for assessing muscle strength to determine changes or unexpected findings are discussed here.

When the plan of care includes goals related to increase in specific muscle grades, the PTA must use the same technique for assessing the muscle strength as the evaluating PT used at the time of the initial examination and evaluation. In general, specific manual muscle testing takes into account the precise attachments, action, and position of a muscle during movements or isometric contractions against gravity. Scales for specific muscle grades are also precise, based on word/letter or number scales with strict definitions for each. A table is an organized and convenient way to record data relating to muscle strength testing; an example of a table format is provided in Box 2-4.

In contrast to specific manual muscle testing, gross manual muscle testing techniques are used to quickly determine a nonprecise, yet objective measurement of functional strength. This technique might be used as an efficient method to determine a patient's readiness to

---

BOX 2-4

Sample Format for Recording Muscle Strength

Joint/Motion	Muscle Test Grade*		
Shoulder	Right	Left	Other Response†
Flexion	4–/5	2+/5	
Extension	4/5	3/5	
Internal rotation	4/5	3–/5	
External rotation	4+/5	3–/5	

*Measurements represent example of ascending 0 to 5 scale.
†"Other responses" could include notation regarding the presence of pain, etc.

progress with exercise or gait activities, for example. This method also may be used to gather data about any changes in the patient's status since the initial examination or last therapy session. In general, movements should be resisted bilaterally and, when possible, simultaneously on both sides for easy comparison. Positions or test movements do not necessarily take gravity into account but focus more on functional positions and movements, such as shaking hands, grasping the therapist's fingers, or lowering and rising to and from a squatting position. In addition to gross strength, the PTA should be alert for any signs of pain or discomfort with resisted muscle testing. Again, the PTA conducting gross manual muscle tests is not attempting to obtain a precise measurement of strength, but is gathering data relevant to the patient's progress toward goals; readiness to progress through the established plan of care; and status, in terms of changes in condition. The PTA must report any unexpected changes or previously undocumented data related to muscle strength to the supervising therapist.

If the PTA observes signs of pain with resisted movements during strength testing, he or she must make certain that the test is being performed in such a way as to avoid causing active insufficiency of muscles being tested. Active insufficiency results from improper positioning of a two-joint or multijoint muscle and causes a cramping type of pain.[15] Pain experienced with muscle testing during a properly performed technique could be indicative of an inflammatory state or strain of the tissues being stressed. Because the musculotendinous tissue is responsible for sustaining joint position during resistance, the presence of pain with muscle testing, even if the result indicates intact strength, points to involvement of the muscle or tendon. Once again, if these data represent a change from the initial examination or evaluation data, the evaluating therapist must be notified.

Another indication of muscle weakness or the possibility of undiagnosed musculoskeletal or neuromuscular pathology is change in muscle mass or tone. Changes in mass may manifest as either atrophy (muscle wasting) or hypertrophy (excessive mass). The PTA should be able to recognize changes in mass as well as make observations about any pattern of these manifestations, such as the involvement of a specific muscle versus a muscle group; the involvement of muscles innervated by common peripheral or spinal nerve segments; and the involvement of unilateral, asymmetric muscles or groups versus bilateral, symmetric involvement.

Tone refers to the state of contractility of a muscle and is determined through observation of movements for quality of motion and control of motion (including grading and coordination) and through palpation. True changes in muscle tone also should be noted in the context of patterns of involvement such as described in the preceding and should be differentiated from a local muscle "guarding" or "splinting" response.

Stretching and Palpation

When contractile tissue (e.g., muscle and tendon) is stretched, pain is reported at the end of the range in the presence of injury or inflammation. An increase in complaints of pain with stretching is reported in the event that a previous stretching or strengthening exercise program has been performed too vigorously or aggressively.

In addition to pain at end range, muscle and tendon tissue that is in a state of inflammation or injury is tender to palpation over the involved area. Trigger points also may be noted upon palpation (see previous discussion of trigger points).

Muscle tenderness or soreness to palpation is not by itself an accurate indicator of the tissues involved because referred pain can also manifest as tenderness. However, the PTA should note the location and degree of tenderness or soreness for purposes of comparison to initial examination findings and possibly as a measure of progress toward goals, if the evaluating therapist addressed this area in the plan of care. A previously unnoticed pattern of tenderness revealed while the PTA is working with the patient should be reported to the evaluating therapist because patterns of the distribution of tender points represent the hallmark characteristic of conditions such as fibromyalgia. It is also important to note how the patient reports tenderness; a response of "painful" versus "tender" is another hallmark feature of fibromyalgia.

As with pain on stretching contractile tissue to end range, palpable tightness or spasm also may occur after exercise or other activity that is too vigorous or aggressive. A muscle may respond to overwork by subconscious "splinting" or "guarding," which results in a feeling of tightness or increased tension to palpation. When increased tightness or spasm is noted upon palpation, modifications to the level of activity or exercise could be warranted within the parameters of the established plan of care.

Flexibility

The loss of the muscle or tendon unit's ability to obtain full length results in decreased flexibility. Decreased flexibility may be differentiated from decreased joint ROM or loss of accessory motions, which may result from involvement of intraarticular structures (discussed in the section on joints).

The end-feel associated with a loss of muscle or tendon flexibility is described as "muscle spasm" end-feel.[11] This end-feel occurs as a result of (subconscious) muscle guarding to avoid movement into a restricted range.

In terms of assessment, the PTA should use a technique consistent with that used by the evaluating physical therapist. Because a loss of flexibility is a problem that may have a significant impact on function, it is an area frequently addressed in the PT plan of care.

Examination techniques and subsequent goals may be addressed in terms of specific quantitative outcomes or more functionally based. An example of a quantitative measurement is the use of goniometric measurements. As with manual muscle testing, detailed instruction in goniometry techniques is beyond the scope of this text. The most important elements of goniometric measurement are accuracy and consistency among testers and testing techniques. PTA educational programs are organized to allow the student to establish a solid foundation in human anatomy, typically including specific emphasis on the musculoskeletal system and structures. To be effective with the application of assessment techniques such as goniometry, the student is strongly encouraged to ensure that he or she possesses this critical knowledge base. In addition to a solid grasp of skeletal and superficial anatomic landmarks, the student must learn other principles associated with goniometric testing, such as the differences among passive, active, and active-assisted ROM. It is common for the novice to document goniometric measurements as an indicator of flexibility, failing to indicate whether the data represent the patient's ability to actively move through the range or whether passive overpressure was applied to obtain the measurement. The functional implications relating to this concept are significant.

Another technique that may be used to obtain and document information related to flexibility is a functional measurement, such as measuring the distance between the patient's fingertips to the floor during forward flexion (e.g., to measure hamstring flexibility). Although this technique may have specific functional implications, many factors may confound the results and make it less specific to the area of focus. For example, forward trunk flexion performed in this manner may be limited by loss of mobility in the lumbar spine, not the hamstring group. Again, for purposes of data collection to accurately assess the patient's progress, the PTA must employ the same technique as the evaluating therapist for each patient case. Furthermore, there should be consistency among therapists within a practice setting to ensure continuity of care for the patients and valid outcome measurements.

Overuse

As in the case with overuse caused by overaggressive or vigorous exercise (active strengthening or passive stretching), the PTA must be alert for signs of overuse or cumulative stress to contractile tissue, particularly tendons. Signs of tendinitis (the inflammatory condition that results from overuse) include painful but strong resisted isometric contraction (e.g., with manual muscle testing techniques), and possibly pain at end range with stretching, as well as tenderness to palpation over the site of irritation, often near or at the tendinous insertion of the involved muscle. The PTA must not dismiss the possibility that a patient progressing through an exercise program may develop signs and symptoms of tendinitis, even if this is not the original reason for referral. As discussed earlier, the long-term effects of inflammation can have serious implications. Therefore it is imperative for the PTA to present this information to the supervising PT and make recommendations for modification to the plan of care to avoid further excessive stresses to these tissues.

BONES

Of primary importance to the physical therapy clinician is the need to rule out conditions or disease processes that are beyond the professional scope of physical therapy, warranting medical diagnosis and treatment. Even without the advent of direct access to physical therapy care, it is possible that a patient may be referred to PT in error for treatment of a condition that in fact requires strict medical attention. The main consideration with bone tissue is fracture. The potential exists for the fracture to be "missed" on initial examination (medical or physical therapy). An existing fracture also may progress, in terms of malalignment, in the case of a "hairline" or "crack" fracture, in which case referral for immobilization may be indicated. Therefore it is critical for the PTA to have an understanding of the signs and symptoms of acute fracture, regardless of the severity.

If the patient exhibits exquisite "point" tenderness over a localized site other than a ligament or other supportive structure, a fracture may be indicated versus other musculoskeletal involvement (e.g., a ligamentous sprain). Another sign of fracture includes localized edema, again in a region not directly associated with joint involvement (e.g., over the midshaft, diaphysis, or body of a long bone or in the area of the body of a flat bone). Furthermore, the patient may complain of a "grinding" or unstable sensation. Pain associated with fracture is described as "bone pain," or "deep" in nature.

Of particular importance to the physical therapy clinician is the rising incidence of osteoporosis, which affects approximately 10 million people currently living in the United States, with an additional 18 million at risk because of low bone mass (osteopenia).[9,20] Fractures, which may be asymptomatic or "silent," most commonly affect the vertebral bodies, hips, ribs, radius, and femur in the presence of osteoporosis.[9] Because of the high prevalence and risk of osteoporosis, the astute PTA must recognize the possibility of vertebral compression fractures in a patient with complaints of mid- or low back pain. The nature of the pain associated with a vertebral compression fracture tends to be exquisite (localized) and tender upon palpation.[9] The patient may report radiating pain to the abdomen or flanks (sides of the trunk); typically the pain is aggravated with exertion or prolonged sitting or standing.[9] The pain associated with vertebral compression fractures may be differentiated from that associated with metastatic disease, which tends to be more diffuse and not clearly related to positions or activities.

A vertebral compression fracture associated with osteoporosis often occurs in the absence of trauma or other fall-related history.[9] On occasion a patient who has been referred to the physician for further evaluation of a possible vertebral compression fracture—the most common osteoporosis-related spinal fracture[9]—is subsequently diagnosed with osteoporosis; in some cases, radiographs also reveal previously undiagnosed, healed vertebral compression fractures. It is beyond the scope of this text to provide a detailed description of osteoporosis, its risk factors, and its treatment. The reader is referred to the National Osteoporosis Foundation for resources and information available to the public (*www.nof.org*).[22]

In the area of a known, healing fracture, the stability of the fracture fragments is one indicator of the stage of healing of the fracture. *It is contraindicated for the PTA to attempt to mobilize fracture fragments to determine the stage of healing.*

JOINTS AND LIGAMENTS
Accessory Joint Motions

As a component of evaluation, the PT assesses ligamentous integrity and accessory joint motions for the purposes of differential diagnosis and making decisions on which to base the plan of care. It is the position of the American Physical Therapy Association that spinal and peripheral joint mobilization techniques are interventions performed exclusively by the PT.[6] Although the PTA is not responsible for these elements of physical therapy patient care, it is nonetheless important that he or she understands the implications of assessment procedures that may reveal problems with structures that contribute to joint integrity. The PTA also must be able to assess to determine progress or changes in condition.

The term **accessory joint motion** refers to those motions that occur simultaneously with movement of the bony lever(s) within a joint to allow normal, functional movement (normal *arthrokinematics*). Accessory joint actions (also referred to as "component motions" and "joint play")[11] include movement such as gliding, sliding, or rotation of bony components during joint motion. The PTA's role is to assess motions for normal arthrokinematics of accessory joint motions. Abnormal findings that may be noted in the presence of impaired accessory motions include decreased joint range of motion, a capsular end-feel during stretching techniques, and substitution or compensatory attempts by the patient to obtain full motion. When the motion of a given joint is limited by the joint capsule, a normal capsular end-feel is noticed; an example of a motion limited by the capsule is shoulder external rotation. In this discussion, "capsular end-feel" is used to describe joint motion that is normally limited by other structures but is exhibiting a capsular end-feel because of the presence of an abnormal condition.

Distraction and Compression

"Distraction" (a manual separating of adjacent joint surfaces) and "compression" (a manual approximation of joint surfaces) are assessment techniques that can provide information about the involvement of tissues or structures that serve to provide support to the joint (ligaments); that lie between the joint surfaces (cartilage); or that are directly affected by joint mechanics (bursae). In the presence of mechanical or structural problems that result in impingement on structures located within or near a joint, distracting the joint may produce a relief of symptoms such as pain (radiating or local) or dysesthesia. The PTA's role in this case is to report any previously undocumented findings that may provide information as to the nature of the patient's problem.

Likewise, if the PTA notices an increase in the patient's symptoms of pain or signs such as **crepitus** (joint noise resulting from changes—usually increased coarseness or roughening—of the joint surfaces) during approximation or weight-bearing activities, he or she should suspect degenerative or inflammatory conditions and should report these incidents to the PT.

Bursae are fluid-filled sacs that are located near tendinous insertions to reduce friction with motion. Bursae also may develop as an adaptive mechanism in the presence of excessive friction. An inflamed bursa sometimes is visible near a joint as a small, soft, encapsulated protrusion that is tender to touch. Any signs of a pathologic or inflamed bursa should be reported to the supervising PT. Changes in exercise programs or functional activities should be incorporated into the plan of care. If a locally enlarged and painful joint also presents with increased local temperature, a report of sudden onset, and extreme tenderness, the patient may be exhibiting signs of gout and requires referral for further medical workup if this condition has not been diagnosed previously.

Ligamentous Integrity

During the course of administering components of the physical therapy plan of care for the patient with history or diagnosis of ligament sprain, the PTA must be able to assess the patient's readiness to progress with interventions that will increase stresses to the healing tissue. Ligamentous laxity or improper healing results in decreased joint stability, which may manifest as complaints from the patient that the joint or weight-bearing extremity feels as if it may "give." In this case the PTA should consult with the PT before initiating progressive activities; failure to modify interventions in this case may result in impaired healing, regression of healing, or permanent tissue damage.

If the PTA notices the sudden onset of increased edema, heat to touch, and extremely painful and limited mobility during the course of treatment of a patient with a ligament sprain, the supervising PT must be consulted to seek medical referral to rule out *hemarthrosis* (bleeding inside the joint capsule).[9]

Gait

For the PTA to be proficient with assessment of gait, he or she must first obtain a solid understanding of the normal mechanics of walking. Once this underlying knowledge is present, the PTA observes the patient walking, compares the pattern against the normal gait pattern, and notes the deviations. As with all assessment procedures, the PTA must ensure that the techniques he or she employs are consistent with those used by the evaluating therapist. Gait assessment should be performed on flat surfaces, as well as uneven when indicated, and with the patient both wearing and not wearing shoes. The shoes also can be examined for signs of abnormal wear, such as scuff marks on the toe of one shoe or flattening of one side of the shoe sole.

Deviations in gait primarily occur as a result of pain, weakness, or other imbalance between muscle strength and flexibility. Typically the short-term goals in the plan of care will address the specific cause of the deviation, with the long-term goal or outcome addressing the overall quality or function of gait. The PTA is responsible for assessing those components of gait that have been specifically addressed in the plan of care. For example, a patient exhibiting an uncompensated Trendelenburg gait during the initial evaluation may have a goal addressing increased gluteus medius strength on the involved side. In this case, the PTA observes the patient's gait to assess for changes in the Trendelenburg pattern and then measures strength of the gluteus medius for comparison to initial evaluation data.

The PTA also plays a role in determining if a patient is ready to progress to gait training activities with a lesser assistive device. To make appropriate recommendations, the PTA must be familiar with advantages and disadvantages of various assistive devices and must understand purposes and limitations of each. The PTA should keep in mind that ultimately the patient will be best served by the least assistive device that allows for maximum safety, independence, and the most normal gait pattern.

Balance

According to the *Normative Model*, the PTA performs components of patient assessment related to static and dynamic balance.[5] Three physiologic systems linked to balance control include somatosensory (musculoskele-tal and neuromuscular components), visual, and vestibular. The vestibular system involves the structures and organs of the inner ear, which play a key role in maintaining upright posture, equilibrium, and orientation, all components of balance. The application of interventions designed to correct problems with alignment or function of vestibular components is beyond the scope of entry-level PTA educational preparation. However, the PTA must be aware that patients who complain of dizziness, headache with dizziness, or nausea with exercise or balance training may need further physical therapy or medical assessment to rule out or confirm involvement of vestibular conditions.

A patient who constantly or frequently looks at the floor during ambulation or other activities that challenge balance is likely excessively depending on visual input to compensate for somatosensory impairment (e.g., weakness, loss of sensation, or limited joint mobility). In this case, ongoing assessment should include these components or musculoskeletal or neuromuscular integrity according to the plan of care as established. Data collection and documentation must relate changes in the musculoskeletal and neuromuscular function (e.g., ROM, loss of sensation, or weakness) to balance.

Likewise, the patient with visual impairment may depend heavily on musculoskeletal and neuromuscular control to compensate for this deficit. In this case the PTA may notice that the patient reaches for props or ambulates with a wide base of support.

DOCUMENTATION

Documentation is a critical element of the patient's physical therapy experience. Unfortunately, all too often in the present health care environment, the focus of documentation emphasizes reimbursement for services at the cost of cutting short other very important purposes of effective record keeping. In addition to serving as a permanent record of the patient's physical therapy episode of care, documentation is used as a communication tool among members of the health care team; it also may be an effective tool for quality assurance or management within a service or department to measure consistency between providers, set standards for assessment and interventions, and measure effectiveness of outcomes.

The *Physical Therapist Assistant Clinical Performance Instrument*[4] lists the following sample entry-level behaviors associated with the criterion, "Produces documentation to support the delivery of physical therapy services":

■ Documents aspects of physical therapy care, including selected data collection measurements, interventions, response to interventions, and communicates with family and others involved in delivery of patient care
■ Produces documentation that follows guidelines and format required by the clinical setting and law

---

BOX 2-5

Sample SOAP Documents

S. c/o UEs feeling "tired" with parallel

Pregait activities

O: Prior to gait training, GMMT reveals overall WFL strength, with the exception of poor hip clearance with WC push-up. 50% of attempts, pt. requires specific instructions and tactile guidance with proper hand placement with sit-to-stand and stand-to-sit; otherwise carries out this task properly. In parallel bars, pt took 3 steps forward and back + mod assist; stand with trunk and (L) LE flexed and does not push adequately with UEs.

A: Concerns re: difficulty maintaining NWB status (R) LE with pre-amb activities because of insufficient shoulder depression strength; as a result, pt. is not ready to begin gait training with walker. Pt. will benefit from ex. To increase shoulder depression strength to enhance use of assistive device for NWB (R) LE.

P: Include push-up blocks with ther ex next visit; progress with gait training with walker, NWB (R) LE as indicated.

Signature, PTA

- Documents patient care consistent with guidelines and requirements of regulatory agencies and third-party payers
- Produces documentation that is accurate, concise, timely, and legible
- Demonstrates technically correct written communication skills

This discussion focuses on the PTA's role in documenting assessment. Even early in his or her educational experience, the PTA student learns to recognize the standard elements of the SOAP format of documentation; this format is effective as a tool to organize one's thoughts and the content of a treatment note, even if it is not the standard format used by a given facility.

Subjective data ("S") include what the patient reports (relevant to the physical therapy plan of care). Pain is recorded as subjective data. Objective data ("O") include what was observed, measured, and done (e.g., what activities the patient participated in during the session and what interventions the PTA applied or used). And, of course, the plan ("P") states what will be done on the next visit or in the future. So how does assessment fit into the PTA's documentation?

The assessment is the key portion of documentation that links subjective and objective data to the PT goals, outcomes, and plan. It may be helpful for the novice PTA to organize his or her thoughts for assessment by considering the following questions that might be addressed in an assessment:

- In my judgment, how is the patient doing in certain areas?
  - How is he or she responding to treatment?
  - How is he or she progressing toward goals?
- If the patient is making progress toward goals, what is effective in my judgment?
  - Should this be continued?
  - Is it time to progress to next level or degree with this activity, device, and so on?

- If the patient is not making progress toward goals, what are factors impeding his or her progress in my judgment?
  - Based on these factors, do I think a reexamination or interim evaluation by the PT is indicated to modify goals or plan of care?
- What remaining needs does this patient have in my judgment?
  - Do these needs suggest that the PT should consider consultation with or referral to another health care discipline?

A carefully thought-out assessment portion of a note will aid the PTA or student PTA to formulate a response to the broad question, "So, where do I go from here?" This may include progressing the patient within the context of the plan of care according to selected activities assigned to the PTA by the physical therapist or referral of the patient to the evaluating PT for further direction. Box 2-5 provides a sample SOAP note, written with the intent of offering an example of an effectively documented assessment by a PTA.

CONCLUSION

This chapter began with reference to the rapid changes occurring in the physical therapy profession today. It is imperative for PTAs just entering the profession to possess an awareness and understanding of the issues surrounding the dynamics of this evolution. As PTA students gain an understanding of the foundational principles and core documents that affect their clinical and professional roles and function, they will be better equipped to be active participants in these discussions. This chapter was designed with this outcome in mind and focused on the PTA's role in the performance and documentation of assessment procedures used in the care of patients with musculoskeletal disorders.

REFERENCES

1. Alvarez DJ, Rockwell PG: Trigger points: diagnosis and management. *Am Fam Phys* 2002;65(4):653–660.
2. American College of Sports Medicine: ACSM's Resource Manual for Guidelines for Exercise Testing and Prescription, 3rd ed. Baltimore, American College of Sports Medicine, 1998.
3. American Physical Therapy Association: Guide to physical therapist practice. *Phys Ther* 1997;77:1163–1650.
4. American Physical Therapy Association: Physical Therapist Assistant Clinical Performance Instrument. Alexandria, VA, American Physical Therapy Association, 1998.
5. American Physical Therapy Association: A Normative Model of Physical Therapist Assistant Education: Version 99. Alexandria, VA, American Physical Therapy Association, 1999.
6. American Physical Therapy Association: Position statement: Procedural interventions exclusively performed by physical therapists. HOD 06-00-36, 2000.
7. Duesterhaus Minor SD, Duesterhaus Minor MA: Patient Care Skills. Stamford, CT, Appleton & Lange, 1999.
8. Fletcher GF, Balady GJ, Amsterdam EA, et al: Exercise standards for testing and training: A statement for health care professionals from the American Heart Association. *Circulation* 2001;104:1694–1740, doi:10.1161/hc3901.095960
9. Goodman CC, Fuller KS, Boissonnault WG: Pathology: Implications for the Physical Therapist, Philadelphia, WB Saunders, 2003.
10. Goodman CC, Kelly Snyder TE: Differential Diagnosis in Physical Therapy. Philadelphia, WB Saunders, 2000.
11. Hertling D, Kessler RM: Management of Common Musculoskeletal Disorders: Physical Therapy Principles and Methods. Philadelphia, Lippincott Williams & Wilkins, 1996.
12. Hillegas EA, Sadowsky HS: Essentials of Cardiopulmonary Physical Therapy. Philadelphia, WB Saunders, 2001.
13. Irwin S, Tecklin, J S: Cardiopulmonary Physical Therapy. St. Louis, Mosby, 1995.
14. Karges JR, Mark BE, Strikeleather SJ, et al: Concurrent validity of upper-extremity volume estimates: Comparison of calculated volume derived from girth measurements and water displacement volume. *Phys Ther* 2003;83(2):134–145.
15. Kendall FP, McCreary EK, Provance PG: Muscles: Testing and Function. Baltimore, Williams & Wilkins, 1993.
16. Kisner C, Colby LA: Therapeutic Exercise: Foundations and Techniques. Philadelphia, FA Davis, 2002.
17. Kloth LC, McCulloch JM: Wound Healing: Alternatives in Medicine. Philadelphia, FA Davis, 2002.
18. Levangie PK, Norkin CC: Joint Structure and Function: A Comprehensive Analysis. Philadelphia, FA Davis, 2001.
19. Magee DJ: Orthopedic Physical Assessment. Philadelphia, WB Saunders, 2002.
20. May BJ: Home Health and Rehabilitation: Concepts of Care. Philadelphia, FA Davis, 1999.
21. McCance KL, Heuther SE: Pathophysiology: The Biologic Basis for Disease in Adults and Children. St. Louis, Mosby, 2002.
22. National Osteoporosis Foundation: Osteoporosis clinical practice guidelines, 2003, *www.nof.org*.
23. Norkin CC, White DJ: Measurement of Joint Motion: A Guide to Goniometry. Philadelphia, FA Davis, 1995.
24. O'Sullivan SB, Schmitz TJ: Physical Rehabilitation: Assessment and Treatment. Philadelphia, FA Davis, 2000.
25. Stith JS, Sahrmann SA, Dixon KK, et al: Curriculum to prepare diagnosticians in physical therapy. *J Phys Ther Ed* 1995;9(50):46–53.
26. Tatro-Adams D, McGann S, Carbone W: Reliability of the figure-of-eight method on subjects with ankle joint swelling. *J Orthop Sports Phys Ther* 1995;22(4):161–163.

REVIEW QUESTIONS

Multiple Choice

1. Which statement describes the term *assessment* best?
   A. Synonymous with examination and evaluation
   B. Judgment of the significance of data
   C. Summary of objective tests and measures
   D. Synonymous with data collection
2. According to the *Normative Model of Physical Therapist Assistant Education*, the PTA's role in the clinic includes which of the following?
   A. Modifying interventions in accordance with the established plan of care
   B. Assisting with data collection
   C. Making appropriate judgments
   D. All of the above
3. Which statement is true about inflammation?
   A. The use of all physical agents is contraindicated in the presence of inflammation, regardless of the stage of inflammation present.
   B. Certain physical agents may result in increased inflammation.
   C. Acute inflammation retards the healing process.
   D. The presence of inflammation is not a factor in the PTA's clinical decision-making process in terms of implementing the plan of care.
4. Congestive heart failure may be present when bilateral lower extremity edema is noted in the presence of which other signs and symptoms?
   A. Fatigue with shortness of breath
   B. Shortness of breath with exercise
   C. Muscle weakness with activity
   D. All of the above
5. Enlarged and tender lymph nodes should be reported by the PTA because of which of the following?
   A. In the event of underlying pathology, certain interventions may be contraindicated.
   B. Enlarged lymph nodes are frequently associated with trigger points in muscles.
   C. The patient's upper extremity ROM is markedly decreased in the presence of enlarged axillary lymph nodes.
   D. Enlarged lymph nodes do not impact a PTA's clinical decision making in a patient with musculoskeletal signs and symptoms.
6. Which of these findings may be noted in the presence of impaired accessory motions of a joint?
   A. Decreased ROM
   B. Capsular end-feel
   C. Substitution or compensation
   D. All of the above
7. Which statement is true about desirable outcomes for use of an assistive gait device?
   A. The device selected always should be the most-assistive device, regardless of changes in the patient's condition (e.g., strength, balance).
   B. The advantages, purposes, and limitations of all assistive gait devices are similar; therefore selection of one device over another will not affect functional outcomes.
   C. In general the goal for selection of a gait device should take into account the least-assistive device that allows for maximum safety, independence, and normal gait pattern.
   D. The PTA is not involved in assessment as far as selection of the appropriate gait device.

8. What may be the likely explanation for a patient looking at the floor during ambulation?
   A. Vestibular dysfunction
   B. Visual impairment
   C. Compensatory dependence on visual input
   D. Pathology affecting inner ear structures

9. Which statement(s) is/are true about assessment of edema in an extremity?
   A. Bilateral LE edema is a symptom associated with systemic pathologies such as congestive heart failure.
   B. It is most important to use surface landmarks such as skin folds as points of reference when measuring edema.
   C. Volumetric measurement of edema in an extremity has been demonstrated to be less reliable than the traditional tape measure technique.
   D. B and C above are true.

10. A patient with a locally enlarged and painful joint who also presents with increased local temperature, extreme tenderness, and a history of sudden onset may be exhibiting signs of which pathologic condition?
    A. Compression fracture
    B. Gout
    C. Bursitis
    D. Ligamentous laxity

Short Answer

11. What is the most basic, effective method of controlling transmission of infectious agents?

12. List typical signs and symptoms of myocardial infarction (heart attack) that may occur concurrently with the pattern of pain identified as early warning signs of a heart attack.

13. What is the term used to describe increasing pain symptoms in the immediate area of the lesion (as opposed to "spreading" pain)?

14. List five factors that affect respiration rate.

15. What is the term used to describe joint noise that results from degenerative joint changes?

16. What are two potential long-term complications of chronic, unresolved inflammation?

True/False

17. Enlarged and tender lymph nodes are a normal and expected localized response to inflammation.
18. Signs of a deep venous thrombosis include pale skin, increased local temperature, edema, and pain.
19. Assessing patients' vital signs is not necessary on a routine basis in the outpatient, orthopedic clinical setting.
20. The Valsalva maneuver should be taught to patients to use during exercise to increase trunk stability.
21. It is contraindicated for the PTA to assess the stage of fracture healing by attempting to mobilize fracture fragments.
22. For accurate data collection related to gait, assessment should be performed only on level surfaces and only while the patient ambulates with shoes on.
23. Examination of the patient's shoes may provide information about the mechanism of a gait deviation.
24. Fractures associated with osteoporosis may be asymptomatic, or "silent," and diagnosed after healing during medical workup for subsequent fractures.
25. The patient does not play an active role in establishing the severity of general fatigue he or she may experience during activity.
26. The PTA is never involved with placing value on the significance of data or exercising judgment about patient data.

Essay Questions

Answer on a separate sheet of paper.
27. Discuss the difference in the way the PTA handles patient-related data from that of the PT.
28. Briefly describe each component of a SOAP note.
29. Explain the difference between acute and chronic inflammation.
30. Explain the difference between pitting and brawny edema.

Critical Thinking Application

Given the following clinical data, compose the assessment and plan components of a SOAP note.

S: Pt. c/o "tight" feeling in leg, indicating posterolateral aspect R calf. Reports stayed in bed most of yesterday to "rest leg muscles" after exercising with PT last visit (2 days previously). C/o tenderness posterior R calf during girth measurement.

O: Pt. observed ambulating with antalgic gait—?WB and ? stance time on R. On observation, note pallor of skin posterolateral aspect of R calf, increased temperature to touch compared with L LE. Girth measurements at midcalf R LE reveal 4 cm > L.

3

Physical Agents Used in the Treatment of Common Musculoskeletal Conditions

SANDRA ESKEW CAPPS

LEARNING OBJECTIVES

1. Relate principles of basic physiology and physics to the application of physical agents.
2. Discuss the use of specific physical agents to desired physiologic effects in the treatment of various types of musculoskeletal conditions and their associated symptoms.
3. Select appropriate physical agents according to their characteristics and clinical applications in treating common musculoskeletal conditions.
4. Discuss elements of proper documentation of treatment sessions that incorporate physical agents as augmentative therapy.

KEY TERMS

Evidence
Empiric
Adjunctive interventions
Thermotherapy
Conductive
Cavitation
Acoustic streaming
Duty cycle
Beam nonuniformity ratio (BNR)
Effective radiating area (ERA)

Phonophoresis
Diathermy
Radiation
Pulsed short wave diathermy (PSWD)
Hunting effect
Cryokinetics
Delayed onset muscle soreness (DOMS)
Cryostretch
Evaporation
Impedance

TENS (transcutaneous electrical nerve stimulation)
Neuromuscular electrical stimulation (NMES)
Maximal volitional isometric contraction (MVIC)
Russian stimulation
Functional electrical stimulation (FES)
Iontophoresis

CHAPTER OUTLINE

Thermal Agents
  Hot Packs
    Indications and Effects
    Techniques of Application
    Precautions and Contraindications
  Paraffin
    Indications and Effects
    Techniques of Application
    Contraindications

Ultrasound
  Indications
  Thermal Effects
  Techniques of Application
  Phonophoresis
  Considerations for Ultrasound with Musculoskeletal Conditions
  Precautions and Contraindications

Continued

CHAPTER OUTLINE—cont'd

Diathermy
  Techniques of Application
  Precautions and Contraindications
Cryotherapy
  Indications and Mechanisms
  Techniques of Application
  Precautions and Contraindications
Contrast Bath
Electrical Stimulation
  Indications
  Considerations for Application
  Techniques of Application
  Precautions and Contraindications
Iontophoresis
Documentation
Conclusion

It is well known that the use of physical agents is commonly included in the plan of care for patients with musculoskeletal conditions. Although the psychomotor skills necessary for proper application of particular physical agents are not exceptional or especially difficult to master, the physical therapist assistant (PTA) must always keep in mind the purpose for including the intervention, in terms of desired effects, physiologic rationale (where evidence exists), and patient and tissue response. In many cases physical agents have not been proved through scientific studies to result in significant alterations in tissue physiology. Where studies are available they are rated for strength of existing **evidence,** which is a measure of the scientific research technique employed, and the reliability and validity of results. **Empiric** (experiential or clinically accepted) substantiation of many commonly employed physical agents is widely recognized as rationale for use of these interventions. So how does a PTA reconcile the frequent lack of evidence with the widespread use of these agents? According to Bélanger in *Evidence-Based Guide to Therapeutic Physical Agents,*[12] "A lack of scientific evidence related to any therapeutic intervention does not constitute evidence for lack of effectiveness. In other words, something that is 'not proven' does not mean that it is 'proven not.'" Therefore when physical agents are employed as **adjunctive interventions,** they should not be used arbitrarily, but should be carefully and thoughtfully employed, keeping in mind the purpose of their use. Specifically, the entry-level PTA is expected to meet the following outcomes related to intervention:[7,*]

- Implement the delegated interventions within the plan of are established by the physical therapist (PT), monitor the patient response, and respond accordingly.
- Adjust interventions within the plan of care established by the PT in response to patient clinical indications and in compliance with state practice acts, the practice setting, and other regulatory agencies.
  - Modify specific components of intervention within the plan of care established by the PT based on clinical indications and information obtained from data collection.
  - Seek out and assist the PT when the patient's response to intervention requires modification.
- Recognize when intervention should not be provided because of changing clinical conditions and defer to the PT.
  - Provide interventions that demonstrate an understanding of the rationale, indications, precautions, contraindications, benefits, and risks.
  - Identify when to apply components of intervention and when not to apply components of intervention and refer back to the PT.
- Complete thorough, accurate, logical, concise, timely, and legible documentation that follows guidelines and specific documentation formats required by state practice acts, the practice setting, and other regulatory agencies.

The American Physical Therapy Association (APTA) also provides further direction for the PT to determine the ". . . appropriate extent of assistance from the physical therapist assistant . . ."[8] Specifically the APTA Policy statement on "Direction and Supervision of the Physical Therapist Assistant" states:

> The physical therapist remains responsible for the physical therapy services provided when the physical therapist's plan of care involves the physical therapist assistant to assist with selected interventions. Regardless of the setting in which the service is provided, the determination to utilize physical therapist assistants for selected interventions requires the education, expertise and professional judgment of a physical therapist as described by the Standards of Practice, Guide to Professional Conduct and Code of Ethics.

In determining the appropriate extent of assistance from the PTA, the physical therapist considers:

- The PTA's education, training, experience, and skill level
- Patient criticality, acuity, stability, and complexity
- The predictability of the consequences
- The setting in which the care is being delivered
- Federal and state statutes
- Liability and risk management concerns
- The mission of physical therapy services for the setting
- The necessary frequency of reexamination[8]

The purpose of this chapter is not to provide detailed instruction in or review of the principles and applica-

---

*This list does not represent all of the expected outcomes included in the *Normative Model,* but a select few that are emphasized throughout the discussion in this chapter.

tion of all of the physical agents available for use in the treatment of patients with musculoskeletal pathology or dysfunction. Rather, this chapter is designed to aid the student PTA develop an enhanced understanding of the specific concepts and evidence related to how commonly used physical agents are incorporated as augmentative interventions for these patients.

THERMAL AGENTS

The term *thermal agents* refers to interventions that are employed to change tissue temperature, either by elevating or lowering it. Thermal agents that increase tissue temperature to be discussed here include hot packs, paraffin applications, ultrasound (US), and diathermy. Thermal agents that lower tissue temperature to be discussed include cold packs and ice massage. Contrast baths, which employ both warm and cold elements, also are discussed.

The argument that thermal agent interventions are simple to prepare, assemble, and apply has been used to justify the application of these agents by unlicensed, on-the-job trained individuals. Some clinicians may even feel that to administer these types of interventions is a waste of the licensed practitioner's time and skills. Third-party payers may have regarded these arguments as valid, conceding that if the use of these physical agents does not require "skill," payment for these types of interventions should be reduced or even eliminated. Although it is true that putting together a hot pack and laying it on a body part is an uncomplicated procedure, any individual who has completed a course of study in physical agents used in physical therapy realizes that the underlying implications of a "simple" hot pack are far more complex.

The generally accepted physiologic effects of heating body tissue include increased blood flow and increased cellular activity; these properties aid in tissue healing by promoting relaxation and increasing nutritional supply to cells in the heated area. In addition, heating agents have an effect on conduction of nerve impulses and activity and connective tissue extensibility; these qualities provide a rationale for the use of heating agents for pain reduction and relaxation, and as a precursor to stretching connective tissue.

Traditionally, agents that heat tissues have been divided according to whether the effects are considered to be "superficial" or "deep." However, the 2002 reference publication *Evidence-Based Guide to Therapeutic Physical Agents* offers that a more accurate term for agents traditionally classified as "superficial" (e.g., hot packs and paraffin wax applications) is **"thermotherapy."**[12] This conjecture is based on evidence that any of the agents included in this category result in changes in temperature increases in deep tissues (e.g., muscles and joint capsules) as well as superficial tissues. Bélanger[12]

further suggests that agents traditionally classified as "deep" should be considered in terms other than effects on tissue temperature because they have effects described as "mixed," including both thermal and mechanical results.

Cold agents, referred to collectively as cryotherapy, also have hemodynamic, neuromuscular, and metabolic effects on tissues. Lowering tissue temperature via the application of superficial cooling agents results in vasoconstriction and decreased metabolic activity, which decreases bleeding and infiltration of inflammatory metabolites in the area of injury or tissue damage. Likewise, cold application decreases conduction of sensory nerve impulses, which aids with increased pain threshold. In addition, cold affects conduction of motor nerve impulses; the clinical application of this principle is the basis for use of cold agents to decrease spasticity resulting from neuromuscular involvement.

Agents that heat tissues by way of direct contact with the skin are **conductive** in nature. Types of conductive heating agents to be discussed in this chapter include hot packs, cold packs, and paraffin.

Hot Packs

Indications and Effects
Hot packs are indicated to promote soft-tissue healing, decrease pain, promote relaxation, and reduce joint stiffness.[12] The rationale for applying hot packs to soft tissue in a subacute phase of healing relates to the increase in blood flow to the area, thus providing increased oxygenation and nutrients to the healing tissue. Hot packs aid in pain control via stimulation of thermoreceptors, which provides a counterirritation effect on pain mechanisms, resulting in decreased pain and increased relaxation of effected tissue.[12] Applying hot packs before or during the application of stretching techniques has been shown to enhance outcomes in terms of increased tissue length.[27,30] (Other techniques that also enhance stretching include active exercise and US.[27]) Just as exposing gelatin to heat increases its liquidity, applying heat over superficial joint structures decreases viscosity of joint fluids and increases extensibility of joint tissue, allowing for more fluent motion.

Techniques of Application
Certain activities must be performed before each application of a hot pack. The treating PTA must complete an assessment of skin integrity, including temperature (relative to surrounding areas or contralateral extremity); observation for any lesions in the area (compared with findings during the initial examination or recorded in the initial evaluation); and sensory integrity, again to determine any changes since the initial evaluation. The PTA also must assess and note the status of the particular component of the patient's physical therapy plan that is being addressed by the use of hot packs. For

example, if a hot pack is being incorporated for the purpose of decreasing pain before the application of exercise, the PTA should obtain a rating of the patient's perceived pain before and after the application of the hot pack.

Hot packs are stored in water temperatures of 158° F to 168° F and therefore must be applied with adequate toweling, generally accepted to be six to eight layers (although no scientific evidence has been produced to support an exact number of layers). More important than an exact number of towel layers is assessing the patient's response to ensure that therapeutic heating is achieved without causing a burn. Rennie and Michlovitz[38] provide guidelines for skin assessment during hot pack application (Box 3-1).

Rennie and Michlovitz[38] also advise that patients should not be positioned lying with full body weight on the hot pack(s) because this position may increase heat transfer beyond therapeutic levels and also may impair local circulation by compression of blood vessels in the treatment area. Of course, all patients also should be provided with a tap bell or some type of alert system that can be activated if necessary during an intervention.

Because heat begins to dissipate 10 minutes or so after application of hot packs, the conventional treatment time of 20 minutes really has no therapeutic basis. The PTA should keep in mind the purpose of including hot packs as an adjunctive intervention for a given patient situation and apply the hot pack for the length of time needed to achieve that effect (within the boundaries of the plan of care established by the evaluating PT). Furthermore, the application of interventions that are enhanced by application to warmed tissues (e.g., stretching or soft-tissue mobilization) should be applied immediately after the hot pack is removed, for the greatest benefit of heat as an augmentative intervention.

Because subcutaneous fat acts as an insulator to heat conductivity, it must be understood that application of a superficial hot pack over an area with significant underlying fat results in decreased heating of deeper structures. Bélanger[12] uses the following example to illustrate this occurrence: ". . . The application of a given hot pack over the dorsal area of the hand or foot is likely to heat those deep tissues (e.g., muscles, ligaments, joint capsules) as opposed to application . . . over the quadriceps or back area." Bélanger[12] also suggests that using prewarmed and moist toweling may accelerate heat transfer to underlying tissues.

The PTA also should participate in monitoring water levels and temperature of the hot pack storage unit (hydrocollator). Some hot packs are designed with tabs of different colors on either end to provide a mechanism for keeping track of which packs have been in the hydrocollator longer, thereby having time to reheat to a therapeutic temperature.

Precautions and Contraindications

Assessing for possible contraindications can be completed in a relatively short period of time before the application of hot packs. The PTA (as well as his or her supervising PT) is held accountable for applying a hot pack to an area with an existing contraindication, even if the initial physical therapy evaluation did not specifically address potential contraindications.

Hot packs should not be used over an area with compromised discrimination to temperature. Hot packs also should not be applied over or near an area where increased blood flow or metabolic activity is undesirable. These circumstances include areas with hemorrhage, vascular compromise, known malignancy, infection, or acute inflammation. If the patient is unable to comprehend or communicate (e.g., would be the case with a confused patient or one who does not understand English), the use of hot packs is contraindicated.[12,35] Bélanger[12] also advises that application of hot packs is contraindicated over the abdominal, pelvic, or low back regions of pregnant women because it is possible that increased temperature may affect the development and growth of the fetus.[12]

Caution must be exercised when hot packs are employed over skin of a healed wound or used with patients with cardiac disease.

Paraffin

Indications and Effects

Paraffin wax also is used as a conductive heating agent to elevate temperature of superficial tissues. This agent is especially conformable to distal extremities, particularly hands and feet. A common application of paraffin is for patients with arthritis (degenerative or rheumatoid) or other joint disorders of the hands or feet, such as impaired mobility after prolonged immobilization. Indications and effects of paraffin essentially are the same as for hot packs. Paraffin should be selected instead of hot packs when the joints of the hands or feet are the target treatment area. Another unique feature of

---

BOX 3-1

Guidelines for Assessing Skin during Hot Pack Application

- Assess skin and patient response after 5 minutes
  - Look at skin color (pinkish/red or reddish/white for fair-skinned individuals and areas of darkened and lightened skin for darker-skinned individuals)
  - Add towel layers or remove hot packs if patient reports feeling too hot or poor tolerance
- Monitor after 9 to 10 minutes, time to peak heating transfer effect

paraffin is that once the paraffin wrap is removed, the oil from the mixture provides a ready medium for soft-tissue massage to the treated area. In addition, the softened wax may be used for hand exercises after removal from the extremity.[35]

Techniques of Application

As with hot packs, the PTA must assess skin integrity and sensation of the area before and after application of paraffin wax. Likewise, the PTA should keep in mind the specific intention of the use of paraffin and conduct appropriate preintervention and postintervention assessments to determine the effectiveness of the paraffin as an adjunct to other interventions. For example, if paraffin is employed as a precursor to massage and range of motion exercise for stiff and painful joints associated with arthritis, the PTA should assess range of motion and obtain subjective measures of pain before and after the application of paraffin and other interventions.

Paraffin wax employs the application of heat through a mixture of paraffin and oil (mineral or paraffin oil), usually administered via a "bath," a container that maintains a temperature of 113° F to 129° F and is sized for immersion of a distal extremity (wrist and hand or ankle and foot). Paraffin also may be applied by brushing the molten mixture over the target treatment area. Once applied, the treated area is wrapped with plastic or toweling for a treatment time of 20 to 30 minutes. This time frame has not been substantially proven by scientific evidence, but is based on empiric data and also on the premise that the medium loses heat by this time, similar to hot packs.

Care must be taken during application to ensure patient comfort, in terms of skin temperature. Basic guidelines relate to ensuring that initially the extremity is dipped slightly past the joint and that subsequent dips do not extend beyond that point. Also, care must be taken that the patient keeps fingers or toes still once the extremity is dipped into the paraffin to avoid cracks in the deeper layers of the protective paraffin "glove."

Precautions and Contraindications

To prepare the area to be treated with paraffin, be sure that all jewelry has been removed and the area is sufficiently exposed. Use of paraffin over open wounds or in the area of active infection is contraindicated. Communicable skin conditions or the presence of viral warts merits special attention. The area should be covered with a plastic film or other appropriate dressing before immersion. The PTA must attend to proper infection control with the use of paraffin as well. This involves routine cleaning of the paraffin bath unit and replacement of the wax. Each facility should have standard procedures relating to reuse or disposal of wax after each treatment.

A disadvantage associated with the use of paraffin is that the area cannot be easily accessed for observation during the application. Nonetheless, the PTA must still check with the patient periodically (at least after the first 5 minutes of the intervention and at appropriate intervals thereafter). The patient also should be provided with a call bell within easy reach and advised to notify the PTA if he or she experiences unexpected results or complications (e.g., intolerance to the heat, weakness, or dizziness).

Ultrasound

Ultrasound (US) is a physical agent commonly incorporated into the treatment plans for patients with musculoskeletal conditions. Traditionally classified as a form of "deep heat," this term is not fully descriptive of therapeutic US, which also provides mechanical and chemical effects (when used for delivery of topical medications).

The commonly accepted reasons for using US for the treatment of musculoskeletal conditions include its theoretical effects of: increasing collagen extensibility (to enhance stretching), increasing circulation and heating (to promote healing), causing changes in nerve conduction (for pain modulation), and increasing tissue temperature (for relaxation and decreasing pain). However, upon reviewing the literature, one finds that actual evidence (data established through scientific research studies) to confirm these beliefs is lacking. Based on a recent review published in *Physical Therapy*,[9] the authors concluded, ". . . The biophysical effects of ultrasound are unlikely to be beneficial . . . based on the absence of evidence for a biological rationale for the use of therapeutic ultrasound." In spite of this lack of evidence, empiric data are largely relied upon for the continued widespread use of this modality. For clinicians who are continuing to rely on traditional protocol-type treatment approaches, certain guidelines for the clinical application of US should be taken into consideration, including indications, parameter selection, and precautions and contraindications.

Indications

Ultrasound and its effects are traditionally considered according to pulsed waveforms (producing nonthermal [nonheating] effects) and continuous waveforms (producing thermal [heating] effects). After examining the literature, Baker and colleagues[9] asserted that both thermal and nonthermal effects occur during any US application (continuous or pulsed). Nonthermal effects include **cavitation,** the formation and effects of vibration of gas bubbles within treated tissue.[15] With pulsed US, nonthermal effects are believed to be achieved through this mechanism.[15] Appropriate therapeutic dosages of US administered properly do not cause tissue damage as the result of cavitation.[14] However, caution is advised if US is used in areas of air-filled body cavities (e.g., lungs and intestines).[15] **Acoustic streaming** is a term that refers to fluid movement along an US-induced wave. It has been postulated that the mechanical effects of this phenomenon may provide healing benefits to tissues via cellular chemical responses and changes in cell membrane permeability (although these effects have not been scientifically established through human model studies).

Thermal Effects

Ultrasound applied via continuous mode is used when a heating effect is desired. In the case of musculoskeletal conditions, US may be used to produce the following physiologic responses associated with heating tissue: increased pain threshold (resulting in decreased pain), decreased muscle guarding spasm (promoting relaxation), and increased collagen tissue extensibility (to enhance stretching).[35]

Modern US devices offer varying frequencies designed to target tissue of different depths. Higher frequency US (3 MHz) affects more superficial tissue (1 to 2 cm deep), whereas lower frequency US (1 MHz) affects tissue up to 5 cm deep.[15]

Techniques of Application

Duty cycle refers to the percentage of time that US energy is being transmitted with a pulsed waveform to achieve the proposed nonthermal effects associated with this intervention. Duty cycle can be demonstrated by the following formula:

Duty cycle = (on time ÷ on time + off time) × 100

Duty cycles of 20% and 50% are commonly available as preset modes on modern US machines. A 20% duty cycle is most commonly used,[35] although there is no research evidence to support a physiologic rationale for this setting.

Currently the accepted technique of US application is via a constantly moving sound head (or "transducer") applied over a coupling medium, thus avoiding potential overheating of underlying tissue. The speed at which the sound head should be moved is approximately 4 cm/s (1.75 in/s) in a pattern of overlapping circular or longitudinal movements directly over the target tissue.[12] Contact between the transducer and the skin (with the interfacing coupling medium) must be maintained consistently, with a relatively light (~1 pound or 450 g) pressure.[12]

Typically employed coupling media include gels and tap water (with the treated area immersed in a suitable container of water). The purpose of the medium is to permit effective transmission of the acoustic waves produced by the US. Air between the medium–sound head interface interferes with this transmission; therefore if underwater application is employed, the PTA must be sure to periodically wipe away air bubbles during the session.

Beam nonuniformity ratio (BNR) is the term used to describe the variable intensity of the US waveform emitted from the sound head. As the term implies, the intensity of the beam is not uniform across the field. The greater the BNR the more varied the intensity, possibly resulting in "hot spots" of intensity, which may cause discomfort from excessive heating of tissues under that area of the sound head.[12] Therefore units with a lower BNR produce more uniform beam intensity and reduced likelihood of "hot spots." Because the role of the PTA may include involvement in equipment purchase decisions, awareness of this type of equipment feature is important. Disclosure of BNR is required of US manufacturers by the Food and Drug Administration.[12,35]

Another feature of therapeutic US that must be considered clinically is the **effective radiating area (ERA).** The ERA is a function of calibration and is a measure of the area of the US head that actually produces the sound wave; this area is consistent with that of the transducer crystal.[37] It should be remembered that the actual diameter of the transducer is not necessarily indicative of the ERA. The ERA must be considered based upon the size of the area to be treated. An accepted guideline is a target area of two to three times the ERA.[37] Because of the relatively small ERA with US, other forms of heat are more appropriate for larger treatment target areas.

Biomedical calibration must be conducted to ensure that the actual energy output of US units (or any electrical equipment, for that matter) is accurate compared with that indicated by the dosage meter. Although US dosage is traditionally documented in terms of w/cm², Bélanger,[12] in *Evidence Based Guide to Therapeutic Physical Agents* emphasizes that the correct and accurate method to measure US must take the following elements into account: total energy, effective radiating area, and size of the area treated. Michlovitz and colleagues[35] emphasize the importance of including frequency (measured in megahertz or MHz), intensity (w/cm²), duty cycle (in percentage, for pulsed US), and total duration when documenting parameters for US treatments. Regardless of the standard used for documentation, the PTA should play a role in ensuring the proper functioning of the equipment and its periodic calibration and safety inspections to maximize effectiveness in terms of safety, efficiency, and patient outcomes.

Examples of musculoskeletal conditions for which US may be appropriate include those conditions with which pain, soft-tissue restrictions, and soft-tissue injury or inflammation are associated. Considering the physical properties of US previously discussed, it is a physical agent best suited for relatively small areas, involving either superficial tissues or tissue as deep as 5 cm. The position of the patient must allow for maximum comfort and access to the body part or target tissue being treated.

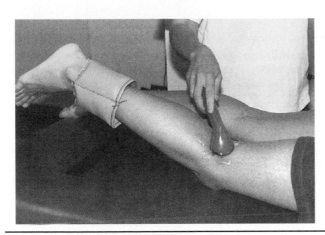

Fig. 3-1 Simultaneous application of stretching with ultrasound. (From Cameron MH: Physical Agents in Rehabilitation, 2nd ed. Philadelphia, WB Saunders, 2003.)

Limited evidence suggests that US may increase extensibility, and therefore the potential for enhanced stretching, of connective tissue.[37] It has also been suggested that US used simultaneously with static stretch produces enhanced tissue length.[48] Figure 3-1 is one example of how to position a patient and apply a passive prolonged stretch during application of US.[15]

Another study examined the benefits of applying US (1.5 w/cm^2 for 7 min) before stretching subjects' ankles.[27] These authors found that US applied before stretching produced beneficial effects.[27]

"Standard" treatment times range from 5 to 8 minutes, although there is no foundational evidence for this range. Another guideline to use for established duration of US application is 5 minutes per two times the area of the sound head. In other words, assuming that the target area measures ~10 cm in diameter; with an US transducer of ~10 cm in diameter, the treatment time would be 5 minutes.

Ultrasound may be used in the treatment of both acute and chronic conditions. For acute conditions in which heating of involved tissues is contraindicated (e.g., with acute inflammation), US may be applied either in continuous mode at a low intensity or on pulsed mode. Suggested guidelines for the total number of treatments are one to two treatments daily for 6 to 8 days for acute conditions, and every other day for 10 to 12 days for chronic conditions.[23,37] The authors of a study published in 1995[39] that was designed to determine the effects of US on tumor growth suggest that discontinuation of US treatment should be considered if no improvement of pain symptoms is noted after two to three treatments.

A critical point for the PTA to keep in mind is that US—as is the case with any physical agent—is an adjunctive intervention and should be used with specific and narrow goals in mind. For example, in the case of a patient who is experiencing limited elbow range

of motion (ROM) because of adaptive shortening (elbow flexion contracture) after prolonged immobilization, one goal of including US as a component of the plan of care may be to mediate pain to allow the patient to tolerate subsequent interventions, such as soft-tissue mobilization or stretching.

Phonophoresis

Phonophoresis is the term used to describe the use of US to enhance the delivery of topically applied medicated creams or gels to the tissues. The theoretic basis for the use of US to deliver topical medications is the increased tissue permeability associated with US. The results of studies to date are equivocal; it has not been demonstrated that phonophoresis is more effective than US alone to achieve better results for treatment of inflammatory or painful conditions. Also, it is suggested that phonophoresis has the greatest potential benefit when used to treat superficial tissue (submuscular or subtendinous levels).[35]

When phonophoresis is included in the plan of care, the PTA should understand the specific indications and desired effects of the medicated solution in each case; furthermore, the PTA should collect and report data to aid with determination of the effectiveness of the intervention in achieving the desired effects. In addition, the PTA should be alert to unusual skin reactions from the drug; naturally the PTA must adhere to all other precautions and skin assessment techniques. According to McDiarmid and colleagues,[33] "Phonophoresis . . . may continue to be the method of choice for patients who are apprehensive about receiving injections." They also suggest that further study is warranted in this area.[33]

Considerations for Ultrasound with Musculoskeletal Conditions

A summary of general considerations and guidelines to use for decision making in the use of US is presented in Box 3-2.

Recall that the role of the PTA includes participating in problem solving, judging the patient's status, and discussing the need for modifications to the plan of care established by the PT.[4] To function in this capacity, the PTA must constantly monitor the response of the target area and the patient as a whole to interventions and be alert for unexpected as well as expected responses to relay these data accurately to the PT.

Precautions and Contraindications

As with any physical agent intervention, the PTA must conduct pretreatment and posttreatment assessment of skin integrity. Changes in sensory integrity (compared with initial examination findings) must be noted also. Caution must be exercised in any area with diminished or impaired circulation or sensation.

BOX 3-2

Guidelines for Application of Ultrasound

- Ensure proper function and safety of equipment
  - Participate in monitoring periodic equipment and safety checks
- Ensure proper positioning of patient
  - Patient comfort
  - Part or tissue exposed and accessible
  - Goal of treatment
- Parameter selection and modification
  - Type or depth of tissue (for proper frequency of sound head)
  - Acuity of injury (for low intensity or pulsed versus continuous waveform)
  - Size of target treatment area (for duration)
  - Total number of treatments to date (for assessing outcomes and determining subsequent plan)

Many commonly accepted precautions and contraindications of US have not been consistently proved to be detrimental. The PTA should always be alert for the presence of these conditions and, any time a question arises, the PTA should ensure that the evaluating PT has considered potential risks versus desired benefits. This principle should be taken into account with the application of *any* physical agent or PT intervention.

Specifically, such precautions include recent fractures and osteoporosis.[23] Ultrasound may be used in areas with metal implants,[12,24] but it is not recommended for use in areas over plastic implants[12,24] or implants that have been fixated with methylmethacrylate cement.[15]

Ultrasound generally is considered to be contraindicated in the presence of known cancer. No definitive evidence exists for the absolute contraindication of US in a body area remote from an area with tumor or history of cancer. Animal model experiments resulted in increased growth of tumors when US was applied directly over the tumor.[39] Because of the heating effect of continuous US, it should not be used any time that the effects of increased heating are not desired. Examples of these circumstances include acute infection, hemorrhage, or signs of DVT. US use should be avoided on pregnant patients because excessive elevation of body temperature or local tissue temperature (in or near the fetus) is not recommended during pregnancy. Because there is no ethical means to determine the potential harmful effects of US during pregnancy, this is a situation where potential risk might be considered to outweigh potential benefits.

Likewise, use of US instead of cardiac pacemakers or implanted neurostimulation devices is not recom-

mended because of the possible resulting malfunction of the electronic devices.[34] Body areas in which US is contraindicated include over or in the areas of male and female reproductive organs, over the lumbar or pelvic regions of menstruating female patients, and over the orbit of the eye.[12,15]

Diathermy

Like US, **diathermy** is a physical agent that offers both thermal and nonthermal effects through application via continuous or pulsed modes. Because it is beyond the scope of this text to discuss detailed biophysical properties of the agents presented, the reader is referred to other resources that provide this information in a format that includes clinically applicable details for the PTA.[11,12,35] A simplified explanation of diathermy is presented here, followed by a discussion of clinical application, indications and contraindications, and advantages and disadvantages. Diathermy (clinically referred to as short wave diathermy, abbreviated as SWD) may be described as a thermal agent that produces therapeutic effects through **radiation.** Thermal effects from diathermy are a result of increased molecular activity in response to exposure to the rapidly oscillating short wave energy produced by the device. The associated rise in temperature produces effects similar to other thermal agents, including increased cell metabolism and subsequent promotion of tissue healing. Thermal effects with diathermy result from both continuous and pulsed modes of application.[12] Preliminary studies with **pulsed short wave diathermy (PSWD)**[19] conclude that PSWD produces thermal effects at tissue depths similar to those of US. However, because of the lessened intensity of thermal effects achieved with PSWD, this mode is recommended when treating tissues in an acute or subacute inflammatory phase of healing.

As stated by Bélanger,[12] "A key biophysical phenomenon associated with SWD therapy is electromagnetic resonance." This phenomenon involves matching the frequency of oscillation between the diathermy unit and the circuit made by the patient's tissue and the electrode interface. When diathermy initially came into use for physical therapy applications, the procedure involved a manual "tuning" process, which is necessary to obtain the therapeutic benefit. Current instrumentation completes this process automatically. If SWD is included in the physical therapy plan of care, the PTA must become familiar with the techniques of setting up this intervention and making adjustments as necessary during the session to maintain effective resonance.

Techniques of Application

Types of diathermy applicators include inductive coil applicators or capacitive plates. Inductive coil applicators are applied either by wrapping coils around the part to be treated or placing coils contained in a drum over the target area. Capacitive plates are applied in pairs to produce a direct electrical field that flows between the two plates through the target tissue. A thin layer of cotton fabric (e.g., a T-shirt or towel) should be used with coil drum and capacitive plate applicators. Thicker toweling or more layers should be used with coil cable applicators.

Diathermy units are equipped with a timer and a dosage meter; however, therapeutic dosage is determined by the patient's perception of heat, with doses ranging from Dose I (no perceived heat, resulting in presumably athermal effects) to Dose IV (maximum tolerable perception of heat). Treatment times are generally from 15 to 30 minutes, taking into account the phase of healing (acute, subacute, or chronic), the frequency of application, and the dose tolerated. As with all thermal (and other) physical agents, careful monitoring of the patient's response, in terms of both expected, desirable effects and unexpected, undesirable effects is an essential element when using this agent.

Given that SWD provides similar effects to tissues at similar depths affected by US, what factors should be taken into consideration of the decision for which agent to use with a given patient? Because US requires constant attendance by the clinician, SWD is a somewhat less time-consuming intervention (although it is understood that constant and careful monitoring is a critical and necessary component to all physical agent applications). Short wave diathermy does not require the application of a conductive medium as does US, and it also is conducive to treating a larger (e.g., the mid-back) or unevenly contoured (e.g., the ankle) body area. Short wave diathermy also is capable of treating "through" a joint (e.g., a hip or shoulder), an application that is frequently indicated in populations of patients with musculoskeletal conditions. Ultrasound equipment is less bulky to store and set up and may be applied with the affected part immersed in water.

Based on the effects and advantages of SWD, it is a useful thermal physical agent that should not be overlooked in the treatment of patients with musculoskeletal conditions.

Precautions and Contraindications

All forms of diathermy are contraindicated for patients with implanted deep brain stimulators.[15] According to Cameron,[15] there have been cases of coma and death resulting from diathermy application to patients with these devices. Particularly in the outpatient clinical setting, detailed medical history is not always provided with each patient referral. The PTA is responsible for confirming the absence of any potential contraindications before applying any physical agent.

Other contraindications for continuous (thermal-level) diathermy include the presence of a pacemaker, malignancy, and pregnancy.[15] Diathermy should not be used over the following areas of the body: eyes, epiphysis of growing bone, or testes.[15] Short wave diathermy also is contraindicated for treatment of internal organs and over internal or external metal implants. In some of these instances, there may not be absolute evidence that diathermy causes deleterious effects; however, it is generally accepted that the *potential* for harmful effects warrants erring on the side of caution.

Caution must be used when applying SWD to an obese patient. Because of the type of energy emitted from diathermy units, care also must be taken to remove potentially conductive objects from the patient and immediate treatment area. This includes jewelry, clothes with zippers, synthetic fabrics, electronic devices, and metal-containing or magnetic equipment.

As with all thermal agents, the patient's sensation to temperature and skin integrity must be assessed before and immediately after application of diathermy. Intact temperature discrimination is critical when considering the use of diathermy because the dosage relies on the patient's perception of warmth during the treatment.

In the past, there had been some concern that clinicians administering SWD might be exposed to hazardous levels of electromagnetic energy. A study published in 1982 measured outputs of several units and applicators and found that if SWD is applied with the operator in the "normal" position (behind the unit console), this risk is unsubstantial.[42]

Cryotherapy

Indications and Mechanisms

Physical agents designed to lower tissue temperature are frequently employed in the PT plan of care for patients with musculoskeletal conditions. Most commonly, methods employed include ice or cold packs and ice massage, all of which cause a change in tissue temperature via conduction. Clinical indications for lowering tissue temperature are primarily related to controlling or alleviating inflammatory responses, particularly pain and edema. Application of cold agents also is used to temporarily reduce spasticity to allow improved mobility.[35]

Techniques of Application

A generally accepted guideline is to apply ice (or cold) immediately after soft-tissue trauma and for 24 to 48 hours after injury (commonly used as the definition for "acute"); however, animal model studies have failed to demonstrate that the application of cold during this period results in significantly reduced development of edema over time.[35]

With reference to the specific application of cryotherapy agents for musculoskeletal conditions, the PTA should keep the preceding characteristics of cold in mind. As with all physical agents applied directly to the skin, a proper pretreatment and posttreatment assessment of skin integrity must be performed. In addition, it may be necessary to establish whether a patient has a hypersensitivity to cold; certain pathologic conditions, such as Raynaud disease, may predispose a patient to intolerance to cold. As with application of heating agents, periodic assessment of the patient's response therefore is necessary.

Common modes of application of cold agents include cold or ice packs, ice massage, and cold compression. Consideration must be made about the depth of target tissue. Deeper tissues and tissues with overlying adipose tissue take longer to cool, as adipose tissue acts as an insulator. Once tissue is cooled to achieve therapeutic effects, the tissue remains cool for longer periods than heated tissue stays warm.[35]

Cold and ice packs are used when a longer-lasting analgesic effect to deeper tissues is desired. Cold packs are commercially available and may be kept in a freezer unit designated for clinical use or in a unit manufactured for the purpose of storing and cooling the packs. Cold packs typically are applied with a layer of toweling as the skin-agent interface. Ice packs are made by placing crushed ice in a bag or towel. Cold packs and ice packs are easy to apply and conform to both smooth and uneven body contours. Because one factor that determines tissue cooling involves the gradient between the tissue temperature and the temperature of the agent applied, ice packs are considered to be a more effective means of achieving cooling of tissue (because ice packs are colder than cold packs).

Ice massage involves freezing water in small paper cups that can be torn away to expose the ice block. Ice massage is indicated for more transient cooling to small areas. The time of application is dependent upon patient response. The PTA instructs the patient that he or she will experience a sequence of responses: cold, burning, aching, and finally numbness. An example of a practical application for ice massage is at the insertion of an inflamed tendon, such as occurs with medial or lateral epicondylitis of the elbow. Ice massage is indicated as a precursor to deep friction massage in such an area as well. An advantage of using ice massage instead of a cold or ice pack is that it is effective in targeting a specific, small, superficial region; results (analgesia) often occur rapidly; it is an inexpensive treatment that can be taught to patients who exhibit good potential for compliance with a home program.

Generally accepted guidelines for treatment times with cold or ice packs describe applications of 20 to 30 minutes to achieve an analgesic effect. Applications of cold for periods longer than this may result in what is referred to as the **hunting effect,** which simply stated is thought to be a protective reflex mechanism resulting in periods of vasodilation during prolonged exposure to cold.

Another factor related to techniques of application for cold agents is whether the material applied to the patient's skin should be wet or dry. Because cold and ice packs transfer heat via a conductive method, a moist interface (most often cotton terry-cloth toweling) enhances conductivity; a plastic bag or dry toweling may serve as more of an insulator, resulting in impedance to tissue cooling. An efficient way to make moist cold or ice packs is to keep a stack of moist towels near the cold pack unit or ice unit for ready access. In facilities with a clothes washer and dryer, this is easily done by stacking towels that have been washed but not placed in the dryer in the area where preparation of cold packs takes place.

In Knight's *Cryotherapy in Sports Injury Management*,[28] the author describes a technique called **cryokinetics,** in which repeated applications of cold are applied, interspersed with periods of active exercise. Specifically, the technique involves an initial application of cold for 20 minutes. This initial application is followed by a 3-minute bout of active exercise, and then a 5-minute application of cold; this 3-minute exercise and 5-minute cold application sequence is then repeated for a total of four cycles. The rationale given for this protocol is accelerated time to return to functional activity after injury.[28]

If cold is applied as a means to decrease or prevent exercise-induced pain in more acute musculoskeletal conditions, the PTA must adhere to precautions for exercising muscles in the acute phase of healing. Throughout this text, guidelines for appropriate exercise and activities based on the stage of tissue healing are provided. Because ice is an effective analgesic, the PTA must err on the side of caution in this case. An example of a safe mode of exercise for muscles in the acute stage of healing is isometric or gentle range of motion. The PTA also should be aware that ice has not been proved to prevent **delayed onset muscle soreness** (commonly referred to as **DOMS**). Delayed onset muscle soreness is caused by performing exercises that are more aggressive than the muscle's current capabilities.

Knight[28] also describes a technique referred to as **cryostretch,** which is similar to the cryokinetics technique described in the preceding. Cryostretch involves the application of the cold agent for an initial 20-minute period followed by alternating periods of stretching (passive stretching with isometric muscle contractions) and renumbing, for a total of three bouts of cold application and stretching.

Cold agents may be applied in conjunction with other interventions. Cold or ice may be used as a precursor to interventions such as exercise or friction massage, as described. Cold is used simultaneously with compression to treat acute conditions resulting in pain and edema. Commercial units designed for this purpose are available. The benefits of this combination of agents relate to the enhanced effects on hemodynamics, through vasoconstriction achieved with cold, and the effect on osmotic pressures and hydrostatic pressures related to lymph and venous flow associated with compression.[34] Limited studies on the efficacy of the application of cold with simultaneous electrical stimulation have produced equivocal results.[35]

Anytime the plan of care established by the evaluating PT calls for the application of combinations of physical agents, the PTA must be diligent in assessing the patient's response and providing the PT with accurate data on which to base decisions for subsequent treatments. It is reasonable to presuppose that any time a number of different agents and interventions are employed in a single patient visit, the beneficial or detrimental effects of any one of the interventions will be difficult to determine. To reiterate an important theme, the PTA should be continually conscientious about the underlying purpose and desired effects of any intervention.

Vapocoolant sprays have been employed as an adjunctive intervention to rapidly and transiently cool superficial tissue via a liquid spray. This method of cooling involves the process of **evaporation** because the cooling occurs with evaporation of the liquid as it comes into contact with the skin. "Spray and stretch" is the term used for a technique that involves passive lengthening of a tight muscle, applying the vapocoolant spray and immediately increasing stretch tension to the muscle. Because the compressed liquid is delivered via chlorofluorocarbons (CFCs), use of this technique declined after manufacture of these substances was banned by the 1990 Clean Air Act.[45] An exception to the ban was made for clinical application of certain products using CFCs; therefore the technique of applying sweeping strokes of the vapocoolant spray along the direction of tight muscles or in the area of trigger points followed by specific stretching techniques is still employed by some therapists. A frequently cited work on this topic is *Myofascial Pain and Dysfunction: The Trigger Point Manual*,[44] by Janet Travell and David Simons, both considered to be pioneers in the field of trigger point therapy. This form of cold agent is designed to provide an immediate numbing effect to the treated tissue. Although the effect is very temporary, a PTA employing this modality as part of a prescribed physical therapy plan of care must be aware of precautions related to stretching anesthetized tissue to avoid causing an increased inflammatory response to already hyperirritable tissues.

Contraindications

Cryotherapy is contraindicated when a patient has a disorder that results in hypersensitivity to cold. Because it is possible that this condition may not have been previously diagnosed, the PTA should be alert to abnormal responses to cold agents; abnormal responses include wheals or swelling in the area of application and unexpected changes in vital signs. A compromise in local circulation in the area to be treated also is a contraindication for cryotherapy.

Contrast Bath

Contrast baths involve immersion of the affected body part (distal extremity) alternately between warm (38°C to 44°F) and cold (10°C to 18°C) water for cycles of: 10 minutes warm; 1 minute cold; and 4 minutes warm (always ending with warm application) for a total of 30 minutes.[46] These time frames represent guidelines; generally, a ratio of hot:cold should be 3:1 or 4:1.[46] The accepted rationale for the contrast bath as an intervention for patients with musculoskeletal conditions is that this intervention offers the beneficial effects of both heat and cold (discussed in the preceding). Another advantage is that water offers a medium that conforms well to unevenly contoured body parts. A disadvantage is that when immersing an extremity in water, the limb must be placed in a dependent position, which could increase edema. Furthermore, there is no substantial evidence demonstrating that contrast bath treatment is particularly effective.[46]

Some specific indications for contrast bath traditionally include arthritis of peripheral joints, joint sprains, and muscular strains.[46] Contraindications for contrast bath include those noted for thermal agents and cryotherapy interventions. Specifically, diabetes-related small vessel disease, arteriosclerotic endarteritis, and Buerger's disease are noted as contraindications for contrast bath.[46] Caution also must be exercised in patients with peripheral vascular disease.[46]

Electrical Stimulation

"It depends." "You *could* use it that way, but you could also do it *this* way." "Any of the waveforms could be used for that problem." "That's not the way I've seen it done in clinic." "What's the difference between 'sweep' and 'scan'?" Just listen to a group of students in a PTA or PT education program, and one quickly senses an atmosphere of frustration with comments such as these related to the theory and application of electrical stimulation agents for the treatment of musculoskeletal conditions.

As in the case of the other physical agents discussed, applying the intervention with attention to the desired tissue effect is of the utmost importance when considering electrical stimulation (e-stim) interventions. In the treatment of common musculoskeletal conditions, e-stim should be employed as an adjunctive intervention to enhance the achievement of goals and outcomes. The proficient PTA focuses on techniques of application and adjustment of parameters according to these desired effects in order to obtain optimal outcomes. Of course, these activities must be carried out within the context of the existing plan of care. As the PT and PTA develop a sound, effective clinical relationship, the PT determines which elements of the plan of care will be administered by the PTA and in what ways (if any) the PTA may modify the interventions. It should be recalled that an expected performance outcome for an entry-level PTA includes recognizing when an intervention is inappropriate or should be modified or discontinued.[7] The significance of this concept is that, as the PTA gains more experience, he or she may be reasonably expected to participate in decisions about application of interventions at a more advanced level than that expected at entry-level. This idea is emphasized here because, to a significant extent, it is these modifications to e-stim interventions that ultimately determine their overall effectiveness.

Many e-stim units that are now commercially available are marketed based on their versatility and countless technologic features. In spite of the "bells and whistles" of current technology, the words of Gad Alon, noted researcher in the topic of e-stim, should be heeded: "No single stimulator is optimally designed to provide all clinical treatments."[2] Much of the confusion, such as that exemplified in the introduction to this section, is the result of inconsistent and often confounding terminology related to the clinical use of e-stim interventions. Because of this, an attempt to use accurately descriptive, noncommercial terms is made throughout this chapter. The PTA student is encouraged to review the APTA document, *Electrotherapeutic Terminology in Physical Therapy—Revision 2000*[5] and Gad Alon's chapter, "Principles of Electrical Stimulation" in *Clinical Electrotherapy*[2] to clarify definitions and commonly used terms. It is only through widespread awareness, acceptance, and application of accurate terminology and descriptions that the use of contradictory and confusing labels and terms will diminish.

The PTA student also is strongly encouraged to learn how to reference specifications of the various e-stim devices employed in laboratory and clinical settings; these specifications can be found in manufacturers' instruction manuals that should be kept with the units themselves or in another readily accessible location in the lab or clinic.

Indications

Clinically, e-stim is employed in the treatment of patients with musculoskeletal conditions for several purposes. Empirically for this patient population, e-stim is used to decrease or control pain, decrease acute edema, treat muscle weakness and denervation, and increase joint range of motion. As with all physical agents used in physical therapy, actual evidence to support the use of e-stim for these indications exists to varying degrees; certainly the need for further research is well established.

Considerations for Application
Impedance
Impedance is the term used to describe resistance to current flow in a biological system (body tissue). Intact, dry skin has high impedance, which, if not addressed, decreases the delivery of therapeutic current to target

tissue. Proper preparation of the skin, which is simply achieved, has direct potential for increasing the effectiveness of the treatment, thereby improving results. In spite of this, students continually report that they do not observe this practice routinely being carried out in the clinical setting. It is hard to believe that one could formulate a rational defense for not applying a quick, easy approach that may significantly enhance outcomes, especially at a time when the profession is striving for recognition as providers of effective and beneficial services.

Having stated a strong argument for addressing skin impedance, how should this be done? The simple process of abrasively cleaning the skin where the electrodes are to be placed is one method. Some sources suggest using alcohol to clean the area; however, because dry skin has higher impedance, the use of alcohol may cause excessive drying and, theoretically, increased impedance. Therefore cleaning with plain water or soap and water may be more effective. Warm, moist skin free from oils or lotions has lower impedance.[21] The presence of any skin lesions, leading to a loss of skin integrity, results in decreased impedance in the area.[21] Body hair also may increase impedance and make electrode removal more uncomfortable. Therefore if there is excessive hair in the area where an electrode should be placed, the hair should be clipped, not shaved, because shaving results in microlesions, lowering the impedance in this area and causing undesirable inconsistencies in current flow.

Other than skin, adipose tissue is another source of high impedance. Theories have been proposed that using higher frequency modes of e-stim will improve current flow through adipose tissue by lowering impedance.[21] This theory is not supported by scientific research but is commonly cited by manufacturers as a selling point for clinical units that offer higher-frequency mode selections. The application of electrical current to the skin also decreases impedance. The implications of this are significant because the PTA must monitor the patient during an e-stim treatment to ensure that, as the impedance decreases during the intervention, any compensating adjustments to the amplitude are made to maintain therapeutic dosages (in terms of amplitude).*

Pain
When e-stim is included in the plan of care with the goal of decreasing pain, the PTA must consider the particular desired outcome, taking into account how the e-stim intervention to decrease pain fits into the plan as

---

*The PTA also should become familiar with constant-voltage and constant-current features of currently available electrical stimulation devices. These features are designed to maintain safe, therapeutic, and comfortable levels of stimulation in spite of changes in tissue impedance or interruptions in power supply.

a whole. Again, the e-stim intervention should not be arbitrarily applied but carefully and thoughtfully integrated into the treatment sessions to maximize desired results and contribute to achieving the ultimate desired outcome—typically improved function or a return to previous function. It should be remembered that with musculoskeletal conditions, e-stim cannot "cure" the primary condition that is resulting in pain.

Pain is a unique and complex problem frequently encountered when one works with patients with musculoskeletal conditions. It is interesting to note that in the Introduction to the *Guide to Physical Therapist Practice*,[6] "alleviating pain" is listed as the first item in a list of general benefits provided by physical therapists. As the PTA is aware, pain in and of itself is not a distinct pathology. Conversely, it may often even be the component of a PT problem list for which it is most difficult to ensure resolution. For example, if a patient presents with a PT problem list that includes pain, decreased ROM, and muscle disuse atrophy after prolonged immobilization, it is likely that goals will be included in the plan of care that address each of these areas. Of these three broad problems, there can be less assurance that physical therapy interventions will result in measurable improvements in the area of pain. This is true in part because of the very nature of pain: It is largely a subjective factor in the presence of musculoskeletal pathology. Pain also is poorly defined and is described differently by individuals based on each person's experience with pain, motivation for improved health, attitudes toward illness, and other unique factors.

Does this mean that we should not address pain in the physical therapy plan of care? Of course, and as stated, the opposite is true. Physical therapists are known for providing interventions to control, decrease, or eliminate pain, and patients with pain typically include this as an important goal of their own when seeking physical therapy services. Furthermore, employing interventions to alleviate pain promotes a feeling of well-being toward physical therapy on the part of the patient and also generally aids with progressing the patient toward achievement of other goals. For example, in the preceding problem list, it may be pain that is preventing the patient from having functional ROM and using the involved extremity. Therefore addressing pain enables one to work toward achieving specific functional goals.

As discussed, terminology related to the various forms and modes of e-stim is often confusing. The term **transcutaneous electrical nerve stimulation (TENS)** is no exception to this issue. This simply refers to e-stim applied superficially. Taken literally, all clinical forms of e-stim could fall under this category. However, the common use of this term refers to e-stim applied when pain management is the primary therapeutic goal.[12] Furthermore, the universal image invoked by the term

TENS usually is that of portable, battery-operated e-stim units that have preset parameter ranges (waveform, pulse duration, pulse/burst frequency, and current amplitude) designed to affect pain relief or control.[12] (Note that other forms of e-stim that are designed to elicit muscle contraction for purposes of muscle reeducation or augmentative muscle strengthening are termed **neuromuscular electrical stimulation [NMES]**).[12] The reader should keep in mind that TENS is a nonspecific term and that many modes of e-stim, available on a variety of clinical units, customarily are used to treat pain.

There are several generally acknowledged theories about the mechanism of pain relief with the use of TENS. Two universally presented and clinically accepted theories propose a "gate" system of pain control, in which the transmission of pain signals is overridden with the TENS stimulus; and an "opiate" system, which presupposes the release of biological (naturally occurring) pain control substances.[12] The PTA student will undoubtedly be exposed to a more thorough explanation and opportunities for enhanced understanding of these mechanisms. Specific applications in the treatment of patients with musculoskeletal conditions are the focus of this discussion.

Because of the availability of many different units claiming the same therapeutic benefits, studies are being conducted to aid clinicians in sorting out this myriad of options for the use of e-stim to treat pain and other conditions associated with musculoskeletal conditions. For example, in a recent study published in the journal, *Physical Therapy*,[25] the authors report similar clinical results in the treatment of pain with both clinical interferential current (IFC) units and portable TENS units. The authors conclude, "If the analgesic effects of IFC are no different than those of TENS, then the practice of short-duration treatment sessions may be of little value. Most TENS machines are portable, and patients can self-administer treatment throughout the day. Thus, the use of TENS may be a more appropriate treatment strategy to control an ongoing pain problem."[25] As with a majority of the studies reviewed, the authors go on to suggest the obvious need for further ". . . well-designed clinical and experimental studies . . ." in this area.[25]

Parameter selection and adjustment for the treatment of pain

John Barr proposes an algorithm as an aid to making clinical decisions about TENS.[10] The use of such a tool helps the PTA to assess outcomes of TENS for pain control and relief and determine if changes in the plan of care are indicated.

In a textbook chapter entitled, "Transcutaneous Electrical Nerve Stimulation for Pain Management,"[10] Barr also provides a table summarizing historical studies conducted to determine TENS effectiveness. Some of these and other studies have examined the specific parameters and the interaction of pulse characteristics that may combine to produce desired therapeutic results. One such study published in the physical therapy literature in 1986[31] examined parameter selection (stimulation characteristics: pulse width, frequency, and amplitude) to determine which variables or interaction among variables may have the greatest effect on pain reduction. These authors determined that amplitude, delivered at a subthreshold level of stimulation, is more effective for pain relief than amplitude delivered to tolerance.[31]

Recently published evidence about optimum treatment times using TENS for pain control suggests that "40 minutes is the optimal treatment duration of TENS, in terms of both the magnitude (visual analog scale [VAS] scores) of pain reduction and the duration of poststimulation analgesia for knee osteoarthritis."[17] This study compared treatment times of 20, 40, and 60 minutes and included a group treated with placebo TENS as well. The group receiving 40-minute TENS applications achieved greater, longer-lasting pain relief, even at the time of follow-up, compared with the other groups.[17] Given the results of this study, the PT and PTA are provided with an evidence-based rationale to prescribe 40 minutes as the initial treatment time for TENS. As always, modifications to this time should be made based on the patient's response.

Instead of the theoretic direct effects on pain mechanisms widely accepted, Gad Alon[1] proposes that e-stim may be used to effectively "mask" pain symptoms to allow a patient to participate more comfortably in other components of the PT plan of care.[1] Specifically, he suggests that using e-stim during simultaneous application of other interventions (e.g., joint mobilization), active exercises, and stretching may provide sufficient pain relief to enable the clinician to apply the optimum intensity with these manual techniques.[1] Clinical data presented by Alon[1] suggest that biphasic waveforms are more comfortable for the patient than monophasic and have less likelihood of resulting in skin irritation under the electrodes.

Electrode placement for the treatment of pain

Generally, three clinically accepted and practiced techniques of electrode placement are employed.[12] Electrodes may be placed in the area of, or in the area surrounding, the painful site. Other methods include placing the electrodes along proximal pathways of nerve distribution (dermatomes) or in areas identified as acupuncture or trigger points. Because of the lack of evidence to support any approach for electrode placement, it is critical once again for the PTA to monitor each patient's response to each intervention and make modifications or recommendations for modification accordingly. It is nonetheless also critical for the PTA to document electrode placements (drawings may be helpful)[15] so that changes in

response can be accurately determined and to serve as a baseline for subsequent trials. In the 2002 reference publication, *Evidence-Based Guide to Therapeutic Physical Agents*,[12] Bélanger refers readers to the PTA textbook, *Physical Agents—Theory and Practice for the Physical Therapist Assistant*[11] for a comprehensive discussion of, and a guide to, electrode placement.

Edema

E-stim may be used in the treatment of acute edema associated with musculoskeletal injuries. Edema, like pain, is a condition that is associated with the presence of inflammation. Also like pain, unresolved or excessive edema may lead to secondary functional impairments such as decreased ROM and decreased strength.

As we know, active motion aids with circulation and promotes fluid movement through lymphatic and circulatory systems.[26] E-stim is believed to have indirect effects on microcirculation.[2] However, a study published in 2000 concluded that a measurable increase in blood flow with TENS was a result of the muscle contraction, not directly because of the e-stim.[36] The TENS-induced increased blood flow, however, did last slightly longer than that produced by active muscle contraction.[36] If a patient with edema is either reluctant or unable to move the involved extremity through a sufficient ROM, e-stim may be an effective adjunct intervention. When e-stim is used for this purpose, parameters that will achieve a muscle contraction must be selected.[12] Alon[1] has also used a monophasic high-rate (100 to 125 pulses/s) sensory stimulation with a negative polarity for a minimum of 2 hours per day to successfully treat acute edema. Guidelines for when to discontinue e-stim for treatment of acute edema include resolution of the edema, after three to five treatments if no response is achieved, when edema reduction is stable for three to four treatments, or in the presence of increased signs and symptoms.[1]

Muscle denervation and disuse atrophy

When muscle becomes partially denervated as a result of musculoskeletal trauma (e.g., an overstretch injury) or pathology (e.g., compartment syndrome), PT interventions are designed to maintain tissue integrity of the weakened muscle and ultimately to return the muscle to functional use. Whether e-stim is an appropriate intervention to employ in this case is debatable. There is speculation that the potential for overwork of electrically stimulated muscles may be harmful.[41] Furthermore, the use of e-stim or partially or completely denervated muscles actually may inhibit the physiologic healing processes involved with nerve degeneration.[41]

In a discussion of the possible benefits or potential deleterious effects of e-stim for denervated muscle, Spielholz[41] presents an interesting case study involving an axillary nerve lesion of a healthy young patient. As nerve healing took place, interventions focused on maintaining ROM and reeducating the deltoid muscle with the use of electromyogram (EMG) biofeedback. Ultimately, full recovery was achieved, including a complete return to all previous functional activities (including sports). The author uses this example to illustrate how healing can occur naturally without the use of multiple complicated interventions.[41] Other examples of nerve conditions that traditionally have been treated with e-stim, but that have an excellent prognosis even without the use of physical agents, include Bell's palsy and "Saturday night palsy" (compression of the radial nerve).[41]

Another common application of e-stim in patients who have orthopedic conditions is to reeducate atrophied muscles or muscles that lack the ability to initiate a normal, functional contraction. Numerous protocols are available to aid with parameter selection for this use of e-stim. As mentioned, little scientific evidence exists to support or refute use of these protocols as guidelines. The PTA should keep that in mind: These protocols serve as *guidelines*; clinical decisions must be based on the plan of care, the PT goals, the patient's response, and the outcomes achieved. The following discussion includes summary findings from research articles and relevant information about the use of e-stim as an adjunct for muscle strengthening.

Researchers have attempted to determine which characteristics or parameters of e-stim actually influence muscle contractions or outcomes, in terms of improved strength. A 1989 study determined that the ". . . torque-generating capability [of a muscle] varies directly with phase charge."[40] Charge is a function of current amplitude and pulse duration; these pulse characteristics are associated with capabilities of equipment. Another study[29] looked at the characteristic of waveform. This study showed that a polyphasic waveform produced a weaker muscle contraction and more rapid fatigue than monophasic and biphasic waveforms. Even though a contraction of similar quality may be produced with different waveforms, waveform may have implications related to the strength of the contraction and fatigue.[41] The study used battery-operated units, suggesting that the power (in terms of output source) of the unit may not be as critical in determining quality of the muscle contraction produced; this has implications for the use of smaller, battery-operated e-stim units for home use. Specifically, patients may be able to achieve the same or better outcomes with more frequent e-stim application (using the proper protocol) between PT sessions. These findings are important to keep in mind if the PTA is involved with making decisions about purchase of equipment. The PTA should be able to assist the PT with these decisions by thinking of appropriate clinical questions for the equipment sales representative, asking for data and evidence to support the need for the various features of the device, and remembering that just because the machine does more or offers more features, actual clinical benefits may not be associated with these attributes.

Techniques of Application

The term neuromuscular stimulation (NMES) refers to stimulation used to produce a muscle contraction (as opposed to TENS, which specifically refers to stimulation of nerves to produce stimulation designed for pain control). A case report published in the PT literature in 2001 suggests that NMES, ". . . offered a safe addition to a traditional, high-intensity volitional strengthening program."[32] The parameters used were an on:off ratio of 10 seconds: 50 seconds with a ramp time of 3 seconds. The amplitude was determined based on a percentage of **maximal volitional isometric contraction (MVIC)** and the patient's tolerance. Duration of treatment was based on 10 repetitions.[32] Note that this results in a total treatment time with e-stim of only 10 minutes; treatment time and number of repetitions was limited to avoid fatigue, an important principle to keep in mind when using e-stim as an adjunct to strengthening weak muscles. The authors of this case report used a percentage of MVIC, which may be a good determinant of intensity because it has functional implications and is not arbitrary. However, determining actual MVIC requires the use of a dynamometer.[32] Also note that, as a result of their findings, the authors support the use of NMES as an *addition* to an exercise program. Once again, it is not suggested that the e-stim in and of itself is sufficient to produce strength increases.

In the preceding study, the authors also address fatigue as a concern.[32] A 1992 study looked at the effects of e-stim in relation to fatigue.[13] Specifically they compared stimulation frequencies and the effect on fatigue; discussion of findings suggests that higher frequencies (>60 pulses/second) used as a muscle fatigues result in maximum force generation; previous studies suggested that lowering the frequency as a muscle fatigues is more effective in retarding the development of fatigue.[13] Once again, the PTA must keep this concept in mind when using e-stim for strengthening. Although the available evidence has produced inconsistent findings, the PTA should understand that frequency of pulses (pulse rate) may have an effect on the quality of the muscle contraction produced with e-stim. The clinical relevance is that the PTA must monitor the patient's response during e-stim used for strengthening and may make adjustments to stimulation frequency as indicated, based on the quality of the contraction desired and signs of muscle fatigue.

A particular mode of e-stim used to augment muscle strengthening that has been popular in orthopedic clinical settings is known as **Russian stimulation.** This title refers to a preset or predetermined combination of waveform characteristics and pulse parameters designed with the premise of enhancing strengthening outcomes.

(The PTA again is advised to refer to manufacturers' instruction manuals for each device for descriptions of each type of current; one finds that terms such as "Russian current" or "interferential current" are actually nonspecific terms used to describe waveforms available with particular units, and not standardized parameters.) A recent perspective[18]* on the historical work of Russian scientist Yakov Kots (to whom the development of Russian stimulation for muscle strengthening has been attributed) suggests that, ". . . the choice of a 10/50/10 [10-s "on" cycle/50-s "off" cycle for 10 repetitions] stimulation regimen to avoid neuromuscular fatigue has a sound physiologic basis."[47] In spite of their belief, the authors report that data are inconclusive relating to both this regimen and the optimum frequency of the pulse current.[47] They conclude that, ". . . 'Russian current' stimulators should provide a choice of 1 kilohertz (kHz) or 2.5 kHz (2500 hertz [cycles/second]) stimulus waveforms."*[47]

As patients progress to the minimum protection phase of healing (the point at which they are working toward their optimum functional outcome), it is beneficial and recommended that function- or activity-specific training be included in the PT program.[20] This training may further be enhanced by using e-stim (if otherwise appropriate and indicated) during the task-specific training. For example, if a patient is having difficulty coming from a sitting to a standing position, e-stim electrodes may be placed on the quadriceps muscles and the parameters adjusted so that the stimulation augments a functional contraction while the patient practices standing after being seated.

A final point from the physical therapy literature is worth noting, although it relates specifically to the use of a mode of e-stim referred to as **functional electrical stimulation (FES),** a mode of stimulation designed with parameters for retraining muscles affected by neuromuscular or central nervous system conditions more so than musculoskeletal conditions. This particular study looked at results of using multichannel FES (MFES) for gait impairments in patients with hemiplegia.[14] The authors contend that MFES combined with traditional therapy was effective.[14] They state, "The MFES method is, however, in no case a comprehensive rehabilitation program; *it serves only as a supplement to all therapeutic methods currently used in every day practice.*"[14]†

Suggested guidelines for discontinuing e-stim for disuse atrophy include the following: strength has returned to normal, strength has plateaued for a period of 2 to 4 weeks, no contraction has been elicited after five to seven treatments, and stimulation causes an increase in any sign or symptom.[1]

Reflex muscle guarding is not an uncommon response of a muscle in a painful state, such as in the presence of a musculoskeletal injury. This response involves a prolonged muscle contraction that serves as a physiologic "splint" to avoid moving the injured area, which would result in more pain.[26] Traditionally e-stim is used to reduce tension in the tight muscle and thus promote relaxation.[11] Artificially stimulated contractions produce fatigue rapidly. Muscle fatigue results in decreased ability of a muscle to generate active tension and decreased force of muscle contraction; although this response is normal in healthy muscle tissue that is being worked to increase strength, it is not desirable when a muscle is in the early stages of recovery after injury. According to Gad Alon,[3] ". . . replacing one undesired phenomenon (spasm) with another (fatigue) may not benefit the patient and . . . there are better ways to achieve reduction of the guarding." He offers contract–relax techniques or using e-stim to mask the pain as alternatives.[3]

Ultimately, it is not human physiology or physiologic responses to e-stim that have changed; the elaborate and sometimes complicated features of modern equipment will still elicit a limited number of physiologic responses. Based on this understanding, it is the responsibility of the PTA to continually monitor the patient's response to e-stim interventions and make recommendations for modifications or possibly to discontinue e-stim when indicated.[7]

Precautions and Contraindications

Because of its effect of increasing cellular activity, e-stim is considered to be contraindicated in the area of a malignancy. Cancer in a site distant from the target treatment area is considered to be a precaution.[43] E-stim is contraindicated in patients with cardiac pacemakers or other implanted stimulators.[22] Because potential effects on a developing fetus cannot be safely measured, pregnancy should be considered a contraindication for e-stim when considering its use for orthopedic conditions. E-stim is considered to be a relative contraindication for patients with cardiac disease; the stability of the patient's condition and the area to be treated must be taken into consideration. In the presence of unstable cardiac disease or an area where current flow could potentially affect heart conduction, e-stim should be considered contraindicated.[22] Thrombophlebitis is a contraindication for e-stim because of its effects on increasing blood flow. Other contraindications include active tuberculosis over the carotid sinus or in areas of active hemorrhage.[22]

Caution must be used when applying e-stim over areas with excessive adipose tissue because of its characteristic of high impedance. As in the case of other superficially applied physical agents, caution must be exercised

---

*This perspective[47] is a document that is not necessarily based on actual available scientific data, but rather one that provides the authors' interpretation—and in this case, translation—of data that the authors claim is attributable to Kots's original work.[18]

†Italics added for emphasis.

with any patient who has loss of skin integrity or compromised circulation. Although metal implants are not considered to be an absolute contraindication for the use of e-stim, if this procedure is employed, the current flow must not flow directly through the area with the metal implant.[22] If the e-stim is being employed to augment active muscle contraction, the PTA must be certain to apply all precautions related to active exercise for each patient.[22]

Iontophoresis

Iontophoresis is a technique that employs electrical stimulation to drive medication into superficial tissue. Typically this agent is used to treat superficial structures (e.g., a tendinous insertion) for pain or inflammation. With this application, the PT or the referring physician selects the medication based on the clinical indication. The role of the PTA with this intervention is to apply the intervention with the prescribed medication, adjusting and modifying parameters according to the patient's response (determined by subjective tolerance and tissue and skin reaction) and the dosage (calculated by the relationship of treatment time and intensity). As with other forms of e-stim, the PTA must monitor these responses closely and assess for effective results on an ongoing basis. Because of the high current density of this application, the PTA also must monitor closely for any signs of burns to the skin under the relatively small treatment electrode. The PTA should also assess for any abnormal responses to the medication, such as rashes or systemic reactions.

DOCUMENTATION

When documenting interventions that include physical agents, the PTA must include details to provide treatment guidelines for those working with the patient on subsequent visits. This information should include the following:

- Preintervention and postintervention status
  - Subjective reports of pain (visual analog scale [VAS], if indicated)
  - Subjective reports related to functional status
  - Skin integrity before and after intervention
  - Objective measurement of any area anticipated to be affected by intervention (strength, edema, ROM, etc.)
- Patient position
- Position or simultaneous activity of treated area (e.g., e-stim applied during active exercise or US applied during positional stretch)
- Parameters of intervention
  - Intensity
  - Duration
  - Characteristics of delivered agent (e.g., duty cycle for US or e-stim or waveform of e-stim)

- Assessment of whether progress toward goals and functional outcomes is being achieved
  - If no progress noted, judgment about cause or factors that may be impeding progress
  - If progress noted, recommendations for any appropriate modifications to subsequent intervention (increase or decrease parameters; continue or discontinue intervention)
- Plan for subsequent sessions
  - Consult with PT, if indicated, about assessment recommendations
  - Modify intervention according to plan of care
  - Progress according to plan of care

CONCLUSION

Because the literature about the use of physical agents for the treatment of musculoskeletal conditions often reflects equivocal or confusing findings, an attempt to summarize it or to draw definitive application guidelines has not been made here. The PTA student is advised to become familiar with suggested clinical protocols available in the clinical setting but always to monitor results and outcomes, keeping in mind the underlying principles of the theoretic physiologic effects of each agent. Also, the PTA should participate in decisions relating to purchase of clinical equipment when given the opportunity. During this process, keep in mind what types of patients will be treated and relate this to the specific capabilities and features of the available equipment.

❖ ADDITIONAL FEATURES

Active Transport: Transmission of topical medications into tissues via acoustic energy of US as a result of increased cell membrane permeability.

Bladder Technique: The therapeutic technique of US transmission applied over a water-filled small balloon placed directly over the injured area, which serves as a coupling medium.

Cryokinetics: Application of cold alternated with therapeutic exercise to induce the physiologic effects of cold and stimulate the effects of exercise to propagate function.

Electric Stimulation for Fracture Repair: Generally used for treatment of nonunion fractures. Constant direct or pulsed electromagnetic fields externally applied stimulation enhances production of insulin-like growth factor (IGF) in osteoblast cells.

Electrically Evoked Muscle Stimulation: Reeducation of asynchronous muscle contraction; elicits muscle vasodilation, reduces muscle atrophy, stimulates muscle strength, and improves joint range of motion. Caution: Electrically evoked muscle contractions potentially create greater fatigue via synchronous muscle firing.

Iontophoresis: The use of electric current to transmit ions into tissues for analgesic and antiinflammatory effects.

Mechanisms of Heat Transmission Conduction: Direct contact with heat or cold, convection–transmission, or air or water over the skin's surface, radiation–transmission of heat source to a cooler area.

Physiologic Effects of Cold: Reduced localized tissue temperature, reduced localized cell metabolism, decreased blood flow via vasoconstriction, reduced nerve conduction velocity, analgesia.

Physiologic Effects of Heat: Increase in localized superficial temperature, increase in localized and superficial cell metabolism, vasodilation and increased blood flow, superficial increase in capillary permeability, increased elasticity of dense connective tissue, reduced muscle spasms, analgesia.

Short Wave Diathermy: Advantages: Able to treat larger areas compared with US, delivers uniform thermal energy effects, able to apply therapeutic stretching techniques for a longer duration posttreatment compared with US, less dedicated clinician treatment time compared with US.

Ultrasound for Fracture Healing: Clinical studies demonstrate that low-intensity pulsed US stimulates bone growth and fracture repair healing in nonunions.

REFERENCES

1. Alon G: Course Notes: Clinical Electrotherapy. Athens, GA, Athens Regional Medical Center, 2003.
2. Alon G: Principles of electrical stimulation. In Nelson RM, Hayes KW, Currier DP, eds. Clinical Electrotherapy, third ed. Stamford, CT, Appleton & Lange, 1999.
3. Alon G: Personal correspondence. March 11, 2003.
4. American Physical Therapy Association: Clinical Performance Instrument for the Physical Therapist Assistant. Alexandria, VA, American Physical Therapy Association, 1998.
5. American Physical Therapy Association: Electrotherapeutic Terminology in Physical Therapy. Alexandria, VA, American Physical Therapy Association, 2000.
6. American Physical Therapy Association: Guide to Physical Therapist Practice. Alexandria, VA, American Physical Therapy Association, 1999.
7. American Physical Therapy Association: The Normative Model for Physical Therapist Assistant Education. Alexandria, VA, American Physical Therapy Association, 1998.
8. American Physical Therapy Association: Policy on Direction and Supervision of the Physical Therapist Assistant, HOD06-00-16-27. Alexandria, VA, American Physical Therapy Association, 2000.
9. Baker KG, Robertson VJ, Duck FA: A review of therapeutic ultrasound: biophysical effects. Phys Ther 2001;81:1351–1358.
10. Barr JO: Transcutaneous electrical nerve stimulation for pain management. In: Nelson RM, Hayes KW, Currier DP, eds. Clinical Electrotherapy, 3rd ed. Stamford, CT, Appleton & Lange, 1999.
11. Behrens BJ, Michlovitz SL: Physical Agents: Theory and Practice for the Physical Therapist Assistant. Philadelphia, FA Davis, 1996.
12. Bélanger A-Y: Evidence-Based Guide to Therapeutic Physical Agents. Philadelphia, Lippincott Williams & Wilkins, 2002.
13. Binder-Mcleod SA, McDermond LR: Changes in the force-frequency relationship of the human quadriceps femoris muscle following electrically and voluntarily induced fatigue. Phys Ther 1992;72:95–104.
14. Bogataj U, Gros N. Kljajic M, et al: The rehabilitation of gait in patients with hemiplegia: a comparison between conventional therapy and multichannel functional electrical stimulation therapy. Phys Ther 1995;75(6):490–502.
15. Cameron MH: Physical Agents in Rehabilitation: From Research to Practice. St Louis, WB Saunders, 2003.
16. Castel JC: Therapeutic ultrasound. In Prentice WE, ed. Therapeutic Modalities for Physical Therapists. New York, McGraw-Hill, 2002.
17. Cheing GL, Tsui AY, Lo SK, et al: Optimal stimulation duration of tens in the management of osteoarthritic knee pain. J Rehab Med 2003;35(2):62–68.
18. Delitto A: Introduction to "Russian electrical stimulation": putting this perspective into perspective. Phys Ther 2002;82:1017–1018.
19. Draper DO, Knight K, Fujiwara T, et al: Temperature change in human muscle during and after pulsed short-wave diathermy. JOSPT 1999;29(1):13–18.
20. Durstine JL, Davis PG: Specificity of exercise training and testing. In Roitman JL, ed. ACSM's Resource Manual Guidelines for Exercise Testing and Prescription, 4th ed. Philadelphia, Lippincott Williams & Wilkins, 2001.
21. Gerleman DG, Barr JO: Instrumentation and product safety. In Nelson RM, Hayes KW, Currier DP, eds. Clinical Electrotherapy, 3rd ed. Stamford, CT, Appleton & Lange, 1999.
22. Gillespie CA: Foundations for electrical stimulation. In Behrens BJ, Michlovitz SL, eds. Physical Agents: Theory and Practice for the Physical Therapist Assistant. Philadelphia, FA Davis, 1996.
23. Harris S, Draper DO, Schulthies S: The effect of ultrasound on temperature rise in preheated human muscle. In Prentice WE, Voight MI, eds. Techniques in Musculoskeletal Rehabilitation. New York, McGraw-Hill, 2001.
24. Hecox B, Mehreteab TA, Weisberg J: Physical Agents: A Comprehensive Text for Physical Therapists. Norwalk, CT, Appleton & Lange, 1994.
25. Johnson MI, Tabasam G: An investigation into the analgesic effects of interferential currents and transcutaneous electrical nerve stimulation on experimentally induced ischemic pain in otherwise pain-free volunteers. Phys Ther 2003;83:208–223.
26. Kisner C, Colby LA: Therapeutic Exercise: Foundations and Techniques. Philadelphia, FA Davis, 2002.
27. Knight CA, Rutledge CR, Cox ME, et al: Effect of superficial heat, deep heat and active exercise warm-up on the extensibility of the plantar flexors. Phys Ther 2001;81(6):1206–1214.
28. Knight KL: Cryotherapy in Sports Injury Management. Champaign, IL, Human Kinetics Publications, 1995.
29. Laufer Y, Ries JD, Leininger PM, et al: Quadriceps femoris muscle torque and fatigue generated by neuromuscular electrical stimulation with three different waveforms. Phys Ther 2001; 81(7):1307–1316.
30. Lentell G, et al: The use of thermal agents to influence the effectiveness of a low-load prolonged stretch. JOSPT 1992:16:200.
31. Leo KC, Dostal WF, Bossen DG, et al: Effect of transcutaneous electrical nerve stimulation characteristics on clinical pain. Phys Ther 1986;66(2):200–205.
32. Lewek M, Stevens J, Snyder-Mackler L: The use of electrical stimulation to increase quadriceps femoris muscle force in an elderly patient following a total knee arthroplasty. Phys Ther 2001;81:1565–1571.
33. McDiarmid T, Ziskin MC, Michlovitz SL: Therapeutic ultrasound. In Michlovitz SL: Thermal Agents in Rehabilitation. Philadelphia, FA Davis, 1997.
34. Medtronic of Canada, Ltd: Medtronic Safety Reminder: Contraindication to Diathermy for Patients Implanted with any Type of Medtronic Neurostimulation System. 2001.
35. Michlovitz SL: Thermal Agents in Rehabilitation. Philadelphia, FA Davis, 1997.
36. Miller BF, Gruben KG, Morgan BJ: Circulatory responses to voluntary and electrically induced muscle contractions in humans. Phys Ther 2000;80:53–60.
37. Prentice WE: Therapeutic Modalities for Physical Therapists. New York, McGraw-Hill, 2002.
38. Rennie GA, Michlovitz SL: Biophysical principles of heating and superficial heating agents. In Michlovitz SL: Thermal agents in Rehabilitation. Philadelphia, FA Davis, 1997.
39. Sicard-Rosenbaum L, Lord D, Danoff JV, et al: Effects of continuous therapeutic ultrasound on growth and metastasis of subcutaneous murine tumors. Phys Ther 1995;75(1):3–13.

40. Snyder-Mackler, Garrett M, Roberts M: A comparison of torque generating capabilities of three different electrical stimulating currents. JOSPT 1989;10:297–301.
41. Spielholz NI: Electrical stimulation of denervated muscle. In Nelson RM, Hayes KW, Currier DP, eds. Clinical Electrotherapy, 3rd ed. Stamford, CT, Appleton & Lange, 1999.
42. Stuchly MA, Repacholi MH, Lecuyer DW, et al: Exposure to the operator and patient during shortwave diathermy treatments. *Health Phys* 1982;42(3):341.
43. Sussman C, Byl NN: Externally applied electric current for tissue repair. In Nelson RM, Hayes KW, Currier DP, eds. Clinical Electrotherapy, 3rd ed. Stamford, CT, Appleton & Lange, 1999.
44. Travell J, Simons D: Myofascial Pain and Dysfunction: The Trigger Point Manual, vol. 2. Philadelphia, Williams & Wilkins, 1993.
45. U.S. Environmental Protection Agency: The Plain English Guide to the Clean Air Act. 2003. *www.epa.gov/air/uaqps/peg_caa/pegcaa06.html*
46. Walsh MT: Hydrotherapy: the use of water as a therapeutic agent. In Michlovitz SL, ed. Thermal Agents in Rehabilitation. Philadelphia, FA Davis, 1996.
47. Ward AR, Shkuratova N: Russian electrical stimulation: the early experiments. *Phys Ther* 2002;82:1019–1030.
48. Wesling KC, DeVane DA, Hylton CR: Effects of static stretch versus static stretch and ultrasound combined on triceps surae muscle extensibility in healthy women. *Phys Ther* 1987;67:674–679.

REVIEW QUESTIONS

Multiple Choice

1. Which statement about evidence for the use of physical agents to treat musculoskeletal conditions is **NOT** true?
   A. There is strong evidence that physical agents play a direct role in healing of tissues affected by musculoskeletal pathologic conditions or injuries.
   B. Physical agents, when appropriately applied, serve as a beneficial adjunctive intervention in the treatment of musculoskeletal conditions.
   C. Evidence for beneficial and detrimental effects of physical agents is limited.
   D. Many contraindications associated with the use of physical agents in the treatment of musculoskeletal conditions have not been scientifically proved, but the potential risks may outweigh possible benefits in some cases.

2. Effects of cold agents include which of the following?
   A. Vasoconstriction and decreased metabolic activity
   B. Decreased conduction of sensory nerve impulses
   C. Decreased conduction of motor nerve impulses
   D. All of the above are effects of cold.

3. Cryokinetics describes which of the following?
   A. Periodic removal and reapplication of cold agents to areas around the target tissue
   B. Interspersing repeated applications of cold with bouts of active exercise
   C. Rapid movement of ice massage application over injured area
   D. Application of simultaneous stretch with therapeutic cold agent

4. Which term is used to describe the area of the US head that actually produces the sound wave?
   A. Duty cycle
   B. Beam nonuniformity ratio
   C. Acoustic streaming
   D. Effective radiating area

5. Of what benefit to a patient with a painful orthopedic condition is the use of a portable TENS unit over a clinical unit with IFC capabilities?

A. The TENS unit may be used more frequently for patient-controlled pain relief treatments because it is portable.
B. TENS has been proved to be more effective than IFC for relieving pain.
C. IFC units have a lower frequency than TENS; therefore, there is less penetration of therapeutic stimulation.
D. There is no particular benefit of TENS over IFC.

6. As a study on the treatment of pain for patients with knee osteoarthritis showed, which duration of TENS treatment was most effective?
   A. 10 minutes
   B. 20 minutes
   C. 30 minutes
   D. 40 minutes

7. Which statement is **NOT** true about guidelines for use of e-stim for edema reduction?
   A. Treatment should be discontinued when edema reduction is stable for three to four treatments.
   B. Treatment should be discontinued when the edema is resolved.
   C. Treatment should be discontinued if no response is noted within three to five treatments.
   D. Strong evidence exists demonstrating the direct effects of edema reduction through the use of e-stim.

8. Which statement **is** true about application of e-stim?
   A. Clinical protocols should be used as final determinants when selecting parameters for e-stim applications.
   B. The effectiveness of an e-stim device is related to its features. The more features and parameter adjustments available on an e-stim unit, the more effective it is.
   C. Waveform is an e-stim parameter that may be associated with the strength of muscle contraction achieved and fatigue.
   D. Russian stimulation has been scientifically proved to be superior for augmenting strengthening programs compared with other modes of e-stim.

9. Which of the following is an effective method of progressing a patient in the minimum protection phase of healing?
   A. Incorporate task-specific activities into the program.
   B. Increase frequency of pulses.
   C. Increase on:off cycle ratios to decrease fatigue.
   D. Incorporate the interferential mode of e-stim into the program.

10. Which of the following contraindicate(s) the use of e-stim?
    A. Malignancies
    B. Pregnancy
    C. Cardiac pacemakers
    D. All of the above

Short Answer

11. Is it appropriate to have a patient lie on top of a hot pack?

12. List the benefits and advantages of paraffin (versus hot pack).

13. Does superficial heat or superficial cold result in longer-lasting effects of tissue once the agent is removed?

14. How does frequency of US affect the depth of heating effect?

15. What is an appropriate guideline to use for determining duration of US application?

True/False

16. Treatments established through empiric data have been proven to be the most effective.
17. Under no circumstances is it appropriate for a PTA to modify components of interventions included in the physical therapy plan of care.
18. "Thermotherapy" is a term that could be used to describe those heating agents traditionally classified as "superficial," because there is evidence that deeper tissues also are affected.
19. Applying heat over superficial joint structures enhances motion by decreasing viscosity of joint fluids and increasing extensibility of joint tissues.
20. Hot packs reach peak of heating intensity through heat transfer within 5 minutes of application, requiring the PTA to check the skin only after the first 5 minutes of application.
21. Ultrasound is preferred to SWD to treat a larger target area because the area can be more readily observed during treatment.
22. US units with a higher BNR are preferred because these provide greater uniformity of heat transmission across the sound head.
23. PSWD offers a mode of heating that results in less intense heating effects than US; therefore it may be a more appropriate choice when treating acute or subacute conditions.
24. A disadvantage of contrast baths is that the involved extremity is place in a dependent position, which may contribute to increased edema.
25. Shaving excessive body hair before applying electrodes increases therapeutic effectiveness of e-stim by lowering impedance.

Essay Questions

Answer on a separate sheet of paper.

26. Explain the rationale for determining the appropriate number of towel layers to use with application of hot packs.
27. Define impedance and discuss ways to address it with application of e-stim.
28. Name and briefly describe the two theories related to pain control through the use of e-stim.
29. Explain why e-stim may not be effective to treat muscles with partial denervation. Give two examples of conditions that have an excellent prognosis for recovery without the use of physical agents.

Critical Thinking Application

Describe a technique for positioning and treating a patient, using a thermal modality while applying a prolonged stretch. Develop an appropriate scenario, including diagnosis and examination findings.

Consider specific parameters for your physical agent of choice:

- Position of patient
- Position of extremity or body part to be treated
- Intensity or amplitude, duty cycle, waveform characteristics (if appropriate)
- Duration of treatment

What other interventions are appropriate to include before or after the application of the physical agent described? Document the objective portion of a SOAP note associated with the setup for the chosen intervention.

4 Flexibility

LEARNING OBJECTIVES

1. Define and discuss range of motion and flexibility.
2. Identify the properties of connective tissue.
3. Explain the differences between stress and strain.
4. Describe plastic deformation and elastic deformation.
5. Discuss how temperature affects connective tissue.
6. Identify and describe various stretching techniques.
7. Define Golgi tendon organs (GTOs) and muscle spindles.
8. Describe the clinical applications for stretching soft-tissue contractures.
9. Describe and contrast the differences and similarities between scar tissue and adhesions.
10. Outline various methods used to measure flexibility.

KEY TERMS

Flexibility
Range of motion (ROM)
Collagen
Stress
Strain
Elastic deformation
Plastic deformation

Static stretching
Ballistic stretching
Proprioceptive neuromus-
   cular facilitation (PNF)
Specificity
Golgi tendon organs
   (GTOs)

Muscle spindles
Scar tissue
Contracture
Adhesions
Low-load, prolonged
   stretch

CHAPTER OUTLINE

Flexibility
Properties of Connective Tissue
Practical Applications
   Static Stretching
   Ballistic Stretching
   Proprioceptive Neuromuscular Facilitation
Stretching of Soft-Tissue Contractures
Measuring Flexibility

FLEXIBILITY

Flexibility can be defined as the ability of a muscle to relax and yield to a stretch force.[12] Kisner and Colby[12] assert that "flexibility exercises are stretching exercises designed to increase range of motion." Therefore flexibility can refer to various measurable components of joint motion. Muscles, tendons, ligaments, skin, joint capsule, and bone geometry all influence the degree of movement in joints. For example, a muscle can stretch or elongate, creating a measurable effect on the joint or joints upon which it acts. If a muscle becomes damaged by trauma or disease or becomes shortened because of immobilization, its ability to stretch and allow freedom of joint motion is affected.

The amount of movement available to a joint moving within its anatomic range is called its **range of motion (ROM).** The stretching or elongating of muscle and joint ROM are two components of flexibility. An understanding of the properties and components of various connective tissues is fundamental in delivering various stretching and flexibility regimens.

PROPERTIES OF CONNECTIVE TISSUE

Just as amino acids are the building blocks of protein, tropocollagen is the building block of **collagen** (Fig. 4-1). Collagen is found in all connective tissues: bone, tendon, muscle, skin, hyaline cartilage, and joint capsule.[4,22] Collagen is a protein building block of connective tissue, and it provides the strength needed to withstand high levels of tension and force during movement and exercise. Five separate types of collagen have been identified: I, II, III, IV, and V. These are found in varying amounts within the different connective tissues. Types I and III collagen are the most common types found within joint capsule and muscle tissue.

Elastin is a structural protein present in tendons in amounts of less than 1%.[4,9] Tissues with greater amounts of elastin usually demonstrate greater degrees of flexibility. Elastin assists collagen in the "recovery" of tissues after stress.[4]

Stress is defined as the amount of tension or load placed on tissues.[4,22,23] **Strain** is the proportional degree of elongation that occurs during stress.[4,23] The ability of tissues to recover after stress is extremely important in relation to flexibility. Woo and colleagues[27] have shown that increasing the levels of stress produces an increase in collagen within ligaments and tendons, whereas reducing the levels of stress causes weakening in connective tissues.

Recovery is the ability of tissues to return to their previous resting state. It does not imply that permanent elongation or microscopic damage has not occurred. Lehman and colleagues[14] and Warren and colleagues[26] have demonstrated that recovery of the tissue's rest-

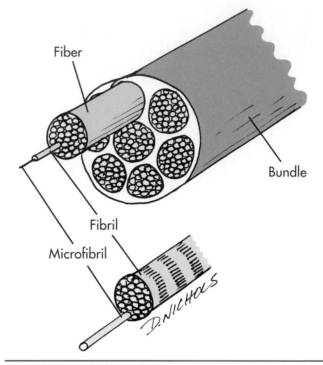

Fig. 4-1 Collagen bundle.

ing length had occurred after microscopic failure had begun.

The rate at which tissues are stretched has a profound effect on the degree or percent of strain. Slower rates of stress produce greater amounts of strain or elongation, whereas faster rates of stretch produce much smaller amounts of elongation.[4,22,23]

Tissues gradually lengthen when they are subjected to constant or repeated stress over a long duration. This slow response to stress is called *creep*.[24]

Two viscoelastic properties of connective tissue are elastic and plastic deformation. **Elastic deformation** is similar to the changes that occur in a rubber band under high rates of strain. The rubber band rapidly conforms to a new length and is able to return to its original resting length when the stress is removed. However, the rubber band breaks if the degree of stress exceeds the strain capabilities (Fig. 4-2). **Plastic deformation** is force dependent under slow rates of stress. For example, when a low degree of stress is applied to a plastic spoon, the spoon slowly deforms to a new shape. The spoon breaks if the stress is applied too fast (Fig. 4-3).

Along with stress and the rate of stress applied to tissues, temperature also affects connective tissue extensibility. Temperatures in the range of 37°C (98.6°F) to 40°C (104°F) affect the viscoelastic properties of connective tissue.[23] The higher the temperature (approximately 45°C [113°F] is the therapeutic upper limit), the greater the degree of elongation with stress before tissue failure.[28] Because connective tissue's viscoelastic and plastic changes occur at higher temperatures, there

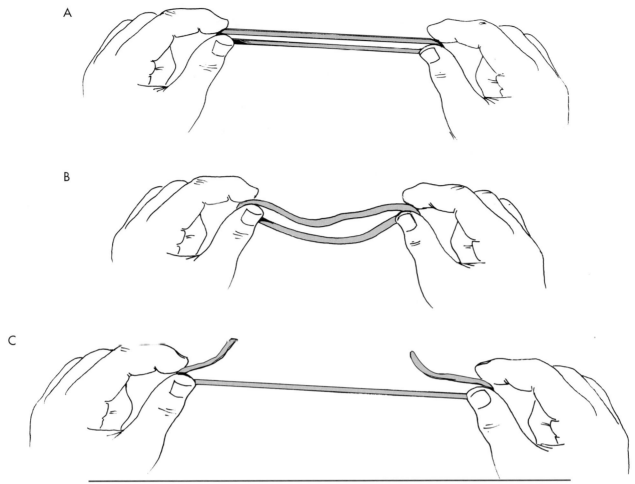

Fig. 4-2 Elastic deformation. **A,** Stress applied to a rubber band. **B,** When stress is removed the rubber band returns to its original length. **C,** If the stress exceeds the strain capabilities of the band, it can break.

is less microscopic damage under stress at these temperatures. Studies by Warren and colleagues[25] have demonstrated that a temperature of 45° C is needed to reduce tissue damage during strains of 2.6% or less.

Muscle or contractile tissue responds to stretch by elastic and plastic deformation properties in ways similar to connective tissue. Obviously the contractile properties of muscle allow for the greatest degree of freedom of movement around a joint. The arrangements and relationships of the microscopic elements of the sarcomere, actin, myosin, A-band, Z-band, I-band, and H-zone are addressed in Chapter 5.

Although connective tissue is considered a passive resistant to joint motion, muscle tissue is considered an active restraint to joint motion by virtue of its elastic and contractile elements.

Active exercise (muscular contractions) affects intramuscular temperature. Increases to approximately 39° C are observed in exercised muscle.[3] Commonly used passive thermal agents that increase tissue temperature are moist heat and ultrasound. The judicious use of active

exercise and passive thermal agents before and during stretching programs enhances the effectiveness of the prescribed program.

PRACTICAL APPLICATIONS

In discussion of flexibility and associated stretching programs, the stretching of nonpathologic muscle must be separated from stretching noncontractile connective tissue. Improving muscle extensibility in nonpathologic conditions and in adaptive muscle shortening after injury or immobilization requires a complement of active exercise techniques and thermal agents.

Types of active stretching exercises are **static stretching,** ballistic stretching, and **proprioceptive neuromuscular facilitation (PNF)** techniques (contract-relax, hold-relax, and slow-reversal-hold).

Static Stretching

Static stretching involves placing a muscle in a fully elongated position and holding that position for a

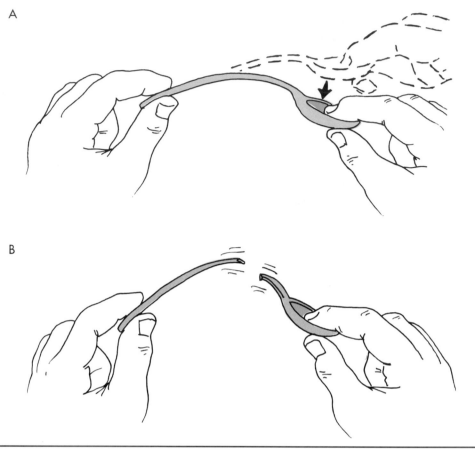

Fig. 4-3 Plastic deformation. **A,** A low degree of stress is applied to a plastic spoon. The spoon will deform slowly and accommodate to a new shape. **B,** If stress is applied suddenly and with great force, the spoon will break.

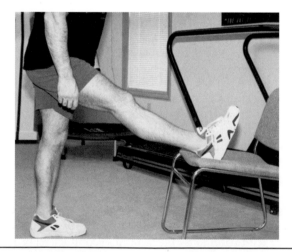

Fig. 4-4 Static stretching. Initial starting position for standing hamstring stretch.

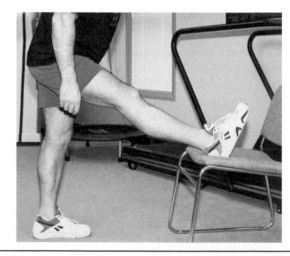

Fig. 4-5 The muscle will slowly conform to an elongated position by maintaining stress on the tissue for a period of time.

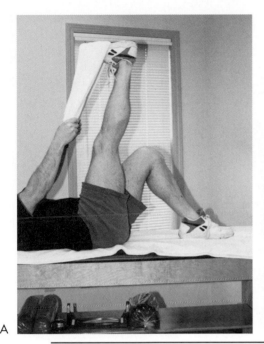
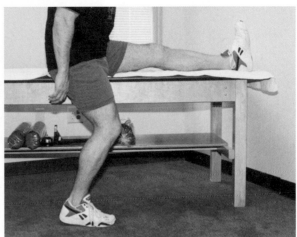

Fig. 4-6 **A,** Supine static hamstring stretch using a towel. **B,** Sitting hamstring stretch.

period of time (Figs. 4-4 and 4-5). Athletes use static stretching before sports activities as part of a warm-up before a workout and as part of a cool-down after a workout. Because intramuscular temperature rises to approximately 39°C during exercise,[3] active general body movements can improve muscle temperature before stretching is done.

Studies on rattail tendons[13] demonstrate that ruptures occur with 31% of normal loads when temperatures are at 25°C, whereas increasing temperatures to 45°C delays tendon rupture until 102% of normal load. This demonstrates that stretching at normal body temperatures damages tissue,[26] but elevating tissue temperature before and during prolonged stretch is less damaging.[25,26]

Static stretching has distinct advantages, such as reduced chance of exceeding strain limits of tissues, reduced energy requirements compared with other forms of stretching, and reduced potential for muscle soreness.[9,23,28] The ease and practicality of teaching patients to perform static stretching is another advantage. For example, hamstring stretches can be taught with the patient in various positions (Fig. 4-6). Outline and describe general and specific goals and expected outcomes for the patient when teaching the proper execution of static stretching programs. The general goals of static stretching are to prevent or minimize the risk of soft-tissue injury from participation in sports or physical activities, improve movement and increase flexibility, and prevent contracture.[1,12]

Generally, static stretches are "held" in a fully elongated position for 10 to 60 seconds.[1,11] After a short rest (5 to 10 seconds), an attempt is made to extend the stretched position farther within tolerable limits (Fig. 4-7). Multiple repetitions are performed (5 to 15), with one "set" of stretches generally equal to 10 repetitions. The limits of motion achieved during a stretching program depend on the patient's tolerance, age, pathologic condition (if any), motivation, and commitment. The muscle's ability to adapt is a prolonged process. Patients must be cautioned not to exceed their pain limits and must receive counseling about the fact that many sessions of stretching are needed to produce change and lasting improvement. Approximately 6 weeks of stretching are necessary to demonstrate significant increases in muscular flexibility.[29] An individual must stretch at least three times per week to improve flexibility. An individual must stretch at least 1 day per week to maintain the flexibility gained during the program.[28]

Ballistic Stretching

Athletes use dynamic, high-velocity, and even violent motions during sporting events and require extraordinary flexibility to prevent or reduce the risk of potential musculoskeletal injury. A concept applicable to conditioning athletes to better defend against injury is specificity. **Specificity** is described as training an organism in a way that most closely duplicates the desired application or functional goal. In other words, if you want to

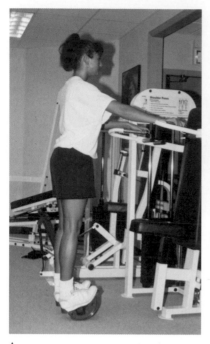 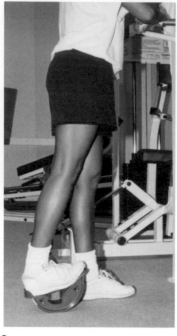 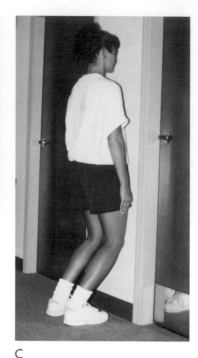

A   B   C

Fig. 4-7 Examples of static stretching positions and techniques for the Gastroc-soleus complex. **A,** Standing bilateral calf stretch. **B,** Single limb static calf stretch. **C,** Gastroc-soleus stretch.

improve an athlete's ability to move dynamically with rapid changes in direction and velocity, you must train and condition the athlete in that manner.

Dynamic or ballistic stretching involves a "bounce" at the end of the ROM (Fig. 4-8). Relatively high-velocity or quick bouncing may not be appropriate for many patients. The potential for tissue damage exists in all forms of exercise, but ballistic stretching may increase the risk of connective tissue and contractile tissue trauma, although a narrow segment of patients may benefit. Ballistic stretching is used as a part of a progression of stretching and never as a single treatment. In training, a general body warmup is needed first. The beneficial effects of a warmup before strenuous activities include the following:

- Blood flow to working muscles is increased.
- Temperature in working muscles is increased.
- Cardiovascular response to sudden, dynamic exercise is improved.
- Breakdown of oxyhemoglobin for the delivery of oxygen to the working muscles is increased.
- The risk of connective tissue and contractile tissue damage is reduced.

A progressive static stretching program is begun after a warmup of 5 or 10 minutes. A gradually increasing period of ballistic stretching is started after a few repetitions of static stretches.

Ballistic stretching does not imply aggressive, violent, high-velocity stretches throughout the ROM; instead it involves a slight but progressively greater bounce at the end of the range achieved through static stretching.

Proprioceptive Neuromuscular Facilitation

PNF stretching techniques have been found to be superior to other forms of active stretching.[5,17-20] They are based on the stretch reflex.[1,20] Two neurophysiologic sensory receptors involved with the stretch reflex are the **Golgi tendon organs (GTOs)** and the muscle spindle. The GTOs are inhibitory sensory receptors located within the myotendinous junction (Fig. 4-9). The GTOs are activated by excessive or prolonged stretches and by muscular contractions. When a muscle is stretched, the GTOs send messages to the spinal cord to inhibit contraction. This causes a reflex relaxation, which protects against damage to the muscle fibers.

Muscle spindles are excitatory specialized fibers within the muscle (Fig. 4-10) that are sensitive to rapid changes in muscle length. When a muscle is stretched quickly, the spindles send messages to the spinal cord, which in turn signals the muscle to contract. The classic clinical demonstration of the stretch reflex is produced by tapping the relaxed patellar tendon, which causes

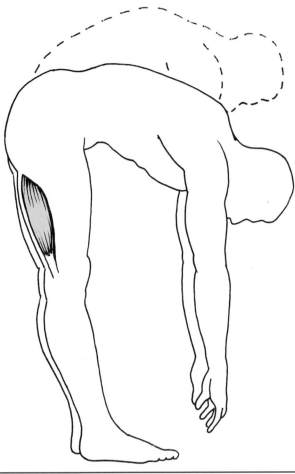

Fig. 4-8 Dynamic or ballistic stretching requires a relatively high velocity "bounce" at the end-range of motion. Typically ballistic stretching techniques are reserved for an athletic population in preparation for high-velocity, ballistic, and sometimes violent physical activity.

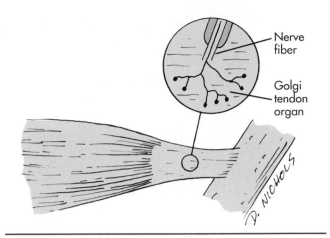

Fig. 4-9 Golgi tendon organ.

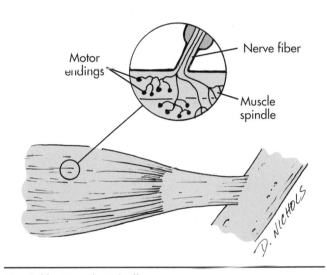

Fig. 4-10 Muscle spindle.

the reflexive contraction of the quadriceps. The muscle spindles within the quadriceps are activated by the quick stretch of the patellar tendon, causing the quadriceps to contract reflexively (Fig. 4-11).

PNF stretching has several drawbacks: it is more time consuming than other methods, requires skillful application by trained professionals to be effective, and may lead to complaints of patient discomfort.[28]

Three effective PNF stretching techniques are contract-relax, hold-relax, and slow-reversal-hold. The *contract-relax* technique involves instructing the patient to relax the affected muscle while the therapist passively moves the limb to the limit of motion. The patient is instructed to actively contract the antagonist against the isotonic, manually applied resistance of the therapist for 10 seconds. The patient is then instructed to relax while the therapist passively moves the limb to the new limits of motion (Fig. 4-12). Relaxation of the

antagonist muscle during contraction is called *autogenic inhibition*.[1,20]

The *hold-relax technique* is similar to contract-relax. However, instead of an active, isotonic contraction of the antagonist, the patient isometrically contracts against the force applied by the therapist at the end of the ROM. After a 10-second isometric contraction, the patient is instructed to relax. The therapist then passively stretches the limb to the new limits of motion (Fig. 4-13).

The *slow-reversal-hold technique* requires the patient to actively move the affected limb to the limits of motion. The patient then applies an isometric 30-second contraction of the antagonist against the force applied by the therapist. The patient is instructed to relax the antagonist, and then actively contract the antagonist to bring the limb to the new limits of motion (Fig. 4-14). The reflexive relaxation of the antagonist during contraction of the agonist is termed *reciprocal inhibition*.[1,20]

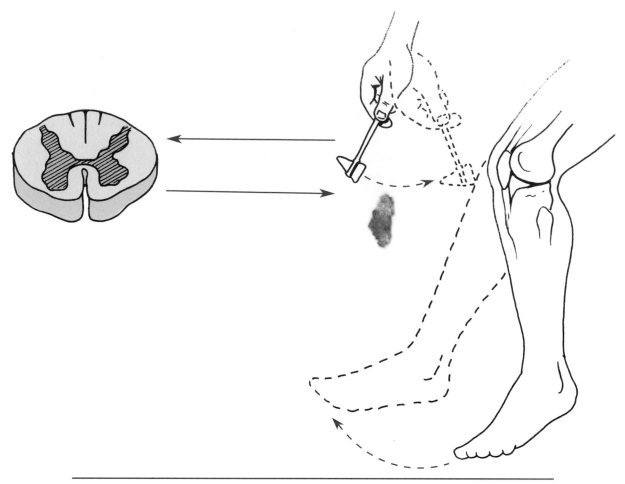

Fig. 4-11 Muscle spindle activation by quick stretch-reflex between the spinal cord and quadriceps.

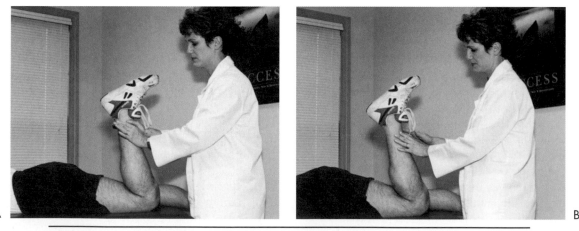

Fig. 4-12 Proprioceptive neuromuscular facilitation, contract-relax technique. **A,** The patient actively contracts against manually applied resistance for 10 seconds. **B,** The patient then relaxes while the therapist passively moves the limb to the new limits of motion.

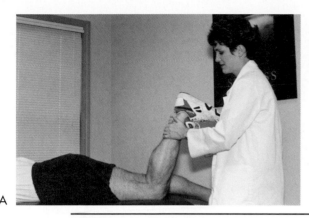
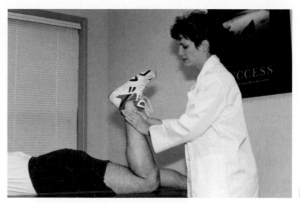

A

B

Fig. 4-13 Proprioceptive neuromuscular facilitation hold-relax technique. **A,** The patient isometrically contracts against the force applied by the therapist for 10 seconds. **B,** The patient relaxes and the therapist passively moves the limb to new limits of motion.

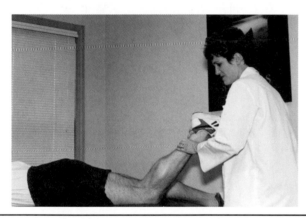

Fig. 4-14 Proprioceptive neuromuscular facilitation slow-reversal-hold technique (see text for description of technique).

STRETCHING OF SOFT-TISSUE CONTRACTURES

The stretching of soft-tissue contractures involves muscle, capsule, tendon, ligament, bursa, and skin. The stretching of joint contractures differs significantly from static, ballistic, or PNF stretching. Many options exist for the therapist when prescribing stretching exercises for patients after immobilization or injury. Long-duration, low-load static stretching has been an effective technique that produces long-lasting connective tissue changes.[8,13,25,26] The physical therapist assistant (PTA) must recognize adaptive changes that occur in various soft tissues after injury or immobility. First, **scar tissue** is formed and a **contracture** develops. In this text a contracture is defined as a permanent or transient limitation of movement or shortening of muscle or other soft tissues.[6] Scar tissue is the same as an adhesion and results from healing or union of two injured or torn

parts (Fig. 4-15). An adhesion involves a limitation of function resulting from scar tissue that forms between structures.[6] For example, when scar tissue forms after knee surgery, it can "bind down" and form **adhesions** among the patella, suprapatellar pouch, and quadriceps tendon (Fig. 4-16).

Generally, immature scar is defined as adaptable for up to 8 weeks and becomes progressively less changeable for up to 14 weeks.[7] Scar becomes quite inextensible at 14 weeks and is termed *unadaptable,* or mature scar.[2] According to Cummings,[7] adaptable scar is highly vascular, with many cells (including myofibrocytes) that give the scar the ability to contract. Immature scar tissue also has a high rate of remodeling,[2,7] which is the process of tissue restructuring in response to stress or immobilization.[8]

Adaptable or immature scar tissue becomes increasingly organized and oriented, with specific directional lines of stress.[7] As new scar tissue is formed, the collagen fibers become highly unorganized and arranged randomly, creating an immobile structure.[16]

Where stretching is concerned, the PTA must be attentive to the following critical components:

■ The time dependent and stress reactive nature of scar tissue

■ The fragility of immature adaptable scar:
  ■ At 5 days, new scar is only 10% of its maximum potential strength
  ■ At 40 days, new scar is 40% of its maximum strength
  ■ At 60 days, new scar is 70% of its maximum strength
  ■ At 12 months, new scar is approximately 100% of its maximum strength

■ New scar tissue organizes and aligns itself along lines of stress; therefore appropriately applied stress helps to remodel unorganized scar

■ Low-load, long-duration stretching of joint contractures in combination with thermal agents to preheat

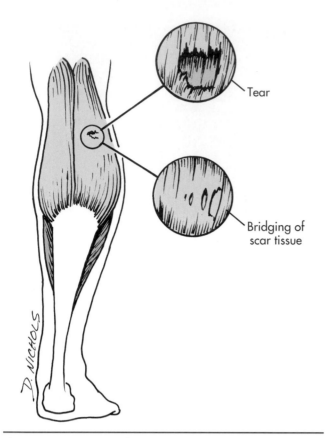

Fig. 4-15 Scar tissue formation.

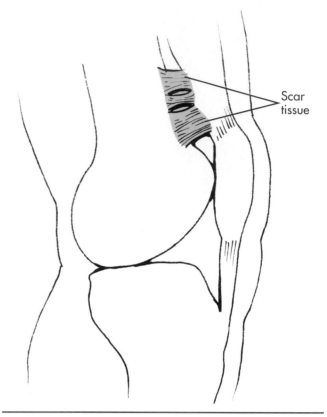

Fig. 4-16 Adhesions formed between quad tendon and underlying bone results in a limitation of function.

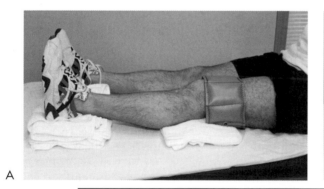

A

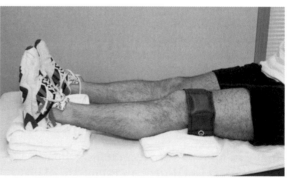

B

Fig. 4-17 External force is applied to enhance passive low-load prolonged stretch. **A,** Excessive weight causes reflexive muscle splinting and guarding. **B,** Only very light resistance is necessary to elicit appropriate relaxation.

extensible connective tissue has proved effective in the treatment of soft-tissue contracture.[10,14,15] Long-duration stretching means stretching over a period of 20 to 60 minutes.[7]

Clinically, the following areas are involved in a **low-load, prolonged stretch** technique:

1. Preheat the involved structures with moist heat or ultrasound.[8]

2. Place the involved structures in a position of comfort, not maximum stretch. This is an extremely important point. To elicit relaxation, the involved structures must be placed in a supported and comfortable gravity-assisted position.

3. Maintain moist heat application during the entire course of treatment (20 to 60 min).

4. Apply stress or load gradually and minimally. With

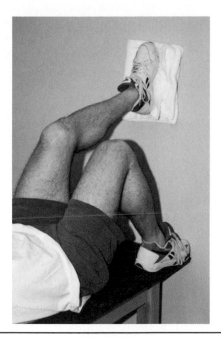

Fig. 4-18   Supine wall slides to gain knee flexion motion.

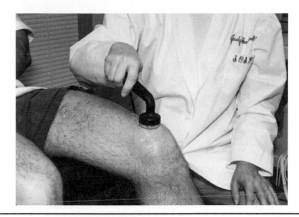

Fig. 4-19   Thermal agents of moist heat and ultrasound applied before passive stretching techniques help elevate tissue temperature and aid in soft-tissue extensibility and patient relaxation.

new immature scar, gravity alone may be enough to clinically effect change. With mature scar, only slightly greater loads should be used. This is a critical point. Lentell and colleagues[14] found that the magnitude of force used in their study (0.5% of body weight) to create a significant long-lasting change in motion fostered such relaxation that many subjects "did not even feel a sensation of stretch during the procedure." In efforts to gain knee extension after surgery, for example, it is wise to use this technique to avoid reflexive splinting or muscle guarding (Fig. 4-17).

5. Allow the patient to rest or recover for a few minutes during the course of treatment if the sensation of stretch becomes too uncomfortable.
6. Maintain heat application for 5 to 10 minutes after removal of the loads. Some researchers[21] have advocated the use of ice packs after stretch in this protocol. Lentell and colleagues[14] did not find cooling to be effective in their study. However, cooling the involved structures after stress may be effective in selected cases where pain and an inflammatory response are present.
7. Initiate isometric contractions after the application of heat and passive stretching to enhance strength gains at the new end of ROM.

Lentell and colleagues[14] demonstrated the effectiveness of applying heat before and during low-load, prolonged stretching and external rotation of nonpathologically involved shoulders. Heat application before and during such stretching was clinically superior to bouts of stretching alone, stretching plus ice, and a heat-stretch-ice protocol. Clinically few contraindications exist when attempting to gain motion after specific surgical procedures.

Adhesions are desirable and, in fact, are a surgical goal in selected cases. Desirable permanent shortening of connective tissue is needed to prevent a functional loss of movement in some knee surgeries and surgical correction of some shoulder instabilities. If an attempt is made to fully regain external shoulder rotation after surgery to correct recurrent dislocation, the intent to "scar down" and protect the joint from further dislocation may be derailed. In this case it is wise to gain functional motion very slowly to allow enough time for a mature scar to form (14 weeks).

The clinical application of low-load, prolonged stretch can be modified to varying degrees depending on the surgical procedure, time constraints of healing, and goals of the rehabilitation program. For example, supine wall slides are a modified technique that uses some of the points of low-load, prolonged stretch (Fig. 4-18). When attempting to gain knee flexion range, it is wise to preheat the quadriceps muscles and suprapatellar pouch before stretching. Next, the patient is placed in a supine position and the foot of the involved limb put on a towel against a wall. To reduce friction against the wall, the contact surface of the towel is lightly coated with baby powder so it will slide more easily against the wall. As the patient relaxes, gravity assists in knee flexion and the foot slides down the wall.

This concept can be modified further. In keeping with the example of gaining knee flexion range, the use of isotonic exercise equipment can be helpful. With the patient in a seated position on a knee extension machine, moist heat or ultrasound can be used before and during the stretch (Fig. 4-19). Many knee extension machines are manufactured with an adjustable range-limiting device that allows the patient to adjust the starting and stopping angle of the exercise. Before the stretch is begun, the patient's hips are secured with straps to keep them from rising during the treatment. An angle is selected that is comfortable to the patient. As the tissues are continually heated, a very gradual increase in the flexion angle is initiated. The angle does not have to be excessive to be effective. Thus the protocol remains essentially the same, but the equipment and the position of the patient are changed.

The knee serves as an excellent example to further describe and clarify methods to improve ROM by prolonged static stretching. To gain knee extension range,

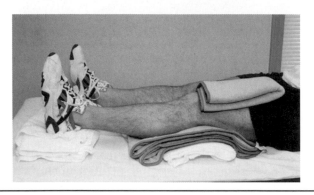

Fig. 4-20   Gaining knee extension using thermal agents (moist heat) and low-load, prolonged stretch.

the patient can be supine with moist heat applied behind the knee (popliteal fossa) and on the hamstring and quadriceps. The heel of the involved limb is placed on a small folded towel (Fig. 4-20). If the knee is contracted to −20°, for example, towels are added under the hot packs under the knee to ensure a very comfortable starting position. During the course of treatment, small layers of towel can be removed gradually to allow for improved range of knee extension. As a progression to this technique, a small vertical force can be applied on the knee. Care should be taken to ensure that this force is sufficiently small (1 to 2 lbs or lighter) and that it is applied superior to the patella to avoid compressive forces between the patella and femur (Fig. 4-21).

The patient is brought to a sitting position to enhance this stretch further. A towel is used to dorsiflex the involved foot, and the patient is instructed to slowly lean forward to stretch the hamstrings (Fig. 4-22). Simultaneous isometric quadriceps sets also are used to improve strength at the new limits of knee extension.

Gaining knee extension can be achieved in a prone position as well (Fig. 4-23). However, care must be taken to elevate the patella off the table and thereby prevent excessive patellofemoral compression. This is done by

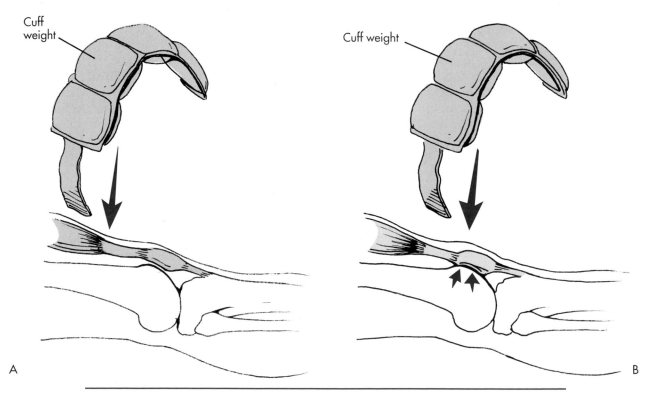

Fig. 4-21   **A,** When applying resistance on the knee to gain extension, it is essential that the resistance be placed superior to the patella. **B,** If resistance is placed directly on the patella, there is a sharp concentration of force, which increases patellofemoral compression.

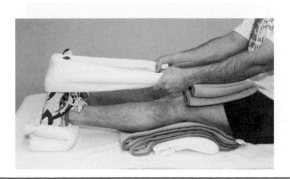

Fig. 4-22 Seated passive towel stretch.

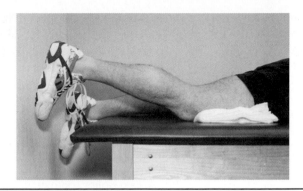

Fig. 4-23 Passive prone knee extension stretch. Note the use of towels placed under the quadriceps to elevate the patella off the table to reduce patellofemoral compression.

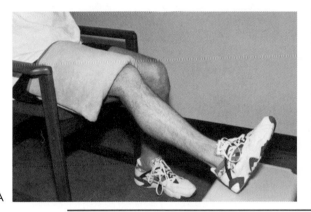

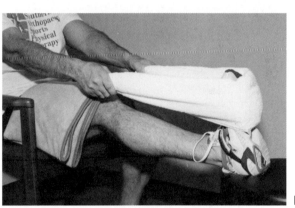

A   B

Fig. 4-24 **A,** Seated knee extension stretch with moist heat application to the quadriceps. **B,** Stretch is enhanced by using a towel to dorsiflex the foot of the involved limbs and to instruct the patient to flex the trunk forward.

placing a small folded towel superior to the patella. This position works well when only slight degrees of motion are needed (5 to 10 degrees of knee extension). This procedure also can be done on an isotonic exercise apparatus following the same process as described with gaining knee flexion on an isotonic exercise machine.

Knee extension range also can be improved in a sitting position with or without the aid of isotonic exercise equipment (Fig. 4-24).

There are many commercially available tools that use the concept of low-load, prolonged stretch. Dynasplint (Dynasplint Systems, Inc.) and Pro-glide (LMB) are two examples of dynamic splints used to progressively "load" selected joints to gain motion (Fig. 4-25). An arrangement of pivot points and incrementally adjustable degrees of tension provides the levels of stress needed to effect change in joint motion.

The selection of patients for use of one of these splints must be made carefully. Skin integrity is an issue that must be addressed in the elderly population. Metal hinges and spring-loaded tension flanges may not be appropriate for this population because of the weight of the devices and the patient's potential for skin breakdown.

Simple tools for dynamic stretching can be used at home. A wand, cane, or shortened broomstick can be used for general shoulder flexibility (Fig. 4-26, *A*). Increased mobility can be gained by using the unaffected arm to assist the affected extremity (Fig. 4-26, *B*).

Codman's pendulum exercises are effective for gaining relaxation and small degrees of motion in the shoulder. Relaxation is paramount to the effectiveness of this exercise. In one exercise technique, the patient is placed prone on a treatment table and a very light weight is held

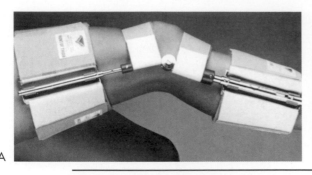
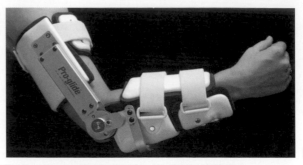

A

B

Fig. 4-25 **A,** Dynasplint commercial appliance for low-load prolonged stretch. (Courtesy of Dynasplint Systems, Inc., Severna Park, MD). **B,** Pro-glide appliance.

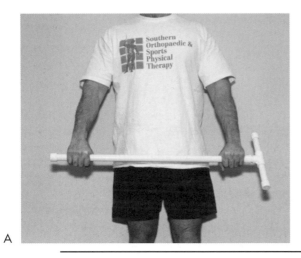
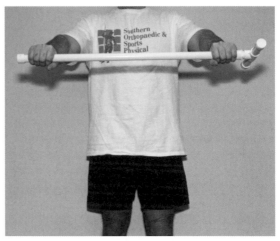

A

B

Fig. 4-26 A wand, **A,** or cane, **B,** can be used to enhance motion of the shoulder.

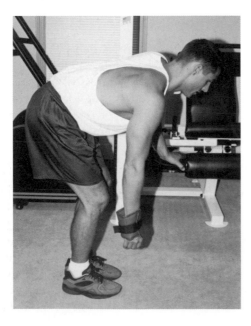

Fig. 4-27 Codman's pendulum exercise. For the exercise to be effective, the patient must relax completely and allow the affected arm to hang and gently oscillate in various directions.

in the hand of the affected extremity. This light distraction force is used in conjunction with gradual, light oscillations in various directions (Fig. 4-27). Relaxation is enhanced by applying moist heat followed by ultrasound to the affected joint before pendulum exercise.

When one is teaching the oscillation component of this exercise, it must be made clear that muscular contractions must not be used to initiate and maintain the prescribed motions. The oscillation movements can be initiated by gently swinging the upper body or torso.

MEASURING FLEXIBILITY

Measuring joint ROM is accomplished by using standard goniometric instruments. Joint stability differs from joint ROM in that the ligaments and surface geometry of joint articulations dictate static joint integrity (stability). A patient may demonstrate limited ROM in knee flexion and extension (by goniometry); however, anterior and posterior joint motion may be excessive and unstable (Fig. 4-28). On the other hand a patient may demonstrate "normal" joint ROM, yet when tested statically the joint may be very stable, "tight," and unyielding to pressure.

The sit and reach test (Fig. 4-29), standing toe touch for back and hamstring flexibility (Fig. 4-30), seated hip external rotation test (Fig. 4-31), and standing knee recurvatum test generally are less specific flexibility tests. These tests and others are used to provide very general assessment of multijoint flexibility. Such tests also can be used as stretching techniques to improve limitations in movement. However, objective clinical documentation of joint ROM is made by joint goniometry.

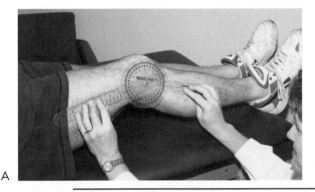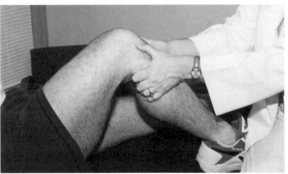

Fig. 4-28 **A,** Measuring joint motion with a goniometer. **B,** Joint stability is measured by manually applied clinical tests. Anterior drawer test of the knee is shown.

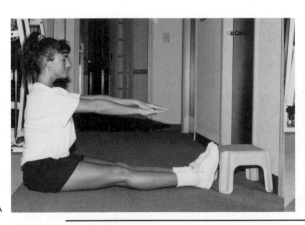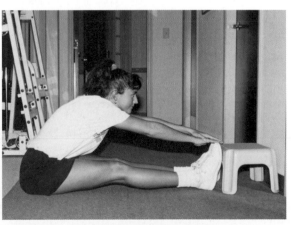

Fig. 4-29 General, nonspecific flexibility test. **A,** Sit and reach test for hamstrings and low-back flexibility, starting position. **B,** End position of sit and reach test.

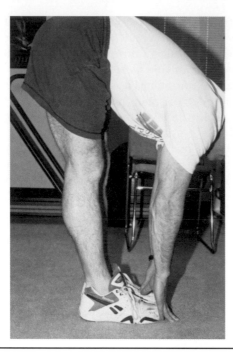

Fig. 4-30 General, nonspecific standing toe-touch flexibility test for the hamstring and lower back.

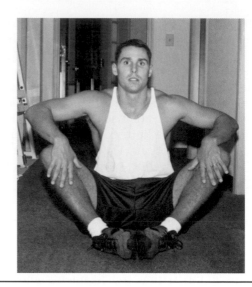

Fig. 4-31 Seated hip external rotation "butterfly" stretch.

✤ ADDITIONAL FEATURES

Breaking Point: The point at which material fails or fractures.

Creep: A viscoelastic property in which there is a change in the shape (deformation) of tissue without actual loss of continuity.

Deformations: Temporary deformations display transient elastic properties. Permanent deformations display plastic properties. Change in loads results in change in deformations.

Fibrotic Adhesions: Chronic inflammation leading to fibrous adhesions in the joint capsule, ligaments, fascia, and tendons.

Hooke's Law: Stress is proportional to strain up to a limit, which is called the proportional limit.

Loads: The force sustained by the body. Types of loads include compression, tension, shear, and torsion.

Neuromuscular Response to Stretch: Golgi tendon organs are stimulated by the presence of muscular tension. Golgi tendon organs act to inhibit tension development in muscle, promoting muscle relaxation. Muscle spindles respond to stretch via stretch reflex and reciprocal inhibition.

Remodeling: A process that alters the structure of connective tissue in response to stress.

Strain: The relative measure of the deformation of a body as a result of loading. Strain equals the change in length or original length of a tissue.

Stress: Intensity of internal force. Stress equals force divided by area. It can be compressive, tensile, or shear.

Ultimate Strength: Maximum strength obtained by a material.

Viscoelastic: Stress or strain behavior that is time rate dependent.

Young's Modulus of Elasticity: A measure of the stiffness of a material or its ability to resist deformation. Elasticity equals stress divided by strain.

REFERENCES

1. Allerheiligen WB: Stretching and warm-up. In Baechle TR, ed. Essentials of Strength Training and Conditioning. Champaign, IL, Human Kinetics, 1994.
2. Aram AJ, Madden JW: Effects of stress on healing wounds: intermittent noncyclical tension. J Surg Res 1976;20:93–102.
3. Asmussen E, Boje E: Body temperature and capacity for work. Acta Physiol Scand 1945;10:12.
4. Best TM, Garrett WE: Basic science of soft tissue. In DeLee JC, Drez D, eds. Muscle and Tendon, in Orthopaedic Sports Medicine: Principles and Practice, vol 1. Philadelphia, WB Saunders, 1994.
5. Cornelius W, Jackson A: The effects of cryotherapy and PNF on hip extensor flexibility. Athletic Training 1984;19:183.
6. Cummings GS, Crutchfield CA, Barnes MR: Orthopedic Physical Therapy Series, vol 1. Soft Tissue Changes in Contractures. Atlanta, Stokesville Publishing, 1983.
7. Cummings GS, Crutchfield CA, Barnes MR: Orthopedic Physical Therapy Series, vol 2. Soft Tissue Changes in Contractures. Atlanta, Stokesville Publishing, 1983.
8. Cummings GS, Tillman LJ: Remodeling of dense connective tissue in normal adult tissues. In Currier P, Nelson RM, eds. Dynamics of Human Biologic Tissue. Philadelphia, FA Davis, 1992.
9. Gelberman R, et al: Tendon. In Woo Savio L-Y, Buckwalter JA, eds. Injury and Repair of the Musculoskeletal Soft Tissues. Park Ridge, IL, American Academy of Orthopedic Surgeons, 1988.
10. Hettinga D: Normal joint structures and their reaction to injury. J Orthop Sports Phys Ther 1979;1:83–88.
11. Knott M, Voss P: Proprioceptive Neuromuscular Facilitation, 3rd ed. New York, Harper & Row, 1985.
12. Kisner C, Colby LA: Therapeutic exercise foundations and techniques. Philadelphia, FA Davis, 1990.
13. Lehman JF, et al: Effect of therapeutic temperatures on tendon extensibility. Arch Phys Med Rehab 1970;50:481–487.
14. Lentell G, et al: The use of thermal agents to influence the effectiveness of a low-load prolonged stretch. J Orthop Sports Phys Ther 1992;16(5):200–207.
15. Light K, et al: Low load prolonged stretch VS high load brief stretch in treating knee contractures. Phys Ther 1984;64:330–333.
16. Longacre JJ: Scar tissue: Its use and abuse in light of recent biophysical and biochemical studies. In Longacre JJ, ed. The Ultrastructure of Collagen. Springfield, IL, Charles C Thomas, 1976.

17. Louden KL, et al: Effects of two stretching methods on the flexibility and retention of flexibility at the ankle joint in runners. *Phys Ther* 1988;65:698.

18. Markos PD: Ipsilateral and contralateral effects of proprioceptive neuromuscular facilitation techniques on hip motion and electromyographic activity. *Phys Ther* 1979;59:1366.

19. Moore M, Hutton R: Electromyographic investigation of muscle stretching techniques. *Med Sci Sports* 1980;12:322.

20. Prentice W: A comparison of static and PNF stretching for improvement of hip joint flexibility. *Athletic Training* 1983;18(1):56.

21. Sapega A, et al: Biophysical factors in range of motion exercise. *Phys Sports Med* 1981;9:57–65.

22. Taylor DC, et al: Viscoelastic properties of muscle-tendon units: the biomechanical effects of stretching. *Am J Sports Med* 1990; 18(3):300–309.

23. Tillman LJ, Cummings GS: Biologic mechanisms of connective tissue mutability. In Currier DP, Nelson M, eds. Dynamics of human biologic tissue. Philadelphia, FA Davis, 1992.

24. Van Brocklin JD, Ellis DG: A study of the mechanical behavior of toe extensor tendons under applied stress. *Arch Phys Med Rehabil* 1965;46:369–370.

25. Warren CG, Lehman, JF, Koblanski JN: Heat and stretch procedures: an evaluation using rat tail tendon. *Arch Phys Med Rehabil* 1976;57:122–126.

26. Warren CG, Lehman, JF, Koblanski JN: Elongation of rat tail tendon: effect of load and temperature. *Arch Phys Med Rehabil* 1971;52:465–484.

27. Woo SL-Y, et al: Connective tissue response to immobility. *Arthritis Rheum* 1975;18:257–264.

28. Zachazewski JE: Improving flexibility. In Scully RM, Barnes MR, eds. Physical Therapy. Philadelphia, JB Lippincott, 1989.

20. Zebas CJ, Rivera ML: Retention of flexibility in selected joints after cessation of a stretching exercise program. In Dotson CO, Humphrey JH, eds. Exercise Physiology: Current Selected Research. New York, AMS Press, 1985.

REVIEW QUESTIONS

Multiple Choice

1. Two components of flexibility are which of the following?
   A. Speed and joint motion
   B. Tension and stretch
   C. Elongation of muscle and range of motion
   D. Range of motion and tension

2. Collagen is which of the following?
   A. Muscle
   B. Protein
   C. Mucopolysaccharide
   D. Carbohydrate

3. Collagen is found in which of the following?
   A. Muscle
   B. Bone
   C. Tendon
   D. Capsule
   E. All of the above

4. The most common types of collagen found in joint capsule and muscle are which of the following?
   A. Types I and II
   B. Types III and IV
   C. Types I and III
   D. Types II and III

5. *Strain* is defined as which of the following?
   A. Too much stress
   B. Tearing of tissue
   C. Painful stretching
   D. Proportional elongation of tissue during stress
   E. All of the above

6. Two viscoelastic properties of connective tissue are which of the following?
   A. Stress and strain
   B. Rate and tension
   C. Plastic and elastic deformation
   D. Speed and tissue failure

7. Goals of static stretching are which of the following?
   A. To improve athletic performance
   B. To increase ligament stability
   C. To reduce contractures; improve motion; minimize risk of soft tissue injury
   D. To decrease muscle tension
   E. All of the above

8. A general body warmup preceding ballistic stretching or static stretching helps to do which of the following? (circle any that apply)
   A. Teach the patient proper form
   B. Duplicate activities of daily living (ADLs)
   C. Increase tissue temperature
   D. Reduce risk of connective tissue damage
   E. Improve sports performance

9. A permanent or transient limitation of movement or shortening of muscle or other soft tissue is called which of the following?
   A. Scar tissue
   B. Joint adhesion
   C. Rupture
   D. Contracture

10. A limitation of function that results from the formation of scar tissue is called which of the following?
    A. Nodule
    B. Adhesion
    C. Contracture
    D. None of the above

11. Long duration static stretching refers to holding the stretch for how long?
    A. 20 seconds
    B. 1 to 5 minutes
    C. 10 to 12 minutes
    D. 20 to 60 minutes

Short Answer

12. Muscle tissue is considered to be (*active* or *passive*) restraint to joint motion.

13. Name three types of active stretching.

14. A(n) _____ is an inhibitory neurophysiological sensory receptor involved with the stretch reflex.

15. The _____ is an excitatory specialized fiber found in muscle.

True/False

16. Stress is the amount of tension or load placed on tissues.
17. Tissue temperature does not affect connective tissue extensibility.
18. Active exercise has an effect on intramuscular temperature and tissue extensibility.
19. PNF stretching is superior to other forms of active stretching.

20. Low-load, long-duration static stretching is a technique used to stretch soft-tissue contractures.
21. Scar tissue is strong and fully mature at 60 days after injury or surgical repair.
22. To effectively stretch scar tissue, maximum stress must be applied.

Essay Questions
Answer on a separate sheet of paper.
23. Define and discuss range of motion and flexibility.
24. Identify the properties of connective tissue.
25. Explain the differences between stress and strain.
26. Describe plastic deformation and elastic deformation.
27. Discuss how temperature affects connective tissue.
28. Identify and describe various stretching techniques.
29. Define Golgi tendon organs and muscle spindles.
30. Describe the clinical applications for stretching soft-tissue contractures.
31. Describe and contrast the differences and similarities between scar tissue and adhesions.
32. Outline various methods used to measure flexibility.

Critical Thinking Application
In small groups, outline and thoroughly describe methods, techniques, and protocols to effectively treat a soft-tissue knee flexion contracture. Which therapeutic agents would you recommend? For how long? Which specific stretching techniques would you use? Would strengthening play a part in overcoming the contracture during the flexibility program? How? Distinguish exactly what you are attempting to correct or enhance. How does scar tissue affect function? How do adhesions affect function? Organize your thoughts and discussion in an orderly, specific sequence that relates to immature and mature scar tissue and details which stretching techniques to use during various phases of recovery. Contrast this discussion with techniques you would recommend for improving muscle extensibility in a patient who demonstrates tight hamstrings and complains of lower back dysfunction. How does ballistic stretching play a role in your program? Does temperature affect soft-tissue extensibility; if so, how would you employ or recommend thermal agents in the treatment of tight hamstrings? Discuss specific examples of PNF stretching, static and ballistic stretching, and the application of each.

5 Strength

LEARNING OBJECTIVES

1. Name the noncontractile and contractile elements of muscle tissue.
2. Describe and contrast muscle fiber types.
3. Define types of muscle contraction.
4. Give examples of concentric and eccentric contractions.
5. State two definitions of strength.
6. Define and clarify terms used to describe muscular performance.
7. List methods used to measure strength.
8. Compare muscle contraction types related to tension produced and energy liberated.
9. Discuss muscle response to exercise.
10. Identify clinical features of delayed onset muscle soreness (DOMS).
11. Discuss velocity spectrum training related to isokinetic exercise.
12. List three clinically relevant exercise programs to enhance strength.
13. Discuss plyometrics.
14. Explain opened and closed kinetic chain exercise.
15. Identify goals and applications of strength training programs for the elderly.

KEY TERMS

Epimysium
Fasciculi
Perimysium
Endomysium
Myofibrils
Actin
Myosin
Slow twitch (ST) (type I, red oxidative) muscle fiber
Fast twitch (FT) (type II, white glycolytic) muscle fiber

Concentric
Eccentric
Isometric
Strength
Tension
Work
Power
Hypertrophy
Atrophy
SAID principle

Delayed onset muscle soreness (DOMS)
Progressive resistance exercise (PRE)
Plyometrics
Closed kinetic-chain exercise (CKC)
Open kinetic-chain exercise (OKC)

CHAPTER OUTLINE

General Muscle Biology
Muscle Fiber Types
Types of Muscle Contractions
Definitions of Strength and Power
Measuring Strength
Comparison of Muscle Contraction Types
Muscle Response to Exercise
Delayed Onset Muscle Soreness
Velocity of Muscle Contractions
Clinically Relevant Exercise Programs
    Plyometrics

Closed Kinetic-Chain Exercise
Periodization of Strength Training Programs
Strength Training for Older Populations
Strength Training for Younger Populations
    Physiologic Adaptations
    Injury Risk
    Relevant Clinical Applications
Therapeutic Exercise Equipment Used in Strength Training

Maintaining, enhancing, and regaining strength are critical for improving body function during all phases of recovery after surgery, injury, or disease affecting the musculoskeletal system. The physical therapist assistant (PTA) must understand the basic foundations of strength development and, more importantly, how to apply strength-gaining principles during recovery after immobilization, surgery, or musculoskeletal injury. In this chapter the PTA is introduced to basic concepts and universally accepted principles that can be applied in numerous clinical situations with various orthopedic pathologies.

The response of human skeletal muscle to intense exercise leads to increased functional performance and morphologic changes (e.g., hypertrophy) within the muscle. A muscle's angle of attachment to a tendon, its fiber length, muscle mass, and cross-sectional area are the primary determinants of its strength and power potential.[18] A basic understanding of muscular composition and gross structure helps clarify concepts of therapeutic exercise and provides a foundation for developing advanced principles and applications of strength.

GENERAL MUSCLE BIOLOGY

The body of an individual muscle is surrounded by noncontractile connective tissue called the **epimysium.** Within the muscle are bundles of fibers called **fasciculi,** which are surrounded by another noncontractile connective tissue called the **perimysium.** The **endomysium** is a noncontractile connective tissue that surrounds each individual muscle fiber. The individual muscle fibers are composed of **myofibrils** that lie parallel to each other and the muscle fiber itself (Fig. 5-1). The structural components of the myofibrils are called myofilaments, and they comprise two predominant proteins, **actin** and **myosin.** The functional, or contractile, unit of a muscle fiber cell is called the sarcomere (Fig. 5-2). Myosin (a thick protein) and actin (a thin protein) are actively involved with the mechanics of muscular contraction, which involves a complex and highly structured series of chemical and mechanical events. The extraordinarily complex biochemical excitation–contraction coupling and mechanical actions of muscular contraction are described in physiology textbooks. In simple terms, the neurologic stimulus to

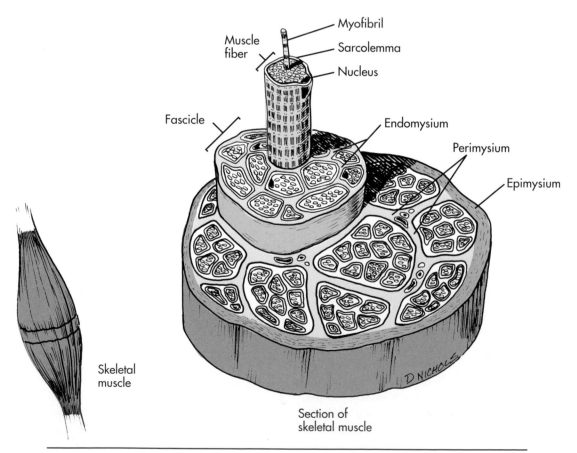

Fig. 5-1 Section of skeletal muscle with contractile and noncontractile connective tissue.

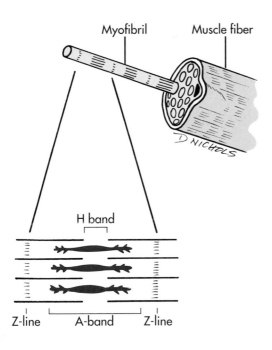

Fig. 5-2 Functional or contractile unit of skeletal muscle fiber cell.

contract a muscle causes the release of acetylcholine, which initiates the release of calcium. The calcium ions bond with troponin and tropomyosin, two proteins within the actin filaments. This allows actin-adenosine triphosphate (ATP) to react with myosin-adenosine triphosphatase (ATPase), producing energy so the thick myosin and thin actin filaments can "slide" past each other, generating tension and producing contraction of the muscle.

MUSCLE FIBER TYPES

Generally two types of muscle fiber have been identified in humans. **Slow twitch (ST) (type I, red oxidative) muscle fibers** possess more mitochondria, triglycerides, and oxidative enzymes (succinic dehydrogenase [SDH]), which allow for aerobic work. This type of fiber is specialized for muscular endurance activities. These fatigue-resistant fibers contract slowly but are highly efficient for prolonged aerobic events.

Fast twitch (FT) (type II, white glycolytic) muscle fibers, by contrast, are anaerobic. These fibers are not as vascular as type I fibers, but they "fire," or contract, at a higher speed than type I fibers and with more force. These fibers have a very high level of myosin-ATPase, which provides energy for speed of contraction and tension; they also have low myoglobin content and very few mitochondria. However, they are larger in diameter

than red fibers. These fibers are used mainly in activities that require speed, strength, and power. Type II fibers can be further broken down into three distinct subclassifications: type II, A; type II, AB; and type II, B.[38,56]

These fiber types differ mainly in terms of endurance and are classified as intermediate fiber types with both aerobic and anaerobic capacities; occasionally they are referred to as *fast-oxidative glycolytic fibers.*

The recruitment of muscle fiber types during strength training programs is determined in part by the size of the motor neuron and the intensity of force production. In general, slow twitch fibers are innervated by smaller neurons. Therefore the orderly recruitment of muscle fibers during contraction proceeds according to increased force requirements, as shown in the following:

Slow twitch (ST) → fast twitch (FT) → fast twitch A (FTA) → fast twitch AB (FTAB) → fast twitch B (FTB)

TYPES OF MUSCLE CONTRACTIONS

The three true types of muscle contractions are **concentric, eccentric,** and **isometric.** In a concentric contraction, tension is produced and shortening of the muscle takes place. The action produced by a concentric contraction brings together or approximates the origin and insertion of the contracting muscle (Fig. 5-3).

An eccentric muscle contraction is sometimes referred to as a "negative contraction" or "negative work." In an eccentric contraction, tension is actually produced, but lengthening of the muscle occurs so that the net action is opposite that produced by a concentric contraction. The origin and insertion of the contracting muscle moves farther apart during the contraction (Fig. 5-4). For example, as one slowly descends to sit in a chair and moves from a standing to a sitting position; the quadriceps muscles must eccentrically contract to control the rate of descent (Fig. 5-5) or one would suddenly fall into the chair.

In an isometric contraction, tension is produced but no joint movement or action takes place. An example is a quadriceps "set" or "quad set." (The word "set" is used to describe an isometric contraction.) If the quadriceps contracts as a knee is held straight, tension is produced within the muscle but no change in joint angle takes place. Clinically, isometric contractions can take place at any joint angle. If the knee is placed at a 90-degree angle and contracts against an object that cannot be moved, tension is produced but no joint motion or change in joint angle occurs.

Two other terms have been used to describe muscle contractions, *isokinetic* and *isotonic.* These are not types of contractions but rather terms used to describe events. In an isokinetic contraction, the speed or velocity of movement is held constant regardless of the magnitude of force applied to the resistance. Examples of

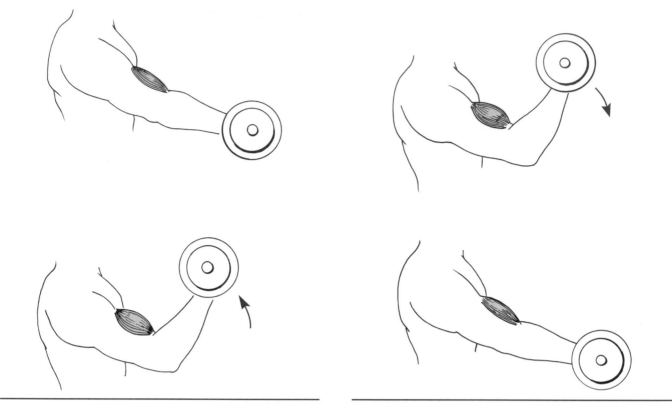

Fig. 5-3 Concentric muscle contraction.

Fig. 5-4 Eccentric muscle contraction.

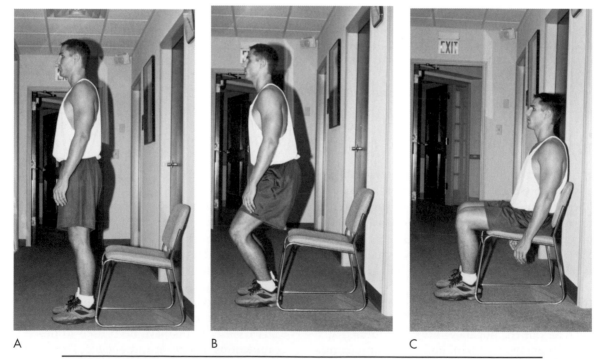

A   B   C

Fig. 5-5 Eccentric muscle contraction of the quadriceps. **A,** Starting position. **B,** Mid-portion of descent. The quadriceps are eccentrically contracting (elongating) to control the velocity of descent. **C,** End phase of descent. Without eccentric muscle contraction of the quadriceps, one would suddenly fall into the chair.

Manual Muscle Testing Grading Scale

–5/5 = *Normal*. Full resistance against gravity

–4/5 = *Good*. Partial resistance against gravity

–3/5 = *Fair*. Unable to provide resistance against gravity

–2/5 = *Poor*. No movement against gravity

–1/5 = *Trace*. Only slight muscle contraction (no joint movement)

–0/5 = *Zero*. No muscle activity

companies that manufacture isokinetic equipment are Cybex, Biodex, Lido, and Kin-Com.

An isotonic muscle contraction is not an accurate name for what happens physiologically. The name implies that the resistance, force, load, or tension remains constant, but actually the tension or force created in a muscle during this type of action must change as the joint angle changes. For example, when one lifts a barbell (constant resistance), the amount of force generated by the contracting muscle varies at different angles during the movement even though the weight itself remains constant. Therefore a more precise and descriptive term, *isoinertial*,[43] can be used in place of *isotonic*. The term *isotonic* is used in this book to describe the action of variable velocities of movement with a constant load. Examples of isotonic resistance equipment are barbells, dumbbells, and ankle weights, which are collectively referred to as "free weights."

DEFINITIONS OF STRENGTH AND POWER

Strength is a notoriously ambiguous term. Generally strength is the ability of a muscle to generate force. **Tension** is described by Soderberg[50] as, "A type of force that tends to pull things apart, it is the only type of force a muscle can generate." In Webster's dictionary,[59] strength is defined as, "The capacity for exertion or endurance." *Exertion* and *endurance* are seemingly contrasting terms that do not clearly relate to strength. Harman[28] defines strength as, "The ability to exert force under a given set of conditions defined by body position, the body movement by which force is applied, movement type, and movement speed." Knuttgen and Kramer[35] offer this definition of strength: "The maximal force a muscle or muscle group can generate at a specified velocity." Without a clear scientific consensus that accurately describes strength, confusion will continue to surround this term.

To help clarify strength clinically, it is perhaps most useful to consider strength in terms that describe perfor-

mance. **Work** is used to describe the result or product of a force exerted on an object and the distance the object moves.[28] This term is expressed as Work = Force × Distance. *Force* can be described as either *linear* or *rotary*.[50] Linear force is described as Force = Mass × Acceleration, whereas rotary force is expressed as Force = Mass × Angular acceleration. *Torque* is clearly defined as Torque = Force × Perpendicular distance from the axis of rotation.

Power is defined as the time rate of doing work, which can be expressed in several ways:[43]

$$\text{Power} = \frac{\text{Work}}{\text{Time}} = \text{Force} \times \frac{\text{Distance}}{\text{Time}}$$

or

$$\text{Power} = \text{Force} \times \frac{\text{Distance}}{\text{Time}}$$

or

$$\text{Power} = \text{Force} \times \text{Velocity}$$

Velocity is defined as a vector that describes displacement. Overall, these terms help describe resultant muscular performance as they relate to the development of strength.

MEASURING STRENGTH

Strength can be measured by five methods: (1) manual muscle testing, (2) cable tensiometry, (3) dynamometry, (4) isotonic one-repetition maximum lift, and (5) isokinetics.

Manual muscle testing describes a muscle or muscle group's ability to isometrically "hold" or resist a force applied by the tester. Therefore it is used to generally grade a muscle's isometric contraction capacity at a specific joint angle against an applied force or gravity. The grading scale for this test is clinically easy to use (Box 5-1). However, the tester must have a comprehensive and detailed understanding of kinesiology to accurately and consistently reproduce manual grading of muscle strength (performance). The results of manual muscle testing cannot be inferred to relate to anything other than a muscle's ability to isometrically resist an applied force.

Cable tensiometry is used to isometrically measure a muscle's strength (Fig. 5-6). Essentially this tool is a mechanical form of manual muscle testing. Clinically, this form of testing is inappropriate for many acute, chronic, or postsurgical orthopedic patients. This method is used primarily to measure strength in normal subjects in research projects. Many tests were developed in the 1950s to describe static force or isometric strength by use of the cable tension method.[11,12]

Dynamometry is used extensively in physical therapy. Hand-held dynamometers (Fig. 5-7) are used to quantify grip strength, and the standing-back dynamometer is used to evaluate back extension strength. In this latter example, many factors contribute to the subject's

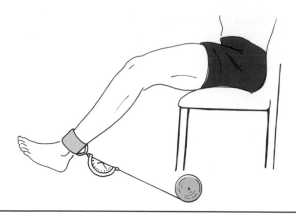

Fig. 5-6 Seated cable tensiometer for quantifying isometric quadriceps strength.

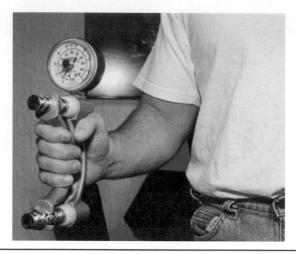

Fig. 5-7 Hand-held grip dynamometer for measuring grip strength.

ability to generate tension or force during the back pull, including the patient's motivation, degree of pain (if any), arm length, leg length, height, weight, and the obvious contribution from other muscle groups. These variables make dynamometry an unreliable, nonspecific testing tool.

Isotonic one-repetition maximum lift is used to test strength using commercially available exercise equipment or barbells and dumbbells. In this method the patient performs a single, full range of motion (ROM) lift, such as a bench press (Fig. 5-8), shoulder press, or arm curl, for a particular muscle group. Applying this method is difficult because the tester and patient must first establish a reasonable starting weight through trial and error, fatigue becomes a factor if many trials are needed, and precise performance or execution of the proper lift is determined subjectively by the tester. This method is best used for normal subjects, in a sports medicine environment, or with uninvolved body parts not necessary for stabilization of a disabled joint.

Perhaps the most widely used and clinically relevant method of objective, reproducible strength testing is through *isokinetics*. The data collected with isokinetic testing document strength (force production), torque, power, and work.[47] As stated, isokinetics employs a fixed speed, or velocity, of movement that allows for maximum loading throughout the full ROM. If a patient experiences pain during any part of the test, or does not apply a maximum force throughout the entire ROM, the velocity remains constant with a variable resistance that is totally "accommodating" to the individual.[15] To test for strength, slow speeds (30 to 60 degrees per second) are generally used.[37] Because isokinetic equipment can be interfaced with computers, a hard-copy graph of the data can be used for evaluation and exercise prescription. In addition to being a valid and reliable tool for strength testing, isokinetics also can evaluate neuromuscular endurance, speed of muscle contraction, and muscular power.[31]

COMPARISON OF MUSCLE CONTRACTION TYPES

Generally, muscle contractions are characterized by the amount of tension the contraction produces and the amount of energy liberated (ATP use) by the contraction. The most common clinically applicable way to strengthen muscle is with concentric and eccentric contractions using isotonic (isoinertial)[43] progressive resistive exercise (PRE). Ankle or cuff weights, hand-held weights (dumbbells), and weight machines are examples of isotonic equipment used in physical therapy practice.* Elftman[19] has demonstrated that the production of maximal force of contraction by various methods occurs in a predictable fashion, as follows:

Eccentrics → Isometrics → Concentric exercises

The force of contraction is expressed as the amount of tension developed per unit of contractile tissue. In terms of energy liberated (ATP use), eccentric muscle contractions use the least ATP, and concentric contractions use the most;[3] therefore:

Concentric exercises → Isometrics → Eccentrics

Based on this information, it appears that eccentric muscle contractions are more energy efficient and produce greater tension per contractile unit than both concentric and isometric contractions. However, Davies[15] points out that much of the tension produced by eccentric muscle contraction results from stress imposed on the noncontractile serial elastic components (perimysium, epimysium, and endomysium) of the muscle. Therefore eccentric muscle contractions stimulate both

---

*Cybex, Nautilus, Rehab Systems, Body Masters, Universal, Paramount.

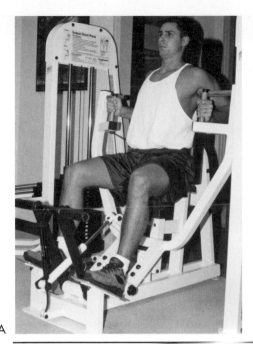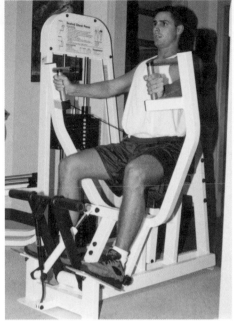

Fig. 5-8 Concentric and eccentric one-repetition maximum lift test. This is a much generalized nonspecific method to determine strength with commercial isotonic equipment. **A,** Starting position. **B,** End position.

contractile and noncontractile elements, whereas concentric contractions and isometrics focus on the contractile elements.[47]

The physical therapist assistant must consider the context in which each muscle contraction type is used clinically. Fundamentally implementing multiple muscle contraction types during all phases of rehabilitation is well supported.[4,27,52] In comparing muscle contraction types, it is best to view the decision concerning which type to use, when to use it, and in what pathologic conditions it should be used as a progression or continuum rather than a choice of one type over another. Davies[15] has described a classic model of exercise progression (Box 5-2) that can be used as a general guide. Certain criteria must be established for the progression from one type of contraction to another.

First, exercise variables and parameters must be understood so that necessary adjustments can be made in a patient's exercise prescription (Box 5-3).

The criteria established for progressing from one exercise mode to another is based on many factors and is patient specific. In general, pain usually dictates the time frame for progression, although swelling also does to a lesser degree. The sequence proceeds from the least intense to more challenging exercises with increased joint forces and metabolic demands.

Some of the advantages and disadvantages of concentric and eccentric isotonic exercise and isokinetic exercise equipment are outlined for general comparison in Box 5-4.

BOX 5-2

Davies Model of Exercise Progression (1985)

Isometric/eccentric contractions, multiple angle
Isometrics (submax effort)
Multiple angle isometrics (max effort)
Short arc concentric-isokinetics (submax effort)
Short arc isotonics-concentric/eccentric
Short arc concentric isokinetics (max effort)
Full ROM concentric isokinetics (submax effort)
Full ROM isotonics-concentric/eccentric
Full ROM concentric isokinetics (max effort)
Full ROM eccentric isokinetics (submax effort)
Full ROM eccentric isokinetics (max effort)

From Davies G: A Compendium of Isokinetics in Clinical Usage and Rehabilitation Techniques. Onalaska, WI, S&S Publishers, 1987.

MUSCLE RESPONSE TO EXERCISE

Muscle tissue morphology is mutable; that is, it has the ability to change. Muscle mutability has two distinct categories, **hypertrophy** and **atrophy.**

Various stimuli are necessary to affect muscle mutability. The **SAID principle** (specific adaptations to imposed demands)[20] is the precursor to overload, specificity, and reversibility as related to strength and reconditioning after injury. In part, the SAID principle defines

BOX 5-3

Therapeutic Exercise Parameters

FREQUENCY
Daily, 3 days a wk, 2 days a wk (QD = once daily, bid = twice daily)

INTENSITY
Amount of resistance, full range of motion, short arc of motion, velocity of contraction (slow, moderate, fast)

DURATION
6 weeks, 8 weeks, 10 weeks

TYPE OF RESISTANCE
Isotonic, isokinetic

MUSCLE CONTRACTION TYPE
Concentric, eccentric, isometric

DEGREE OF RESISTANCE
Total amount of weight or force applied

NUMBER OF REPETITIONS
1 to 15

NUMBER OF SETS
1 to 5

LENGTH OF REST BETWEEN SETS
Short rest for aerobic-metabolic pathway, long rest (2 to 3 min) for anaerobic pathways

ORDER OF EXERCISE
Exercise large muscle groups first, progress to smaller muscle groups

DEGREES OF EFFORT
Low intensity (submax effort), high intensity (max effort)

BOX 5-4

Comparison of Isotonics versus Isokinetics

Commercially available machines and free weights	Isokinetics
ADVANTAGES	
▪ Low cost (relative)	▪ Can exercise over a wide velocity (0 degrees to 300 degrees)
▪ Has both concentric and eccentric components	▪ Accommodates to pain and fatigue
▪ Easy to instruct patients	▪ Low compressive forces at high speeds
▪ Objective increase in muscle performance by increasing weight	▪ Provides objective permanent record of data
▪ Can perform static or isometric contractions	▪ Valid and reliable
DISADVANTAGES	
▪ Cannot exercise at high speeds (functional)	▪ Very expensive
▪ Momentum is involved	▪ Some models do not provide eccentrics
▪ Not safe if patient has pain during the motion of lifting	▪ Takes time to switch machine for other body parts (time consuming)

specific adaptations and alterations in response to highly specific demands. After injury, muscle reeducation helps the patient adapt and prepare for return to function.

Strength training must be individually tailored to meet the goals of recovery. As stated by DeLee and colleagues,[16] "Function increases with use; functions we do not use, we lose. The intensity, duration, and frequency of activity are all related to the functional capacity that is developed."

The stimuli for adaptive changes in skeletal muscle are described as frequency, intensity, and duration.[8] Human skeletal muscle responds and adapts to these stimuli and is characterized by the nature, rate, magnitude, and duration of the stimulus.[4] In a clinical situation, the stimulus provided to human muscle is the conditioning or training program. These programs are based on certain principles that lead to the necessary adaptive changes, which in turn affect function. The principles of overload, specificity, and reversibility[20] provide the foundation for the strength training programs used in physical therapy and are as follows:

Overload principle: For performance and morphologic changes to occur, a stimulus (load, tension) must progress and exceed the normal functional capabilities of the muscles being trained.

Specificity: The specific and predictable adaptations a muscle goes through in response to specific training.

Reversibility: Adaptive changes in response to specific training are reversible;[20] if the stimulus used to elicit morphologic changes is removed the changes revert to the pretraining state.

In general, type I muscle fibers (red [high myoglobin content] and oxidative) respond more favorably to low-intensity (low tension), high-volume (sets and repetitions) exercise than type II (white [low myoglobin content] and glycolytic) muscle fibers. High-volume, low-intensity exercise is repetitive, and gross muscle movements occur (e.g., bicycling, running, swimming, and rowing). In this type of training, oxidative capabilities increase and relative percent increases in type I muscle fibers occur in the specific muscle or muscle groups used.

In strength training programs, a desirable and predictable morphologic adaptive change is *hypertrophy*, which is the compensatory increase in individual muscle fiber size as a result of increases in and synthesis of the contractile proteins actin and myosin.[25] Type II muscle fibers increase more than type I fibers do. This can be observed in comparing the body types of long-distance runners with the larger, more muscular physiques of sprinters. The physiques of long-distance runners and most aerobic athletes are thinner, possess less body fat, and have smaller muscles that are more adapted to endurance activities. Highly specific or "absolute strength" programs use a high-tension (heavy loads) and low-volume protocol. This type of training program requires relatively short bouts of progressive overload to stimulate the type II muscle fibers.

Biochemical adaptations of muscle occur in specifically applied strength training programs. After intense strength training, significant increases appear in glycogen, ATP, and creatine phosphate; increased activity and quantity of enzymes involved with anaerobic glycolysis, creatine kinase, and myokinase also are seen.[13]

Hyperplasia (the development of new muscle fibers) or longitudinal fiber splitting may occur in response to high-intensity strength-training programs. Gonyea and colleagues[26] reported in animal studies that an increase of 19% of the total number of muscle fibers occurred in cat forelimb muscles after weight lifting. This phenomenon has not been proved in humans. The predominant change in response to high-intensity strength-training programs is hypertrophy of existing skeletal muscle fibers. The relative contribution (if any) of hyperplasia or muscle fiber splitting has not been determined.[8] Induced hypertrophy in injured or postoperative muscle tissue is important because hypertrophy relates to a potential to generate greater tension.

It is interesting to note that passive stretching of innervated muscle tissue creates tension and also results in fiber hypertrophy. The change in fiber size associated with this stretch-induced hypertrophy results from increased protein turnover.[8] This feature has clinical relevance in muscle recovery during immobilization.

DELAYED ONSET MUSCLE SORENESS

The clinical features of exercise-induced muscle soreness are diffuse and general, occurring in the absence of specific, intense injury.[45] Acute muscle strain can be differentiated from exercise-induced soreness primarily by the history leading to the injury. With an acute strain, the patient is able to relate a specific event or episode that caused the injury.[45]

Based on this distinction, the PTA can identify complaints of diffuse muscle soreness resulting from new or unaccustomed exercise.[45] However, if the patient can describe a history of local, intense pain after a specific episode, an acute muscle strain must be considered.[45]

Although the PTA does not interpret and define complaints of pain without consulting with the physical therapist (PT), the assistant must be able to accurately identify and describe the nature and disposition of any pain based on the patient's complaints and relevant history and be able to communicate this information to the PT.

After a specific exercise program, muscle soreness is an anticipated byproduct of intense eccentric exercise.[22,23,31,40,49,51] The degree and presence of after-exercise muscle soreness appear to be greater with these eccentric programs than with concentric exercise programs.[7,31,40,42,49,55]

Symptoms of **delayed onset muscle soreness (DOMS)** include pain, swelling, tenderness, reduced ROM, and stiffness.[3,31,40,49] Albert[3] reports five general theories concerning the process of DOMS:

1. Lactic acid theory
2. Torn tissue theory
3. Tonic muscle spasms theory
4. Connective tissue damage theory
5. Tissue fluid theory

The lactic acid and tonic muscle spasms theories do not appear to be related to DOMS.[1,2,48,58] Studies[38,39] show evidence that the primary cause of muscle soreness

Table 5-1	*Suggested Treatment Techniques for Delayed On-set Muscle Soreness*
Type	**Efficacy**
Rest	None
Nonsteroidal antiinflammatory	Highly successful
Steroidal antiinflammatory	Moderately successful
Electrical stimulation	Proposed only
Exercise	Highly successful
Transcutaneous electrical nerve stimulation	Highly successful
Stretching	Mixed success
Iontophoresis	Not successful
Cryotherapy	Not successful
Calcium antagonists	Proposed only

From Albert M: Eccentric Muscle Training in Sports and Orthopaedics. New York, Churchill Livingstone, 1991.

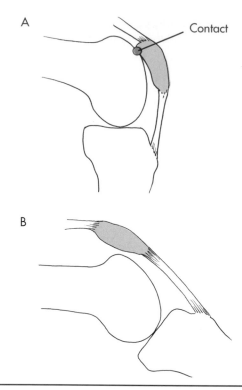

Fig. 5-9 **A,** With the knee flexed to 90 degrees there are resultant increases in patellofemoral compression with excursion of the knee (leg) into extension. **B,** With the knee in extension there is less patellofemoral compression.

after exercise is skeletal muscle damage. Greater tensions produced by eccentric exercise contribute to the initial muscle damage, although isometric and concentric contractions are not absolved of producing latent muscle soreness. In fact, isometric exercise and concentric exercise can produce DOMS even in well-trained athletes. The treatment of DOMS is outlined in Table 5-1.

VELOCITY OF MUSCLE CONTRACTIONS

Muscle contraction velocity and speed of limb movement are not the same. If two arms are bending at the same speed but one arm is holding a weight, the muscle bending the arm with more weight must produce a greater speed of contraction to overcome the resistance. Therefore more tension is developed in the muscle lifting the heavier arm, even though the speed of limb movement is the same.

Slower speeds of muscle contraction can produce greater force and tension than the same muscle moving at a higher rate of speed. A slower contracting muscle moving a heavy resistance can produce greater tension than a faster contracting muscle lifting a lighter resistance.[41] When slow speeds of full arc resistance exercise are used to generate greater tension and strength, greater joint compression forces and torque are increased as well. Therefore to minimize the negative or unwanted effects of joint compression (Fig. 5-9), a program of isometric exercise may be more appropriate in some instances.

Initially strength programs focus on using slow-speed tension to produce isometric contractions and spare the negative effects of excessive joint motion, torque, and compressive forces found in full ROM slow-speed isotonic (concentric and eccentric) exercises. Fast

and slow contraction speeds can be distinguished with isokinetic exercise. By controlling the speed of limb movement with an isokinetic apparatus, better control of joint compression forces can be achieved. (*Speed* is defined isokinetically as control of limb movement, not necessarily the actual speed of muscle contraction.) A slow speed of limb movement using an isokinetic apparatus may be 60 degrees per second, and a fast speed may be 300 degrees per second.

Higher speeds of limb movement require the resistance to be lighter than in a slower moving limb with greater resistance. Isokinetic testing and exercise use the concept of velocity spectrum training, which is the ability to control limb speeds within a range of slow to fast speeds. Higher speeds of limb movement produce less joint compression and lower forces relative to slow-speed, high-resistance training.

Functionally, human limbs move at various speeds and with various degrees of motion. Velocity spectrum training allows a patient to train at speeds of motion that more closely approximate normal human limb speeds.[6,46,61] For example, a training program using the velocity spectrum concept may include submaximal contractions at slow speeds (60 to 90 deg/s) for two sets of 8 to 12 repetitions, then contractions at incrementally increasing speeds up to 240 degrees per second or higher for two or three sets of 15 repetitions.

In a comparison of isokinetic and isotonic exercise, most isotonic exercise is performed at approximately 60 degrees per second,[15] whereas isokinetic exercise can be adjusted specifically to train the affected area at speeds more closely duplicating normal functional speeds of movement. The higher velocity contractions used with isokinetic exercise allow for the following:

- Improved functional speeds of contraction
- Reduced joint compression forces
- Accommodation of patient's pain (the patient will not undergo more force than he or she can safely produce)

Using velocity spectrum training with isokinetics allows the progression from multiangle isometrics (0 deg/s) to slow speeds (60 deg/s) for greater tension and torque, to higher speeds (240 deg/s and faster) for functional activities and lower compressive forces.

CLINICALLY RELEVANT EXERCISE PROGRAMS

Three broad fundamental strength protocols are used extensively in physical therapy. The DeLorme[17] **progressive resistance exercise (PRE)** protocol is still used widely for strength training programs after injury to the musculoskeletal system. This program uses the classic and well-recognized exercise of three sets of 10 repetitions of resistance. Its protocol states that the patient must establish a maximum weight that can be lifted for 10 repetitions. This is termed the *10 RM* (repetitions maximum). To initiate the program the patient performs 10 repetitions at half (50%) of the predetermined 10 RM. The next set of exercise is performed at three fourths (75%) of the 10 RM. Finally, the third set is performed for 10 repetitions at the established 10 RM (100%).

The DeLorme protocol calls for an arbitrary increase in resistance each week. It allows for a systematic and gradual progression during each exercise session by providing a warmup period using submaximal contractions before the 10 RM.

The Oxford program[62] is the opposite of the DeLorme protocol. Although it begins by establishing the individual's 10 RM, the second set is performed at three fourths (75%) of the 10 RM and the following set at half (50%) of the established 10 RM. Each set involves 10 repetitions. The method reportedly takes advantage of the muscle's fatigue during exercise.

There are fundamental differences in philosophy between the DeLorme PRE protocol and the Oxford technique. The DeLorme program calls for a progressive overload during each session by *adding* resistance while the muscle fatigues. The Oxford technique calls for *reducing* resistance as the muscle fatigues. Both programs were developed in the 1950s, and since then many variations and combinations have been used to discover the most effective and efficient means to regain strength after an injury.

To objectively control the progression or resistance with exercise programs, Knight[34] established the daily adjustable progressive resistance exercise technique (DAPRE). Instead of using three sets of 10 repetitions like DeLorme and Oxford did, Knight's program calls for four sets with variable repetitions. The protocol calls for establishing the patient's six RM instead of 10 RM, with the number six based on research by Berger[5] as the optimum number of repetitions for developing strength.

The first set is performed at half (50%) of the established working weight for 10 repetitions. The second set is performed at three fourths (75%) of the six RM for six repetitions. The third set is performed at the full previously established maximum weight, but the patient is asked to perform as many repetitions as possible with this weight. The number of repetitions performed in this set is used to determine the weight used in the fourth set. The goal of this technique is to establish a maximum resistance that can be performed for six repetitions.

As the individual's strength increases, the number of repetitions in the third set increases, which increases the weight in the fourth set. The hallmark of this program is understanding the guidelines used to adjust the working weight of the third and fourth sets.[16] The DAPRE adjusted working weight guide is as follows:

Third Set Number of Repetitions	Fourth Set Change
0 to 2	Reduce weight 5 to 10 lb
3 to 4	Reduce weight 5 to 10 lb
5 to 7	Keep weight the same
8 to 12	Increase weight 5 to 10 lb
13 or more	Increase weight 10 to 15 lb

The rationale for the weight adjustments described in the preceding list is to modify resistance during the fourth set to maintain the goal of keeping repetitions between five and seven, whereas encouraging maximum resistance to influence strength increases and morphologic changes, such as hypertrophy.

In this protocol, the exact amount of weight used by the patient is highly specific and tailored to the individual and goals of recovery. Adjustments in weight are made to accommodate the specific healing constraints of the injury and the individual tolerance level of the patient. Thus extremely close communication and supervision of the patient are necessary. With the DeLorme PRE program and Oxford program the patient works with a percentage of an established weight each session and advances in resistance once each week. The DAPRE protocol requires daily adjustments; it takes advantage of the fact that submaximal work does not provide the necessary stimulus for maximal gains in strength. By reducing the volume of repetitions to six and adjusting the weight so that a maximal load is used for six repetitions, the intensity of work is increased.

Other protocols have suggested[53] that by initially focusing on muscular hypertrophy, a greater potential for strength would exist. Because the cross-sectional area of muscle would be increased by a program of higher volume, the potential to develop greater amounts of tension is increased by reducing the volume of exercise and increasing the loads used.

The rule of tens is followed in isometric exercise protocols that are commonly used in rehabilitation.[47] This rule states that the patient must perform 10-second contractions for 10 repetitions with a 10-second rest between each repetition.[15] The patient is taught to perform isometric contractions by gradually developing

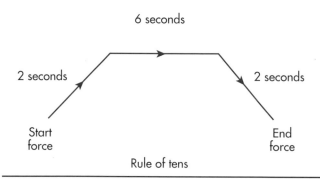

Fig. 5-10 Isometric contractions by rule of tens. (From Davies G: A Compendium of Isokinetics in Clinical Usage and Rehabilitation Techniques. Onalaska, WI, S&S Publishers, 1987.)

tension for 2 seconds, maintaining a maximal contraction for 6 seconds, then gradually decreasing tension for 2 seconds (Fig. 5-10).

While one is performing isometric exercise, an "overflow" of strength occurs approximately 10 degrees above and below the angle (Fig. 5-11) at which the exercise is occurring.[33] Multiple-angle isometrics are taught at 10-degree increments to achieve strength gains throughout a described range of motion.

A circuit training program is a predetermined, organized sequence of exercise. Traditionally, this type of program is used for general body conditioning and total fitness. A general circuit program calls for the performance of one or two exercises for each body part in sequence (Table 5-2). Usually a rest period of 30 seconds to 1 minute is allowed between sets. If resistance exercise equipment is used, circuit weight-training programs also tax the aerobic metabolic pathway to a degree. The movement from one station to another does not allow for maximum recovery and high-intensity loads, but it does provide an adequate stimulus for both aerobic and anaerobic work.

The clinical delivery of specific exercise protocols depends on many factors. The patient's pathologic condition; time constraints for healing of specific tissues; and degree of swelling, pain, function, and motivation all play a role in determining the most appropriate program to use and when to use it. In making an organized, systematic progression from one program to

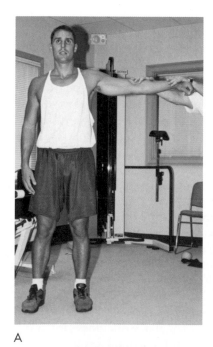
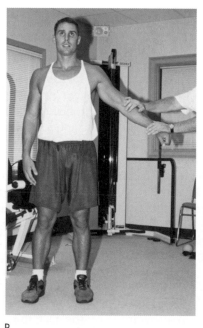
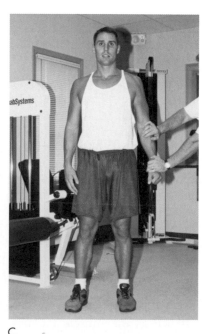

A B C

Fig. 5-11 Multiangle isometric shoulder abduction. **A,** Isometric hold in approximately 90 degrees of abduction. **B,** Midrange isometric shoulder abduction. **C,** Isometric "set" in 0 degrees of abduction.

another, following specific guidelines is a responsible and appropriate plan for strength training programs for a wide variety of musculoskeletal system injuries.

Plyometrics

Plyometric exercises are intense power-generating exercises that are traditionally confined to sport-specific functional training near the end of a rehabilitation program. *Plyo* comes from the Greek word *plythein*, meaning to increase, and *metric* refers to measure. **Plyometrics** is a system of exercising that uses the stretch reflex to develop muscle contraction speed.[60]

Plyometric exercises are also highly adaptable for use with the general orthopedic patient population. However, the inherent nature of plyometrics requires the patient to be prepared for high-intensity, task-specific, dynamic exercise.

The principles behind plyometrics are based on the neurophysiologic responses from the Golgi tendon organs (GTOs) and muscle spindles.[60] The most rudimentary example of plyometrics is the depth jump (Fig. 5-12). As the foot of the patient contacts the ground (amortization phase), the muscle spindles respond by causing a reflex muscular contraction. Albert[3] states, "The greater and more quickly a load is applied to a muscle, the greater the firing frequency of the muscle spindle with a corresponding stronger muscle contraction." The fundamental goal of plyometric exercise is to minimize the amortization phase of the exercise, which, in this example, is contact with the ground.

All forms of jumping, skipping, and hopping can be used in a plyometric exercise program.[60] Upper body exercises, such as throwing and catching a weighted object, are examples of plyometrics. An isotonic supine leg press "hop" is an example of plyometrics used to develop rapid, eccentric loading with a corresponding rapid, concentric contraction.

Table 5-2	Sample Circuit Weight Training Program		
Exercise	**Repetitions**	**Sets**	**Rest**
Leg press	10	2	30 s between each set
Leg extension	10	2	30 s between each set
Leg curl	10	2	30 s between each set
Bench press	10	2	30 s between each set
Supine fly	10	2	30 s between each set
Shoulder press	10	2	30 s between each set
Lateral pull-down	10	2	30 s between each set
Bent over row	10	2	30 s between each set
Bicep curl	10	2	30 s between each set
Tricep press-down	10	2	30 s between each set

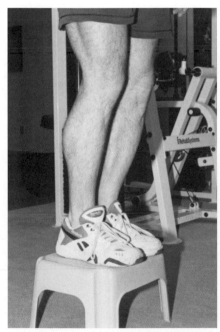 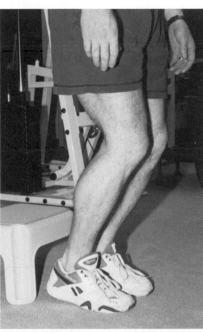 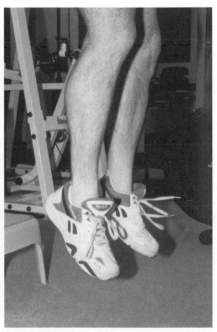

A   B   C

Fig. 5-12 Plyometric "depth jump." **A,** Starting position on a short stool. **B,** Without jumping up, the patient steps off the stool down to the ground with both feet simultaneously. The time spent on the ground is called the amortization phase. **C,** Rapid concentric contraction follows the amortization phase, which results in a powerful leap.

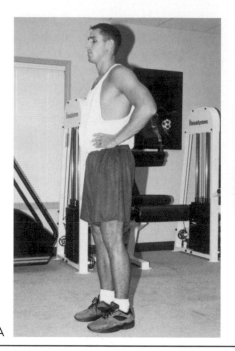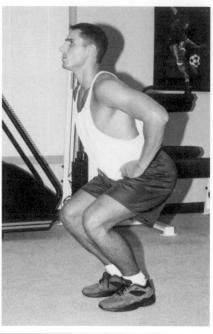

Fig. 5-13 A closed kinetic chain. **A,** Starting position of a standing squat or leg bend maneuver. **B,** Motion of the knee produces predictable motion in all joints within the kinetic chain. With knee flexion the resultant change in joint position of the ankle, hip, and spine is noticeable.

Plyometrics must be used judiciously and principally as an end component in a phase progression program. The fundamental concept of plyometrics involves ballistic, high-velocity movement patterns, which cannot be used during early rehabilitation when tissues are still healing. Plyometrics can be added to increase function as the patient progresses from one program or phase to another.

Many isotonic strength training programs involve lifting a load from a seated, supine, or standing position. These exercises are meant to isolate and strengthen specific muscle groups throughout a single plane of motion. Plyometrics, on the other hand, focus on weight-bearing functional activities that duplicate high-velocity, multiplane, normal human movement.[60] Therefore the physical therapist assistant must recognize that the value of plyometrics is primarily to prepare the patient to return to function. Naturally not all patients recovering from an orthopedic injury require an intense plyometric exercise program. If, however, the patient desires to return to dynamic sporting activities, or his or her job requires dynamic or ballistic physical labor, then plyometrics are appropriate conditioning to enable one to withstand high levels of both eccentric and concentric loads.

CLOSED KINETIC CHAIN EXERCISE

During any exercise, if the distal portion of the exercising segment is weight bearing or "fixed," it is called a **closed kinetic-chain exercise (CKC).** An **open kinetic-chain exercise (OKC)** involves the distal segment moving freely in space, such as a seated knee extension. A CKC is best described as a system of interdependent articulated links. For example, with a weight-bearing leg (Fig. 5-13), as the knee is flexed, the entire chain or link system joining the ankle to the knee and to the hip is affected. In an OKC system, such as the arm (Fig. 5-14), the shoulder and elbow are fixed, whereas the distal wrist segment moves freely in space. Davies[14] states, "In a closed kinetic chain, motion at one joint will produce motion at all of the other joints in the system in a predictable manner."

The human body functions as a combination of both open- and closed-chain activities such as walking and stair climbing. The primary advantage of CKC exercises is the highly functional nature of the exercises, which use concentric and eccentric muscle contractions synchronously to produce functional movement. In a strength-training program, combinations of OKC and CKC exercises should be used to condition the patient to perform purposeful, functional activities.

In knee rehabilitation programs,[10,44] for example, quadriceps strengthening can be achieved through knee extension exercises (which are open chain), or leg press exercises or squats (which are closed chain). In many cases, patients are introduced to therapeutic exercises by way of submaximal isometric muscle contractions. More intense and demanding exercises are added as pain, strength, and function allow. Open kinetic chain resistance exercises can be employed to further stimu-

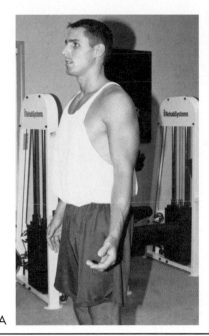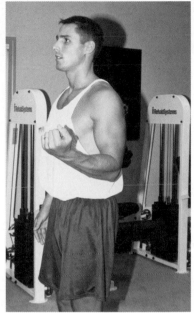

A   B

Fig. 5-14 An open kinetic chain. **A,** Beginning position of elbow flexion. **B,** The distal arm and wrist segments move freely in space.

late growth in strength. In some cases, the PT institutes CKC exercises early in the recovery phase of rehabilitation. For example, CKC exercises are frequently used within the first few weeks after anterior cruciate ligament reconstructive surgery. In addition, select open-chain exercises (those that do not place unwanted forces on the newly repaired tissues) are used. Closed-chain exercises may not be appropriate for some patients with osteoarthritis or other conditions where vertical, compressive loads would exacerbate the condition.

The general rationale for using closed-chain exercises in rehabilitation programs are as follows:

■ CKC exercises are more functional than OKC exercises
■ Loading of the affected joint(s) produces an increase in kinesthetic awareness
■ Improved neuromuscular coordination is achieved
■ CKC exercises are nonisolation exercises that produce muscular co-contractions

Caution must be used when prescribing CKC activities during rehabilitation when pain, swelling, dysfunction, or muscle weakness is present.[14] Because an articulated joint system is being exercised under these conditions (limited ROM, pain, swelling, etc.), unpredictable compensation may occur in the joint(s) superior and inferior to the affected joint.[14] Therefore OKC exercise must be used to isolate and strengthen the weakened area before progressing to CKC exercises.

PERIODIZATION OF STRENGTH TRAINING PROGRAMS

Periodization involves a predictable pattern of exercise volume, intensity, and rest periods that enhance strength-developing capabilities.[54] Its main components are "cycles" or periods of strength training. Many fundamental strength programs call for a progressive resistance exercise system without consideration for variations in frequency, intensity, duration, and recovery. The periodization model takes into consideration progressive cycles of various training loads and degrees of intensity during strength programs.[54]

Periodization can involve any of three cycles: microcycle, mesocycle, or macrocycle. The *microcycle* is the smallest unit of time (usually weeks), and accumulated microcycles form a mesocycle. The *mesocycle* is traditionally a few months long and consists of multiple microcycles that vary in volume, frequency, and intensity. The *macrocycle* is the largest segment of time (it can be a year long) and involves a collection of mesocycles.

Periodization of strength training programs in the clinical rehabilitation setting was originally designed for and used extensively in athletics and is justified by following a series of defined protocols directed specifically at developing strength while minimizing fatigue and overtraining of the recovering orthopedic patient.

The fundamental goals and objectives of a classic periodization program are outlined in Figure 5-15. This is only a basic example, which must be modified to meet the specific rehabilitation goals for recovering patients. It can be adapted for many patients who require strength as part of their rehabilitation program.

In a periodization program, instead of constantly striving to increase resistance during each treatment or each week by use of the same system of sets and repetitions for a recovering patient, an attempt should be made to cycle the program into specific phases. In

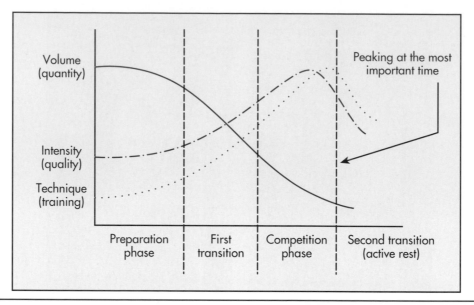

Fig. 5-15 Classic periodization model. (From *Natl Strength Cond Assoc J* 1993;15:64–66.)

general the first phase (microcycle) strives to develop basic strength and muscular hypertrophy. There are small alterations in sets (between three and six sets) and repetitions (between 8 and 12) in each week of rehabilitation, and a high volume of exercise is used, dictating a lower intensity level (~65% to 70% of the one RM). This phase can be called the preparatory phase, or initial rehabilitation protocol. The second phase (mesocycle) is designed to enhance strength by increasing the loads used (85% of one RM) and decreasing the volume of exercise to three to five sets of four to six repetitions. This mesocycle, as well as the first, may last for 2 or 3 months. Remember that during each mesocycle there are numerous microcycles (weeks) where various changes are made to reduce chronic overwork. The second phase of this basic example is called the *first transition phase* or *active rehabilitation phase*.

The traditional athletic model for this modified periodization program is described in Figure 5-16. The strength protocol should be modified to fit the specific needs of each individual.

STRENGTH TRAINING FOR OLDER POPULATIONS

Strength training programs for the geriatric population include special considerations. In an elderly population, declines in muscle performance, force-generating capabilities, and concomitant muscle mass are well documented.[30,36] Therefore strength training programs for the elderly are focused on delaying muscle atrophy, improving function, and increasing force-generating capabilities by stimulating muscle hypertrophy. Note that resistance exercise programs for healthy, older populations show significant improvements in muscle strength, muscle volume (hypertrophy), and other parameters of muscle structure and function.[57] Thompson[57] reports that studies show that "Given an adequate training stimulus, older men and women show similar gains compared to young individuals after resistive training." In addition, McCartney and colleagues[39] report that "Long term resistance training in older people is feasible and results in increases in dynamic muscle strength, muscle size, and functional capacity."

In addition, multiple conditions and degenerative joint disease must be considered in strength training programs for the disabled elderly. Unstable, chronic, and complex medical problems may preclude certain types of strength-training programs. For example, in cardiovascular disease, chronic obstructive pulmonary disease, and other conditions, a protocol of general, very low-intensity gross body movement may be more beneficial and safer than isometric or isotonic resistance exercise. In advanced cases of osteoarthritis of the knee and hip, it is prudent to avoid vertical compression loads and full ROM-heavy isotonic exercise. Pain and swelling from osteoarthritic lesions, bone spurs, and osteophytes (Fig. 5-17) can be exacerbated by the tibiofemoral vertical compressive loads involved in leg press or squatting exercises.

In general, studies support the fact that high-intensity resistance training promotes force-generating capabilities in aged muscle[32] and that resistance training enhances muscle hypertrophy in elderly people.[9,24] In one study,[21] a very small population of very old (89- to 90-year-old) men and women showed the beneficial effects of isotonic resistance exercise for this age group. When they trained for 8 weeks, three times per week,

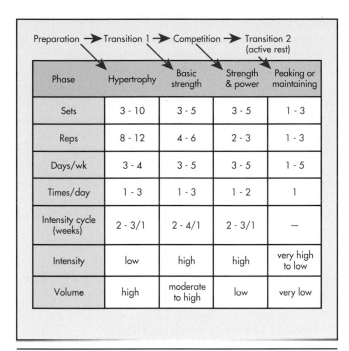

Phase	Hypertrophy	Basic strength	Strength & power	Peaking or maintaining
Sets	3 - 10	3 - 5	3 - 5	1 - 3
Reps	8 - 12	4 - 6	2 - 3	1 - 3
Days/wk	3 - 4	3 - 5	3 - 5	1 - 5
Times/day	1 - 3	1 - 3	1 - 2	1
Intensity cycle (weeks)	2 - 3/1	2 - 4/1	2 - 3/1	—
Intensity	low	high	high	very high to low
Volume	high	moderate to high	low	very low

Fig. 5-16 Traditional athletic model of a modified periodization program. (From *Natl Strength Cond Assoc J* 1993;15:64–66.)

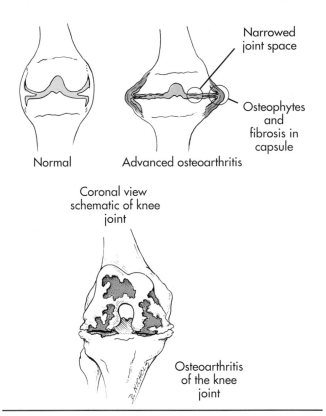

Fig. 5-17 Advanced osteoarthritis of the knee. Joint space narrowing and osteophytic bone spurs. Vertical compressive loads may not be indicated with osteoarthritic lesions.

the force-generating capacity of the trained muscles increased 174% ± 31%. The muscle mass of this group increased 9% ± 4.5%. In addition, two subjects improved in ambulation, no longer requiring the use of a cane. A hypothesis drawn from these findings suggests that increased force-generating capacity can be correlated to increased function.[29]

The previously outlined resistance exercise protocols (DeLorme, Oxford, and Knights DAPRE protocols) may be inappropriate for disabled elderly persons. However, modifications of these programs have provided some guidance in developing strength programs for elderly persons.[29] Frontera[24] states, "The isotonic resistance protocol that produced the greatest increases in force-generation capacity and attenuated atrophy to the greatest extent in older human muscle was three sets of eight repetitions of exercise performed at an intensity of 80% of a muscle's one RM, 3 days a week for 12 weeks."[24] Studies also support the need to closely monitor heart rate, blood pressure, respirations, and subtle signs of distress during any exercise program for elderly persons.[29]

As with any resistance program to elicit strength, intensity of effort is the key element in the magnitude of functional or morphologic change in muscle tissue.[9,24] In the elderly population, intensity of effort must take into account age, history of cardiovascular or pulmonary disease, history of orthopedic pathologic conditions, present disease states, osteoarthritis, and multiple medical conditions present.

STRENGTH TRAINING FOR YOUNGER POPULATIONS

A clear definition of the age range of this special population must be made at the outset to clarify and define the application of resistance exercise and the physiologic adaptation to the precise mode of training. "Prepubescent" and "child" are synonymous terms used to describe both boys and girls before the onset of secondary sex characteristics.[63] The general range of prepubescence is 11 years for girls and 13 years for boys.[63] The term pubescent or adolescent are synonymous descriptive terms related to girls 12 to 18 years and for boys 14 to 18 years of age.[63]

In general, these definitions correspond to the classic Tanner stage classification system. Tanner stage I represents preadolescence or prior ages before the onset of secondary sex characteristics. Tanner stages II through IV describe various levels of development of secondary sex characteristics within adolescence. Tanner stage V is defined as adulthood.[63] Other definitions that must be clarified are strength, weight training, resistance training, and weight lifting. The use of the terms strength training, weight training, and resistance training are used to describe submaximal progressive resistance exercise to improve strength, whereas weight lifting describes an attempt to lift maximum weight for a single repetition as a competitive sporting event. Examples are Olympic weight lifting (e.g., clean and jerk, snatch lift) and power lifting (e.g., bench press, squat, dead lift). The appropriate terminology must be specific to denote the precise intent of the mode of exercise.

The use of the terms progressive resistance exercise, weight training, resistance training, or strength training are both appropriate and practical in the context of orthopedic rehabilitation.

Physiologic Adaptations

Preadolescent children (Tanner stage I) do not possess circulating androgenic-anabolic hormones (testosterone) that act to stimulate hypertrophy, muscular strength, and secondary sex characteristics. Historically this single irrefutable fact has led many researchers to state, "prepubertal boys do not significantly improve strength or increase muscle mass in a weight training program because of insufficient circulating androgens."[63] However, the complexity of strength acquisition is dependent on many factors, including hypertrophy, increases in muscle cross-sectional area, motor activation, central nervous system stimulation, genetic control, and psychologic drive, as well as circulation levels of endogenous hormones.[63]

Several leading researchers and scientists have identified that preadolescent children can significantly increase strength with appropriately applied resistance exercise protocols.[63] However, current evidence strongly suggests that neuromuscular activation, motor coordination, and intrinsic muscular adaptations contribute to preadolescent strength gains.[63] In fact, when investigating the effectiveness of nine studies supporting strength gains in children younger than 13 years of age, researchers found a 71.6% increase in strength versus control group.[27]

Injury Risk

In nonpathologic conditions, progressive resistance exercise for preadolescent and adolescent children is both safe and effective, providing a few conditions are strictly followed. Also the nature of the specific type of training is directly related to the risk of injury. Namely, unsupervised weight training poses no greater risk for injury when compared with other sports or recreational activities common to this age group.[63]

Injuries specific to this age group include disruption of the primary growth centers of ossification, the physeal plates. The secondary growth centers, the apophyses, are at risk of injury from traumatic and chronic traction at these sites.

Specific sites of injury occurring from nonsupervised "weight lifting" include the wrist, shoulder, elbows,

lumbar spine, and knee. Estimates are more than 17,000 injuries occur annually to adolescents participating in nonsupervised "weight lifting" or "power lifting."[63]

Other researchers have found no evidence of subclinical or clinical manifestations of musculoskeletal injury in prepubertal boys participating in 20 weeks of resistance training on the basis of bone scans and serum extraction of creatine phosphokinase (a marker of muscle damage).[63]

Therefore well-supervised, submaximal resistance exercise with use of nonballistic, slow, controlled motions is both effective and safe for preadolescent and adolescent children. The mechanism of physiologic adaptations of resistance exercise for this population is primarily a result of motor unit recruitment, motor control, and neuromuscular activation. Morphologic changes via hypertrophy do not play a role in strength development in preadolescent children.[63]

Relevant Clinical Applications

The specific therapeutic intervention of strength development in children follows a parallel progression of bone and soft-tissue healing. Each contraction type (isometric, concentric, eccentric) is appropriately used during the defined stages of tissue healing (acute inflammatory, stage I; fibroplasia, stage II; and maturation, stage III), depending on radiographic confirmation of osseous union and stability, as well as soft-tissue healing constraints. In concert with specifically applied flexibility techniques (autogenic and reciprocal inhibition, covered in "flexibility"), strength acquisition in children using the foundation of therapeutic exercise parameters—frequency, intensity, duration, muscle contraction type, degree of resistance, number of repetitions, number sets, length of rest between sets, speed of contraction, and order of exercise—as well as a clearly defined model of exercise progression (see Davies model of exercise progression), the preadolescent can be expected to develop strength primarily by neurogenic activation.

THERAPEUTIC EXERCISE EQUIPMENT USED IN STRENGTH TRAINING

The most commonly used strength training tools are ankle or cuff weights. These extremely versatile pieces of equipment are easily adapted to many programs, body parts, and age groups. Thera-Band, surgical tubing, or latex rubber bands are popular, inexpensive, highly adaptable, very portable (for home use), and effective tools. They allow for diagonal patterns of resistance, as well as those involving a single plane. Some manufacturers have added handles to ends of thick rubber cords to enhance the versatility of this equipment.

Dumbbells also are used extensively in physical therapy. Inexpensive, portable, and versatile, dumbbells also can be used to develop excellent ROM and unilateral or bilateral motions. Barbells also can be used but are cumbersome; barbells are effective in sports medicine practices where young athletes should develop overall strength and fitness, not usually in acute rehabilitation environments or hospital physical therapy departments.

Wall pulleys or cable column systems are used in most rehabilitation departments. The amount of resistance used with pulleys can vary from a few to more than 100 pounds. Cable columns are extremely useful for both upper extremity and lower extremity strength training and can be used for many age groups and conditions.

There are many commercially available isotonic exercise systems.* Generally, isotonic exercise machines are fairly adaptable, provide a wide range of resistance (5 to 500 lb for some leg machines), and are mechanically adjustable to accommodate different body types. Individual pieces can be expensive ($3000 or more for a single leg press machine), and a full system may cost $20,000 or more. Various types of muscle contractions can be used with isotonic exercise machines, including concentric and eccentric contractions, isometric static holds, and unilateral or bilateral movements; these exercises can be done using a wide degree of contraction velocities. As discussed, one RM testing can be performed on isotonic systems.

Space availability also is a consideration when one acquires exercise equipment. Whereas the "footprint" of many of these machines is small, a space of several hundred square feet to a few thousand feet may be needed for complete systems. Most of these systems use weight stacks, cables, straps, cams, and chains, but some use pneumatic (air), hydraulic, or electromagnetic resistance.

Isokinetic exercise systems are used extensively in physical therapy practices for testing, documentation, medicolegal presentations, rehabilitation, and velocity spectrum training. These systems generally are very expensive, with a single multijoint system costing $40,000 or more.†

These systems are extremely adaptable to most major body parts (knee, ankle, hip, wrist, elbow, shoulder, and back attachments are available with most systems), and therapeutically these systems are perhaps the most versatile of all strength-training tools. Protocols and training modes that are generally available with most isokinetic systems are as follows:

- Passive
  - Continuous passive motion
  - Active assistive range of motion
- Isometric
  - Multiangle isometrics
- Isotonic
  - Types of contraction modes:
    - Concentric/eccentric
    - Concentric/concentric
    - Eccentric/concentric
    - Eccentric/eccentric
- Isokinetic
  - Types of contraction modes:
    - Concentric/eccentric
    - Concentric/concentric
    - Eccentric/concentric
    - Eccentric/eccentric

Isokinetic systems typically function from 0 degrees per second to 350 to 400 degrees per second. These systems are designed to isolate, test, and rehabilitate single joints. Unfortunately, it is very time consuming to change from one leg to another or from one joint (knee) to another (ankle). The versatility of these systems is presented in Box 5-5.

BOX 5-5

Example of Knee Rehabilitation

PROTOCOL VERSATILITY USING ISOKINETIC TECHNOLOGY
To Gain Knee Motion
Continuous passive motion
To initiate muscle contractions
Use isometric mode. Progress to multiangle isometric, from 0 degrees to 120 degrees of knee motion at 20-degree increments.

To Progress Strength
Use isotonic modes. For example, knee extension (concentric)
Quads followed by knee flexion (eccentric)
Quads from 60 deg/s to 180 deg/s (five sets: 60, 90, 120, 150, and 180 degrees).

Progress to
Isokinetics.
Knee extension (concentric)
Quads followed by concentric hamstrings velocity spectrum training: (eight sets: 30, 60, 90, 120, 150, 180, 210, and 240 degrees).

---

*Some of the more common systems are the Universal, Paramount, Nautilus, Body Masters, and Cybex systems.

†Some common multijoint systems are the Cybex, Lido, Kin-Com, Biodex, Isotechnologies, and Ariel systems.

BOX 5-6

Application for Inertial Training

CONDITIONS

Submaximal plyometrics

Neuromuscular training

Training of tendon tissue

Alteration of electromechanical delay

Physiologic crossover effects

INDICATIONS

Painful arc remediation

Mechanical, reproducible joint pain

Capsular afferens and coordination

Proposed prevention of bone loss

From Albert M: Eccentric Muscle Training in Sports and Orthopaedics. New York, Churchill Livingstone, 1991.

The impulse inertial exercise apparatus is a system used for submaximal plyometric training. The impulse system provides limited ROM (by design), high-velocity, low-intensity, concentric, and eccentric loading. The application of inertial exercise involves rapid, coordinated, cyclic, and dynamic motions with reduced loads or resistance. The impulse system can be used for upper and lower extremity exercise. Extremely adaptive components with various handles allow for the duplication of sports such as tennis, racquetball, and golf. Clinically, this system is used mainly for neuromuscular coordination and strength in limited degrees of motion. The clinical delivery of inertial exercise is shown in Box 5-6.[3]

❖ ADDITIONAL FEATURES

ATP Use in Muscle Contractions: Concentric contractions use more ATP than isometric contractions. Eccentric contractions use the least.

Closed Kinetic Chain: Resistance exercise—a system of predictably interdependent articulated biomechanical "links," a system that stimulates joint afferent neuromechanoreceptor input, highly functional, proprioception, and kinesthetic awareness—nonisolation exercise.

Components of Muscle Contraction and Strength Development: Calcium, potassium, and sodium ions; axoplasmic transport; efficient neuromuscular activation; muscle contraction types; activation of motor units; modes of exercise frequency-intensity and duration of contraction types, rest recovery, adaptation.

Contractile Tissue: Myofibril—two basic proteins, myosin and actin.

Contraction Types: Concentric, eccentric, and isometric.

Exercise and Program Design Variables: Choice of exercise, metabolic demands, order of sequence of exercises, sets, and repetitions (Consider Delorme protocol, Oxford protocol,

or DAPRE), loads used, ratio of rest to exercise, frequency of exercise, and progression.

Exercise Modifications: Precise identification of anatomic pathology; limit ROM to accommodate pain and biomechanical limitations; adjust resistance; use slow, controlled precision movements; control velocity.

Force Production: Eccentric contractions create more force than isometric contractions. Concentric contractions produce the least force.

General Adaptation Syndrome: Alarm stage, resistance stage, exhaustion stage, and adaptation.

Increase in Blood Flow to Exercising Muscle: Immediate blood flow response may increase vascular supply tenfold.

Muscle Fiber Types: Fast twitch (type II)—white, glycolytic, speed, strength, and power; slow twitch (type I)—red, oxidative, fatigue resistant.

Noncontractile Tissue: Epimysium, perimysium, and endomysium.

Periodization: Microcycle—daily or weekly changes in intensity, frequency, duration of exercise; mesocycle—monthly changes; macrocycle—annual adaptations.

Reactive Hyperemia: Further blood flow increase occurs in muscle as contraction stops via endothelial relaxation.

SAID Principle: Specific adaptation to imposed demands.

Specific Proprioceptive Closed-Chain Neuromuscular Training: Multiangle, closed-chain functions; reciprocal, coordinated, balanced, full body, or joint-specific dexterity, considering joint position, movement, direction, speed, amplitude, and deceleration.

Strength Adaptations: Early increases in strength do not parallel increases in hypertrophy. Early increases in strength are caused by increased neuromuscular activation and efficiency. Evoked hypertrophy is a time-dependent adaptive response to increased loads.

Vascular Response to Exercise: At rest, blood flow is estimated at 2 to 3 mL per 100 mL of muscle per minute.

REFERENCES

1. Abraham WM: Exercise induced muscle soreness. *Phys Sports Med* 1979;7:57.
2. Abraham WM: Factors in delayed muscle soreness. *Med Sci Sports Exer* 1977;9:11.
3. Albert M: Eccentric Muscle Training in Sports and Orthopaedics. New York, Churchill Livingstone, 1991.
4. Belka D: Comparison of dynamic, static, and combination training on dominant wrist flexor muscles. *Res Exerc Sport* 1968;39:244.
5. Berger RA: Optimum repetitions for the development of strength. *Res Q Exerc Sport* 1962;33:334–338.
6. Brinkman JR, et al: Rate and range of knee motion in ambulation. *Phys Ther* 1982;62(5):632.
7. Byrnes WC, et al: Delayed onset muscle soreness following repeated bouts of downhill running. *J Appl Physiol* 1985;59:7109.
8. Caplan A, et al: Skeletal Muscle. In Woo SL-Y, Buckwalter J, eds. Injury and Repair of the Musculoskeletal Soft Tissues. Rosemont, IL, American Academy of Orthopaedic Surgeons, 1988.
9. Charette SL, et al: Muscle hypertrophy response to resistance training in older women. *J Appl Physiol* 1991;70:1912–1916.
10. Chu DA: Rehabilitation of the lower extremity. *Clin Sports Med* 1995;14(1):205–222.
11. Clarke HH, et al: New objective strength tests of muscle groups by cable tension methods. *Res Quart* 1952;23:136.
12. Clarke HH: Improvements of objective strength tests of muscle groups by cable tension methods. *Res Quart* 1950;21:399.

13. Conroy BP, Earle RW: Bone, muscle and connective tissue adaptations to physical activity. In Baechle TR, ed. Essentials of Strength Training and Conditioning. Champaign, IL, Human Kinetics, 1994.

14. Davies GJ: Course notes. Open and Closed Kinetic Chain Exercises and Their Application to Testing and Rehabilitation: Advances on the Knee and Shoulder. Cincinnati Sports Medicine and Orthopaedic Center, 1993.

15. Davies GJ: A Compendium of Isokinetics in Clinical Usage and Rehabilitation Techniques, third ed. Onalaska, WI, S&S Publishers, 1987.

16. DeLee J, et al: Therapeutic exercise modalities. Am Orthop Soc Sports Med, St Louis, Mosby, 1989.

17. DeLorme TL, Watkins A: Progressive Resistance Exercise. New York, Appleton-Century, 1951.

18. Edgerton VR, et al: Morphological basis of skeletal muscle power output. In Jones NL, McCartney N, McComas AJ, eds. Human Muscle Power. Champaign, IL, Human Kinetics, 1986.

19. Elftman H: Biomechanics of muscle. J Bone Joint Surg 1966; 48:363.

20. Faulkner JA: New perspectives in training for maximum performance. JAMA 1986;205:741–746.

21. Fiatarone MA, et al: High intensity strength training in nonagenarians: effects on skeletal muscle. JAMA 1990;263:3029–3034.

22. Francis KT: Delayed muscle soreness: a review. J Orthop Sports Phys Ther 1983;5:10.

23. Friden J, Sjostrom M, Ekblom B: Myofibrillar damage following intensive eccentric exercise in man. Int J Sport Med 1983;4:170–176.

24. Frontera WR, et al: Strength conditioning in older men: skeletal muscle hypertrophy and improved function. J Appl Physiol 1988; 64:1038–1044.

25. Gollnick PD: Fiber number and size in overloaded chicken anterior latissimus dorsi muscle. J Appl Physiol 1983;54:1292.

26. Gonyea W, Ericson GC, Bonde-Peterson F: Skeletal muscle fiber splitting induced by weight-lifting exercise in cats. Acta Physiol Scand 1977;99:105–109.

27. Hakkinen K, Komi PV: Effect of different combined concentric and eccentric muscle work regimes on maximal strength development. J Hum Mov Stud 1981;7:33.

28. Harman E: Strength and power: a definition of terms. J NSCA 1993;15(6):18–20.

29. Hopp JF: Effects of age and resistance training on skeletal muscle: a review. Phys Ther 1993;73(6):361–373.

30. Jzankoff SP, Norris AH: Effect of muscle mass decreases on age-related BMR changes. J Appl Physiol 1977;43:1001–1006.

31. Kellis E, Baltzopoulos V: Isokinetic eccentric exercise. Sports Med 1995;19(3):202–222.

32. Klitgaard H, et al: Function, morphology and protein expression of aging skeletal muscle: a cross-sectional study of elderly men with different training backgrounds. Acta Physiol Scand Suppl 1990; 140:41–54.

33. Knapik JJ, et al: Angular specificity and test mode specificity of isometric and isokinetic strength training. J Orthop Sports Phys Ther 1983;5(2)58–65.

34. Knight KL: Quadriceps strengthening with the DAPRE technique: case studies with neurological implications. Med Sci Sport Exerc 1985;17(6):646–650.

35. Knuttgen H, Kramer W: Terminology and measurement in exercise performance. J Appl Sports Sci Res 1987;1:1–10.

36. Kuta I, Parizkova J, Dycka J: Muscle strength and lean body mass in old men of different physical activity. J Appl Physiol 1970; 29:168–171.

37. Mangine R, Heckman TP, Eldridge VL: Improving strength, endurance and power. In Scully RM, Barnes MR, eds. Physical Therapy. Philadelphia, JB Lippincott, 1989.

38. McAllister RM, Amann JF, Laughlin MH: Skeletal muscle fiber types and their vascular support. J Reconstr Microsurg 1993; 9(4):313–317.

39. McCartney N, et al: Long-term resistance training in the elderly: effects on dynamic strength, exercise capacity, muscle, and bone. J Gerontol Appl Biol Sci Med Sci 1995;50(2):97–104.

40. Miles MP, Clarkson PM: Exercise-induced muscle pain, soreness, and cramps. J Sports Med Phys Fitness 1994;34(3):203–216.

41. Newham DJ, et al: Ultrastructural changes after concentric and eccentric contractions of human muscle. J Neurol Sci 1983; 61:109–122.

42. Newham DJ, et al: Pain and fatigue after concentric and eccentric muscle contractions. Clin Sci 1983;64:55.

43. Norkin CC, Levangie PK: Joint Structure and Function: A Comprehensive Analysis, 2nd ed. Philadelphia, FA Davis, 1992.

44. Nyland J, et al: Review of the afferent neural system of the knee and its contribution to motor learning. J Orthop Sports Phys Ther 1994;19(1):2–11.

45. Page P: Pathophysiology of acute exercise induced muscular injury: clinical implications. J Ath Train 1995;30(1):29–34.

46. Palmieri G: Weight training and repetition speed. J Appl Sport Sci Res 1987;1(2):36–38.

47. Rothstein JM, Lamb RL, Mayhew TP: Clinical uses of isokinetic measurements: critical issues. Phys Ther 1988;67:1840.

48. Schwane J, et al: Blood markers of delayed onset muscle soreness with downhill treadmill running. Med Sci Sports Exer 1981;13:80.

49. Smith LL, et al: Impact of a repeated bout of eccentric exercise on muscular strength, muscle soreness and creatine kinase. Br J Sports Med 1994;28(4):267–271.

50. Soderberg G: Kinesiology: Application to Pathological Motion. Baltimore, Williams & Wilkins, 1986.

51. Stauber WT: Eccentric action of muscles: physiology, injury and adaptation. Exerc Sport Sci Rev 1989;19:157.

52. Steadman JR: Rehabilitation of athletic injury. Am J Sports Med 1979;7:147.

53. Stone M: Literature review: explosive exercise and training. NSCA J 1993;15(3):6–19.

54. Stone MH, et al: Periodization. NSCA J Part I reprinted 1993; 15(1):29.

55. Talag TS: Residual muscular soreness as influenced by concentric, eccentric and static contractions. Res Q Exerc Sport 1973;44:458.

56. Talmadge RJ, Roy RR, Edgerton VR: Muscle fiber types and function. Curr Opin Rheumatol 1993;5(6):695–705.

57. Thompson LV: Aging muscle: characteristics and strength training. Issues Aging 1995;18(1)25–30.

58. Waltrous B, Armstrong R, Schwane J: The role of lactic acid in delayed onset muscular distress. Med Sci Sports Exer 1981;13:80.

59. Webster's New Collegiate Dictionary. Springfield, MA, G&C Merriam Co, 1981.

60. Wilk KE, et al: Stretch-shortening drills for the upper extremities: theory and clinical application. J Orthop Sports Phys Ther 1993; 17(5):225–239.

61. Wyatt MP, Edwards AM: Comparison of quadriceps and hamstring torque values during isokinetic exercise. J Orthop Sports Phys Ther 1981;3(2):48–56.

62. Zinowieff AN: Heavy resistance exercise: the Oxford technique. Br J Phys Med 1951;14:129.

63. Guy JA, Michel LJ: Strength training for children and adolescents. J Am Acad Orthop Surg 2001;9:26–31.

REVIEW QUESTIONS

Multiple Choice

1. An individual muscle's potential to gain strength and power is determined by which of the following?
   A. Muscle fiber length
   B. Mass of the muscle
   C. Angle of attachment of the muscle to a tendon
   D. All of the above

2. Red muscle fibers are also identified as which of the following?
   A. Slow-twitch
   B. Type I fibers
   C. Oxidative
   D. All of the above

3. White muscle fibers have which of the following characteristics? (Circle any that apply.)
   A. Have more mitochondria
   B. Contain succinic dehydrogenase
   C. Are larger in diameter than red fibers
   D. Have low myoglobin
   E. Are recruited for endurance activities

4. White, fast-twitch, glycolytic type II muscle fiber can be further classified into how many subclassifications?
   A. Two
   B. Three
   C. Five
   D. Four
   E. None of the above

5. Circle the examples of muscle contractions.
   A. Isotonic
   B. Concentric
   C. Isokinetic
   D. Eccentric
   E. Isometric

6. Which testing tool affords the clinician the greatest degree of evaluating muscular performance?
   A. Hand dynamometers
   B. Cable tensiometry
   C. One-repetition maximum lifts
   D. Isokinetics

7. The data collected from an isokinetic dynamometer measure which of the following?
   A. Strength (force)
   B. Torque
   C. Power
   D. Work
   E. All of the above

8. The foundations of all clinically applied strength programs involve which of the following principles? (Circle any that apply.)
   A. Overload
   B. Duration
   C. Specificity
   D. Reversibility
   E. Order

9. To best stimulate type I fibers, which program would be most appropriate? (Circle any that apply.)
   A. High intensity, short duration
   B. Low intensity, long duration
   C. Stationary cycle ergometer
   D. Upper body ergometer
   E. One repetition max on the leg press

10. High-intensity resistance exercise leads to increases in which of the following? (Circle any that apply.)
    A. ATP
    B. Creatine kinase
    C. Creatine phosphate
    D. Succinic dehydrogenase
    E. Type I muscle fibers

11. Which of the following more accurately describe the symptoms of delayed onset muscle soreness (DOMS)? (Circle any that apply.)
    A. Local muscle pain
    B. Diffuse muscle soreness
    C. Specific intense injury
    D. General muscle soreness
    E. Radiating pain

12. Which of the following muscle contraction types result in the greatest occurrence of DOMS?
    A. Isometric
    B. Eccentric
    C. Concentric
    D. Isokinetic
    E. Isotonic

13. When full arc motions of slow-speed, high-resistance exercise are used to generate greater tension and strength, the joint compression forces and resultant torque are affected in which way?
    A. Reduced
    B. The same as with high-speed, low-resistance exercise
    C. Increased
    D. Greatly reduced

14. To minimize joint compression forces during the initial stages of recovery, the most appropriate muscle contraction to use to develop or maintain strength is which of the following?
    A. Short arc eccentrics
    B. Isokinetic full arc high-speed concentric
    C. Isometrics
    D. Slow-speed short arc isokinetic concentric

15. The angular velocity of the human knee during normal walking is approximately how much?
    A. 60 degrees per second
    B. 240 degrees per second
    C. 180 degrees per second
    D. 200 degrees per second

16. To recover functional use of the knee after injury, which of the following best describes the most appropriate selection of muscle contraction types to regain strength?
    A. Isometrics, isotonic (concentric)
    B. Isometrics, isotonic (eccentric)
    C. Isometrics, isotonic (concentric and eccentric)
    D. Isotonic (concentric and eccentric), isokinetic slow speed (concentric and eccentric)

17. High-velocity isokinetic exercise can allow for which of the following?
    A. Accommodation of the patient's pain
    B. Reduced compression forces
    C. Improved functional speeds of contraction
    D. All of the above

18. Which PRE program does the following describe: three sets of 10 repetitions of exercises, with the first set performed at 50% of 10 RM, the second set at 75% of 10 RM, and the third set at 100% of 10 RM?
    A. Oxford
    B. Regressive resistance exercise program
    C. DeLorme PRE
    D. DAPRE

19. Which of the following describes the rule of tens when applied to isometric exercise?
    A. 10 body parts must be exercised
    B. 10 exercises must be used
    C. 10-second contractions, 10 repetitions, 10-second rest
    D. None of the above

20. When instructing a patient to perform isometric contractions, which of the following best describes the most appropriate sequence?

A. 8-second contraction, 2-second rest
B. 10-second maximal contraction
C. 5-second contraction, 5-second rest
D. Gradual 2-second development of tension, 6-second maintenance of maximum contraction, gradual 2-second decrease in tension

21. Which of the following best describes an open kinetic chain?
    A. Wall squats
    B. Supine leg press
    C. Biceps curls
    D. Stair steppers

22. A closed kinetic chain exercise for the knee is which of the following?
    A. Short arc quads
    B. Isometric quad sets
    C. Seated knee extension
    D. Supine leg press
    E. All of the above

23. Climbing stairs is an example of which of the following?
    A. Open kinetic chain exercise
    B. Closed kinetic chain exercise
    C. Open and closed chain exercise
    D. Plyometric exercise
    E. All of the above

24. The general rationale for utilizing CKC exercises in rehabilitation is which of the following?
    A. To improve neuromuscular coordination
    B. To stimulate muscular co-contractions
    C. Joint approximation leads to increases in kinesthetic awareness
    D. CKC exercises are more functional than OKC exercises
    E. All of the above

Short Answer

25. How many muscle fiber types have been identified in humans?

26. Aerobic exercises require muscle fibers that are primarily _____ . (*oxidative* or *glycolytic*)

27. Organize the following five muscle fiber types into a numeric sequence of recruitment, proceeding from the lowest force requirements (1) to the greatest (5):

    _____ Fast twitch (type II) _____ Fast twitch (type II, AB)

    _____ Slow twitch (type I) _____ Fast twitch (type II, A)

    _____ Fast twitch (type II, B)

28. List the five ways muscular strength is measured.

29. Organize the following muscle contraction types in orderly sequence from greatest (3) to least (1) use of ATP:

    _____ Eccentrics _____ Concentrics _____ Isometrics

30. Organize the following muscle contraction types in orderly sequence from greatest (3) to least (1) force production:

    _____ Concentrics _____ Isometrics _____ Eccentrics

31. Name the two categories of muscle mutability.

32. What does *SAID* stand for?

33. Name the three stimuli for adaptive changes in skeletal muscles.

34. A patient returns to the outpatient physical therapy department and reports localized, specific muscle pain and describes an isolated event of lifting a box, which immediately increased pain. Describe the appropriate course of action the PTA will take to manage this patient's complaints of increased pain.

True/False

35. *Isokinetic* and *isotonic* do not describe muscle contractions but rather are terms used to define and describe events utilizing true muscle contractions.

36. Manual muscle testing can be used to determine a muscle's power, work capacity, and force production.

37. Clinically it is important to choose one contraction type throughout the course of recovery from injury.

38. In terms of muscle hypertrophy, type I fibers hypertrophy more than type II fibers.

39. Stretching an innervated muscle creates tension, which results in muscle hypertrophy.

40. Muscle soreness is never an anticipated byproduct of new or more intense exercise.

41. Plyometric exercises are functionally appropriate exercises to use for all orthopedic patients.

42. Plyometrics are most often used to develop strength.

43. Plyometrics is a "system" of exercises that utilizes the myotatic stretch reflex and neurophysiologic responses from the Golgi tendon organs and muscle spindles to create high-speed reaction forces and power.

44. Closed kinetic chain exercises always must be deferred until the final phase of recovery.

45. The human body functions as a combination of both open and closed kinetic chain activities.

46. High intensity strength training for the elderly is not safe or effective and does not lead to improved function.

47. Studies demonstrate that muscle size (hypertrophy), strength (force-generation), and function (gait and balance) can be improved in elderly people with appropriately applied high-intensity resistance exercise.

Essay Questions
Answer on a separate sheet of paper.

48. Name the noncontractile and contractile elements of muscle tissue.
49. Describe and contrast muscle fiber types.
50. Define types of muscle contraction.
51. Give examples of concentric and eccentric contractions.
52. Give two definitions of strength.
53. Define and clarify terms used to describe muscular performance.
54. List methods used to measure strength.
55. Compare muscle contraction types in relation to tension produced and energy liberated.
56. Discuss muscle response to exercise.
57. Identify clinical features of delayed onset muscle soreness.
58. Discuss velocity spectrum training related to isokinetic exercise.
59. List three clinically relevant exercise programs used to enhance strength.
60. Discuss plyometrics.
61. Explain open and closed kinetic chain exercise.
62. Identify goals and applications of strength training programs for the elderly.

Critical Thinking Application

In small groups, discuss and develop specific sequential sets of exercises and identify types of muscle contractions that will enhance quadriceps strength and power after a rectus femoris muscle strain. Which muscle contraction type would you recommend initially? Why? Which types of exercises would you encourage to stimulate type I muscle fiber? Which exercises would you encourage to stimulate type II muscle fiber? Develop a continuum of exercises that appropriately addresses isometrics, concentric and eccentric contractions, and isokinetics. Give three clinically relevant examples of each contraction type and explain when and why you would use each. What is an anticipated byproduct of your exercise continuum as you progress your patient from one contraction type to another? What modifications, if any, would you recommend to prevent or minimize patellofemoral compressive loads during quad-strengthening activities? Describe the appropriate application of closed kinetic chain exercises and plyometrics after recovery from a rectus femoris muscle strain.

6

Endurance

LEARNING OBJECTIVES

1. Define VO_2 max.
2. List adaptive physiologic changes related to aerobic exercise.
3. Describe the age-adjusted maximum heart rate.
4. Discuss several guidelines for the development of aerobic fitness related to frequency, intensity, duration, and mode of activity.
5. Outline methods of aerobic training.
6. Identify orthopedic considerations during aerobic exercise.
7. Discuss two hypotheses that attempt to clarify peripheral neuromuscular fatigue as a result of prolonged or strenuous muscle activity.
8. Compare endurance training alone with the effects of a combined program of aerobic training and strength training.

KEY TERMS

Aerobic capacity

Cardiovascular endurance

Maximal oxygen uptake (VO_2 max)

Age-adjusted maximum heart rate (AAMHR)

Karvonen method

Borg scale

Frequency

Intensity

Duration

Mode of activity

Continuous aerobic activity

Discontinuous aerobic activity

Muscle fatigue

Local muscular endurance

Circuit training

CHAPTER OUTLINE

Adaptive Physiologic Changes with Aerobic Exercise

Measuring and Prescribing Aerobic Exercise

Methods of Aerobic Training

Orthopedic Considerations During Aerobic Exercise

Muscle Fatigue and Local Muscular Endurance

Combining Endurance and Strength Training

Endurance activities can be classified as either those affecting the muscular system or those affecting the cardiovascular system. During endurance exercises the body relies on aerobic activity, which involves those metabolic pathways that use oxygen to provide energy for muscle contractions.[14,24] Aerobic metabolism takes place in structures called mitochondria. In this metabolic process the breakdown of protein, fats, and carbohydrates forms energy-rich adenosine triphosphate (ATP), a process known as oxidative phosphorylation.[14,24] This aerobic energy system (oxidative capacity) can produce approximately 19 times the ATP produced by the anaerobic adenosine triphosphate-phosphocreatine (ATP-PC) energy system.[15,24]

The degree of aerobic fitness or the ability to do work (see definition of work in Chapter 3), one possesses is expressed as **aerobic capacity, cardiovascular endurance,** cardiovascular fitness, or cardiorespiratory fitness. The efficiency of the aerobic system is measured by the maximum volume of oxygen consumed during exercise, termed **maximal oxygen uptake (vo_2 max).**[14,24] Activities that stress long-duration, low-intensity exercise enhance aerobic fitness. The main rationale for aerobic conditioning is to improve the body's aerobic capacity. Researchers have established guidelines for prescribing aerobic exercise for untrained, moderately trained, trained, and highly trained individuals (Box 6-1).[8,21] In general, long-term aerobic training can improve aerobic fitness approximately 10% to 20%.[1,2]

ADAPTIVE PHYSIOLOGIC CHANGES WITH AEROBIC EXERCISE

The most notable changes in the oxygen transport system after long-term aerobic exercise training are as follows:[3,12,24]

- Increased size and number of mitochondria
- Increased myoglobin content
- Improved mobilization and use of fat and carbohydrates
- Selective hypertrophy of type I slow-twitch oxidative muscle fibers
- Decreased resting heart rate and submaximal heart rate
- Increased blood volume and hemoglobin
- Reduced systolic and diastolic blood pressure
- Significantly improved oxygen extraction rates from the blood

MEASURING AND PRESCRIBING AEROBIC EXERCISE

Perhaps the most clinically relevant and practical way to prescribe aerobic fitness programs for healthy adults (those without chronic or unstable complicated medical conditions) involves the **age-adjusted maximum heart**

BOX 6-1

Exercise Prescription Recommendations for Untrained, Moderately Trained, Trained, and Highly Trained Individuals

FREQUENCY

3 to 5 days per week for untrained to moderately trained; 5 to 7 days per week for highly trained

INTENSITY

60% to 90% of maximum heart rate (MHR): untrained, 60%; highly trained, 90%

DURATION

15 to 60 minutes or more (continuous)

---

rate (AAMHR). The American College of Sports Medicine (ACSM)[22] defines the minimal training intensity threshold for improved vo_2 max as approximately 60% of the maximum heart rate (MHR). An individual's MHR is determined by the following equation:

$$220 - Age = MHR$$

The recommended intensity level (ACSM)[22] range is 60% to 90% of MHR. The individual's target or training heart rate (THR) is established as follows:

$$THR = MHR \times \text{Intensity level range (60\% to 90\%)}$$

For example, if

$$MHR \text{ is } 180, THR = 180 \times 70\%^{70}$$
$$= 126 \text{ or } 180 \times 80\%^{80}$$
$$= 144$$

Another method for establishing a THR is with the **Karvonen** formula. The training intensity range for this formula is 50% to 85% of vo_2 max. The Karvonen method uses the difference between the MHR and the resting heart rate (RHR), which is called the maximum heart rate reserve (MHR reserve). The following are examples of the Karvonen formula:

$$MHR \text{ (in beats per minute)} = 180$$
$$RHR = 180 - 60 = 120$$
$$\text{Intensity level} = 70\%$$
$$120 \times 0.70 = 84$$
$$RHR = 60$$
$$RHR + \text{Intensity level} = \text{Maximum training heart rate}$$
$$60 + 84 = 144$$

13

Black

7½

The Ring 2

——

Mexico "soccer."

The range of intensity using the Karvonen method is expressed as follows:

$$\text{Low THR} = (50\% - \text{MHR reserve}) + \text{RHR}$$
$$\text{High THR} = (85\% - \text{MHR reserve}) + \text{RHR}$$

Clinically, the intensity of exercise can be monitored using a subjective estimate of exercise stress. The relative perceived exertion scale is used to prescribe exercise intensity based on an individual's perception of exertion. The classic **Borg Scale**[4] is used to describe perceived exertion (Box 6-2).

BOX 6-2

Borg Scale of Relative Perceived Exertion

6
7　Very, very light
8
9　Very light
10
11
12
13　Somewhat hard
14
15　Hard
16
17　Very hard
18
19　Very, very hard

The **frequency, intensity, duration,** and mode of activity recommended by the ACSM[22] are as follows:

Frequency of training: 3 to 5 days per week

Intensity of training: 60% to 90% of age-adjusted MHR or 50% to 85% of MHR

Duration of training: 20 to 60 minutes of continuous aerobic activity

The mode of activity is any activity that uses large muscle groups, can be maintained continuously, and is rhythmic and aerobic. Examples include walking, bicycling, jogging, stair climbing, rowing, and swimming.

When initiating or intensifying an aerobic conditioning program with any patient, one should recognize that greater levels of intensity have been associated with higher cardiovascular risk,[23] increased rates of orthopedic injury,[19,20] and reduced compliance with exercise as compared with lower levels of intensity.[7,19]

METHODS OF AEROBIC TRAINING

Aerobic conditioning programs are either continuous or discontinuous. **Continuous aerobic activities** provide no rest interval during the entire bout of exercise, and generally little variation in heart rate occurs. Examples of continuous activities are jogging, walking, running, cycling, and stair climbing. As with all forms of exercise, the benefits obtained are specific to the type, quality, and quantity of exercise undertaken.

For clinical purposes, stationary bicycle ergometers and treadmills are commonly used (Fig. 6-1). Continuous aerobic activities that use more muscles burn more calories and consume more oxygen than continuous

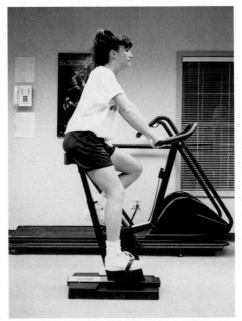
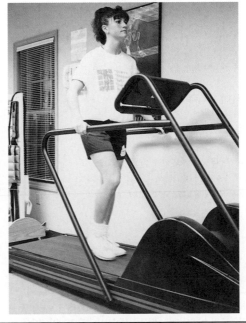

Fig. 6-1 **A,** Seated stationary bicycle ergometer. **B,** Standard treadmill.

activities that use fewer muscles. For example, jogging on a treadmill burns more calories and uses more muscle than pedaling a seated bicycle ergometer.

Discontinuous aerobic activities are also called interval training activities. They can involve the same activities as continuous aerobic programs, but in interval training, repeated exercise bouts are interspersed with rest intervals. One advantage of interval training over continuous aerobic activities is that interval training provides large amounts of high-intensity work in a relatively short amount of time. However, interval training tends to develop strength and power more than endurance.[5]

Adjusting the ratio of work (aerobic) to rest (recovery) is the foundation of interval training.[14] For aerobic fitness, a work:rest ratio of 1:1 or 1:1.5 is advised. The rest or recovery interval can be passive (total rest) or active (active recovery). Active recovery involves reducing the intensity of work, which allows the individual to continue the activity for long periods of time. It is most appropriate for stressing the aerobic metabolic pathways and minimizing the capacity to develop strength and power through use of high-intensity interval training.

ORTHOPEDIC CONSIDERATIONS DURING AEROBIC EXERCISE

The use of endurance activities for orthopedic patients is challenging. Acute injury or surgery requires a period of rest so that the injured part can heal properly.

Aerobic endurance activities are essential after a back injury.[26] However, sitting on the saddle seat of a stationary ergometer may not be appropriate for many patients with back problems. A recumbent cycle has a large bucket car seat (Fig. 6-2) to provide lumbar support so that the patient can comfortably perform the aerobic exercise. In some cases back patients may tolerate treadmill activities more than seated aerobic activities. If treadmill walking is not tolerated, an underwater treadmill can provide enough buoyancy during walking to allow patients to do aerobic activity (Fig. 6-3).

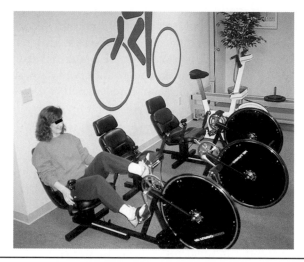

Fig. 6-2 Recumbent bicycle ergometer. Large bucket seat used in a recumbent position may allow some patients to tolerate seated aerobic activities.

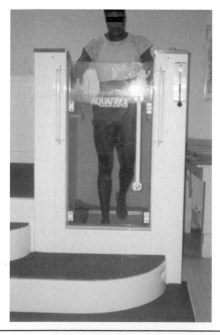

Fig. 6-3 Underwater treadmill. The buoyancy of the water may allow early vertical loading and the initiation of normalized gait mechanics.

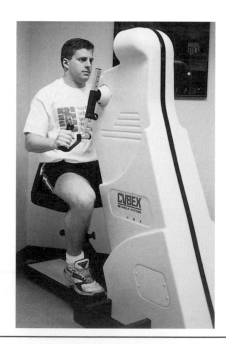

Fig. 6-4 For patients with lower extremity injuries, an upper body ergometer allows continued aerobic activities during periods of immobilization.

Patients who have a lower extremity injury or surgery can maintain or improve cardiorespiratory fitness using an upper body ergometer (UBE) (Fig. 6-4). This is an effective tool for continuous or interval training when patients cannot perform lower body endurance activities. Older patients with hip, knee, or ankle osteoarthritis (degenerative joint disease) may not tolerate the vertical compressive loads developed during treadmill walking, stair climbing, or even stationary cycling; therefore, a UBE may provide an effective aerobic activity for these individuals. Patients who have a lower extremity injury can be instructed in how to do a single-leg stationary bicycle ergometer exercise (Fig. 6-5).

Patients with upper extremity conditions can use a stationary cycle or treadmill for endurance training. Patients also can be instructed to use one-arm cycling on a UBE (Fig. 6-6) to maintain upper body aerobic fitness.

Many throwing athletes and industrial workers require specific aerobic fitness, strength, and power in their shoulders and arms. During recovery after injury or surgery to the shoulder, elbow, arm, or hand, the patient can maintain a certain level of specific fitness by using a one-arm aerobic activity.

Modifications can be made on stationary cycles to allow for continued aerobic conditioning after an ankle injury or surgery. Typically the seat height should allow for slight knee flexion (~10 degrees) at the end of the pedal stroke. With the seat in normal position, the foot generally plantar flexes toward the end of the pedal stroke, causing stress to the anterior talofibular ligament.

Therefore the seat height is lowered for a patient with a severe ankle sprain to allow for a complete pedal stroke and keep the ankle joint in neutral (Fig. 6-7).

Stair climbing, seated rowing, and cross-country ski machines are popular aerobic tools but must be used judiciously. Stair climbers require the patient to be correctly positioned vertically and maintain balance (holding the hand rails) to perform the exercise correctly. Therefore stair climbers are difficult for many patients in the acute or immediate post-orthopedic surgery period to use. Rowing machines require both a pulling motion with the arms and hip and knee flexion and extension. These simultaneous motions make modifications for use with specific orthopedic problems quite difficult. Cross-country ski machines require bilateral, reciprocal leg and arm motions and are also difficult to modify for orthopedic patients with acute disorders. However, stair climbers, rowing machines, and cross-country ski machines can be effective tools in aerobic conditioning programs after the acute phase of recovery from injury or surgery.

MUSCLE FATIGUE AND LOCAL MUSCULAR ENDURANCE

Two hypotheses attempt to clarify peripheral neuromuscular fatigue as a result of prolonged or strenuous muscle activity.[9,16] One states that **muscle fatigue** results from decreasing amounts of the energy substrates, ATP, glycogen, and phosphocreatine. The other states that

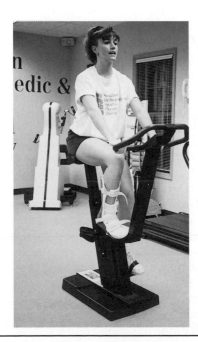

Fig. 6-5 In some cases, a single-leg stationary cycle ergometer can be used for cardiovascular fitness during periods of immobilization.

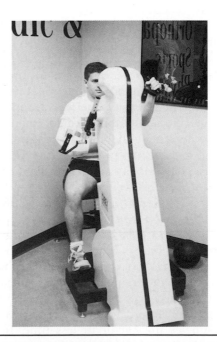

Fig. 6-6 A one-arm, upper body cycling activity with an upper body ergometer is also an effective aerobic exercise activity.

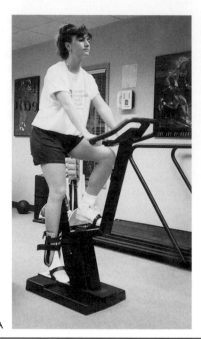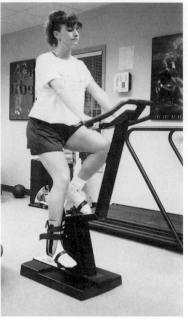

A   B

Fig. 6-7 **A,** Normal seat elevation for the performance of a seated bicycle ergometer allows for greater plantar flexion motion. Plantar flexion may be contraindicated with acute and subacute sprains of the lateral ligament complex of the ankle. **B,** With the saddle seat lowered, the affected ankle can be maintained in a more appropriate neutral position during periods of aerobic activity on the cycle ergometer.

muscle fatigue occurs when noxious metabolites (hydrogen ions and ammonia) accumulate. Either of these events may occur as a result of high-intensity or prolonged muscular effort.

The ability to perform repeated submaximal bouts of physical activity is a vital and critical component of recovery after injury or surgery.[26]

Circuit training, in effect, is a combination of resistance and aerobic exercise. Its goal is to improve **local muscular endurance,** cardiorespiratory fitness, and muscular strength. The intensity of **circuit training** directly affects the specific adaptations desired. Intensity can be increased by decreasing the amount of time allowed to perform the exercise, keeping the time constant but increasing the repetitions or sets of desired exercise, or decreasing the time allowed for rest between exercises.

Generally a circuit may contain 12 to 15 exercise stations that offer various levels of resistance. Typically the resistance is 40% to 50% of the predetermined 1 RM (repetitions maximum). The patient performs each exercise in sequence.

The two types of circuits are fixed-load and target circuits.[25] In a fixed-load circuit, the load or resistance remains constant. Improved fitness occurs as the individual completes the circuit in less time. In a target circuit, the time required to complete the program is constant, and the individual is required to complete as many repetitions as possible during the prescribed time.

Generally the exercises are performed in 15- to 20-second bouts in a nonstop sequence. Another way to structure a target circuit is to perform each exercise in 30-second sets with a short 15-second rest between sets.

An important metabolic adaptation that occurs with muscular endurance exercise is a significant increase in oxidative enzyme levels. High-volume aerobic exercise increases the oxidative enzymes succinic dehydrogenase (SDH) and malate dehydrogenase (MDH).[6,11]

COMBINING ENDURANCE AND STRENGTH TRAINING

Recovering from orthopedic trauma or disease frequently involves rehabilitation programs that stress endurance, strength, and flexibility. Strength may be inhibited to some degree during simultaneous endurance training[10] because of the intensity of each program.[13,18] If the major goal of training is to improve strength, a program of strength training should be combined with a moderate, long-duration endurance program. Conversely, if the rehabilitation goal is to primarily improve endurance, then a program of strength and high-intensity interval training should be used.[10,18]

The adaptations to specific training modes are highly selective and relate to the metabolic pathways stressed and the muscle groups used, as well as the intensity of the programs prescribed. Modest gains in both strength and endurance can occur during combined programs.[17] The therapeutic exercise program emphasizes the intensity of the specific mode of training to obtain the desired physiologic adaptation.

❖ ADDITIONAL FEATURES

Blood Pressure Adaptations: Resistance exercise leads to decreased heart rate, reduced blood pressure, and decreased double product.

Double Product: Refers to heart rate × systolic blood pressure. Elevation of double product indicates an increase in myocardial oxygen consumption.

Histochemical Changes: Increase in motoneuron metabolism and efficient activation with endurance training, pronounced increase in oxidative enzymes, and improved supply of adenosine triphosphate.

Intrathoracic Pressure: Tendency to increase with resistance exercise; intrathoracic pressure limits venous return.

Muscle Fatigue: Failure to maintain a required or expected repetitive force.

Muscle Fiber Changes with Fatigue: Declined force production; reduced relaxation of fatigued muscle. Reduced impulse conduction, decreased electromyographic activity, increased sodium (Na^+), decreased potassium (K^+), reduced phosphocreatine (PCr).

Neuromuscular Fatigue: Acetylcholine is reduced with repetitive activation of motor neuron terminals. May be a contributory factor in local muscle fatigue.

Oxygen Consumption and Circuit Training: Circuit exercise training may increase peak oxygen consumption 4% in men and 8% in women.

Reduced Muscle Fatigue: Partly caused by relative increase in mitochondria, as well as capillary neovascularization from specific high-volume training.

Reducing Acute Cardiovascular Responses to Resistance Exercise: Minimize Valsalva maneuver, reduce or minimize large muscle group exercise; use submaximal repetitions. Avoid near-maximum or maximum resistance.

Stroke Volume: Cardiac output and muscle contraction. There is an acute response, including elevation of both cardiac stroke volume and cardiac output during concentric phase of progressive resistance exercise.

Vascular Changes with Local Muscle Fatigue: Local and diffuse ischemia creates a decrease in force production, which may prolong fatigue.

REFERENCES

1. Astrand PO, Rodahl K: Textbook of Work Physiology, 2nd ed. New York, McGraw-Hill, 1977.
2. Astrand PO: Physical performance as a function of age. *JAMA* 1968;205:105–109.
3. Barnard RJ, Edgerton VR, Peter JB: Effects of exercise of skeletal muscle. I. Biochemical and histochemical properties. *J Appl Physiol* 1970(6);28:762.
4. Borg GAV: Psychophysical bases of perceived exertion. *Med Sci Sports Exerc* 1982;14:377.
5. Burnett CN: Principles of aerobic exercise. In Kisner C, Colby LA, eds. Therapeutic Exercise: Foundations and Techniques, 2nd ed. Philadelphia, FA Davis, 1990.
6. Costill DL, et al: Adaptation in skeletal muscle following strength training. *J Appl Physiol* 1979;46:96–99.
7. Dishman RK, Sallis J, Orenstein D: The determinants of physical activity and exercise. *Public Health Rep* 1985;100:158–180.
8. Fardy PS: Training for aerobic power. In Burke E, ed. Toward an Understanding of Human Performance. New York, Movement Publications, 1977.
9. Fitts RH, Metzger JM: Mechanisms of muscular fatigue. *Med Sport Sci* 1988;27:212–229.
10. Hickson RC: Interference of strength development by simultaneous training for strength and endurance. *Eur J Appl Physiol* 1980;45:255–263.
11. Holloszy JO: Biochemical adaptations to exercise: aerobic metabolism. *Exerc Sport Sci Rev* 1973;1:45–71.
12. Kiessling K: Effects of physical training on ultra structural features in human skeletal muscle. In Pernow B, Saltin B, eds. Muscle Metabolism During Exercise. New York, Plenum Press, 1971.
13. Kraemer WJ, et al: Compatibility of high-intensity and endurance training on hormonal and skeletal muscle adaptations. *J Appl Physiol* 1995;78:376–989.
14. Kraemer WJ: General adaptations to resistance and endurance training programs. In Baechle TR ed. Essentials of Strength Training and Conditioning. Champaign, IL, Human Kinetics Books, 1994.
15. Lamb DR: Physiology of Exercise: Responses and Adaptations. Indianapolis, Macmillan, 1978.
16. Maclaren DPM, et al: A review of metabolic and physiological factors in fatigue. *Exerc Sport Sci Rev* 1989;17:29–66.
17. McCarthy JP, et al: Compatibility of adaptive responses with combining strength and endurance training. *Med Sci Sports Exerc* 1995;27:329–436.
18. Nelson AG, et al: Consequences of combining strength and endurance regimens. *Phys Ther* 1990;70:287–294.
19. Pollock ML: Prescribing exercise for fitness and adherence. In Dishman RK, ed. Exercise Adherence: Its Impact on Public Health. Champaign, IL, Human Kinetics Books, 1988.
20. Pollock ML, Wilmore JH: Exercise in Health and Disease: Evaluation and Prescription for Prevention and Rehabilitation, 2nd ed. Philadelphia, WB Saunders, 1990.
21. Pollock ML, Wilmore JH, Fox III SM: Health and Fitness Through Physical Activity. New York, John Wiley & Sons, 1978.
22. The Recommended Quantity and Quality of Exercise for Developing and Maintaining Cardiorespiratory and Muscular Fitness in Healthy Adults. Position Stand, Indianapolis, American College of Sports Medicine, 1990.
23. Siscovick DS, et al: The incidence of primary cardiac arrest during vigorous exercise. *N Engl J Med* 1984;311:874–877.
24. Stone MH, Conley MS: Bioenergetics. In Baechle TR, ed. Essentials of Strength Training and Conditioning. Champaign, IL, Human Kinetics Books, 1994.
25. Totten L: General physical training for the weightlifter. In United States Weightlifting Federation Coaching Manual, vol 2. Colorado Springs, United States Weightlifting Federation, 1986.
26. Trafimow JH, et al: The effects of quadriceps fatigue on the technique of lifting. *Spine* 1993;18:364–367.

REVIEW QUESTIONS

Multiple Choice

1. Oxidative phosphorylation is capable of producing how many more times the amount of ATP than the anaerobic ATP-PC energy system?
   A. 5
   B. 10
   C. 40
   D. 19
   E. 15

2. The measurement of the efficiency of the aerobic system is called which of the following?
   A. Aerobic efficiency
   B. Vital capacity
   C. Maximum oxygen uptake (VO_2 max)
   D. Cardiovascular fitness

3. The capacity of an aerobic system to perform work is called which of the following?
   A. Aerobic capacity
   B. Cardiovascular fitness
   C. Cardiovascular endurance
   D. Cardiorespiratory fitness
   E. All of the above

4. Which of the following describes the changes that occur as a result of long-term aerobic exercise training? (Circle any that apply.)
   A. Increase in myosin ATPase
   B. Increase in mitochondria
   C. Selective hypertrophy of type II muscle fibers
   D. Blood volume and hemoglobin increased
   E. Atrophy of red muscle fiber

5. Which of the following describes the AAMHR?
   A. 120 − age = MHR
   B. 220 − age = MHR
   C. 220 + age = MHR
   D. 150 + age = MHR

6. The ACSM recommends the following intensity level for aerobic exercise in healthy adults:
   A. 50% to 80% of MHR
   B. 60% to 75% of MHR
   C. 60% to 90% of MHR
   D. 75% to 100% of MHR

7. The Borg scale is used to describe which of the following?
   A. Perceived exertion
   B. Actual, objective aerobic stress
   C. Exercise intensity
   D. None of the above

8. To elicit aerobic fitness a person must train how much?
   A. 2 to 3 days per week
   B. 1 to 3 days per week
   C. 3 to 5 days per week
   D. 2 to 4 days per week

9. To affect physiologic aerobic adaptations, the duration of exercise must be how much?
   A. 5 to 10 minutes
   B. 20 to 60 minutes
   C. 15 to 20 minutes
   D. 10 to 20 minutes

10. Aerobic exercise can be divided into two categories:
    A. Rapid and slow
    B. Long duration and short duration
    C. Continuous and discontinuous
    D. Intense and brief

11. If a patient is recovering from a lower extremity injury (with a cast), which of the following aerobic exercises can be safely employed? (Circle any that apply.)
    A. Underwater treadmill
    B. Single leg stationary cycle ergometer
    C. Stair stepper
    D. UBE
    E. Slide board

12. For patients recovering from an injury to one upper extremity, which of the following aerobic exercise tools is most appropriate? (Circle any that apply.)
    A. One arm UBE
    B. Stationary cycle
    C. Treadmill
    D. Upper extremity slide board
    E. Swimming

13. Aerobic conditioning is an important factor when recovering from injury or surgery of the lumbar spine. Which of the following may be most appropriate in this type of recovery? (Circle any that apply.)
    A. Saddle seat stationary cycle ergometer
    B. Recumbent seat ergometer
    C. Treadmill
    D. Underwater treadmill
    E. Long distance running

True/False
14. Aerobic exercise is ill advised for patients recovering from orthopedic injury or surgery.

Essay Questions
Answer on a separate sheet of paper.
15. Define VO_2 max.
16. List adaptive physiologic changes related to aerobic exercise.
17. Describe the age-adjusted maximum heart rate.
18. Discuss several guidelines for the development of aerobic fitness related to frequency, intensity, duration, and mode of activity.
19. Outline methods of aerobic training.
20. Identify orthopedic considerations during aerobic exercise.
21. Discuss two hypotheses that attempt to clarify peripheral neuromuscular fatigue as a result of prolonged or strenuous muscle activity.
22. Compare endurance training alone with the effects of a combined program of aerobic training and strength training.

Critical Thinking Application
Describe various activities you would recommend to stimulate cardiovascular fitness for a patient recovering from a lower back injury. Design an aerobic fitness program using three different modes of training that would be appropriate for this patient. Which methods would you use to prescribe and measure aerobic exercise? How would you determine the intensity and subsequent progression of the aerobic activities? Describe the frequency, intensity, and duration of cardiovascular exercise you would recommend in this case. How do progressive increases in the intensity of aerobic conditioning affect cardiovascular risk, orthopedic injury, and general exercise compliance? In prescribing aerobic conditioning programs, name 10 adaptive physiologic changes you would hope to affect. By contrast, list three modes of cardiovascular fitness training for a patient with a knee joint replacement. What considerations are there when identifying the most appropriate mode of training for patients with various orthopedic conditions or limitations? Rarely are strength and cardiovascular fitness prescribed independently of one another. Discuss the concept of specificity and the SAID principle and how they relate to the development of strength and aerobic fitness.

7

Balance and Coordination

LEARNING OBJECTIVES

1. Define and contrast balance and coordination.
2. Discuss the mechanoreceptor system and define four mechanoreceptors.
3. List static and dynamic balance and coordination tests and activities.
4. Define proprioception and kinesthetic awareness.
5. Discuss several factors that contribute to balance dysfunction.
6. Identify functional closed kinetic chain proprioceptive exercises.
7. Discuss the rationale for proprioceptive training for the upper extremity.

KEY TERMS

Balance
Coordination
Kinesthesia
Proprioception
Joint displacement
Velocity and amplitude
  of joint motion
Pressure

Stretch and pain
Ruffini mechanoreceptors
Pacinian mechanoreceptors
Free nerve endings
Mechanoreceptor feedback
  system
Afferent neural input
Minitrampoline

Biomechanical ankle
  platform system (BAPS)
Wobble board
Kinesthetic ability training
  (KAT) device
Physioball

CHAPTER OUTLINE

Exercise in Orthopedic Disorders
Definition of Balance and Coordination
  The Mechanoreceptor System
  Balance and Coordination Tests
  Functional Balance Training in Orthopedics
  Specific Balance Tasks in Orthopedics
  Proprioceptive Training for the Upper Extremity

EXERCISE IN ORTHOPEDIC DISORDERS

Rehabilitation after an acute injury, surgery, immobilization, or chronic orthopedic condition must address all the components of normal function. Regaining lost strength, reducing pain and swelling, improving flexibility, enhancing local muscular endurance, and building cardiovascular fitness are obvious and vital areas requiring specific therapeutic interventions. Optimal recovery from orthopedic injury requires normalized sequencing and patterns of movement that produce synchronous, fluid, and stable motor function.

The interdependence of gait, posture, and coordinated functional movements must be restored for complete recovery from injury. Long-term convalescence reduces strength, flexibility, and cardiorespiratory fitness, as well as the vestibular and afferent neural input needed for balance and coordination.

DEFINITION OF BALANCE AND COORDINATION

Balance is "the ability to maintain equilibrium; that is, it is the ability to maintain the center of body mass over the base of support."[6] *Static balance* refers to the ability to maintain posture during nonmovement activities,[10] whereas *dynamic balance* relates to the ability to maintain body mass over the base of support while the body is in motion.[6,10] Balance is one component of **coordination,**[6] which is the ability to perform fine motor skills, tasks requiring postural control, and reciprocal motions such as walking and performing functional activities.[6]

Terms related to balance and coordination are *position sense,* kinesthesia or *kinesthetic sense,* and *proprioception.* Brunnstrom[4] classifies position sense as static balance or "awareness of static position." **Kinesthesia** deals with sensory receptor signals from muscle, tendons, and joints, and relates to an awareness of joint motion.[4] **Proprioception** is the function of joint receptors (sensory and mechanoreceptors) to deliver input concerning joint position, movement, direction, speed, and amplitude.[4]

The Mechanoreceptor System

In addition to muscle spindles and Golgi tendon organs, joints are innervated with various types of specific mechanoreceptors that provide the central nervous system with information concerning **joint displacement, velocity and amplitude of joint motion, pressure,** and **stretch and pain.** Four types of mechanoreceptors have been classified.[8,17] Type I mechanoreceptors, or **Ruffini mechanoreceptors,** respond slowly to static joint position.[17] **Pacinian mechanoreceptors,** type II, adapt very quickly to changes in joint position. These highly sensitive receptors detect ligament tension and

velocity of motion.[13] Type III mechanoreceptors are active at "extremes of joint motion, such as motions that produce joint injury."[12] **Free nerve endings** are type IV mechanoreceptors and transmit information related to pain and inflammation.[12]

The **mechanoreceptor feedback system (afferent neural input)** is vital in regulating adaptive changes related to joint movement and body position.[9]

Balance and Coordination Tests

To prescribe appropriate balance and coordination exercises, it is essential to have data related to present balance and coordination status. Various simple, clinically applicable coordination tests are used to assess a patient's ability to replicate accurate reciprocal motions. Box 7-1 outlines common coordination tests.

Interestingly, balance tests and specific balance treatment activities are rarely separated, with the same movements used for fundamental balance exercises and clinically relevant balance tests. The double-leg stance test (DLST), for example, is a static test first performed with the eyes open. The amount of postural sway and amount of time the patient can maintain static equilibrium are recorded. This very simple test is made more challenging by having the patient maintain balance on

---

BOX 7-1

Coordination Tests

Finger to nose: A reciprocal motion test in which the patient touches the tip of the index finger to the tip of the nose.

Finger opposition: A reciprocal motion test in which the patient alternately touches the tip of each finger with the tip of the thumb.

Fixation-position hold: A static position test in which the arms are held horizontal or the knees extended.

Heel on shin: A reciprocal motion and accuracy test in which the patient is supine and is asked to slide the heel of one leg from the ankle to the knee of the opposite leg.

Pronation-supination: A reciprocal motion test in which the palms are rotated up and down.

Tapping foot or hand: A reciprocal motion test in which the patient is asked to repeatedly tap the ball of one foot while keeping the heel in contact with the floor. With the hand, the patient is asked to tap hand on knee.

Throwing and catching a ball: A reciprocal motion test in which the patient is asked to receive and deliver a ball.

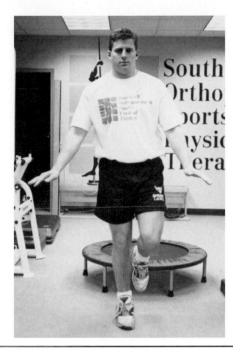

Fig. 7-1   Single-leg stance test.

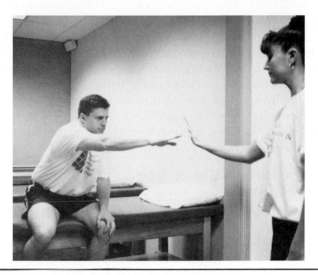

Fig. 7-2   Seated reach test. The clinician offers the patient a target to reach for, which tests the patient's margin of support while seated.

both legs with his or her eyes closed. Obviously this test easily can be used as a static balance training drill, with visual, vestibular, and proprioceptive afferent neural input all contributing to the maintenance of balance.[5] Balance tests frequently call for a progressive battery of specific tasks of incremental difficulty that attempt to eliminate visual input.

Another progressive test also used as an exercise is the single-leg stance test (SLST) (Fig. 7-1). Functionally this test is perhaps more practical to administer because walking, turning, climbing stairs, and so on, all have components of single-leg standing. Progressive training is needed to master single-leg stance equilibrium. The SLST can be made more difficult by asking the patient to close his or her eyes while documenting the degree of postural sway and amount of time equilibrium is maintained, then providing a manual external force to stimulate a quick-balance response.

Another balance test is tandem walking (straight line, heel-to-toe sequencing). This test is graded in distance (feet). The patient is asked to maintain equilibrium for a prescribed distance while walking heel-to-toe, first with the eyes open, then with the eyes closed. In the foam test, the patient is asked to maintain equilibrium while standing on unstable foam padding. First, high-density padding is used to provide a relatively stable, unyielding surface. Then the surface is progressively changed until it is a low-density unstable foam padding, creating a task demanding a high level of balance.

Close observation of the patient's protective reactions during loss of balance is a critical component of all balance tests and training activities. Immediate corrective action by the patient to maintain balance is necessary to move the patient from low-level balance activities to more challenging, complex maneuvers.

Automatic activities, such as catching a ball, can be performed in sequence from a seated to a standing position. The velocity, angle, and direction of throwing the ball to the patient challenge the patient's ability to rapidly move arms and trunk out of a static balance state, and then back to equilibrium.

Other tests use pulley systems and sophisticated computerized machinery. Wolfson and associates[16] designed the postural stress test (PST) to help quantify static balance. This test measures a patient's ability to maintain balance during a series of progressive "graded destabilizing forces."[5] It is clinically cumbersome in that it involves applying a belt to the patient's waist and attaching a weight-pulley system behind the patient. Without the patient's knowledge, a weight is applied to the pulley system, which provides a sudden posterior force necessitating rapid correction of the postural interference. The test is graded on a scale from 0 to 9, with 0 representing a total inability to correct balance, and 9 representing no loss of balance. Sophisticated computer systems such as NeuroCom's Balance Master (Clackamas, OR) manipulate visual, vestibular, and proprioceptive input, specifically, by grading postural sway as the patient stands on a force plate.

The reach test (Fig. 7-2) is a very practical and functional test that determines a patient's ability to perform simple daily tasks. The test can be performed with the patient seated or standing. The patient is offered a target that is slightly out of reach to test the diagonal component of reaching.

Dynamic balance tests require the patient to maintain a base of support, negotiate a single plane or multidirectional movement, and keep the body in motion. Walking in a straight line for a prescribed functional distance (e.g., from a chair to the bathroom) is a simple test to administer. Adding directional changes, such as turning a corner or negotiating a random series of obstacles, provides information concerning the patient's dynamic balance.

Functional Balance Training in Orthopedics

In concert with regaining strength and motion, specific functional tasks must be incorporated into the rehabilitation plan to accentuate muscular coordination, equilibrium, and dynamic stability. Progressive static and dynamic balance exercises exploit the proprioceptive-afferent neural input system to improve static and dynamic task-specific equilibrium. Duncan* has identified several factors that may significantly contribute to balance dysfunction:

a. Perception
b. Behavior
c. Range of motion
d. Biomechanical alignment
e. Weakness
f. Sensory
g. Synergistic organization strategy
h. Coordination
i. Adaptability

Many unique studies[1-3,7,11] have demonstrated how injury, surgery, immobilization, and rehabilitation programs without specific proprioceptive training can have a profound negative effect on joint receptors. One study shows that patients with anterior cruciate ligament injuries suffer from a significantly lower perception of joint position compared with healthy subjects.[2] Other studies report that patients complain of perceived joint instability, weakness, and specific fatigue after rehabilitation programs devoid of balance training.[1,3,11]

It can be concluded from these studies that the physical therapist assistant must clearly recognize that injury, surgery, and non–weight-bearing immobilization negatively affect the proprioceptive feedback system, and that when balance training to improve proprioception is neglected, function is affected and reinjury is likely. Therefore functional balance and coordination training combined with closed kinetic chain (CKC) resistive exercises allows for afferent neural input from peripheral joint mechanoreceptors, which may enhance the perception of joint stability, joint position, and proprioception.

*From Duncan PW: Balance dysfunction: Implications for geriatric and neurological rehabilitation. Course Notes, Nov. 1994, Advanced Educational Seminars, Inc.

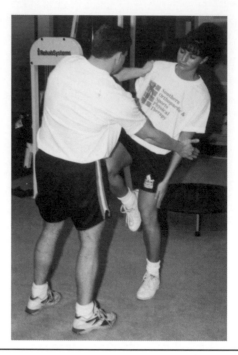

Fig. 7-3 To test and challenge a patient's protective reactions, the clinician can apply a sudden external force while the patient's eyes are closed. Close protection and support must be provided by the clinician during this activity.

Specific Balance Tasks in Orthopedics

In cases of lower extremity injury with long-term, bedbound convalescence, manual resistive hip and knee extension may be appropriate to initiate CKC proprioceptive feedback. Progressive balance training is initiated by vertical weight bearing (double-leg standing) or seated weight bearing. For proper gait mechanics, weight shifting (changing base of support from one leg to another) is critical.

After the patient masters double-leg standing static balance, the physical therapist assistant should begin training the patient to shift balance from one leg to the other. Progressing along an increasingly difficult sequence, the patient can begin single-leg static balance training. Generally the length of time the patient can maintain equilibrium on one leg is recorded. As balance and strength improve, the time the patient is able to maintain equilibrium increases.

Because considerable perceptual awareness is gained by visual input, progressive balance training involves eliminating this sensory input system. Single-leg standing with eyes closed is a challenging task. Progressively more difficult tasks can be initiated in which the clinician applies sudden force to the patient while the patient is standing on one leg with the eyes closed (Fig. 7-3). For teaching and safety purposes, all balance drills should be initiated on the uninvolved limb. As confidence and motor learning progress, the patient then

BOX 7-2

Progressive Balancing Exercises

Seated: Eyes open, eyes closed, manually applied postural stress. Throwing and catching a ball.

Seated: Uneven surface, physioball (Swiss ball). Eyes open, eyes closed.

Standing: Double-leg standing—eyes open, eyes closed, manually applied postural stress, weight shifting

Single-leg standing—eyes open, eyes closed, postural stress

Surface changes: All standing drills can be advanced by changing the inclination and type of surface:
- Concrete
- Carpet (short, dense, thick)
- Asphalt
- Tile (slick), linoleum
- Grass, loose gravel, dirt

Minitrampoline: Double-leg standing—eyes open, eyes closed, hopping

Single-leg standing—eyes open, eyes closed, hopping

Foam padding: Double- and single-leg standing, ambulation, eyes open, eyes closed

Balancing devices: BAPS board, KAT, balance board, seated position, standing position, double-leg and single-leg standing-eyes open, eyes closed

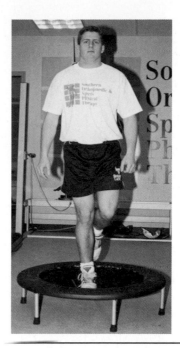

Fig. 7-4 A minitrampoline provides a unique, challenging, and "forgiving" surface to encourage balance and proprioception while hopping or standing.

performs the balance activity on the involved limb. In all cases of balance training, manual support is provided as required.

Static balance drills can be initiated with the patient seated. Similar progressive sequencing can be used, with the patient first attempting to maintain balance with the eyes open, then with the eyes closed. Manually applied external force can be applied while the patient's eyes are closed. Standing or seated, manual postural stress applied in different directions and with varying degrees of force can enhance the patient's ability to "right" or correct balance. Box 7-2 describes various static and dynamic balance activities.

Dynamic balance activities involve progressively challenging tasks that stimulate the patient's ability to safely and accurately negotiate obstacles and make multidirectional changes while in motion. Forward and backward gait, sidestepping (lateral steps), and braiding steps (carioca) are examples of dynamic gait exercises.

Other functional CKC proprioceptive exercises can replicate the specific demands of daily activities or athletic skills. Frequently, progressively demanding tasks are omitted from rehabilitation programs, with

reliance put on increased clinical strength tests, greater range-of-motion grades, and reduced pain and swelling, as objective data leading to discharge from formal therapy. Functional balance drills, such as hopping, increase muscle strength, power, coordination, and balance. Hopping drills can be rather simple vertical leaps or quite challenging combinations of vertical and horizontal patterns. Hopping is useful with an athletic population and can be done on a flat, hard surface or on a **minitrampoline** (Fig. 7-4).

Using the minitrampoline after hip, knee, or ankle injury for static standing balance and for dynamic single-leg or double-leg hopping is unique and challenging for many patients. As with other balance drills, single-leg or double-leg standing or hopping can progress from eyes open to eyes closed. The forgiving, uneven rebound surface of the minitrampoline adds an appropriate challenge for progressive balance training.

Various training devices have been developed to assist with proprioceptive training, including the **biomechanical ankle platform system (BAPS).** The name is misleading because this unit can be used for a wide variety of lower extremity conditions. The generic names for this tool are **wobble board** and balance board (Fig. 7-5). This device is very adaptable, portable, and affordable for many physical therapy environments. Initially, double-leg support progresses to single-leg standing. One of the most challenging balance drills is to perform single-leg standing on a balance board with the eyes closed.

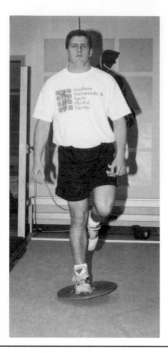

Fig. 7-5 A wobble board or biomechanical ankle platform system board can be used to challenge single- or double-leg proprioception and balance.

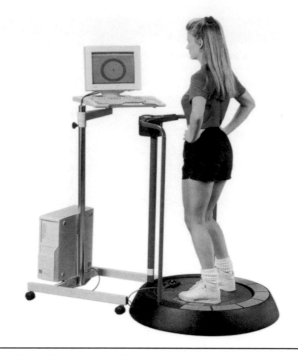

Fig. 7-6 Kinesthetic ability trainer. (Courtesy of Breg, Inc., Vista, CA).

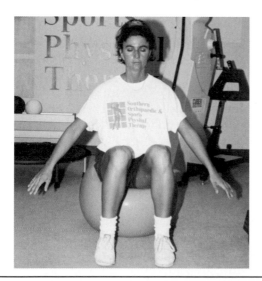

Fig. 7-7 Sitting trunk balance can be progressed using a physioball (Plyoball) to challenge and test a patient's ability to demonstrate protective reactions and appropriate muscular corrective action while seated.

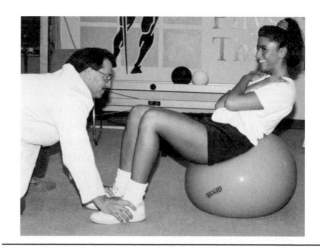

Fig. 7-8 Supported partial direct sit-ups for improving trunk balance and strength on a large diameter physioball (Plyoball).

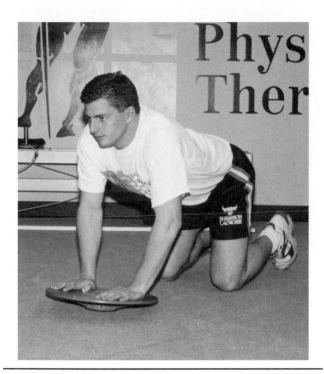

Fig. 7-9 For upper extremity proprioception and balance training, a wobble board can be used; initially, both arms are involved. As the patient gains strength, balance, and confidence, one arm can be used.

Another device used for balance training is the **kinesthetic ability training device (KAT)** (Breg, Vista, CA). This tool is similar to the BAPS board or balance boards. The KAT is unique (Fig. 7-6) in that an air-filled bladder under the standing platform provides various degrees of stability under manual control of the inflation and deflation of the bladder. When the bladder is fully inflated, the balancing surface is stable. As the bladder deflates, the standing surface becomes unstable, requiring greater degrees of balance. Measurements are taken by documenting the pounds-per-square inch (PSI) the patient is able to deflate the bladder while maintaining equilibrium. Specific manual control of incremental degrees of surface stability can be used to document subjective and objective data for patients on a firm stable surface versus a highly random unstable surface.

A rehabilitation protocol rarely suggests a comprehensive, specific sequence in use of each balance activity just described. Generally, drills are initiated and progressed according to the abilities of the patient and the desired goals of the patient and clinician. For example, one patient may progress from double-leg standing to single-leg hopping on a minitrampoline, whereas another patient may progress from single-leg balancing with eyes closed to braiding steps. No particular sequence of balancing is used for every patient.

Often balance training begins with the patient in a seated position, as mentioned. A large **physioball** or Swiss ball can be used as part of a static and dynamic trunk-balancing program (Fig. 7-7). The physioball, which is a rather demanding exercise apparatus, has many applicable and creative uses in balancing and strengthening programs for various orthopedic patients. One very challenging test is the performance of support sit-ups on the physioball (Fig. 7-8). Obviously this particular exercise is for a rather active population, and not for all patients.

Generally, adaptive balance changes and improvements in equilibrium occur with consistent and practiced bouts of CKC, proprioceptive training drills.

Proprioceptive Training for the Upper Extremity

Many household chores involve the repetitive use of the arms and shoulders to lift, pull, and carry. Industrial workers, manual laborers, and assembly line workers all use their arms and shoulders in vigorous weight-bearing positions (weight bearing in these instances refers to overhead lifting, pulling, and climbing maneuvers). Athletes in particular use their arms and shoulders to perform sports skills. Gymnasts require extraordinary flexibility, strength, and glenohumeral stability during demanding upper-body, weight-bearing activities.

As mentioned, injury, surgery, and immobilization lead to significant loss of proprioceptive awareness. Specific proprioceptive exercises have been proposed that, when used in conjunction with proprioceptive neuromuscular facilitation exercises, rhythmic stabilization strengthening exercises, and general range of motion, may contribute to improved proprioception in the upper extremity.[14,15]

The upper extremities can be progressed in much the same way as the lower extremities. Using the balance board, the patient balances with both arms and eyes open (Fig. 7-9). This exercise can be intensified by having the patient use one arm with the eyes closed. The minitrampoline can also be used as a balance training device for upper extremity injuries (Fig. 7-10). The patient begins the exercise using both arms with eyes open and progresses to single-arm balancing with eyes closed. Global stability of the glenohumeral joint can be enhanced effectively with the use of a physioball (Fig. 7-11). The patient begins the progression of this exercise by kneeling in front of the ball and placing both hands on the ball. As the exercise progresses, extraordinary joint stability, strength, and balance are required to maintain equilibrium. Stone and associates[14] proposed these exercises specifically for an athletic population. However, they can be adapted to the general orthopedic population who must rely on dynamic vigorous weight-bearing shoulder and arm activities to accomplish tasks of daily living.

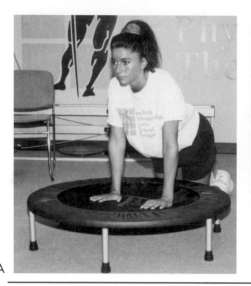
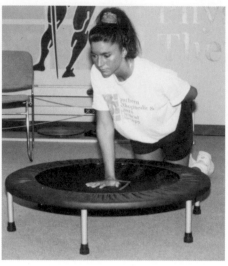

Fig. 7-10 A, The minitrampoline also can be used to encourage closed chain proprioception for the upper extremities. **B,** Progressing this activity will have the patient perform one-arm balancing, push-ups, and hopping maneuvers on the "forgiving" surface of the minitrampoline.

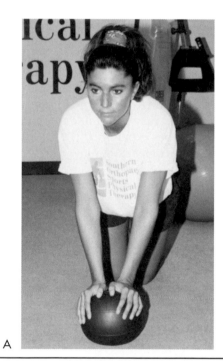
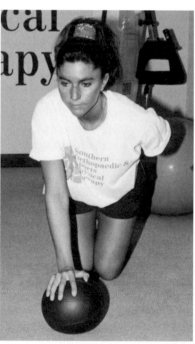

Fig. 7-11 A, A small physioball (Plyoball) also can be used to encourage dynamic closed-chain proprioception for the upper extremities. **B,** Closed-chain, weight-bearing activities can be progressed by having the patient balance and support on one arm on a Plyoball.

❖ ADDITIONAL FEATURES

Afferent Receptors: Five classes—mechanoreceptors, thermoreceptors, nociceptors, chemoreceptors, and electromagnetic receptors.

Balance: The ability to maintain equilibrium with gravity, both statically and dynamically.

Base of Support: The area over which the center of gravity widens or narrows in response to maintain balance in relation to the center of gravity.

Center of Gravity: Anterior to the second sacral vertebra. However, the center of gravity is not constant but varies in location with reference to changes in movement and position.

Coordination: The production of volitional accurate, smooth, purposeful, controlled, dynamic movements.

Mechanoreceptors: Mechanical deformation stimulates free nerve endings, Ruffini endings, Pacinian corpuscles, muscle spindles, and Golgi tendon organs.

Mobility: Complex volitional, high-level gross motor and sophisticated fine motor activity.

Proprioception: Afferent information sense of anatomic location or position. It is either static (proprioception) or dynamic (kinesthesia).

Stability: Bodies that have a wide base of support and a center of gravity that is relatively caudal and is close to the base of support demonstrate the greatest stability. Equilibrium is a form of stability.

REFERENCES

1. Barber SD, Noyes FR, Mangine RE, et al: Quantitative assessment of functional limitations in normal and anterior cruciate ligament-deficient knees. *Clin Orthop* 1990;255:204–214.
2. Barrack R, Skinner H, Buckley S: Proprioception in the anterior cruciate deficient knee. *Am J Sports Med* 1989;17:1–6.
3. Bonamo J, Fay C, Firestone T: The conservative treatment of the anterior cruciate deficient knee, *Am J Sports Med* 1990; 18:618–623.
4. Lemkuhl DL, Smith LK: Brunnstrom's Clinical Kinesiology, 4th ed. Philadelphia, FA Davis, 1983.
5. Chandler JM, Duncan PW, Studenski SA: Balance performance on the postural stress test: comparison of young adults, healthy elderly, and fallers. *Phys Ther* 1990;70:410–415.
6. Crutchfield CA, Shumway-Cook A, Horak FB: Balance and coordination training. In Scully RM, Barnes MR, eds. Physical Therapy. Philadelphia, JB Lippincott, 1989.
7. Freeman MAR, Dean MRE, Hanham WF: The etiology and prevention of functional instability of the foot. *J Bone Joint Surg* 1985;473:678–685.
8. Freeman MAR, Wyke BD: The innervation of the knee joint: an anatomical and histological study. *J Anat Cat* 1967;101:505–532.
9. Gentile A: Skill acquisition: action, movement, and neuromotor processes. In Carr JH, Shepherd RB, Gordon J, eds. Movement Science: Foundations for Physical Therapy in Rehabilitation. Gaithersburg, MD, Aspen Publishers, 1987.
10. Meyer TJ: Coordination. In Review Book for the Physical Therapist Assistant. Herman, MO, Midwest Hi-Tech Publishers, 1993.
11. Noyes F, Barber S, Mooar L: A rationale for assessing sports activity levels and limitations in knee disorders. *Clin Orthop* 1989; 246:238–249.
12. Nyland J: Review of the afferent neural system of the knee and its contribution to motor learning. *J Orthop Sports Phys Ther* 1994; 19:2–11.
13. Schutte M, et al: Neural anatomy of the human anterior cruciate ligament. *J Bone Joint Surg* 1987;69A:243–247.
14. Stone JA, et al: Upper extremity proprioceptive training. *J Ath Train* 1994;29:15–18.
15. Wilk KE, et al: Stretch-shortening drills for the upper extremities: theory and clinical application. *J Orthop Sports Phys Ther* 1993; 17:225–239.
16. Wolfson LI, et al: Stressing the postural response: quantitative method for testing balance. *J Am Geriatr Soc* 1986;34:845–850.
17. Wyke BD: Articular neurology: a review. *Physio Ther* 1972;58:94–99.

REVIEW QUESTIONS

Multiple Choice

1. Proprioception and the mechanoreceptor system provide information concerning which of the following?
   A. Joint displacement
   B. Joint position, direction, and speed
   C. Pressure and stretch
   D. Pain
   E. All of the above

2. Pacinian mechanoreceptors are involved with which of the following:
   A. Pain detection
   B. Muscle tension
   C. Ligament tension and velocity of motion
   D. Vestibular input
   E. All of the above

3. Free nerve endings are type IV mechanoreceptors and are involved with which of the following?
   A. Pain and inflammation
   B. Posture
   C. Muscle stretch
   D. Ligament tension
   E. None of the above

4. Type I mechanoreceptors are called Ruffini mechanoreceptors and are responsible for which of the following:
   A. High-speed position sense
   B. Muscle tension
   C. Static joint position
   D. Direction of joint motion
   E. None of the above

5. A critical safety component to all balance and proprioception activities is the patient's ability to demonstrate which of the following?
   A. Increased ROM
   B. Improved strength
   C. Protective reactions
   D. Faster gait
   E. All of the above

6. A challenging dynamic balance test and activity requires the patient to do which of the following:
   A. Maintain balance with eyes closed while standing
   B. Ambulate and negotiate obstacles
   C. Maintain balance while seated, performing trunk rotation
   D. Maintain balance while seated, performing marching

7. Which of the following factors contributes to balance dysfunction?
   A. Perception
   B. Weakness
   C. Range of motion
   D. Coordination
   E. All of the above

8. Which of the following devices represents challenging tasks to improve balance and proprioception?
   A. KAT
   B. BAPS
   C. Minitrampoline
   D. Wobble board
   E. All of the above

9. Which of the following exercises can be used for closed chain-proprioception activities after upper extremity injuries? (Circle any that apply.)
   A. Push-ups
   B. Minitrampoline
   C. Physioball, or Plyoball
   D. Biceps curls
   E. Pendulum exercises

Short Answer

10. Name two ways to increase the intensity of the double-leg stance test.

11. Studies have demonstrated that many elderly people fall during walking, ascending and descending stairs, and turning. Which activity or test is most appropriate for developing single-leg stance equilibrium?

12. Organize the following balance and proprioception activities from the simplest[1] to the most challenging.[5]

    _____ Double-leg standing-eyes closed

    _____ Standing-weight shifting

    _____ Single-leg standing-eyes closed

    _____ Sitting balance-eyes open

    _____ Single-leg standing-eyes closed with manual resistance

13. List three Plyoball exercises that can be used to increase dynamic trunk balance, proprioception, and strength.

True/False

14. The joint mechanoreceptor system (afferent neural input system) is important in regulating changes related to joint movement and body position.

15. SLST and DLST are examples of balance tests and are never used as treatment activities.

16. High-density foam padding is used for patients to stand and walk on during the final phase of balance training.

17. A high degree of balance is necessary to maintain equilibrium while standing and walking on low-density foam.

18. The reach test shows the patient's ability to reach and challenge the limits or borders of the base of support.

19. Injury, surgery, immobilization, and non–weight-bearing convalescence have a profoundly negative effect on the afferent neural input system.

20. Rehabilitation programs that do not address balance, coordination, and proprioception can result in poor restoration of function and increase the risk of reinjury.

21. Postoperative shoulder patients do not require proprioception exercises because the shoulder is a non–weight-bearing structure.

Essay Questions

Answer on a separate sheet of paper.

22. Define and contrast balance and coordination.
23. Discuss the mechanoreceptor system and define four mechanoreceptors.
24. List static and dynamic balance and coordination tests and activities.
25. Define proprioception and kinesthetic awareness.
26. Discuss several factors that contribute to balance dysfunction.
27. Identify functional closed kinetic chain proprioceptive exercises.
28. Discuss the rationale for proprioceptive training for the upper extremity.

Critical Thinking Application

To test and apply the principles of progressive balance tasks as described, perform the following activity: Stand on one leg with your eyes open. Now close your eyes. What effect does visual input have on static balance? How does the mechanoreceptor system play a role in static and dynamic balance? What happens to a patient's balance and proprioception after major ligament reconstruction of the knee? Outline and describe a specific sequence of progressively challenging and demanding balance and proprioception activities that would stimulate the afferent neural input system after knee ligament reconstructive surgery. Discuss how range of motion, weakness, and sensory input all contribute to balance dysfunction. Describe the goals of closed chain proprioception activities after injury or surgery to the upper extremity. Analyze why proprioception activities are encouraged for non–weight-bearing structures such as the shoulder, elbow, and wrist. Develop a progressive series of proprioception activities that would follow glenohumeral dislocation.

PART II

REVIEW OF TISSUE HEALING

The physical therapist assistant (PTA) must understand the general healing mechanisms of specific tissues to make sound clinical recommendations, develop a progression of rehabilitation exercises, and readily identify problems associated with immobilization, surgery, or injury. Trauma and immobilization (usually longer than 4 weeks) profoundly affect bone and soft tissues. To understand the events and factors that negatively influence healing, the PTA must be aware of the tissue response to injury, surgery, and immobilization. Different tissues (ligament, tendon, bone, muscle, and cartilage) heal or remodel at different rates.[2]

When beginning therapeutic exercises after ligament surgery, cast removal, or an acute traumatic injury, initial clinical information must include which specific tissues are involved, length of time immobilized, weight-bearing status during immobilization, and which surgical procedure, if any, was performed. These points help the clinician recognize healing constraints of specific tissues, as well as indications and contraindications for modifying therapeutic interventions and functional activities. This section provides information concerning immobilization, stress, exercise, joint protection, inflammation, repair, and remodeling, as well as outlines the clinical foundations for specific exercises and progressions.

Three overlapping, interrelated series of events initiate healing: phase I, the inflammatory response; phase II, the repair sequence; and phase III, connective tissue formation or remodeling (Fig. II-1).[3]

The five cardinal signs of inflammation are: redness, swelling, pain, heat, and loss of function. (These are all present with acute inflammatory reactions.) The acute phase of inflammation lasts 24 to 48 hours, with the entire inflammatory response generally complete after 2 weeks.[3,8]

Immediately after injury, vasoconstriction, stimulated by serotonin,[1,7] limits blood and fluid loss for a few minutes. A platelet plug occludes small vessels surrounding the injury site, blocking the flow of blood and fluids away from the site. Other strong chemical mediators responsible for vascular constriction and later tissue permeability are histamine (permeability), serotonin (vasoconstriction), bradykinin (permeability), and prostaglandins (inflammatory regulation, permeability, and pain) (Fig. II-2).[2]

A principal feature of the inflammatory response to injury is the process of ridding the injured area of tissue debris (autolytic wound débridement). This occurs

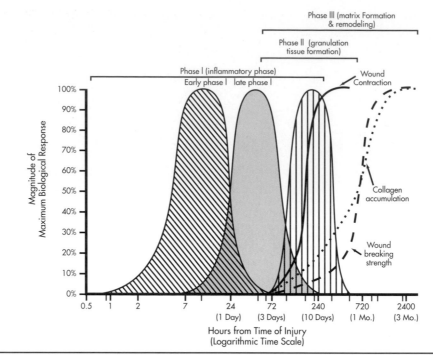

Fig. II-1 The three overlapping phases of wound repair. (From Kloth LC, McCulloch JM, Feedar JA: Wound Healing: Alternatives in Management. Philadelphia, FA Davis, 1990.)

via neutrophils that migrate to the injury site.[3] Other phagocytic cells, macrophages, and lymphocytes help produce enzymes that foster this process.[4]

The repair phase is characterized by fibroplasia, myofibroblast activity, and the organization and production of **collagen** (Fig. II-3).[3] Collagen formation begins about 5 days after injury.[3] Type III immature collagen predominates, providing very limited structural strength to the injury site. The synthesis, orientation, and deposition of new collagen are random, which reduces scar formation strength. After approximately 21 days, the strength of the new collagen is only 20% of its original strength.[5]

Phase III, the remodeling phase, begins about 2 weeks after injury and can last from a few months to as long as a year or more.[1] In remodeling, as the name implies, new collagen and connective tissue gradually reorient along the lines of physical stress imposed on the injured site (Fig. II-4).[1] If tissues are immobilized for prolonged periods, new collagen becomes highly disorganized and is laid down randomly. Active stress or muscular contractions with progressive joint motion promotes longitudinally organized, stronger, more functional collagen arrangements.[1]

Box II-1 outlines basic healing mechanisms.

The inflammatory process

After bleeding is stopped, cellular and vascular responses to the injury are initiated. This is the body's natural damage-control mechanism: it protects the body from foriegn objects at the wound site, cleans the site and brings cells necessary for directing healing in the next stage to the site.

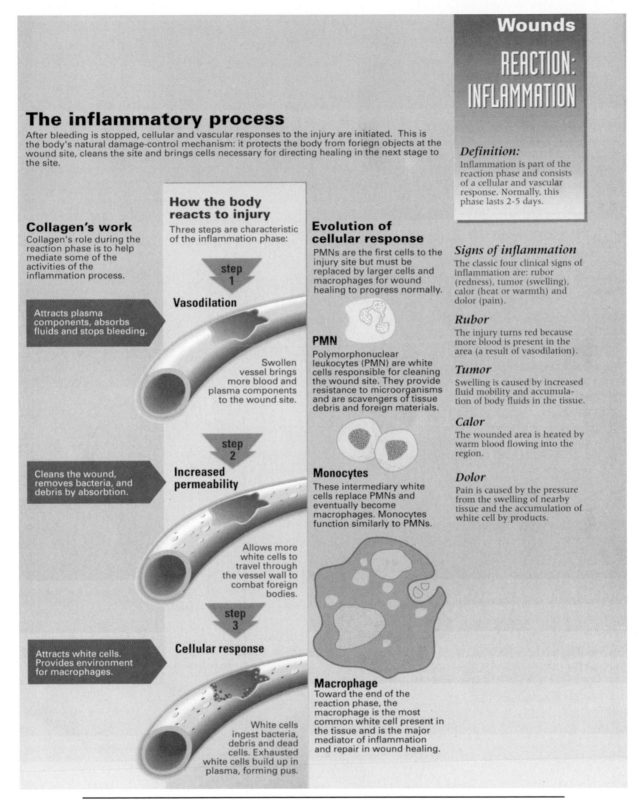

Wounds

REACTION: INFLAMMATION

Definition:
Inflammation is part of the reaction phase and consists of a cellular and vascular response. Normally, this phase lasts 2-5 days.

Collagen's work
Collagen's role during the reaction phase is to help mediate some of the activities of the inflammation process.

Attracts plasma components, absorbs fluids and stops bleeding.

Cleans the wound, removes bacteria, and debris by absorbtion.

Attracts white cells. Provides environment for macrophages.

How the body reacts to injury
Three steps are characteristic of the inflammation phase:

step 1

Vasodilation

Swollen vessel brings more blood and plasma components to the wound site.

step 2

Increased permeability

Allows more white cells to travel through the vessel wall to combat foreign bodies.

step 3

Cellular response

White cells ingest bacteria, debris and dead cells. Exhausted white cells build up in plasma, forming pus.

Evolution of cellular response
PMNs are the first cells to the injury site but must be replaced by larger cells and macrophages for wound healing to progress normally.

PMN
Polymorphonuclear leukocytes (PMN) are white cells responsible for cleaning the wound site. They provide resistance to microorganisms and are scavengers of tissue debris and foreign materials.

Monocytes
These intermediary white cells replace PMNs and eventually become macrophages. Monocytes function similarly to PMNs.

Macrophage
Toward the end of the reaction phase, the macrophage is the most common white cell present in the tissue and is the major mediator of inflammation and repair in wound healing.

Signs of inflammation
The classic four clinical signs of inflammation are: rubor (redness), tumor (swelling), calor (heat or warmth) and dolor (pain).

Rubor
The injury turns red because more blood is present in the area (a result of vasodilation).

Tumor
Swelling is caused by increased fluid mobility and accumulation of body fluids in the tissue.

Calor
The wounded area is heated by warm blood flowing into the region.

Dolor
Pain is caused by the pressure from the swelling of nearby tissue and the accumulation of white cell by products.

Fig. II-2 The inflammatory process and cellular response to injury. (Courtesy of BioCore, Inc., Topeka, KS).

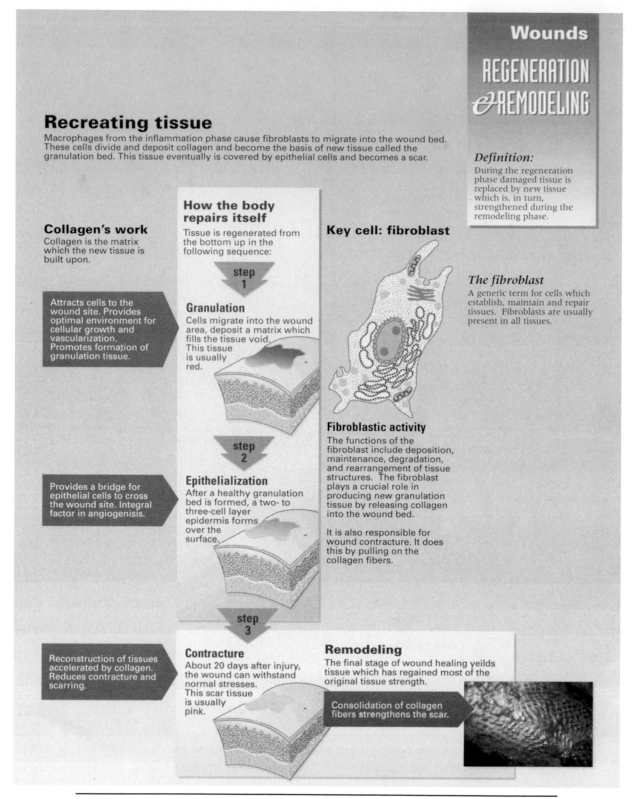

Wounds
REGENERATION *&* REMODELING

Recreating tissue

Macrophages from the inflammation phase cause fibroblasts to migrate into the wound bed. These cells divide and deposit collagen and become the basis of new tissue called the granulation bed. This tissue eventually is covered by epithelial cells and becomes a scar.

Definition:
During the regeneration phase damaged tissue is replaced by new tissue which is, in turn, strengthened during the remodeling phase.

Collagen's work
Collagen is the matrix which the new tissue is built upon.

How the body repairs itself
Tissue is regenerated from the bottom up in the following sequence:

Key cell: fibroblast

The fibroblast
A generic term for cells which establish, maintain and repair tissues. Fibroblasts are usually present in all tissues.

Attracts cells to the wound site. Provides optimal environment for cellular growth and vascularization. Promotes formation of granulation tissue.

step 1

Granulation
Cells migrate into the wound area, deposit a matrix which fills the tissue void. This tissue is usually red.

Fibroblastic activity
The functions of the fibroblast include deposition, maintenance, degradation, and rearrangement of tissue structures. The fibroblast plays a crucial role in producing new granulation tissue by releasing collagen into the wound bed.

It is also responsible for wound contracture. It does this by pulling on the collagen fibers.

Provides a bridge for epithelial cells to cross the wound site. Integral factor in angiogenisis.

step 2

Epithelialization
After a healthy granulation bed is formed, a two- to three-cell layer epidermis forms over the surface.

step 3

Reconstruction of tissues accelerated by collagen. Reduces contracture and scarring.

Contracture
About 20 days after injury, the wound can withstand normal stresses. This scar tissue is usually pink.

Remodeling
The final stage of wound healing yeilds tissue which has regained most of the original tissue strength.

Consolidation of collagen fibers strengthens the scar.

Fig. II-3 Remodeling and regeneration. Collagen and fibroplasia provide key functions that characterize this phase of tissue healing. (Courtesy of BioCore, Inc., Topeka, KS).

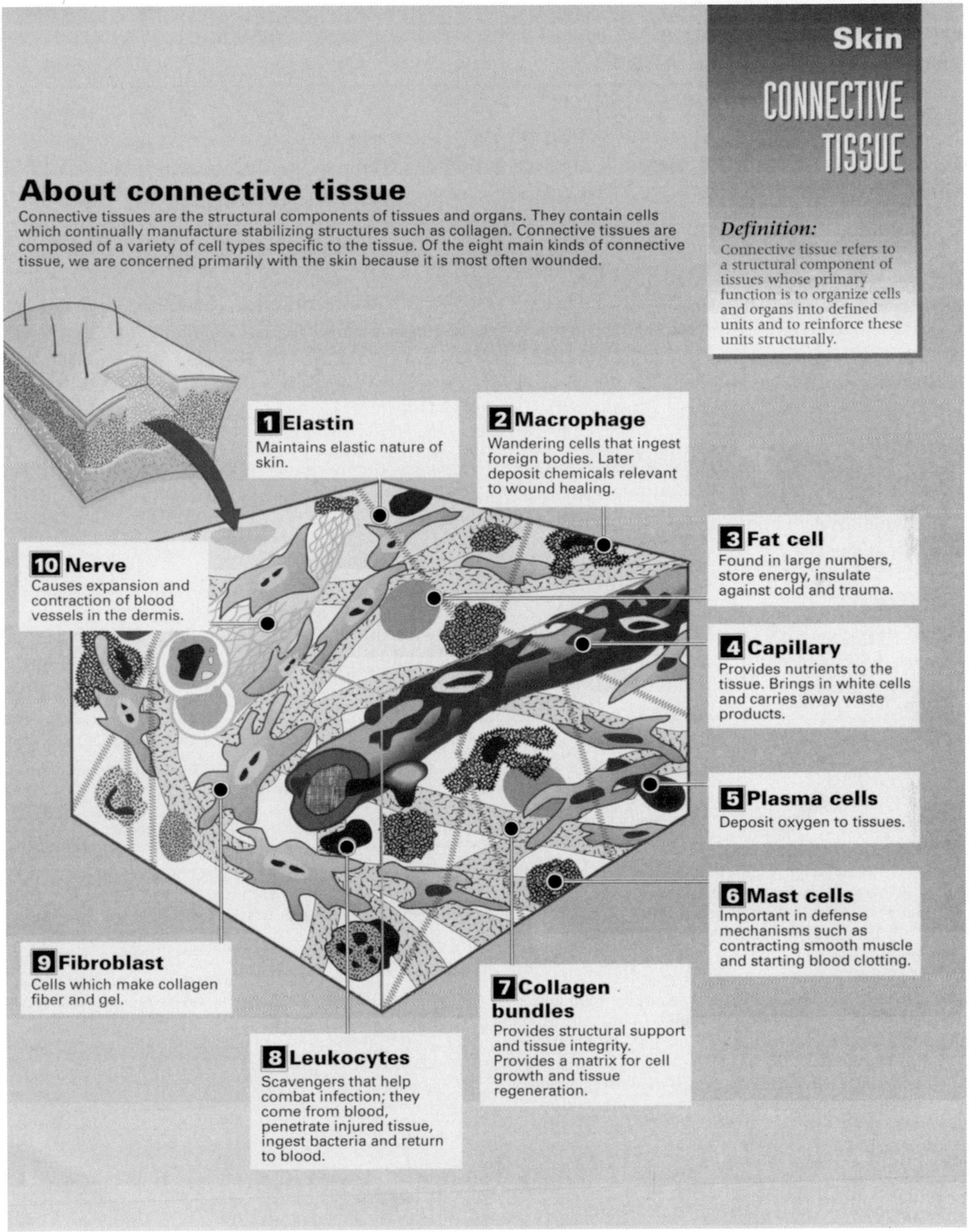

Skin
CONNECTIVE TISSUE

Definition:
Connective tissue refers to a structural component of tissues whose primary function is to organize cells and organs into defined units and to reinforce these units structurally.

About connective tissue

Connective tissues are the structural components of tissues and organs. They contain cells which continually manufacture stabilizing structures such as collagen. Connective tissues are composed of a variety of cell types specific to the tissue. Of the eight main kinds of connective tissue, we are concerned primarily with the skin because it is most often wounded.

1 Elastin
Maintains elastic nature of skin.

2 Macrophage
Wandering cells that ingest foreign bodies. Later deposit chemicals relevant to wound healing.

10 Nerve
Causes expansion and contraction of blood vessels in the dermis.

3 Fat cell
Found in large numbers, store energy, insulate against cold and trauma.

4 Capillary
Provides nutrients to the tissue. Brings in white cells and carries away waste products.

5 Plasma cells
Deposit oxygen to tissues.

6 Mast cells
Important in defense mechanisms such as contracting smooth muscle and starting blood clotting.

9 Fibroblast
Cells which make collagen fiber and gel.

7 Collagen bundles
Provides structural support and tissue integrity. Provides a matrix for cell growth and tissue regeneration.

8 Leukocytes
Scavengers that help combat infection; they come from blood, penetrate injured tissue, ingest bacteria and return to blood.

Fig. II-4   Components of connective tissue. (Courtesy of BioCore, Inc., Topeka, KS).

BOX II-1

Review of Basic Healing Mechanisms

DAYS 2–4

Scar tissue composition: A clot forms in the wound. Connective tissue cells infiltrate the area, with macrophages attracting fibroblasts. In this initial stage of scarring, the tissue is very fragile and easily disrupted because of the predominance of weak and unstable type III collagen. Adhesion is by cellular attachments, and stretching of the scar causes tearing of the cells.

DAYS 5–21

Fibroplasia and contraction: This stage is very cellular. The scar increases in bulk because of fibroplasia, with an increase in the quantity of collagen fibers. This is a highly active stage of collagen synthesis and degradation. Treatment to increase range of motion and function of a joint can be very effective during this stage because of the collagen remodeling process.

DAYS 21–60

Consolidation: The scar contains well-organized collagen. The tissue gradually changes from predominantly cellular to fibrous, with a large amount of collagen fibers. There is a gradual increase in strength of the scar because of an increased stable covalent bonding. During this time, there will be a continuous decrease in the ability of the scar to respond to treatment.

DAYS 60–360

Maturation: Type I collagen fibers are compact and large. The fully mature scar is only 3% cellular and almost totally collagenous. Response to treatment is poor, and hypertrophic and keloid scar tissue increases when stretched in multiple directions.

From Currier D, Nelson R: Mechanisms of connective tissue. In Currier D, Nelson R, eds. Dynamics of Human Biologic Tissues. Philadelphia, FA Davis, 1992.

REFERENCES

1. Bushbacher R: Tissue injury and healing. In Musculoskeletal Disorders: A Practical Guide for Diagnosis and Rehabilitation. Boston, Andover Medical Publishers, 1994.
2. Cummings GS, Tillman LJ: Remodelling of dense connective tissue in normal adult tissues. In Currier DP, Nelson RM, eds. Dynamics of Human Biologic Tissues. Philadelphia, FA Davis, 1992.
3. Kloth LC, Miller KH: The inflammatory response to wounding. In Kloth LC, McCulloch JM, Feedar JA, eds. Wound Healing: Alternatives in Management, Contemporary Perspectives in Rehabilitation. Philadelphia, FA Davis, 1990.
4. Laub R, Huybrechts-Godin G, Peeters-Joris C, et al: Degradation of collagen and proteoglycan by macrophages and fibroblasts ACTA Biochem Biophys 1982;721:425.
5. Levenson SM, et al: The healing of rat skin wounds. *Ann Surg* 1965; 161:293–303.
6. Tillman LJ, Cummings GS: Biologic mechanisms of connective tissue mutability. In Currier DP, Nelson RM, eds. Dynamics of Human Biologic Tissues. Philadelphia, FA Davis, 1992.
7. Vander AJ, Sherman JH, Luciano DS: Human Physiology: The Mechanisms of Body Function, 3rd ed. Minneapolis, McGraw-Hill, 1980.
8. Zarro V: Mechanisms of inflammation and repair. In Michlovitz S, ed. Thermal Agents in Rehabilitation. Philadelphia, FA Davis, 1986.

8

Composition and Function of Connective Tissue

LEARNING OBJECTIVES

1. Outline components of connective tissue.
2. Discuss the sequence of overlapping events of inflammation.
3. Define fibroplasia.
4. Identify the sources of coagulation.
5. Describe and discuss the various cells of inflammation and their function.
6. Discuss the molecular cascade of arachidonic acid metabolic pathways of lipoxygenase and cyclooxygenase.
7. Define cytokines and growth factors, and discuss their various functions.

KEY TERMS

Extracellular matrix
Elastin
Collagen
Proteoglycans
Glycosaminoglycans
Keratan sulfate
Chondroitin sulfate
Hyaluronic acid
Coagulation

Inflammation
Fibroplasia
Remodeling
Cytokines
Smooth endoplasmic
    reticulum
Rough endoplasmic
    reticulum
Golgi apparatus

Lysosomes
Peroxisomes
Polymorphonuclear
    leukocytes
Mononuclear phagocytes
Arachidonic acid
Prostaglandins
Thromboxanes
Leukotrienes

CHAPTER OUTLINE

Review of Tissue Healing
    Coagulation
    Inflammation
    Fibroplasia
    Remodeling and Tissue Maturation
General Cell Types Involved in
        Injury Repair
    Cellular Structure
    Proteoglycans and Glycoproteins

Cells of Inflammation and Repair
    Polymorphonuclear Leukocytes
    Mononuclear Phagocytes
    Fibroblasts
    Prostaglandins, Thromboxanes, and
        Leukotrienes
    Cytokines
General Cell Injury and Repair
General Repair and Regeneration Process

The functions of various connective tissues are to bind cells together to organize and form tissues, organs, and systems and to provide a mechanical link system between musculoskeletal junctions and articulations of joints. Generally, all connective tissues consist of cells with various amounts of **extracellular matrix,** which are produced by the cells. Extracellular matrix is defined as the noncellular components of connective tissue.[3]

Two classic functions of connective tissues are mechanical support for bone and soft tissues, and intercellular exchange of oxygen, blood, water, gases, cells, and wastes.

The basic mechanical support functions of connective tissues (bone, ligament, tendon, muscle, and cartilage)[1] are to provide stability and shock absorption in joints,[2] provide a mechanical link system between bones, and transmit muscle forces.[3]

Intracellular exchange involves relying on circulating blood to supply tissues with nutrients and oxygen, and provide removal of extracellular waste and gases.

The basic aggregate components of extracellular matrix of connective tissues are I-**elastin,** II-**collagen,** III-ground substance, IV-**proteoglycans** and **glycosaminoglycans,** and V-lipids, phospholipids, proteins, and glycoproteins.

Elastin is a noncollagenous glycoprotein whose molecules are arranged randomly as a constituent of extracellular connective tissue matrix. Elastin is found in varying amounts in tissues requiring high levels of physiologic motion (elasticity). Two special amino acids, desmosine and isodesmosine, are found in elastin that are directly responsible for the cross-linking arrangement of elastin fibers and its unique ability to deform under stress then return to its original orientation and shape. Primarily, elastin fibers contain the amino acids glycine, proline, alanine, and valine. Characteristically, elastin fibers can elongate about 70% without undergoing fiber disruption.[3]

In contrast to elastin, collagen is the most abundant component of connective tissue matrix. Various sources identify 12 to 19 distinct types of collagen.[3] Generally, types of collagen are classified according to their structure and tissue distribution. Biochemical properties of connective tissues (ligament, cartilage, tendon, bone, and muscle) are dependent on the specific predominant type of collagen found in the extracellular matrix. The characteristic extensive network of cross-links in collagen significantly contributes to the stability and strength of the extracellular matrix. The basic histochemical profile of collagen includes amino acids of glycine, hydroxyproline, proline, and hydroxylysine. Proline generally is responsible for resisting tensile forces in collagen.[3] Fibroblasts stimulate collagen synthesis through assembly of polypeptide chains of proline and lysine, which aggregate into a triple helix monomer.[3]

Ground substance is an amorphous nonfibrous aqueous–gel component of connective tissue matrix. Generally this substance is responsible for facilitating intercellular exchange of water, oxygen, cells, and gases, as well as providing mechanical support between various tissues.

Proteoglycans are protein and mucopolysaccharide macromolecules subclassified as glycosaminoglycans (GAGs). Generally, GAGs are responsible for the compressive strength of the cartilage matrix. Proteoglycans are extremely hydrophilic, so they attract and bind water. The major and distinct types of GAGs found in cartilage are chondroitin sulfate, **keratan sulfate,** and dermatan sulfate. **Chondroitin sulfate** represents almost 90% of all GAGs in cartilage. These large proteoglycans, specifically chondroitin and keratan, bind together to form a distinct type of GAG referred to as aggrecan. Various types of connective tissues (e.g., ligament, cartilage, tendon, and muscle) contain varying amounts of these large proteoglycans that relate directly to the specific biomechanical and biochemical nature of all connective tissues. The networking capacity of proteoglycans and collagen within all forms and types of connective tissue contributes to the classically distinct nature of strength, stiffness, rigidity, and flexibility of connective tissues.[3] Noncollagenous proteins and glycoproteins are relatively minor constituents in terms of volume in the extracellular matrix of connective tissues. Generally, these molecules function in matrix organization and cell matrix interactions, and help with orientation and maintenance of matrix structure. Two important glycoproteins found in the extracellular matrix are fibronectin and laminin. Fibronectin regulates the spread of cells and has strong chemotactic properties that attract and bind various connective tissue cells. Fibronectin is synthesized by many connective tissue cells, including osteoblasts and may play a role in cell matrix interactions during osteoblast maturation. Laminin is a multifunctional glycoprotein found in the extracellular matrix that is important in establishing epithelial tissue and basement membranes during wound healing.

Lipids represent less than 1% of human articular cartilage matrix. The specific function of lipids and phospholipids is not clearly known. However, the presence of lipids in extracellular connective tissue matrix varies with the onset of osteoarthritis (OA).[3]

REVIEW OF TISSUE HEALING

Healing of biologic tissue is characterized by predictable, orderly, and sequential phases of repair. In essence, healing can be broadly classified in four overlapping series of events: I-**coagulation,** II-**inflammation,** III-**fibroplasia,** and IV-**remodeling** and tissue maturation. All musculoskeletal tissue proceeds to heal and repair by these individually unique processes.

Coagulation

Directly after trauma, platelets migrate to the injury site and release specific growth factors and chemical mediators, which stimulate homeostasis and initiate the repair process. A fibrin scaffold structure is formed within the trauma bed, creating a matrix that allows for platelet aggregation and adherence to the injury site. This process of platelet activation stimulates synthesis of thrombin, fibrin, and the random organization of clot formation. Platelet plug formation is essentially a four-step process: I-adhesion, II-aggregation, III-secretion, and IV-procoagulant activity (Fig. 8-1).

Adhesion of platelets is the deposit of these cells on the subendothelial matrix. Platelets have a surface receptor glycoprotein that binds to a sticky protein substance referred to as von Willebrand factor (vWF) found in the subendothelial matrix. Endothelial cells synthesize vWF, which is released into the circulating plasma, then deposited in the subendothelial matrix in response to exposure from injury.[1]

Aggregation is actually platelet–platelet cohesion from the platelets' surface fibrinogen receptor complex.

Secretion is the release of a number of platelet-derived growth factors (PDGFs) by stimulated platelets. Aggregate stimulators of serotonin, thrombospondin, and thromboxane also are secreted. Procoagulant activity refers to the process of thrombin formation and ensures that coagulation occurs at the site of the platelet plug.

Angiogenic growth factors involved with the stimulation of neovascularization are fibroblast growth factor (FGF), tumor necrosis factor-β (TNF-β), and wound angiogenesis factor (WAF). The end stages of angiogenesis signal vascular capillary and network tube formation, creating new vascular basement membranes that directly communicate with the injury site.[1,3]

Several days (5 to 7) after the injury, the relative population of fibroblasts increases, whereas inflammatory cells and proinflammatory factors decrease. At this stage fibroblasts stimulate PDGF and TGF-β among others to synthesize and deposit extracellular matrix constituents of collagen and glycosaminoglycans.[1,3]

Inflammation

The acute inflammatory process is activated within hours of tissue trauma. This necessary transient initial phase of injury repair lasts approximately 5 to 7 days. The predominant cell types are the **cytokines** (soluble peptide-signaling molecules) that are activated by lymphocytes and monocytes involved with phagocytosis of cellular debris. The intense magnification and amplification of the inflammatory response is mediated by proinflammatory cytokine, interleukin-1 (IL-1), and tumor necrosis factor (TNF). These molecules stimulate vascular permeability and also act to mobilize mononuclear cells to proliferate and differentiate lymphocytes at the injury site.

Regulation of this stage is mediated by macrophages that serve as a rich source of antiinflammatory cytokine growth factors. Platelet-derived growth factor, insulin-like growth factor (IGF), and transforming growth factor-β (TGF-β) help organize the specific sequence of migration of cytokines (neutrophils, macrophages, and then fibroblasts) to the injury site.

Fibroplasia

The proliferation of reparative cells is the hallmark of this stage of injury repair. The general character of this highly vascular stage is the synthesis and proliferation of fibroblastic cells, which form the extracellular matrix constituents of fibronectin, laminin, GAGs, and collagens.

Angiogenesis refers to neovascular budding that helps reestablish oxygen- and growth factor–rich blood to new, fragile healing tissue. Endothelial cells from intact vascular membranes are mobilized to form new tissue from the secretion of specific enzymes and collagens.

Specific connective tissue organization of muscle fibers is systematically arranged by endomysium connective tissue. Muscle fibers collectively are bound together to form fascicles. These fascicles are supported by perimysium connective tissue. The connective tissue membrane surrounding the entire muscle is called epimysium. Muscle tissue is unique in that it consists of contractile elements that respond to stimuli, as well as passive or elastic elements that resist stretching. Muscle tissue and noncontractile connective tissues (endomysium, perimysium, and epimysium) demonstrate characteristic load deformation viscoelastic properties in response to specific stimuli. Human skeletal muscle exhibits the same viscoelastic properties as other dense connective tissues. In fetal development, the connective tissues (endomysium, perimysium, and epimysium) act as tissue scaffolds to hold, support, and provide continuity of gross form and structure of the muscle's belly. In addition, loose connective tissue of the perimysium serves as a channel for nutrient arteries and vessels, as well as nerves that supply the muscle fibers.[3]

As stated, human skeletal muscle connective tissue provides passive resistance to external applied stress, forces, and stretch to dissipate and distribute forces from muscle fibers.

Remodeling and Tissue Maturation

The remodeling phase of injury repair is essentially a balance between enzymatic (proteolytic) degradation of excess collagen and the deposition, organization, modification, and maturation of collagen, as well as a systematic regression of inflammatory cells (Fig. 8-2).

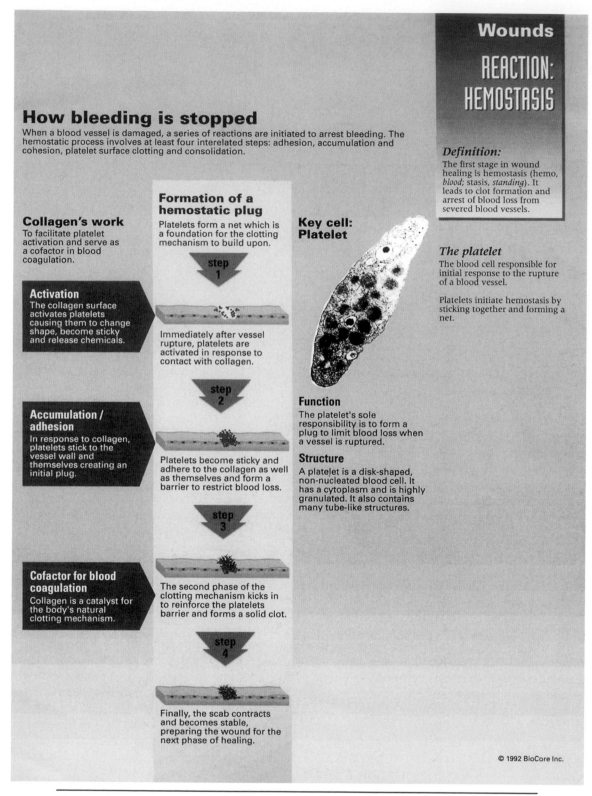

How bleeding is stopped

When a blood vessel is damaged, a series of reactions are initiated to arrest bleeding. The hemostatic process involves at least four interelated steps: adhesion, accumulation and cohesion, platelet surface clotting and consolidation.

Collagen's work
To facilitate platelet activation and serve as a cofactor in blood coagulation.

Formation of a hemostatic plug
Platelets form a net which is a foundation for the clotting mechanism to build upon.

Key cell: Platelet

The platelet
The blood cell responsible for initial response to the rupture of a blood vessel.

Platelets initiate hemostasis by sticking together and forming a net.

Activation
The collagen surface activates platelets causing them to change shape, become sticky and release chemicals.

step 1

Immediately after vessel rupture, platelets are activated in response to contact with collagen.

step 2

Accumulation / adhesion
In response to collagen, platelets stick to the vessel wall and themselves creating an initial plug.

Platelets become sticky and adhere to the collagen as well as themselves and form a barrier to restrict blood loss.

Function
The platelet's sole responsibility is to form a plug to limit blood loss when a vessel is ruptured.

Structure
A platelet is a disk-shaped, non-nucleated blood cell. It has a cytoplasm and is highly granulated. It also contains many tube-like structures.

step 3

Cofactor for blood coagulation
Collagen is a catalyst for the body's natural clotting mechanism.

The second phase of the clotting mechanism kicks in to reinforce the platelets barrier and forms a solid clot.

step 4

Finally, the scab contracts and becomes stable, preparing the wound for the next phase of healing.

Fig. 8-1 Wound hemostasis. (Courtesy of BioCore, Inc., Topeka, KS).

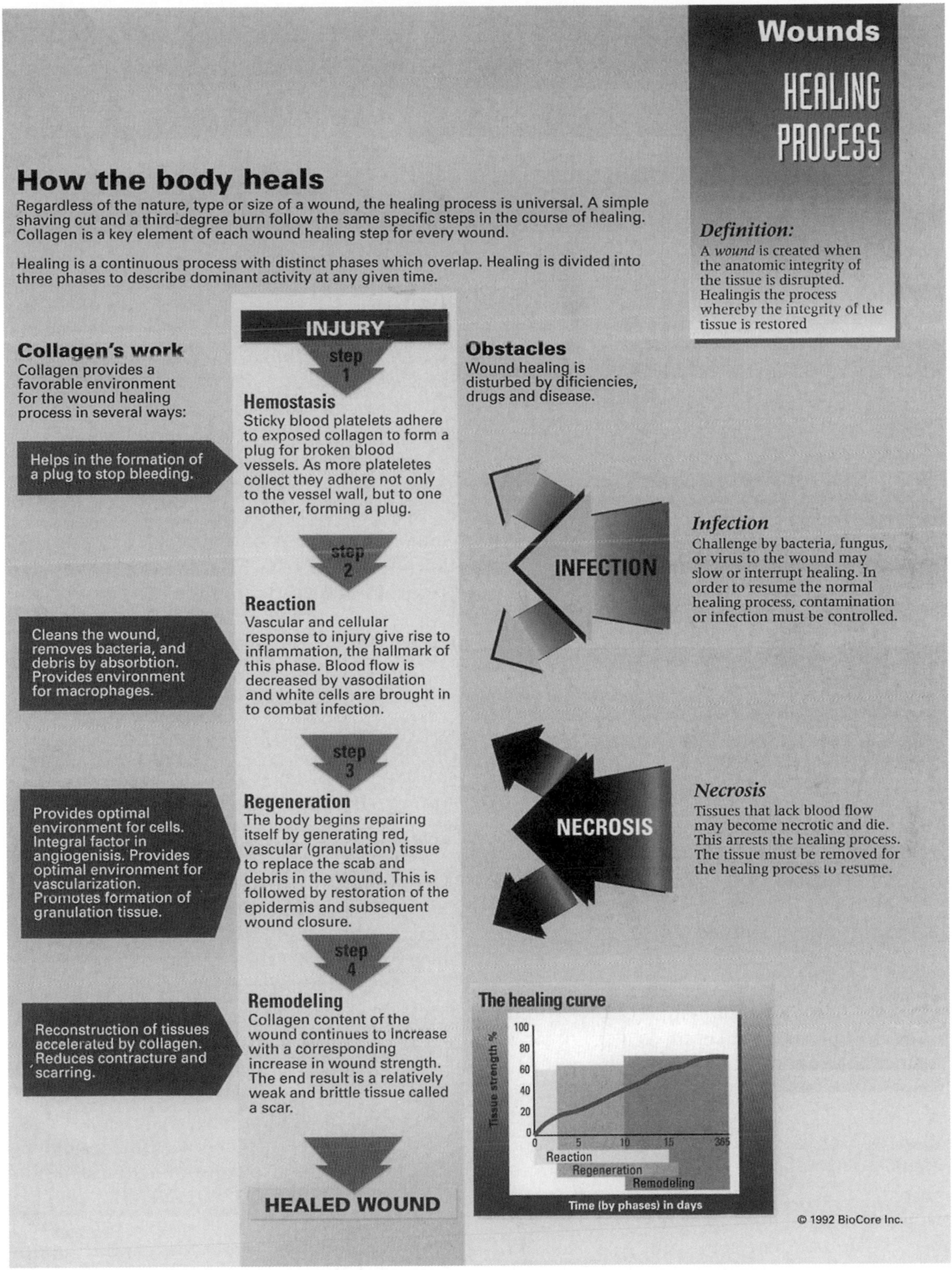

Wounds

HEALING PROCESS

How the body heals

Regardless of the nature, type or size of a wound, the healing process is universal. A simple shaving cut and a third-degree burn follow the same specific steps in the course of healing. Collagen is a key element of each wound healing step for every wound.

Healing is a continuous process with distinct phases which overlap. Healing is divided into three phases to describe dominant activity at any given time.

Definition:
A *wound* is created when the anatomic integrity of the tissue is disrupted. Healing is the process whereby the integrity of the tissue is restored

Collagen's work
Collagen provides a favorable environment for the wound healing process in several ways:

Helps in the formation of a plug to stop bleeding.

Cleans the wound, removes bacteria, and debris by absorbtion. Provides environment for macrophages.

Provides optimal environment for cells. Integral factor in angiogenisis. Provides optimal environment for vascularization. Promotes formation of granulation tissue.

Reconstruction of tissues accelerated by collagen. Reduces contracture and scarring.

INJURY
step 1

Hemostasis
Sticky blood platelets adhere to exposed collagen to form a plug for broken blood vessels. As more plateletes collect they adhere not only to the vessel wall, but to one another, forming a plug.

step 2

Reaction
Vascular and cellular response to injury give rise to inflammation, the hallmark of this phase. Blood flow is decreased by vasodilation and white cells are brought in to combat infection.

step 3

Regeneration
The body begins repairing itself by generating red, vascular (granulation) tissue to replace the scab and debris in the wound. This is followed by restoration of the epidermis and subsequent wound closure.

step 4

Remodeling
Collagen content of the wound continues to increase with a corresponding increase in wound strength. The end result is a relatively weak and brittle tissue called a scar.

HEALED WOUND

Obstacles
Wound healing is disturbed by dificiencies, drugs and disease.

INFECTION

Infection
Challenge by bacteria, fungus, or virus to the wound may slow or interrupt healing. In order to resume the normal healing process, contamination or infection must be controlled.

NECROSIS

Necrosis
Tissues that lack blood flow may become necrotic and die. This arrests the healing process. The tissue must be removed for the healing process to resume.

The healing curve

Tissue strength %
100
80
60
40
20
0
0   5   10   15   365
Reaction
Regeneration
Remodeling
Time (by phases) in days

© 1992 BioCore Inc.

Fig. 8-2 Remodeling and tissue maturation. (Courtesy of BioCore, Inc., Topeka, KS).

Collagenases are enzymes of the metalloproteinase (MMP) family that act to fragment collagen. The regulation of the rate of collagen synthesis and degradation (turnover) is mediated by specific growth factors such as PDGF, IL, TGF-β, and TNF-β.[3]

Cummings and Reynolds[2] describe remodeling as, "the process by which the architecture of connective tissue alters in response to stress. Physiologic loads cause collagen fibers to align parallel to the direction of applied stress, increasing the strength of the scar tissue union. Remodeling simultaneously causes absorption of collagen fibers that lie in other directions. The combined effect of well-controlled remodeling is that the fibrous union becomes simultaneously stronger and suppler with fewer adhesions.

"New scar remodels rapidly because of three properties of the tissue: I-its vascularity, II-the dense cell population of myofibroblasts, and III-the nature of its small, fragile collagen fibers. New collagen fibers are small and randomly aligned, forming a spongy unorganized tissue. As larger, more parallel fibers replace the smaller fibers, they orient across the wound, forming a stronger yet supple union (Fig. 8-3)."[2]

GENERAL CELL TYPES INVOLVED IN INJURY REPAIR

Various cells with complex interactions are involved with tissue homeostasis and injury and repair processes. Generally, cell membranes are "plasma based" with a relatively selective permeable barrier, which promotes bidirectional flow of molecules. Organelles of cells are defined by differences of internal membrane systems. The major components of cellular plasma membranes are proteins and lipids. The major relevant class of cell membrane lipids is phospholipids.

Cellular Structure

Organelles define various component structures within cells. **Smooth endoplasmic reticulum** as a cell organ is involved with the synthesis of steroid hormones, particularly cholesterol. **Rough endoplasmic reticulum** organelles are actively involved with protein synthesis and secretion. Within cells the **Golgi apparatus** functions primarily as a storage and modification organ for various proteins that have been synthesized in the rough endoplasmic reticulum. **Lysosomes** and **peroxisomes** are cellular compartment structures that are involved with enzymatic degradation and oxidation of protein and fatty acids. Mitochondria are actively involved with adenosine triphosphate (ATP) production and protein synthesis.[1]

Proteoglycans and Glycoproteins

Proteoglycans are macromolecules consisting of a protein core and bound polysaccharide units referred to as GAGs. GAGs are major components of ground substance within the extracellular matrix of various connective tissues (ligament, capsule, muscle, tendon, cartilage, nerve, vessel, and bone). GAGs are synthesized in fibroblast cells in connective tissues within the endoplasmic reticulum and Golgi apparatus. Several GAGs are identified in musculoskeletal tissues, which significantly contribute to structure, composition, and function of the extracellular matrix (ECM) of tissues: I-chondroitin sulfate, II-dermatan sulfate, III-keratan sulfate, IV-hyaluronate, V-aggregen, VI-decorin, and VII-biglycan.[1]

Generally, GAGs carry a high negative charge that renders GAGs hydrophilic. Within articular cartilage, proteoglycans (GAGs) are continuously synthesized (by chondrocytes), assembled, degraded, and secreted by the ECM to establish a relative homeostatic environment. Enzymatic degradation of GAGs occurs within lysosome organelles of chondrocytes.[1,3]

Glycoproteins are molecules that organize and maintain the structure of the ECM. Fibronectin, laminin, anchorin, and tenacin are glycoproteins and noncollagenous proteins within the ECM of articular cartilage.

CELLS OF INFLAMMATION AND REPAIR

The complex cascade of molecular events during inflammatory arachidonic acid pathways are mediated by cytokine growth factors acting through endocrine (distant cells), paracrine (adjacent cells), or autocrine (same cells) stimulation.

Polymorphonuclear Leukocytes

Granulocytes, when stimulated by cytokine growth factors and colony-stimulating factors (CSF) differentiate into neutrophils, basophils, and eosinophils. In terms of percentage of white blood cells, neutrophils represent 60%, lymphocytes 30%, eosinophils and basophils 5%, and monocytes 5%. Neutrophils are leukocytes that migrate to damaged tissue after mediation and activation of cytokine factors, platelet factor-IV (PF-IV), and TGF-β that are released by platelets. Primary function of neutrophils includes phagocytosis of foreign matter, bacteria, and cellular debris from the damaged tissue site. Neutrophils also contribute to the immune system inflammation process by stimulation, vasodilation, and vascular permeability assisting with transportation and migration of molecules and cytokine growth factor–PDGF propagating events to further minimize intense inflammatory reactions.

Mononuclear Phagocytes

These single-nucleus cells are derived from pluripotent hematopoietic stem cells, which differentiate into monocytes. Circulating monocytes are mobilized to damaged tissue, where they are activated and become

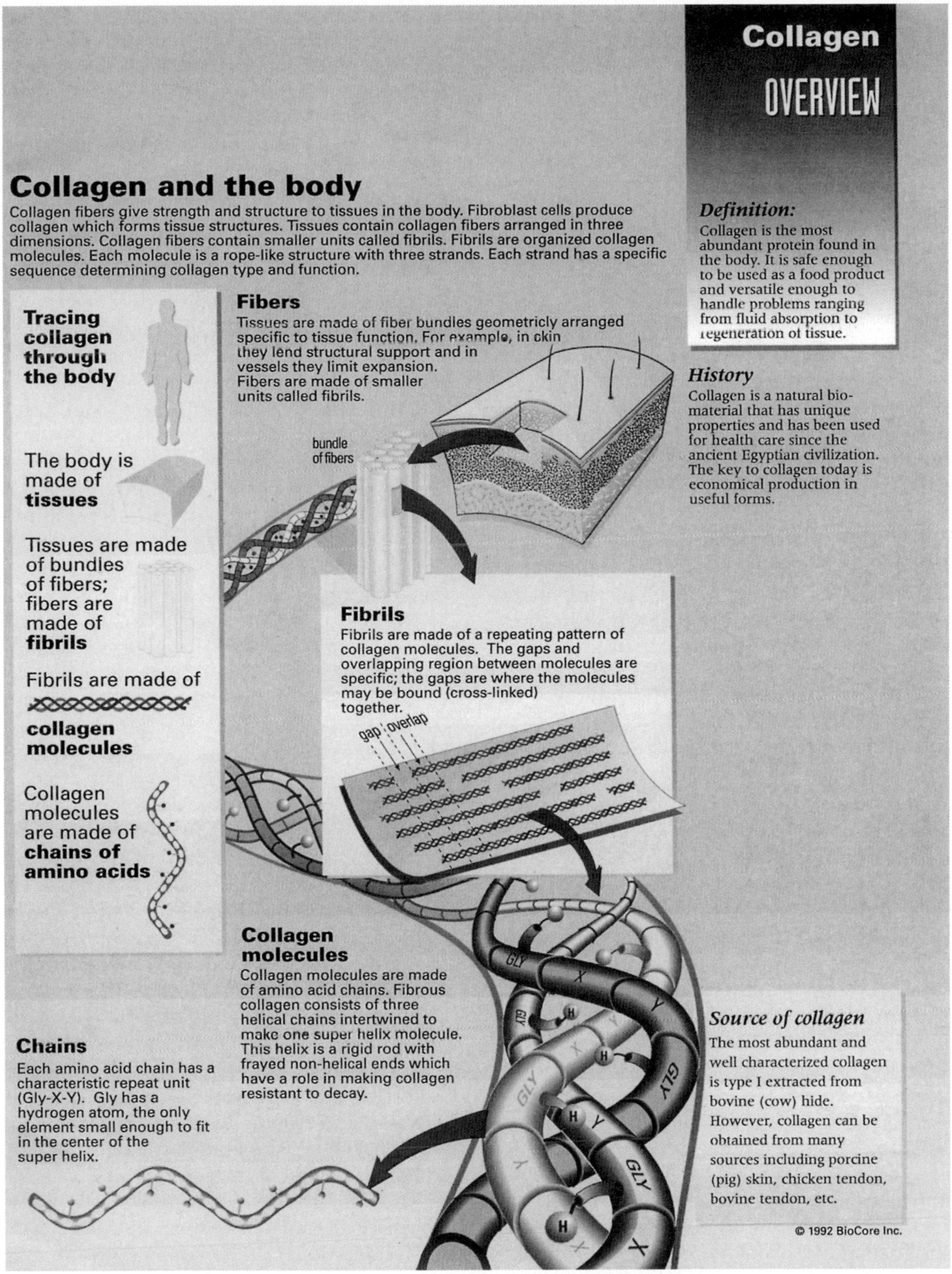

Collagen and the body

Collagen fibers give strength and structure to tissues in the body. Fibroblast cells produce collagen which forms tissue structures. Tissues contain collagen fibers arranged in three dimensions. Collagen fibers contain smaller units called fibrils. Fibrils are organized collagen molecules. Each molecule is a rope-like structure with three strands. Each strand has a specific sequence determining collagen type and function.

Collagen OVERVIEW

Definition:
Collagen is the most abundant protein found in the body. It is safe enough to be used as a food product and versatile enough to handle problems ranging from fluid absorption to regeneration of tissue.

History
Collagen is a natural bio-material that has unique properties and has been used for health care since the ancient Egyptian civilization. The key to collagen today is economical production in useful forms.

Tracing collagen through the body

The body is made of **tissues**

Tissues are made of bundles of fibers; fibers are made of **fibrils**

Fibrils are made of

collagen molecules

Collagen molecules are made of **chains of amino acids**

Fibers

Tissues are made of fiber bundles geometricly arranged specific to tissue function. For example, in skin they lend structural support and in vessels they limit expansion. Fibers are made of smaller units called fibrils.

bundle of fibers

Fibrils

Fibrils are made of a repeating pattern of collagen molecules. The gaps and overlapping region between molecules are specific; the gaps are where the molecules may be bound (cross-linked) together.

gap overlap

Collagen molecules

Collagen molecules are made of amino acid chains. Fibrous collagen consists of three helical chains intertwined to make one super helix molecule. This helix is a rigid rod with frayed non-helical ends which have a role in making collagen resistant to decay.

Chains

Each amino acid chain has a characteristic repeat unit (Gly-X-Y). Gly has a hydrogen atom, the only element small enough to fit in the center of the super helix.

GLY X Y H

Source of collagen
The most abundant and well characterized collagen is type I extracted from bovine (cow) hide. However, collagen can be obtained from many sources including porcine (pig) skin, chicken tendon, bovine tendon, etc.

© 1992 BioCore Inc.

Fig. 8-3 Collagen overview. (Courtesy of BioCore, Inc., Topeka, KS).

macrophages. Noted as "scavenger cells," macrophages display three essential functions during the inflammatory process: I-phagocytosis, II-antigen presentation, and III-production of cytokine growth factors.[1,3]

Macrophages synthesize and secrete numerous cytokines such as TGF-β, PDGF, TGF-α, and IL-1. The release of these cytokines stimulates proliferation of fibroblasts and collagen deposition and degradation of collagen by secreting enzymes (collagenases) also, which denatures collagen during the inflammatory and remodeling phases.[1,3]

Fibroblasts

These important and highly specialized cells are actively involved with collagen production of various stages of injury repair. Fibroblastic cell proliferation is activated by cytokine growth factors released by platelets. PDGF is responsible for the stimulation of fibroblast proliferation. Fibroblasts serve a critical function in wound healing mechanics. Fibronectin is a glycoprotein produced by fibroblasts, which act to bind collagen within the extracellular matrix of healing tissue. Myofibroblasts are specialized contractile cell types that are important during the later stages of wound repair, which requires contraction, remodeling, and maturation of tissue.

Prostaglandins, Thromboxanes, and Leukotrienes

Arachidonic acid metabolism is initiated by the enzymatic degradation of cell membrane phospholipids. Prostaglandins and thromboxanes are lipid-derived powerful and important mediators of inflammatory reactions (Fig. 8-4). Phospholipase-induced cell membrane release of **arachidonic acid**–synthesized cyclooxygenase (COX-1, COX-2) results in metabolic conversion to prostaglandins and thromboxanes. **Prostaglandins** are generally of three forms:[1] I-prostaglandin E_2 (PGE_2) stimulates smooth muscle relaxation and vasodilation; II-prostaglandin I_2 (PGI_2) is synthesized in endothelial cells, and incites vascular dilation and inhibition of platelet adhesion; and III-prostaglandin F_2 (PGF_2) is a potent vasoconstrictor and stimulates smooth muscle contractions. These molecules are capable of producing pain and stimulating synthesis of pain-producing chemicals.[1]

Thromboxanes are synthesized by platelets and are products of the COX pathway along with prostaglandins. These cell-signaling molecules are potent vasoconstrictors and smooth muscle contractors. **Leukotrienes** are products of an alternate arachidonic acid metabolic pathway. In this pathway, lipoxygenase is converted to leukotrienes, which act as smooth muscle contractors; it also stimulates bronchoconstriction and is a strong mediator of other various inflammatory chemicals (chemotactic).[1]

Various pharmacologic agents involved with antiinflammatory action, namely, corticosteroids and non-steroidal antiinflammatory drugs (NSAIDs), target arachidonic acid for the inhibition of prostaglandins, thromboxanes, and leukotrienes. Specifically, corticosteroids inhibit production of arachidonic acid metabolites (cyclooxygenase and lipoxygenase) by inhibiting the conversion of cell membrane phospholipids to arachidonic acid. Conversely, NSAIDs are postarachidonic acid inhibitors of the specific cyclooxygenase (COX-1, COX-2) metabolic pathway.

Cytokines

Cytokines, or growth factors, are a large and complex group (more than 100 identified) of protein-soluble peptide molecules synthesized and secreted by all musculoskeletal tissues, which stimulate and induce cell proliferation, differentiation, and regulation of normal growth, homeostasis, injury, disease, and repair (Table 8-1). Generally referred to as mitogenic, cytokines are powerful and important immunologic mediators that coordinate and amplify various repair processes of injured musculoskeletal tissues.[1]

Cytokines are named for either the biologic effects they perform or the tissue on which they exert action. TNF-α is a proinflammatory cytokine synthesized and secreted by macrophages, lymphocytes, and monocytes. The biologic effects and anatomic target tissues are varied and diverse. General target tissues include stimulation of leukocytes, mononuclear phagocytes, vascular endothelial cells, fibroblasts, chondrocytes, and synovial macrophages. TNF-α activates granulocytes and stimulates other proinflammatory cytokines, which are also important regulators of bone resorption. IL-1 is also proinflammatory cytokine with many isoforms (IL-1-17). Specifically, IL-1 is synthesized by various cells; monocytes and macrophages are major sources. Tissue "targets" include monocytes, synovial macrophages, fibroblasts, chondrocytes, and endothelial cells. Biologically mediated effects include inhibition of ECM synthesis within chondrocytes, stimulation of fibroblast proliferation, proliferation of T cells, and stimulation of other proinflammatory cytokine synthesis. IL-7 is also a proinflammatory growth factor responsible for additional cytokine secretion and stimulation of prostaglandins in epithelial, endothelial, and fibroblastic cells.

TGF-β is a potent immunosuppressive cytokine with strong anabolic activity in cartilage. TGF-β also reduces enzymatic degradation activity specifically within cartilage. In addition, TGF-β promotes wound healing, bone formation, and neovascular activity.[1,3]

IGF regulates many musculoskeletal functions. Generally, IGF stimulates proteoglycan synthesis, chondrocyte proliferation, and osteoblast matrix synthesis. Target cells for neovascularization include platelets and endothelial cells.

PDGF contributes significant stimulation toward the repair process of musculoskeletal and vascular tissue. Cell types activated by PDGF include platelets, neutrophils,

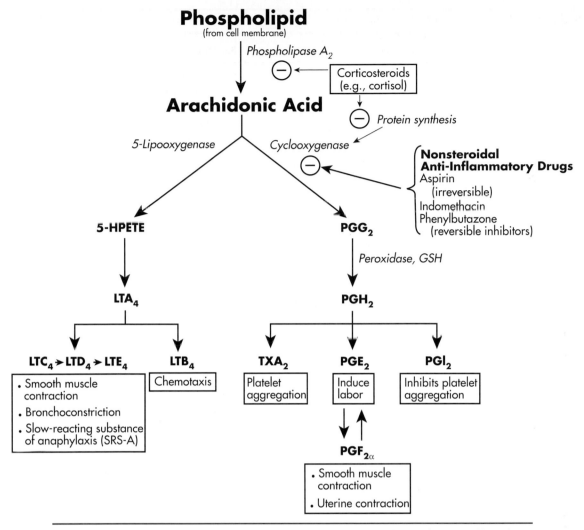

Fig. 8-4 Schematic of prostaglandin and thromboxane synthesis. (From Cell Biology. In *United States Medical Licensing Examination, Step I. The Princeton Review,* 3rd ed. Random House, 2000.)

Table 8-1	*Cytokines*	
Name	**Produced by**	**Function**
Interleukin 1 (IL-1; lymphocyte-activating factor)	Activated mononuclear phagocytes	Similar properties to tumor necrosis factor (TNF)
		Immunoregulatory effects at low concentrations, activation of CD4 cells, and B-cell growth and differentiation
		At high systemic concentrations, causes fever, induces synthesis of acute phase plasma proteins by the liver, and initiates metabolic wasting (cachexia)
IL-2 (T-cell growth factor)	CD4⁺ T cells	Major autocrine growth factor for T cells
		Amount of IL-2 produced by CD4⁺ T cells is a principal factor in determining the strength of an immune response
		Stimulates the growth of NK cells and stimulates their cytolytic function
		Acts on B cells as a growth factor and a stimulus for antibody production

Continued

Table 8-1	Cytokines—cont'd	
Name	Produced by	Function
IL-3 (multilineage colony-stimulating factor)	CD4⁺ T cells	Stimulates growth and differentiation of bone marrow stem cells
IL-4 (B-cell growth factor)	CD4⁺ T cells	Regulates allergic reactions by switching B cells to IgE synthesis and enhancing IgE production
		Inhibits macrophage activation and stimulates CD4⁺ cells
IL-5 (eosinophil differentiation factor)	CD4⁺ T cells and mast cells	Facilitates B-cell growth and differentiation
		Stimulates growth and activation of eosinophils and renders them capable of killing helminths
IL-6 (B-cell differentiation factor/B-cell-stimulating factor II)	Mononuclear phagocytes, vascular endothelial cells, fibroblasts, activated T cells, and other cells	Synthesized in response to IL-1 or TNF
		Serves as a growth factor for activated B cells late in the sequence of B-cell differentiation
		Induces hepatocytes to synthesize acute-phase proteins, such as fibrinogen
IL-7	Bone marrow stromal cells	Facilitates lymphoid stem cell differentiation into progenitor B cells
IL-8 (neutrophil-activating protein 1)	Macrophages and endothelial cells	Powerful chemo-attractant for T cells and neutrophils
IL-10 (cytokine synthesis inhibitory factor)	T cells, activated B cells, macrophages, and some nonlymphocytic cell types (e.g., keratinocytes)	Inhibits T cell-mediated immune inflammation by inhibiting monokine production and inhibiting the accessory functions of macrophages in T-cell activation
		Also inhibits cytokine production and development of T_h-1 cells and drives the system toward a humoral immune response
IL-12	Activated monocytes and B cells	Potent stimulator of NK cells; stimulates the differentiation of CD8⁺ T cells into functionally active CTLs
		Regulates the balance between T_h-1 cells and T_h-2 cells by stimulating the differentiation of naive CD4⁺ T cells to the T_h-1 subset
IL-13	Produced by activated T cells	Has a pleiotropic action on mononuclear phagocytes, neutrophils, and B cells, which produces an anti-inflammatory response and suppresses cell-mediated immunity

macrophages, fibroblasts, and endothelial cells. Biologic activity activated by PDGF includes homeostasis, initiation of wound repair cascade phagocytic activity, synthesis, and deposition of ECM constituents and angiogenesis activity. Vascular endothelial growth factor (VEGF) is an important angiogenic cytokine that stimulates endothelial cell proliferation. VEGF significantly contributes to neovascularization. In addition, VEGF has been identified in the hypertropic zone of calcified cartilage in the epiphyseal plate. VEGF stimulates endothelial cell ingrowth in this area, possibly enhancing cartilage conversion to bone. VEGF also is responsible for the release of degradative enzymes in the ECM. FGF stimulates cell proliferation of cartilage matrix and bone tissue. FGF is also an effective angiogenic stimulant for revascularization after injury. FGF promotes epithelial cell activity during remodeling and neovascular growth.

Overall, tissue disruption and subsequent repair processes initiate and propagate complex cellular events mediated by soluble peptide molecules or cytokines (growth factors). Cytokines regulate, stimulate, and express other growth factors to synthesize, proliferate, excrete, and mobilize numerous molecules involved with ECM deposition, cartilage synthesis, vascular growth, enzymatic degradation, and modulation of inflammatory immune reactions during injury and repair of musculoskeletal and neurovascular repair (Fig. 8-5).[1]

Table 8-1	*Cytokines—cont'd*	
Name	**Produced by**	**Function**
Interferon γ (IFN-γ)	CD4+ T cells, CD8+ T cells, and NK cells	A potent activator of mononuclear phagocytes Facilitates differentiation of T and B cells, activates vascular endothelial cells and neutrophils, stimulates the cytolytic activity of NK cells, up-regulates HLA class I expression, and induces many cell types to express HLA class II molecules
TNF-α	Mainly, macrophages stimulated with bacterial endotoxin but also activated T cells, NK cells, and other cell types	Principal mediator of the host response to gram-negative bacteria At low concentrations, it stimulates leukocytes, mononuclear phagocytes, and vascular endothelial cells At high concentrations, it induces fever, cachexia, and septic shock
TNF-β (lymphotoxin)	Activated T cells	Has similar actions to TNF-α and binds to the same cell surface receptors, although it is usually a locally acting paracrine factor and not a mediator of systemic injury Like TNF-α, a potent activator of neutrophils and an important regulator of acute inflammatory reactions
Transforming growth factor β (TGF-β)	Activated T cells and endotoxin-activated mononuclear phagocytes	Acts as an "anticytokine," which antagonizes many responses of lymphocytes Inhibits T-cell proliferation and maturation and macrophage activation Acts on other cells, such as polymorphonuclear leukocytes and endothelial cells, to counteract the effects of proinflammatory cytokines Promotes wound healing, synthesis of collagens, bone formation, and angiogenesis
Granulocyte-macrophage colony-stimulating factor (GM-CSF)	Produced by activated T cells, activated mononuclear phagocytes, vascular endothelial cells, and fibroblasts	Promotes growth of undifferentiated hermatopoietic cells and activates mature leukocytes Recombinant GM-CSF is administered clinically to promote hermatopoiesis

NK – natural killer; T$_h$ – helper cells; CTL = cytotoxic lyphocyte. (From Cell Biology. In *United States Medical Licensing Examination, Step I. The Princeton Review,* 3rd ed. Random House, 2000;252–253.)

GENERAL CELL INJURY AND REPAIR

Cellular hypertrophy is an adaptive response to a specific applied stimulus when cells and tissues are able to physiologically "cope" with unusual or stressful demands that do not rupture the cell's phospholipid membrane or damage the mitochondria. This situation is essentially a reversible cell injury.[1]

However, cells also can become irreversibly damaged. Hypoxia, caused by ischemia, is the most common cause of irreversible cell injury. Tissue or cellular necrosis refers to the aggregate morphologic changes after irreversible cell injury. When cells are damaged, specific organelles (lysosomes) are involved with autolysis, or "self-killing," leading to tissue necrosis. Cells of the immune system are involved with the process of heterolysis through phagocytosis and degranulation from active circulating T cells. Apoptosis refers to programmed, cellular, organelle, and nuclear disassembly and death. Contrasted with necrosis, in which organelles rupture, cell phospholipid membrane tear from intracellular swelling and inflammatory reaction occurs from cell debris. Apoptosis is somewhat more organized and systematic without inducing an inflammatory response. Apoptosis is an efficient, controlled process of orderly cellular, organelle, and nuclear shrinkage and disassembly of intracellular structures.[1]

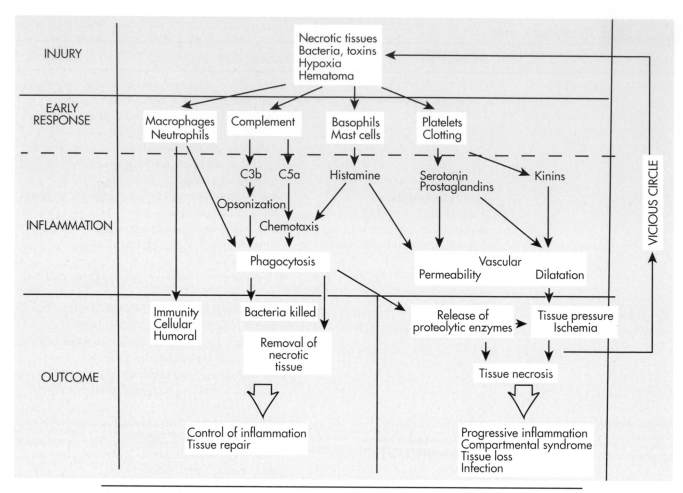

Fig. 8-5 Results of the necrotic process: cellular, hematologic, and immunologic responses to injury lead to repair or further destruction. (From Browner BD, Jupiter J, Levine A, et al: Skeletal Trauma, 2nd ed. Philadelphia, WB Saunders, 1998.)

GENERAL REPAIR AND REGENERATION PROCESS

The term *regeneration* specifically refers to injured tissue being replaced with identical or similar tissue. The process occurs from the activation of various cytokine growth factors that stimulate the synthesis, differentiation, and proliferation of specialized cells that regenerate the damaged tissue. Repair processes involve adaptive scar tissue replacement within the damaged musculoskeletal tissue rather than regenerative similar tissue. Fibroplasia, ECM synthesis, deposition, and collagen formation serve as the foundation for intrinsically repaired tissue.

Specific cells are subclassified according to identified healing characteristics. Labile cells refer to cells that are proliferative and capable of regeneration after injury. Epithelial cells are labile, requiring continued proliferation and regeneration throughout life. Stable cells typically are not continuously regenerating. However, they are capable of regeneration after injury with appropriate stimulation from various cytokines. Permanent cells are

those cells that cannot regenerate after surgery. Permanent cells require fibroplasia, matrix synthesis, and collagen formation with adaptive scar tissue.

✥ ADDITIONAL FEATURES

Cell Apoptosis: Programmed cell death; no inflammation reaction; cell shrinkage with maintenance of organelles.
Cell Necrosis: Cell swelling, loss of organelle structure, rupture of cell membrane, breakdown of cell nucleus, and inflammation.
Connective Tissue, Pathophysiology and Classification of Overuse Injury:
 Grade I—Micro breakdown of noncontractile or contractile tissue, minor soft-tissue inflammatory reaction.
 Grade II—Moderate contractile and connective tissue inflammation.
 Grade III—Severe contractile and connective tissue trauma with periosteal and bone microtrauma.
Connective Tissue, Treatment Strategy:
 Grade I—Connective Tissue Overuse Injury (Transient Pain and Minor Inflammation): Ice, elevation, "active" rest, and general, nonspecific exercises.
 Grade II—Connective Tissue Overuse Injury (Longer Stand-

ing Pain, Moderate Tissue Inflammation): Ice, compression, elevation, "relative" rest, possible NSAIDs, controlled specific exercise, reduce activity 10% to 25%.

Grade III—Connective Tissue Overuse Injury (History of Pain, Reduced Function, and Inflammation Lasting 3 to 4 Weeks, Major Connective Tissue and Contractile Tissue Inflammation): Ice, complete rest, compression, elevation, reduced weight bearing with assistive devices, analgesics (NSAIDS), muscle relaxants, 50% to 75% activity reduction.

Demolition: Inflammation with phagocytosis of cell debris, fibrin, and blood clots.

Ehlers-Danlos Syndrome: Many types of collagen disorders caused by inherited lysine hydroxylation defect.

Glycosaminoglycans: Most common GAGs are hyaluronic acid, chondroitin sulfate, heparan sulfate, dermatan sulfate, and keratan sulfate.

Granulation Tissue: Stimulation, proliferation, and migration of neovascularization and fibroblasts.

Ground Substance: Space between cells and collagen fibers composed of water, salts, and proteoglycans.

Maturation: Process of maturing of granulation tissue to relative avascular fibrous tissue.

Regeneration: Traumatized tissue is replaced by biochemically similar tissues resulting from stimulation, and proliferation of local specialized cells.

Remodeling: Collagen and fibrous tissue organization and orientation to a stable scar.

Repair: Traumatized tissue is replaced with scar.

Systemic Inflammation: Fever caused by acute phase reactants, interleukins and tumor necrosis factor (IL-TNF), action on hypothalamus, thermoregulatory system, hypotension, decreased appetite, and increased sleep.

REFERENCES

1. Cell Biology. In United States Medical Licensing Examination, Step I. The Princeton Review, 3rd ed. New York, Random House, 2000.
2. Cummings GS, Reynolds CA: Principles of soft tissue extensibility of joint contracture management. In Wadsworth C, ed. Strength Conditioning. Applications in Orthopaedics. LaCrosse, WI, APTA, Inc., 1998.
3. Mankin HJ, Mow VC, Buckwalter JA, et al: Articular cartilage structure, composition, and function. In Buckwalter JA, Einhorn TA, Simon SR, eds. Orthopedic Basic Science, Biology, and Biomechanics of the Musculoskeletal System, 2nd ed. Rosemont, IL, American Academy of Orthopedic Surgeons, 2000.

REVIEW QUESTIONS

Multiple Choice

1. The extracellular matrix is defined as which of the following?
   A. Vascular supply of connective tissue
   B. Fibroblasts
   C. Noncellular components of connective tissue
   D. Osteoclasts
2. Elastin fibers can elongate which percentage without undergoing disruption?
   A. 30%
   B. 70%
   C. 90%
   D. 20%
3. The most abundant glycosaminoglycan found in cartilage is which of the following?
   A. Keratan sulfate
   B. Hyaluronic acid
   C. Chondroitin sulfate
   D. Heparin
4. Intense magnification and amplification of the inflammatory response is mediated by which of the following?
   A. von Willebrand factor (vWF)
   B. Insulin-like growth factor (IGF)
   C. Platelet-derived growth factor (PDGF)
   D. Interleukin-1 (IL-1) and tumor necrosis factor (TNF)
5. Which of the following is not an example of a cellular structure or organelle?
   A. Smooth endoplasmic reticulum
   B. Peroxisomes
   C. Leukotrienes
   D. Lysosomes
6. Neutrophils represent what percentage of polymorphonuclear leukocytes?
   A. 10%
   B. 60%
   C. 30%
   D. 90%
7. The cyclooxygenase metabolic pathway of arachidonic acid degradation synthesizes which mediators of inflammation?
   A. Leukotrienes
   B. Thromboxanes only
   C. Prostaglandins and thromboxanes
   D. Prostaglandins only
8. Programmed cellular disassembly, orderly nuclear shrinkage, and controlled cell organelle cell death is referred to as which of the following?
   A. Cell necrosis
   B. Inflammation
   C. Apoptosis
   D. Phagocytosis
9. Labile cell healing characteristics are identified in which cell type?
   A. Skeletal muscle
   B. Epithelial cells
   C. Cardiac muscles
   D. Chondrocytes

Short Answer

10. Healing of biologic tissue is characterized by predictable, orderly, and sequential phases of repair. These phases are broadly classified into four overlapping series of events: coagulation, _____, _____, and remodeling and tissue repair.
11. Angiogenic growth factors involved with the stimulation of neovascularization are _____, _____, and _____.

True/False

12. Elastin is a collagenous proteoglycan.
13. There are essentially three types of collagen found in musculoskeletal tissue.
14. Glycosaminoglycans are responsible for the tensile strength of cartilage matrix.

15. Proteoglycans are hydrophilic.
16. Chondroitin sulfate represents approximately 90% of all glycosamino-glycans in cartilage.
17. Fibroplasia does not represent proliferation of reparative cells.
18. Angiogenesis is synonymous with the term neovascular budding.
19. During coagulation, platelets bind to a sticky protein found in the subendothelial matrix known as von Willebrand factor (vWF).
20. Tissue remodeling is a balance between degradation of excess collagen and the deposition, organization, modification, and maturation of collagen, as well as the systematic regression of inflammatory cells.
21. New collagen fibers are organized and firmly and rigidly attached to damaged and healing tissue.
22. Chondroitin sulfate, dermatan sulfate, keratan sulfate, and hyaluronic acid are examples of GAGs found in musculoskeletal tissues.
23. Prostaglandins and thromboxanes are products of the lipoxygenase metabolic pathway of arachidonic acid metabolism.
24. Nonsteroidal antiinflammatory drugs (NSAIDs) are used to affect the cyclooxygenase pathway of arachidonic acid.
25. Apoptosis is programmed cell death, which results in inflammation.

Essay Questions

Answer on a separate sheet of paper.
26. Discuss two classic functions of connective tissue.
27. Name five basic aggregate components of the extracellular matrix of connective tissue.
28. Identify and discuss the four overlapping series of events that are characteristic of biologic tissue healing.
29. Outline and describe the four organized processes of coagulation.
30. Discuss six cell organelles involved with steroid hormone synthesis, protein synthesis, protein storage and modification, enzymatic degradation and oxidation of protein and fatty acids, and ATP production.

Critical Thinking Application

The patient you are treating in the hospital has a distal femur fracture and quadriceps tendon rupture. The patient demonstrates classic signs of acute inflammatory response secondary to overt musculoskeletal trauma, followed by surgical open reduction and internal fixation of the fracture fragments, as well as soft-tissue surgical repair. In small groups, identify the orderly sequence of intense inflammatory response to injury. Describe the arachidonic acid metabolic pathway and the various other pathways leading to the production of prostaglandins, thromboxanes, and leukotrienes. Identify various cytokines and list the target tissues, cells, and response for each. Outline and describe the fibroplasia phase of repair after soft-tissue injury. In this patient's case, list all of the tissues involved in the repair process (e.g., bone and tendon).

9

Ligament Healing

LEARNING OBJECTIVES

1. Define and discuss the inflammatory response to injury.
2. Describe the phases of healing and sequence of events characteristic of each phase.
3. Identify the five cardinal signs of inflammation.
4. Describe the effects of immobilization on ligaments.
5. Discuss the effects of stress and exercise on ligaments.
6. Identify and discuss practical clinical applications of stress deprivation and protected motion during phases of ligament healing.

KEY TERMS

Inflammatory reaction
Collagen
Ligament

Sprain
Grades of injury
Immobilization

Continuous passive
motion (CPM)

CHAPTER OUTLINE

Ligament Anatomy
Mechanical Properties
Injury and Repair
  Nonsurgical Repair versus Surgical Repair
  Repair versus Nonrepair
  Effects of Immobilization
  Exercise
Effects of Remobilization and Exercise
  Continuous Passive Motion
  Practical Considerations

LIGAMENT ANATOMY

Ligaments are uniformly classified as dense connective tissue. Macroscopic gross examination reveals ligaments to be opaque, white band or cordlike tissue. Ligaments contain primarily type I collagen, fibroblasts, extracellular matrix, and varying amounts of elastin.

Interestingly, certain ligaments (e.g., ligamentum nuchae) contain greater amounts of elastin, which in turn contributes to different mechanical properties than those ligaments with similar amounts of elastin. Although considered hypovascular, ligaments demonstrate relative uniform microvascularity that originates from their origin and insertion sites.[23]

Ligaments have a rich sensory innervation of specialized mechanoreceptors and free nerve endings that contribute to proprioception and pain, respectively. Ligament attachment to bone is by direct or indirect transition. Direct ligament insertion into bone represents a gradual change from specific ligament fiber to fibrocartilage to calcified fibrocartilage to bone. With indirect insertion, the superficial layers of ligament fibers attach directly in the periosteum, whereas the deep fibers transition to bone by way of Sharpey's perforating fibers.[23]

MECHANICAL PROPERTIES

Characteristic behavior of ligament substance (e.g., stress–strain, tensile loading) is directly influenced by collagen composition, proteoglycans, glycosaminoglycans, orientation of fibers, and actions between extracellular matrix and ground substance. It should be recognized that anatomic location of various ligaments (extraarticular versus intraarticular), as well as cellular, histologic, ultrastructural, and biochemical differences strongly influence ligament mechanical and viscoelastic behavior. These unique differences between various ligaments influence intrinsic healing abilities, physical therapy procedures, and surgical intervention.

INJURY AND REPAIR

As with other vascular tissues, extraarticular ligaments heal in a highly structured, organized, and predictable fashion. Generally the sequential cascade of events overlaps four stages of repair.

In contrast, intraarticular ligaments, although demonstrating an intense vascular response to injury, do not heal spontaneously. The environment of intraarticular synovial fluid tends to dilute hematoma formation between the ends of the injured ligaments while preventing fibrin clot organization and ultimately limiting the intrinsic healing mechanism.[23]

The **inflammatory reaction** to trauma represents Phase I of the injury and repair cascade. Initially the injured ends of ligament retract and usually demonstrate a highly disorganized appearance. As the ligamentous microvascularity is disrupted, a hematoma forms between the damaged ends of tissue. Extremely potent chemical mediators of vasodilation, cell wall permeability, and pain are released in response to fibrin clot formation. Prostaglandins, histamine, bradykinins, and serotonin are mobilized to the trauma site to increase capillary permeability and profuse dilation of blood vessels. This action allows migration of specific inflammatory polymorphonuclear cells and lymphocytes to the injured tissue to initiate the action of phagocytosis. The predominant cell types present during the acute inflammatory phase are neutrophils and lymphocytes. Monocytes are referred to as macrophages as they become phagocytes.[23]

The production of type III **collagen,** extracellular matrix, and proteoglycans by fibroblasts initiate the beginning of Phase II matrix and cellular proliferation. Fibroblasts rapidly synthesize new extracellular matrix containing high concentrations of water; glycosaminoglycans; and relatively weak, fragile, and immature type III collagen. Neovascularization (angiogenesis) begins as granulation tissue tenuously attaches to the damaged gap. Gradually the concentration of water, glycosaminoglycans, and type III collagen decreases over several weeks. Inflammatory cytokines are slowly removed from the injured site. Fibroblastic activity synthesizes type I collagen during this highly cellular phase of repair. There is a marked decrease in vascularity within the repair tissue as the collagen concentration increases. Matrix organization continues as the fibrils of type I collagen slowly arrange and align in response to appropriately applied stress. As the density of collagen, elastin, and proteoglycans increase, the tensile properties of repaired tissue also increase.[23]

Remodeling and maturation of intrinsically repaired ligament tissue is a slow process that characteristically lasts a year or more. This Phase III tissue repair process is an overlapping transition from the matrix and cellular proliferation phase of tissue healing. During this final phase, active matrix synthesis decreases while type I collagen content increases toward normal. The hallmark of Phase III remodeling is collagen organization and increases in tensile strength of the repair tissue.

Important consideration must be given to the fact that intrinsically repaired extraarticular ligament does not return to normal biochemically or biomechanically. Even after considerable time and remodeling of dense connective tissue, ultimate tensile strength may approach only 50% to 70% of normal ligaments.[23]

The most common injury of joints are **sprains,** which are injuries involving ligaments. The knee and ankle joints are common areas of ligament sprains, with the incidence of knee ligament sprains, particularly those of the medial collateral ligament (MCL), occurring in as many as 25% to 40% of all knee injuries.[6,17]

Not all ligaments heal at the same rate or to the same degree.[2] For example, the anterior cruciate ligament (ACL) does not appear to heal as well as the MCL of the knee.[21] Factors affecting ligament healing include blood supply and function.[10,21]

Ligaments heal through the three phases of inflammatory response, with Phase I lasting approximately 48 hours after injury; Phase II lasting 48 to 72 hours or more after injury; and Phase III lasting 1 year or more. It is estimated that ligament–tensile strength is only 50% to 70% of its original strength 1 year after injury.[15]

Three key conditions must be present for ligaments to properly remodel or heal:[2]
1. Torn ligament ends must be in contact with each other.
2. Progressive, controlled stress must be applied to the healing tissues to orient scar tissue formation.
3. The ligament must be protected against excessive forces during the remodeling process.

The continuum of the healing process outlined here is ligament specific, and healing is related to blood supply, degree of injury, and mechanical stresses applied to the ligament.[2]

Nonsurgical Repair versus Surgical Repair

Ligaments can be repaired surgically or allowed to heal without surgery, depending on the degree of injury and involvement of supporting tissues. In addition, investigators have shown that untreated ligaments heal by way of scar tissue proliferation rather than true ligament regeneration.[7] Untreated ligament tears are biochemically inferior, possessing a large portion of type III immature collagen, and generally are not healed even at 40 weeks after injury.[7]

The following is a list of **grades of injury** occurring to ligament tissue. They are graded by severity:

Grade I   Microscopic tearing of the ligament without producing joint laxity

Grade II   Tearing of some ligament fibers with moderate laxity

Grade III Complete rupture of the ligament with profound instability and laxity

Grade I and II ligament sprains are most common, with only 15% of all knee ligament sprains classified as grade III.[3] Generally, grade I and II ligament sprains can be treated with protective bracing and comprehensive and progressive rehabilitation with appropriate strengthening to provide dynamic muscular support. With grade I and II ligament sprains of the knee (ACL, MCL, posterior cruciate ligament [PCL], and lateral collateral ligament [LCL]), good to excellent results can be anticipated in 90% of those cases treated nonsurgically.[2]

Surgical repair of a grade III ligament injury frequently involves repair of associated tissues. Cartilage (meniscus) and MCL-, LCL-, or PCL-related injury often is seen with primary ACL grade III injury.

Repair versus Nonrepair

The decision to surgically repair a torn ligament is based on several intrinsic and extrinsic factors. The most clinically relevant example is to contrast the differences between tears of extraarticular MCLs with those of intraarticular (ACL) anterior cruciate ligament tears. Not only must the severity of injury (grade) be considered, but also the anatomic location (biomechanical influences) and vascular supply.

By virtue of its extracapsular anatomy, the MCL provides for a greater periarticular vascular response and the ability to protect the ligament from unwanted forces (e.g., varus, valgus, and internal and external rotation), and allows for an appropriate environment to stimulate healing and propagation of motion, collagen synthesis organization and orientation, proteoglycan concentration, and joint function. Therefore all three distinct grades (grades I, II, and III) of isolated MCL tears appear to heal uneventfully without surgical repair. Even though a fibrous repair gap may exist between torn ends of the ligament, resulting in inferior mechanical resistance to tensile loads, the greater cross-sectional area of the healed ligament provides for biochemical properties (e.g., ultimate tensile load to failure) that more closely resemble injured ligament.[23]

Conversely, the relative pristine environment of the ACL is not conducive to intrinsic repair. In addition, the difficulty of protecting the injured ACL from unwanted deforming forces by using commercial or custom braces contributes to and maintains a high-stress force environment of the ACL that limits healing.

Effects of Immobilization

Immobilization, surgery, injury, and rehabilitation of ligaments must take into consideration not only the healing response of the ligament itself, but also that of the ligament–bone interface. Stress deprivation of the ligament and ligament–bone complexes resulting from prolonged **immobilization** after injury or surgery can have significant and profound negative effects. Joint stiffness after immobilization is related to adhesion formation, active shortening of dense connective tissue (ligament),[2] and decreases in water content. Studies show a gradual deterioration in ligament strength, loss of bone, weakening of cartilage and tendons, significant muscle atrophy, and negative effects on joint mechanics[1] after periods of immobilization (Box 9-1). Immobilization also affects ligament–bone complexes. Studies report that loss of bone directly beneath the junction of ligament and bone reduces the strength of both the insertion site and entire ligament–bone complex.[13]

Rigidly immobilized joints produce chemical and morphologic changes in ligaments 2 and 4 weeks after injury.[8] After 8 weeks of immobilization, ligaments lose 20% of their weight; significant atrophy results, and marked infiltration of connective tissue is

---

BOX 9-1

Effects of Immobilization on Ligament Tissue and Associated Structures

Reduced physiologic motion
Decreased afferent neural input
Muscular atrophy
Ligament shortening
Reduction of water content, proteoglycans and glycosaminoglycans
Bone loss, periosteal bone reabsorption
Articular (hyaline cartilage) erosion
Reduced ligament weight
Reduced ligament size
Reduced ligament strength
Adhesion formation
Increased ligament laxity
Joint stiffness related to synovial membrane adherence

From Kloth LC, McCulloch JM, Feedar JA: Wound Healing: Alternatives in Management. Philadelphia, FA Davis, 1990.

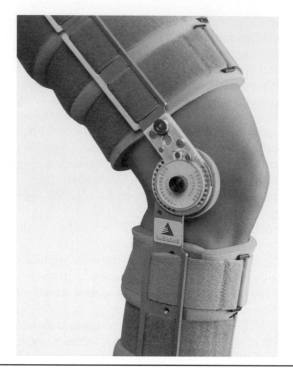

Fig. 9-1 Limited range of motion long leg brace.

observed surrounding the ligament.[8] Although immobilization may be needed to promote healing of damaged tissues, the extended use of rigid cast immobilization should be limited. As an alternative, limited range of motion braces (Fig. 9-1) can be used to protect healing structures and decrease unwanted external forces, as well as allow for progressive motion of involved joints to minimize the negative effects of immobilization.

The biochemical, histochemical, and morphologic changes that occur in ligament and dense connective tissue in response to immobilization are related to the length of time tissues are immobilized. In addition, both structure and mechanical function of ligament substance, as well as ligament–bone insertion complexes (direct insertion and indirect periosteal insertion with Sharpey's perforating fibers), are significantly affected in response to the quality and duration of immobilization.

The effects of immobilization on dense connective tissue have been described by Cummings and Reynolds as follows:

> Following only two weeks of immobilization, animal studies noticed increased GAG synthesis and concentration, decreased water content, thickening of the joint capsule and ligaments, adaptive muscle shortening and adhesion formation of unopposed articular surfaces. After four weeks of immobilization, the biochemical and morphologic changes become more pronounced with a reduction of GAGS, fissures in articular cartilage, a decrease in ligament stiffness, and capsular remodeling. After six weeks of immobilization,

joint mobility becomes significantly limited with thickening noted in the joint capsule, ligaments, and cartilage and decreased ligamentous compliance. In summary, joint immobilization causes a progression of dense connective tissue remodeling, resulting in joint stiffness.[24]

During the first 2 weeks, adaptive muscle shortening appears to be the primary limiting factor in joint mobility. As immobilization extends to 4 weeks, changes in GAGs synthesis and water concentration become more pronounced, resulting in a loss of normal fiber lubrication, spacing, and connective tissue disorganization. As the immobilization period approaches 6 weeks, morphologic and biochemical changes become more evident as the dense connective tissue remodels in a shortened position.[23]

Specifically, immobilization causes more pronounced mechanical and biochemical changes in ligament–bone complex insertion sites compared with ligament substance alone. Generally the area of bone directly beneath the ligament–bone insertion site becomes osteoporotic with osteoclastic activity, resulting in pronounced bone resorption, loss of cortex, and reduced strength of the entire ligament–bone insertion complex.[23]

Exercise

As stated, stress deprivation of ligaments, because of immobilization, results in atrophy.[2,7,8,15,16,21] Conversely, motion, stress, and general physical activity prescribed for healing ligaments produce hypertrophy and increased tensile strength.[2,8] Research shows that ligament and ligament–bone complex strength is related to the type and duration of exercise used during rehabilitation.[2] Tipton[20] has shown that endurance-type exercise is more effective in producing larger diameter collagen than nonendurance-type exercise. In addition, the long-term detrimental effects of prolonged immobilization on ligament–bone insertion sites are reversible.[2] The effects of mobilization and exercise are seen 4 months to 1 year after immobilization.[2]

EFFECTS OF REMOBILIZATION AND EXERCISE

The negative biomechanical, biochemical, and morphologic changes incurred with immobilization generally are reversible. However, there are therapeutically relevant differences between ligament substance and ligament–bone insertion complexes after immobilization.

As stated, ligament substance once injured may regain only 50% to 70% of normal tensile strength after 1 year or more of remodeling.[23] Ligament–bone insertion complexes tend to remodel and regain tensile strength more slowly than ligament tissue after immobilization and therapeutically directed reconditioning.

The clinical significance of delayed ligament–bone insertion healing compared with midsubstance tissue repairs is manifested by the relative increase in avulsion injury during this protracted healing interval.[23]

Generally, ligament substance and ligament–bone complexes are sensitive to exercise. These tissues become stronger depending on the type and duration of exercise prescribed. The orientation, composition, synthesis, and concentration of type III collagen and ultimate load to failure, increase in tensile strength, and stiffness of ligament and ligament–bone complexes are observed with appropriately directed exercise.[23]

It is interesting to note that dense fibrous tissue (e.g., tendon or ligament) not only responds to frequency, intensity, and duration of exercise, but also to the specific type of load applied to the tissue. The structural and biochemical adaptation of dense, fibrous tissue varies according to compressive or tensile loads. Tissues subjected to repeated compressions respond by synthesizing larger and greater amounts of proteoglycans than those tissues exposed to tension loads.

Generally, after injury to ligaments, appropriate controlled motion and exercise stimulates ligament repair by improving matrix organization and composition, increasing the weight of injured ligaments, and promoting normalized collagen synthesis and strength.[23]

Continuous Passive Motion

Motion, exercise, and protected progressive stress can influence and determine the degree and type of healing

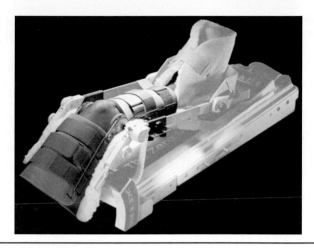

Fig. 9-2 Continuous passive motion machine.

that occur after trauma and subsequent immobilization.[14] Studies have demonstrated that healing is dramatically different in immobilized joints compared with those moved passively through limited motion.[9] Gelberman and colleagues[9] have shown that joints moved passively have well-organized, longitudinally oriented collagen fibers in which no adhesions are present. Conversely, joints that were immobilized demonstrated scar tissue and adhesions.

The concept of early protected motion applied to healing soft tissues has resulted in the development of a technique termed **continuous passive motion (CPM)** (Fig. 9-2). CPM is used in the treatment of the following: knee joint contractures; postoperative ACL reconstructions; joint effusions; knee, elbow, and ankle fratures (after immobilization); joint arthrosis; and total knee arthroplasty.[12] Early motion after surgery or immobilization acts to enhance and facilitate connective tissue strength, size, and shape; evacuate joint hemarthrosis (bloody effusion within the joint space); improve joint nutrition; inhibit adhesions; initiate normal joint kinematics; reduce articular surface changes; and minimize other deleterious effects of prolonged immobilization.[12] Many studies report that the use of CPM can significantly improve joint range of motion, reduce joint swelling, allow patients to ambulate and perform straight leg raises earlier, and promote the healing of hyaline articular cartilage. With postoperative ACL reconstruction, no stretching out of the graft occurs when CPM is used.[4,5,14,18] CPM can be used postoperatively; applied in the operating room; or be done a few days after surgery, immediately upon cast removal, or during the early phases of rehabilitation.

CPM devices have been designed for use on many body parts.[12] The knee is the most common, with the ankle, shoulder, elbow, wrist, hand, and hip joints also benefiting from CPM. The CPM machine is calibrated in cycles per minute and degrees of motion. Progressive increases in the cycle mode and degrees of motion are made gradually so as not to initiate pain or increase the time necessary for healing.

The clinical applications of CPM vary greatly. Protocols range from 24 hours a day for as long as 1 month, to as little as 6 hours a day after surgery. The speed of movement, cycles (rate), and total volume of repetitions depend on patient comfort, surgical procedure, and structures involved. Generally, one cycle (flexion and extension) per minute is well tolerated. The degree of motion should allow for the greatest amount of pain-free or tolerable motion. A reduction is necessary if the degree of motion or speed causes distress; pain inhibits relaxation and causes reflexive muscle guarding or splinting.

CPM usually is used in conjunction with other agents to reduce swelling and pain. Among these are ice packs, oral or intravenous analgesics, antiinflammatory medications, transcutaneous electrical nerve stimulators (TENS), and joint compression bandages.

When not using CPM, the patient performs active and passive range of motion exercises, as well as active assisted exercises to gain motion. Gentle, progressive strengthening exercises, functional electrical stimulation, scar massage, and joint mobilization also are used.

Practical Considerations

The time constraints and healing mechanics of ligaments are well documented.[2,3,7,11,13,15,19,21,22] Careful consideration must be given to the progression of therapeutic exercises and functional activities for patients with ligament injuries. Usually the absence of pain and swelling is an exceedingly poor indicator of healing tissue. With an ACL reconstruction, pain and swelling normally subside within a few weeks, but return of functional joint motion requires a couple of months. Strength values gradually increase, with muscle hypertrophy following slowly.

As the outward clinical signs point to healing, the ligament, being a dynamic tissue, continues to remodel and mature for up to 1 year. Protection of the joint is critical during healing. Functional knee braces with range-limiting devices protect healing ligaments during the various phases of rehabilitation. Initiating progressive resistance exercises after knee ligament injury or surgery, while maintaining joint protection, can be challenging. Placing the resistance (weight) above the joint line during straight leg raises (Fig. 9-3) after ACL surgery can be the first phase of progressive resistance while protecting the healing ligament.

To strengthen hip adduction with an MCL sprain, resistance initially is applied above the joint line so as not to stress the MCL (Fig. 9-4). As the time constraints of healing allow, progressive strengthening of the adductors can involve loading the joint more distally, if joint protection is applied. Awareness of the time necessary for healing and duration of immobilization after

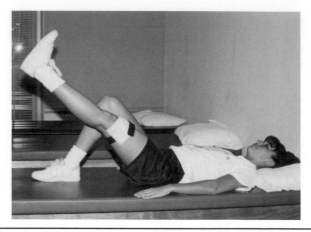

Fig. 9-3 Supine straight leg raises with the resistance placed proximal to the knee joint to reduce anterior translatory forces after anterior cruciate ligament reconstructive surgery.

trauma, weight bearing status, and degree of injury guide the physical therapist assistant (PTA) in making clinical recommendations about the progression of exercise and the placement of force during rehabilitation.

Developing a progressive therapeutic exercise and functional activities program with ankle sprains is similarly challenging. Generally a grade II anterior talofibular ligament sprain does not produce significant pain or functional limitations after a few weeks of conservative treatment involving splinting, crutch walking (non–weight bearing progressing to full weight bearing), ice, compression, and elevation. The PTA should protect the ligament for many weeks after injury because the process of ligament healing occurs slowly (Fig. 9-5).

As pain subsides, the patient may begin to stress the injured ligaments too soon. Encouraging weight bearing as soon as tolerated, while protecting the joint, helps to establish normal joint kinematics and gait.

Protecting the ligaments from further stress not only involves external bracing, but also avoidance of motions that place unwanted force on the healing ligaments. For example, the anterior talofibular ligament of the ankle is stressed with plantar flexion and inversion. To protect the ligaments, these two motions should be avoided during the early (postacute) and middle phases of rehabilitation.

Early protected motion is encouraged after ligament injury, repair, or immobilization, but caution should be taken to avoid overstressing the ligament or duplicating motions that place unwanted strain on the ligament too soon after injury. The acute and postacute phases of rehabilitation after ligament injury or repair usually involve pain management techniques, swelling reduction, muscle reeducation (isometric muscle contraction and functional muscle stimulation), CPM, active range of motion, ligament protection devices via range-adjustable bracing, and weight bearing gait maneuvers

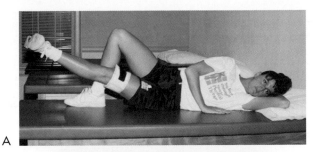

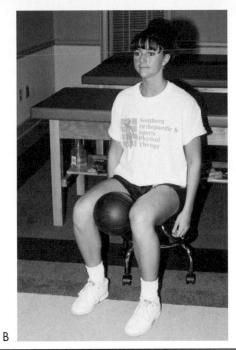

Fig. 9-4　**A,** Side-lying hip adduction exercise with the resistance placed proximal to the knee joint to protect the healing medial collateral ligament. **B,** Isometric hip adduction with the use of a ball placed proximal to the joint line.

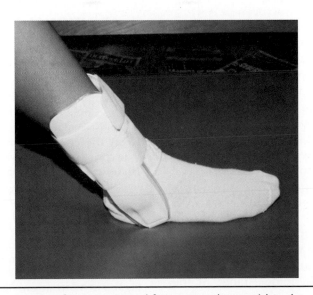

Fig. 9-5　Joint protection from unwanted forces must be considered essential for many weeks after ligament injuries. Air–stirrup brace for lateral ligament complex sprain of the ankle.

Table 9-1	*Therapeutic Considerations During Stages of Ligament Healing*		
DAY 2–4	**DAY 5–21**	**DAY 21–60**	**DAY 60–360**
Acute fibroblast stage. Weak, fragile tissue. Unstable type III collagen.[19]	Highly cellular stage. Scar formation. Active collagen synthesis and remodeling process.	Consolidation. Very gradual changes in collagen strength. Tissue changes from cellular to fibrous.[19]	Maturation.
TREATMENT Rest, ice, compression, elevation, pain management techniques (TENS, Oral-IV analgesics). Non–weight bearing or weight bearing as tolerated. Can initiate CPM *(within limited range of motion)* *Protection of Ligaments* from unwanted stress—usually adjustable range braces or hinged casts. Strict, rigid, long-term cast immobilization should be minimized. Isometric muscle contractions. Contralateral limb exercise as tolerated.	**TREATMENT** Continue RICE. Progressive (CPM). Active-progressive motion. Continued *ligament protection.* Progressive weight bearing. Protected, controlled, active resisted exercise. Cycling (for motion). Isometric exercise progression. Electrical muscle stimulation. Initiate gentle multiangle static holds (isometrics). Avoid excessive motion.	**TREATMENT** Continue RICE as needed. Begin low-load static stretch if needed. Preheating tissues if needed. Continue CPM. Full weight bearing. Isokinetic exercise with continued *ligament protection* with *bracing.* Eccentric isotonic exercise. Progressive concentric isotonic exercise. Hydrotherapy—swimming. Progressive cycling. Initiate closed kinetic chain exercise.	**TREATMENT** Prolonged low-load static stretching. Thermal modalities (heat, US), ice as necessary. Progressive advanced isokinetic and isotonic exercise. Cycling—stairclimbs. Proprioception—balance—coordination exercise. Advanced CKC exercise, progressing to plyometric exercise. Jogging, running, jumping, *maintain joint protection* with functional bracing as needed.

CKC, Closed Kinetic chain; *CPM,* continuous passive motion; *RICE,* rest, ice, compression, elevation; *TENS,* transcutaneous electrical nerve stimulator; *US,* ultrasound.

with crutches as needed. During this early phase of recovery, it is particularly important to avoid excessive motions that may disrupt the intentional scar formation needed for joint stability. The degree of motion, direction of forces, and velocity of joint movement applied during this early postacute phase must be joint specific, functional, and *protected.* For example, with a cruciate ligament sprain, movements that are allowed include knee flexion and extension (within limits), but no rotary or torque-producing motions. After an MCL sprain, knee flexion and extension motion can be initiated in the postacute phase (within limits); however, no valgus stress should be applied. As stated, the reason for ligament protection, maintenance of joint stability, and improved motion is that collagen fiber growth and parallel alignment are stimulated by early tensile loading within the normal physiologic range of the healing ligament.

Table 9-1 outlines the stages of ligament healing and subsequent therapeutic interventions that enhance the healing of ligament tissues.

❖ ADDITIONAL FEATURES

Collagen in Ligaments: Collagen represents 70% to 80% of the dry weight of ligament. Ninety percent of collagen in ligament is type I; about 10% is type III.

Criteria for Ligament Healing: Torn ligament fibers must be in continuity and confined in a well-vascularized soft-tissue bed; control stress to stimulate healing. Continuously protect against inappropriate stress.

Gross Dissection: The ligament is surrounded by loose connective tissue or synovium if the ligament is intraarticular.

Histology and Biochemistry of Ligament Healing: Acute inflammation—Phase I, erythrocytes, cytokines, and other inflammatory cells.

Inflammation: Leukocytes, lymphocytes, monocytes, and macrophages. Active phagocytosis, fibroblasts, and random collagen fibrils produce ECM.

Ligament Gross Morphology: Ligament has a dense, white, hypovascular, homogenous appearance.

Ligament Maturation: This level of healing takes 12 months or longer. Increased ligament contraction and increased tensile strength. Maturation is not achieved before 12 months. After 1 year, ligament tensile strength is between 50% and 70% of normal.

Matrix and Cellular Proliferation: Phase II—neovascular granulation tissue visible at torn ends of ligament at 2 weeks post injury. Fibroblasts are the predominant cell type. Ligament scar is very cellular. There is an increase in collagen content.

Remodeling (Phase III): Decreasing fibroblasts and macrophages. Markedly decreased vascularity and increased density of collagen, with improved alignment.

Remodeling and Maturation (Phases III and IV): Decreased cellularity; water content declines toward normal; collagen concentration and proportion of type III to I declines toward normal.

Summary of Ligament Biochemistry: Dense, regular connective tissue, cells, water, collagen, proteoglycans, fibronectin, elastin.

REFERENCES

1. Akeson WH: An experimental study of joint stiffness. *J Bone Joint Surg* 1961;43A:1,022–1,034.
2. Andriacchi T, et al: Ligament: injury and repair. In Woo SL-Y, Buckwalter J, eds. Injury and Repair of the Musculoskeletal Soft Tissues. Rosemont, IL, American Academy of Orthopaedic Surgeons, 1988.
3. Buschbacher R: Tissue injury and healing. In Musculoskeletal Disorders: A Practical Guide for Diagnosis and Rehabilitation. Boston, Andover Medical Publishers, 1994.
4. Coutts RD, Toth C, Kaita JH: The role of continuous passive motion in the rehabilitation of the total knee patient. In Hungerford DS, Krackow KA, Kenna RV, eds. Total Knee Arthroplasty: A Comprehensive Approach. Baltimore, Williams & Wilkins, 1984.
5. Davis D: Continuous passive motion for total knee arthroplasty. *Phys Ther* 1984;64:709.
6. DeHaven KE, Lintner DM: Athletic injuries: comparison by age, sport and gender. *Am J Sports Med* 1986;14:218–224.
7. Frank C, et al: Medial collateral healing: a multidisciplinary assessment in rabbits. *Am J Sports Med* 1983;11:379–389.
8. Gamble JG, Edwards CC, Max SR: Enzymatic adaption in ligaments during immobilization. *Am J Sports Med* 1984;12:221–228.
9. Gelberman RH, et al: Flexer tendon healing and restoration of the gliding surface: an ultrastructural study in dogs. *J Bone Joint Surg* 1983;65:70–80.
10. Inoue M, et al: Treatment of the medial collateral ligament I: the importance of anterior cruciate ligament on the varus-valgus knee laxity. *Am J Sports Med* 1987;15:15–21.
11. Kloth LC, Miller KH: The inflammatory response to wounding. In Kloth LC, McCulloch JM, Feedar JA, eds. Wound Healing: Alternatives in Management, Contemporary Perspectives in Rehabilitation. Philadelphia, FA Davis, 1990.
12. McCarthy MR, et al: The clinical use of continuous passive motion in physical therapy. *J Orthop Sports Phys Ther* 1992;15:132–140.
13. Noyes FR, DeLucas JL, Torvik PJ: Biomechanics of anterior cruciate ligament failure: an analysis of strain-rate sensitivity and mechanisms of failure in primates. *J Bone Joint Surg* 1974;56A:236–253.
14. Noyes FR, Mangine RE: Early motion after open arthroscopic anterior cruciate ligament reconstruction. *Am J Sports Med* 1987;15:149–160.
15. Noyes FR, et al: Advances in the understanding of knee ligament injury, repair and rehabilitation. *Med Sci Sports Exerc* 1984;16:427–443.
16. O'Donoghue DH, et al: Repair and reconstruction of the anterior cruciate ligament in dogs: factors influencing long-term results. *J Bone Joint Surg* 1971;53A:710–718.
17. Powell J: 636,000 injuries annually in high school football. *Athl Train* 1987;22:19–22.
18. Salter RB, et al: The effects of continuous passive motion on the healing of articular cartilage defects: an experimental investigation in rabbits. *J Bone Joint Surg* 1975;57A:570–571.
19. Tillman LJ, Cummings GS: Biologic mechanisms of connective tissue mutability. In Currier DP, Nelson RM, eds. Dynamics of Human Biologic Tissues. Philadelphia, FA Davis, 1992.
20. Tipton CM, et al: Influence of exercise on strength of medial collateral knee ligaments of dogs. *Am J Physiol* 1970;218:894–902.
21. Woo SL-Y, et al: New experimental procedures to evaluate the biomechanical properties of healing canine medial collateral ligaments. *J Orthop Res* 1987;5:425–432.
22. Zarro V: Mechanisms of inflammation and repair. In Michlovitz S, ed. Thermal Agents in Rehabilitation. Philadelphia, FA Davis, 1986.
23. Woo SL-Y, An K-N, Frank CB: Anatomy, biology, and biomechanics of tendon and ligament. In Buckwalter JA, Einhorn TA, Simon SR, eds. Orthopedic Basic Science, Biology, and Biomechanics of the Musculoskeletal System, 2nd ed. Rosemont, IL, Amercian Academy of Orthopedic Surgeons, 2000.
24. Cummings GS, Reynolds CA: Principles of soft tissue extensibility and joint contracture management. In Wadsworth C, ed. Strength and Conditioning Applications in Orthopedics. Orthopedic Section. LaCrosse, WI, APTA, Inc., 1998.

REVIEW QUESTIONS

Multiple Choice

1. Which type of collagen is predominantly produced after injury?
   A. Type I
   B. Type III
   C. Type II
   D. Type IV
2. Long-term immobilization allows type III collagen to be which of the following?
   A. Arranged randomly
   B. Produced quickly
   C. Highly organized
   D. Quite strong
3. Active stress, muscular contractions, and joint motion allow collagen to be which of the following?
   A. Organized
   B. Stronger
   C. Functional
   D. All of the above
4. A sprain involves:
   A. Muscle
   B. Tendon
   C. Cartilage
   D. Ligament
   E. All of the above
5. Partial tearing of ligament fibers with resultant moderate joint laxity defines which of the following?
   A. Grade II sprain
   B. Grade I sprain
   C. Grade III sprain
   D. None of the above
6. Which of the following are the most common of all ligament sprain classifications?
   A. Grades II and III
   B. Grades I and II
   C. Grades I and III
   D. Grades I, II, and III equally
7. Untreated ligament tears are which of the following?
   A. Composed primarily of type III collagen
   B. Biochemically inferior to ligaments treated with mobilization

C. Generally not healed even 40 weeks after injury
D. All of the above

8. Stress deprivation to ligaments leads to which of the following? (Circle any that apply.)
    A. Improved healing
    B. Secure collagen formation
    C. Ligament atrophy
    D. Reduced ligament strength
    E. Hypertrophy of ligament tissue

9. Some degree of immobilization generally is necessary to promote ligament healing. However, which of the following methods also is appropriate for ligament healing without promoting the negative effects of immobilization? (Circle any that apply.)
    A. Limited range of motion braces
    B. Gentle, protected motion
    C. Rigid, secure plaster casting for 6 to 8 weeks
    D. Full range of motion closed kinetic chain resistance exercise

10. Motion, stress, and general physical activity for healing ligaments (within defined and prescribed limits that do not adversely affect healing) result in which of the following? (Circle any that apply.)
    A. Reduced ligament weight
    B. Increased tensile strength of the ligament
    C. Arthrofibrosis
    D. Hypertrophy
    E. Random collagen alignment

11. Which type of exercise has been shown to be more effective in producing larger diameter collagen in ligaments?
    A. Isometric
    B. Concentric
    C. Endurance type exercises
    D. Eccentric

12. Studies show that joints that are moved passively (within carefully defined limits of motion that do not adversely affect healing) have which of the following?
    A. More adhesions
    B. More bleeding
    C. Well-organized, longitudinally oriented collagen without adhesions
    D. Reduced ligament strength
    E. None of the above

13. Continuous passive motion (CPM) is used for which of the following conditions?
    A. ACL reconstructions
    B. Total knee arthroplasty
    C. Knee, elbow, and ankle fractures
    D. After long-term immobilization
    E. All of the above

14. The concept of early protected motion after immobilization or surgery is to enhance and facilitate which of the following? (Circle any that apply.)
    A. Muscular strength
    B. Reduced bloody effusion within the joint
    C. Increase connective tissue strength
    D. Inhibit adhesions
    E. Organized collagen alignment

Short Answer

15. Name the three phases of tissue healing.

16. Name the five cardinal signs of inflammation.

17. Organization and production of collagen occur during which phase of healing?

18. For torn ligaments to heal properly, the torn ends must be in _____ to one another. To orient collagen fibers and promote a "functional" scar, _____ must be applied. In addition, after injury or surgery to a ligament, protection against _____ must be strictly enforced.

19. Discuss the rationale for continuing or discontinuing external support as it relates to the healing constraints of ligament tissue after 2 weeks of progressive rehabilitation for a ligament sprain of the ankle.

True/False

20. Ligaments heal through a process of tissue regeneration.
21. Strict, long-term, rigid cast immobilization is necessary to allow for proper ligament healing.
22. The specific type and duration of exercise used during rehabilitation is not related to ligament and ligament–bone complex strength.
23. The long-term detrimental effects of immobilization on ligament and ligament–bone complex are not reversible.
24. Pain is an excellent guide to judge the degree of healing a ligament has achieved.
25. Ligaments may take 1 year or more to remodel and mature after surgery or injury.

Essay Questions

Answer on a separate sheet of paper.

26. Define and discuss the inflammatory response to injury.
27. Describe the phases of healing and the sequence of events characteristic to each phase of healing.
28. Identify the five cardinal signs of inflammation.
29. Describe the effects of immobilization on ligaments.
30. Discuss the effects of stress and exercise on ligaments.
31. Identify and discuss practical clinical applications of stress deprivation and protected motion during phases of ligament healing.

Critical Thinking Application

Develop your own "case study" concerning a patient who has a grade II MCL sprain of the knee. Based on your knowledge of the mechanisms of ligament healing, recommend the application of rehabilitation procedures (immobilization, protected motion, bracing, resistance exercise, aerobic conditioning, proprioception, balance training, etc.) in an orderly sequence consistent with the inflammatory response, repair phase, and remodeling phase of tissue healing. In doing so, ask these questions: How do stress and stress deprivation affect collagen? How long should external bracing or support be considered and why? How does immobilization affect ligament tissue? What does protected motion refer to?

10 Bone Healing

LEARNING OBJECTIVES

1. Identify and describe the phases of bone healing.
2. Discuss the objectives that serve as the foundation of fracture management and bone healing.
3. Define osteoblasts, osteoclasts, and osteocytes.
4. Define and discuss Wolff's law.
5. Discuss stress deprivation, immobilization, and normal physiologic stress as they apply to fracture healing.
6. Define three complications of bone healing.
7. Outline and describe six areas of descriptive organization of classifying fractures.
8. Describe the five types of pediatric fractures defined by Salter-Harris.
9. Define pathologic fractures and list four types.
10. Discuss how osteoporosis affects fractures.
11. Define osteomalacia.
12. List common methods of fracture fixation, fixation devices, and fracture classifications.
13. Discuss clinical applications of rehabilitation techniques used during bone healing.

KEY TERMS

Salter-Harris fractures
Pathologic fractures
Osteoporosis
Osteomalacia
Spongy bone
Compact bone
Cancellous bone
Cortical bone

Osteoblasts
Osteocytes
Osteoclasts
Remodeling
Wolff's law
Piezoelectric effect
Bone callus
Immobilization

Delayed union
Nonunion
Malunion
External fixation devices
Internal fixation devices
Open reduction with
   internal fixation (ORIF)

CHAPTER OUTLINE

Structure and Function
Bone Cells
Types of Bone
Macroscopic Structure of Bone
Bone Architecture
Bone Remodeling
Vascular Supply to Bone
Classifications of Fractures
  Osteoporosis
Components of Bone Healing
Bone Injury and Repair

Phases of Fracture Repair
Process of Bone Healing
Effects of Immobilization on Bone Tissue
Complications
Fracture Fixation: Biology and Biomechanics
External Fixation and Fracture Repair
Bone Fixation Devices
Factors Influencing Bone Healing
Stimulation of Fracture Repair
Clinical Application of Rehabilitation
   Techniques during Bone Healing

Orthopedic conditions involving bone tissue are extremely common ailments treated in physical therapy. Therefore the physical therapist assistant (PTA) must appreciate the organized, dynamic nature of bone healing and must recognize the various methods of treating fractures. As with other tissues and injuries, not all fractures heal the same way or to the same degree;[3] bone healing varies greatly, depending largely on which methods of treatment are used.[13] In general, three basic objectives have been identified that serve as the foundation of fracture management and bone healing:

Fragment reduction: The approximation of bone fragments. It is essential to place the bone fragments in anatomic alignment and apposition.

Maintenance of alignment: Securing fracture fragments over time maintains proper anatomic alignment and promotes healing. External fixation devices, traction, or internal fixation may be used.

Preservation and restoration of function: Rehabilitation after the initial phases of fracture management involves regaining lost mobility, improving muscular strength and function, restoring balance and coordination (proprioception and kinesthetic awareness), and teaching proper gait mechanics (for lower extremity injuries).[3]

STRUCTURE AND FUNCTION

Bone is an intense metabolically active tissue. Chemically complex, bone tissue is approximately 65% mineral and 35% organic matrix. The major organic constituent of bone is type I collagen, representing about 90% of the dry weight of bone.[20] The remaining 10% is composed of noncollagenous matrix proteins, lipids, phospholipids, proteoglycans, and phosphoproteins. The principal inorganic component of bone is a crystalline calcium phosphate hydroxyapatite.[20]

BONE CELLS

There are three types of bone cells. Osteoblasts are functionally distinct cells that form bone matrix (osteoid) and synthesize type I collagen.[20] These cells are unique in that they have a large volume of endoplasmic reticulum, Golgi apparatus, and mitochondria to synthesize collagen and secrete matrix proteins.[20]

Osteocytes actually are osteoblasts that are embedded within newly formed mineralized bone matrix.[20] Chemically, osteocytes differ from osteoblasts in that they demonstrate fewer organelles and a greater nucleus to cytoplasmic ratio.[20] These cells represent approximately 90% of mature skeletal tissue and metabolically function to control extracellular concentrations of calcium and phosphorus.[20]

Osteoclasts are giant cell multinucleated bone resorption cells. Osteoclasts synthesize a specific acid phosphatase enzyme and also produce hydrogen ions, which in turn lower the pH environment.[20] The reduced pH increases the solubility of the crystalline phosphate-hydroxyapatite that functions to remove the organic matrix crystals via acid proteolytic degradation.[20]

TYPES OF BONE

The microscopic organization and classification of bone tissue involves two distinct forms: I-normal, mature lamellar bone and II-weak, fragile, immature woven bone (Fig. 10-1).

Woven bone is structurally immature, embryologically (primary) fragile, and weak with a random disorganized collagen arrangement.[2] This specific type of bone is commonly seen in fracture repair callus, newborns, embryos, bone tumors, and various bone pathologies.[20]

Very early after birth (approximately 2 months to 4 years), woven bone slowly remodels into organized structurally mature lamellar bone. A clinically relevant feature of woven bone is that its specific mechanical behavior is termed *isotropic;* that is, woven bone does not respond to Wolff's law, so its biomechanical reactions to applied forces and stress is similar in all planes.[2] The disorganized arrangement of collagen fibers in woven bone strongly contributes to this unique characteristic (Fig. 10-2).[2]

Lamellar bone refers to mature remodeled woven bone. The collagen arrangement in lamellar bone is highly structured and organized. This gives normal mature lamellar bone anisotropic mechanical properties that are stress oriented, which characteristically respond to Wolff's law.[2]

MACROSCOPIC STRUCTURE OF BONE

Osseous tissue is structurally organized as either cancellous (trabecular bone) or cortical (compact bone). Cancellous bone is located at the metaphysis of long bones, as well as the vertebra and other cuboid bones.[2]

Cortical bone is located in the diaphyseal portion of long bones. The major structural subunit of cortical-compact bone is the osteon. As described by Bostrom, Bosky, Kaufman, and Einhorn,[2] the osteon is a central component of the haversian system:

Haversian bone is the most complex type of cortical bone. It is composed of vascular channels circumferentially surrounded by lamellar bone. This complex arrangement of bone around the vascular channel is called the osteon. The osteon is an irregular, branching and anastomosing cylinder composed of a more or less centrally placed neurovascular canal surrounded by cell permeated layers of bone matrix.[2]

Conversely, trabecular or cancellous bone is uniformly less dense with a large surface area and is significantly metabolically more "active" than cortical bone.[2] In fact,

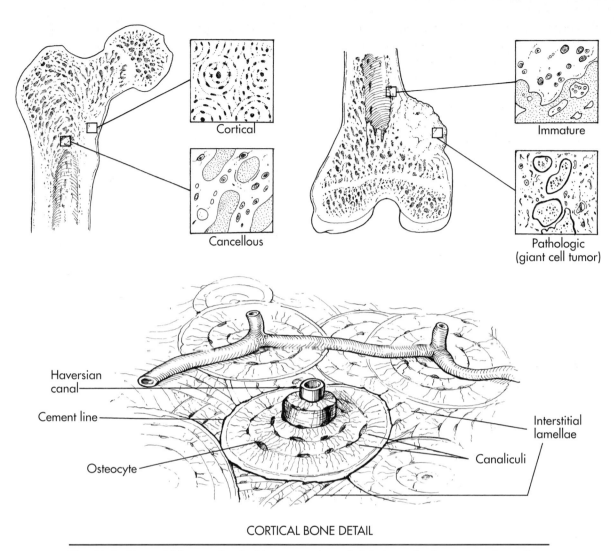

Cortical

Cancellous

Immature

Pathologic
(giant cell tumor)

Haversian
canal

Cement line

Osteocyte

Interstitial
lamellae

Canaliculi

CORTICAL BONE DETAIL

Fig. 10-1 Types of bone. *Cortical* bone consists of tightly packed osteons. *Cancellous* bone consists of a meshwork of trabeculae. In *immature* bone, there is unmineralized osteoid lining the immature trabeculae. Atypical osteoblasts and architectural disorganization are seen in pathologic bone. (From Brinker MR, Miller MD, eds: Fundamentals of Orthopaedics. Philadelphia, WB Saunders, 1999.)

even though cortical bone (compact bone) has four times the mass of trabecular bone, the metabolic activity of trabecular bone is eight times greater than that of cortical bone.[2]

Because bone turnover is a surface-oriented event, the profound surface area of trabecular bone explains the greater cellular exchange of cancellous bone.[2]

BONE ARCHITECTURE

Characteristic differences between cortical bone and trabecular bone are best distinguished by the density and porosity of these two bone types.

Visually, trabecular bone appears as a complex lattice of bone matrix fibers or "spicules" that orient along specific lines of stresses, strains, and compressive forces.

Cortical bone is dense in appearance and is also subject to bending, torsion, and compressive forces. Cortical bone also is defined as bone with less than 30% porosity. Conversely, trabecular bone is generally 50% to 90% porous. Therefore the structure and material characteristics of both cortical and trabecular bone are distinguished by the relative density of each.

BONE REMODELING

The phenomenon of cellular turnover or remodeling of bone is a process that occurs on the surface of various portions of bone (periosteal, endosteal, trabecular, and haversian canal).[20] Generally, bone remodeling is a lifelong activity that responds to mechanical stress (torsion bending, compression, tension) according to Wolff's law.[2] In simplified terms, Wolff's law states that

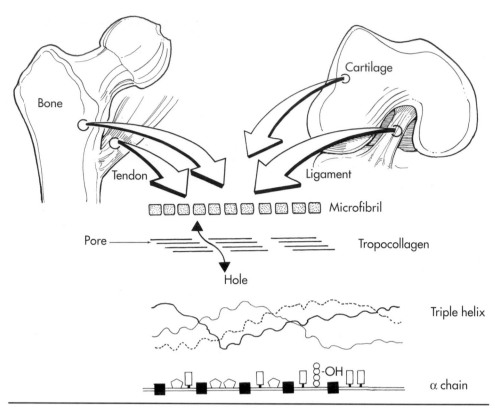

Fig. 10-2 Microstructure of collagen. Collagen is composed of microfibrils that are packed in a quarter-standard fashion to form tropocollagen. Note hole and pore regions for mineral deposition (for calcification). Tropocollagen, in turn, is made up of a triple helix of chains of polypeptides. (From Brinker MR, Miller MD, eds: Fundamentals of Orthopaedics. Philadelphia, WB Saunders, 1999.)

intermittent physiologic loads applied to bone stimulate adaptive responses. Removal of mechanical forces on the bone has the opposite effect. That is, when bone does not receive appropriate physiologic stress, osteoclastic activity overwhelms osteoblast production, which in turn reduces bone mass. The Hueter-Volkmann law is the reverse of Wolff's law and is more specifically applied to compression and tensile forces acting on physeal growth plates. Simply stated, this law suggests that compression forces limit bone growth, whereas tensile stress stimulates growth.[2]

Osseous tissue also is responsive to piezoelectric charges. In conjunction with mechanical forces strengthening compression and tensile stress, compression produces an electronegative charge that acts to stimulate osteoblast activity. Tensile stress produces an electropositive charge that stimulates osteoclastic activity. Therefore mechanical laws of stress (Wolff's law) produce electromechanical changes that act to maintain equilibrium between bone formation and bone resorption.

VASCULAR SUPPLY TO BONE

The adult skeletal system receives between 5% and 10% of the body's total cardiac output.[20] Bone receives blood supply from three distinct but interconnected systems: I-the nutrient artery, II-metaphyseal–epiphyseal system, and III-periosteal systems (Fig. 10-3).

The arterial vascular system provides the origin of the nutrient system via a nutrient foramen in the diaphysis of long bones. The total number of nutrient vessels and foramen varies with each bone.[2] The nutrient arteries enter the medullary space, then ascend and descend into the arterioles within the endosteal surface supplying the diaphyseal area of long bones.[2] The metaphyseal–epiphyseal system is supplied by a periarticular complex system of the genicular arteries that penetrates the thin cortices of the metaphysis of long bones.[2] Muscular attachment to the periosteal cortical sites of bone provides nutrition through the periosteal capillary system.[2]

Fractures, internal fixation devices, external fixation, and prosthetic joint implants devitalize the microcirculation of the cortical–periosteal and endosteal portion of the bone. The resultant ischemia of bone can lead to nonunion and bone infections.[2] These important clinical ramifications of bone circulation disruption are evident when initiating therapeutic interventions of early weight bearing and closed chain resistance exercise after fractures or joint replacement.

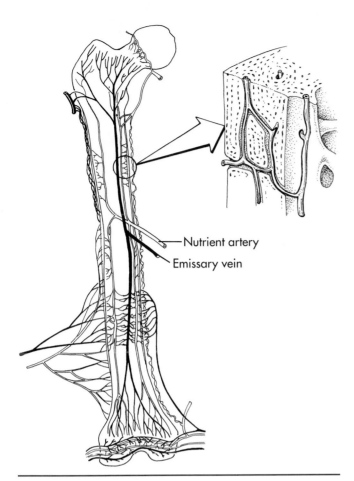

Nutrient artery

Emissary vein

Fig. 10-3 Blood supply to the bone. (From Brinker MR, Miller MD, eds: Fundamentals of Orthopaedics. Philadelphia, WB Saunders, 1999.)

CLASSIFICATIONS OF FRACTURES

By definition a fracture is any abnormal disruption in the normal anatomic continuity of bone. Therefore the classification of fractures takes into account the following criteria:[17,18]

Site of injury: The area of insult on the bone itself. An epiphyseal fracture describes the site, as does an intraarticular fracture or diaphyseal (shaft) fracture. Generally the site is described as the proximal, middle, or distal portion of a bone (Fig. 10-4).

Extent of injury: Complete or incomplete (Fig. 10-5). As the name implies, a complete fracture traverses the bone entirely. Incomplete fractures are commonly described as hairline cracks or greenstick fractures.

Configuration or direction of abnormality: The direction of the fracture. In a transverse fracture, the fracture line goes straight across (horizontally) through the bone; an oblique fracture crosses the bone diagonally. A spiral fracture describes a torsion or rotational injury where the fracture line literally spirals through the bone. An impacted fracture is a long-axis compression injury where the fracture fragments are forced together. The fracture is classified as comminuted when more than two fragments are present.

Relationship of fracture fragments to each other: Can be displaced, nondisplaced, angulated, twisted, rotated, or overriding. An example is an avulsion fracture where a portion of bone is pulled away as part of a musculotendinous attachment or ligament–bone attachment.

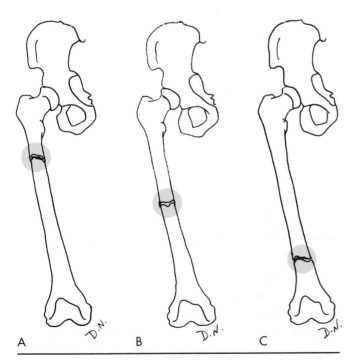

Fig. 10-4 Fracture classification site of injury. **A,** Proximal fracture of the femur. **B,** Middle fracture of the femur. **C,** Distal femur fracture.

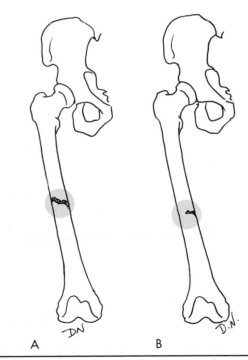

Fig. 10-5 Fracture classification, extent of injury. **A,** Complete fracture of the femur. **B,** Incomplete femur fracture.

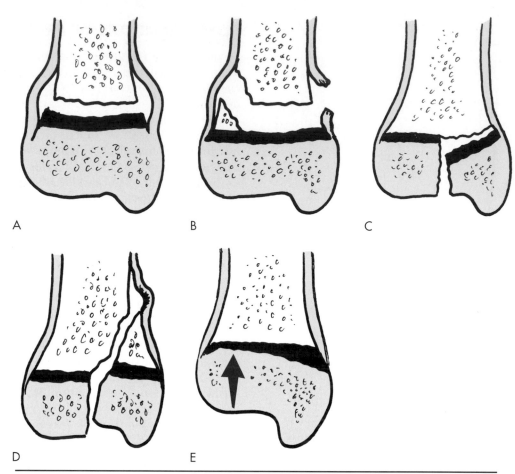

Fig. 10-6 Salter-Harris fracture classification. **A,** Type I—transverse fracture through the physis; **B,** Type II is same as Type I but also has metaphyseal fragment; **C,** Type III—intraarticular fracture. Involves both the physis and the epiphysis; **D,** Type IV—same as Type III, also involves the metaphysis; **E,** Type V—crush injury to the physis.

Relationship of fracture fragments to the environment: Whether the injury is open (compound fracture) or closed (simple).

Complications: Resulting in delayed union, nonunion, or malunion of the fracture fragments. An uncomplicated course of healing is called uneventful.

Pediatric fractures have a special classification of injuries involving the epiphysis. Depending on the type of epiphyseal fracture, the eventual growth of the bone can be profoundly affected.

Salter's fracture classification is outlined in Figure 10-6. Type I **Salter-Harris fractures,** modified by Rang,[13,16–18] are transverse fractures through the physis. Type II fractures are the same as type I, but also have a metaphyseal fragment. Type III fractures involve both the physis and epiphysis. Typically these are intraarticular fractures. Type IV fractures are the same as type III but include the metaphysis. These are significant injuries that can lead to a reduction in bone growth. Type V fractures are severe injuries classified as crush injuries to the physis. This type of fracture also can lead to the arrest of growth.

The PTA should also be aware of the Arbeitgemeinschaft für Osteosynthesefregen (AO) classification system, which is universally applied to both fracture patterns and the devices used for internal fixation. This system will be discussed later in this chapter.[12]

Pathologic fractures are caused by tumors[13] (malignant or primary bone disease), osteoporosis (most common), microtrauma from repetitive overload (stress fractures), or metastatic bone disease (second most common). These usually occur in the elderly person secondary to osteoporosis and can happen spontaneously or with very minor trauma.[13]

Osteoporosis

Osteoporosis is an age-related heterogeneous bone disease characterized by decreased bone tissue. Osteoporosis occurs when osteoblast (bone formation) activity is surpassed by osteoclast (bone resorption) activity.[10] It involves an overall decrease in the quality of bone, not necessarily the quality of bone tissue.[13] This creates weaker bones that are subjected to greater rates of fracture. More than 1 million fractures a year can be attributed to osteoporosis;[13] vertebral body compression fractures are the most common.

Women are at greater risk for developing osteoporosis for several reasons. One reason is related to bone loss. Age-related cortical bone loss generally begins at about age 40,[10] with the rate thereafter being approximately 0.5% annually for both men and women. However, because of lowered estrogen during menopause,[10] women lose bone at a rate of 2% to 8% annually, resulting in a much greater total loss.

Poor absorption of calcium that leads to decreased bone mineralization is called **osteomalacia.**[13] Causes include calcium-deficient diet, accelerated calcium loss, and malabsorption of calcium.[10] Femoral neck fractures are common in patients with osteomalacia.[13]

To appreciate the fragile nature of fractures that occur as a result of osteoporosis or osteomalacia, the following case should be considered:

A frail, elderly woman with osteoporosis suffers resultant multilevel thoracic vertebral body compression fractures. Bed rest with relative immobilization is ordered. She suffers further decrease in bone strength caused by immobilization. Rehabilitation is complicated by osteoporosis and fractures. Combined with the general overall negative effects of immobilization on the body's systems, the effects of immobilization on the remaining skeletal tissue interfere with exercise, sitting, progressive ambulation, and functional activities.

COMPONENTS OF BONE HEALING

Most of the adult skeleton (80%) is composed of compact, cortical bone. Approximately 20% of the skeleton is cancellous or **spongy bone. Compact bone** is extremely dense and unyielding to bending, whereas **cancellous bone** is more elastic and less dense than **cortical bone.**[13]

Three types of cells take part in the highly dynamic, reparative process in bone. **Osteoblasts** help form and synthesize bone. **Osteocytes** are mature bone cells that account for approximately 90% of all bone tissue. **Osteoclasts** are active in bone resorption.

The normal dynamic process of bone synthesis and resorption is termed **remodeling.** Remodeling and stress occur together, which profoundly influences bone shape, density, internal architecture, and external configuration.[1,6,8,13] With normal bone remodeling, weight bearing forces and muscular contractions provide the stress needed for bone formation and adaptation. The absence of physiologic loading, or stress, is detrimental to bone, ligament, cartilage, muscle, and tendons, as well as the cardiorespiratory system. **Wolff's law**[1] states that intermittently applied stress, as well as changes in function of bone, causes definite changes.[3,6] After a fracture, treatment may involve rigid cast immo-

bilization and non–weight bearing over a period of weeks. This decreased stress on the bone causes rapid osteoclast activity (bone resorption) and decreased osteoblast activity.[14] Therefore although the removal of stress is paramount for healing, the decrease in external force also causes significant bone loss.[13] Bone loss caused by immobilization is reversible after progressive weight bearing, active motion, resistive exercise, and vertical loading (closed kinetic-chain exercise).[13] It is recommended that strict, long-term, rigid cast immobilization be minimized whenever possible.

Although normal stresses promote bone development, excessive stress also can lead to gradual bone resorption.[6] Stress that is unrelenting and does not allow for osteoblastic repair of bone can lead to pathologic accelerated bone resorption and eventual stress fracture.[1,6,8]

Bone remodeling is also influenced by electrical charges when forces are applied to bone. The **piezoelectric effect** describes a negative electric charge toward the concave, or compression, side of a force applied to a bone. An electropositive charge is seen on the tension, or convex, side of the bone. The negative-charge side responds by stimulating osteoblasts, whereas the positive-charge side (tension side) responds by increasing osteoclast activity.[13]

BONE INJURY AND REPAIR

Injury repair and eventual regeneration of osseous tissue is a complex process that involves the bone marrow, bone cortex, periosteum, and external soft tissues.

Trauma to the bone disrupts the biological, mechanical, structural, architectural, and histochemical environment of bone. Classic descriptions of fracture healing are divided into primary (direct) cortical healing and secondary (indirect) fracture healing.

The spontaneous natural course of fracture repair can be described as interfragmentary stabilization by periosteal and endosteal callus formation and by interfragmentary fibrocartilage differentiation, restoration of continuity and bone union by intramembranous and endochondral ossification, substitution of avascular and necrotic areas by haversian remodeling, modeling of the fracture site, and functional adaptation.[1-5,9]

Fracture healing responses differ according to the nature of stabilization provided (direct, internal, compression–appositional, alignment fixation, versus cast immobilization). That is, rigid internal fixation results in primary–direct cortical healing, which is an attempt by the cortex of bone to reestablish mechanical and anatomic continuity. This type of fracture healing response usually is devoid of periosteal soft callus formation. Secondary or indirect fracture repair is noted for external periosteal soft-tissue callus bridging between fracture fragments.

PHASES OF FRACTURE REPAIR

In general terms most fractures heal with a combination of primary cortical healing and secondary–indirect healing. The phases of fracture repair are divided into six sequences of events that ultimately lead to functional remodeling of the injured bone.[9] Phase I is inflammation and hematoma formation, Phase II is chondrocyte formation and angiogenesis, Phase III is cartilage and calcification, Phase IV is cartilage removal, Phase V is bone formation, and Phase VI is bone remodeling.[9]

Phase I is characterized by fibrin clot formation. The presence of the fibrin clot between fracture fragments acts as a rich source of activating inflammatory molecules essential to the complex cascade of intense cellular activity required of fracture repair. Many cellular processes are involved during this phase that are responsible for attracting, regulating, and differentiating cells that serve to propagate the development of cartilage and revascularization of bone. Animal models demonstrate intramembranous and endochondral bone formation during the first 2 weeks after fracture.[9] The presence of cartilage within the fracture repair matrix at this point is the hallmark of Phase II repair. Calcification of chondrocytes (cartilage) requires specific enzyme release for phosphate and calcium interactions. During Phase III, there is a gradual decline in proliferative cell activity and an increase in chondrocyte deposition and release of proteolytic enzymes. The calcification process of fibrocartilage is essential before the substitution of woven bone within the fragment gap. Once fibrocartilage is calcified, the ultimate integrity and development of woven bone with resultant remodeling to lamellar bone is dependent on revitalization (vascularity) of injured bone.

Angiogenesis (neovascularization) is critical for delivering oxygen, nutrients, inflammatory cells, and fibroblasts to stimulate and support the healing fracture. The vascular response to a healing fracture varies over time. Initially, the three distinct vascular systems of bone are disrupted significantly, reducing blood flow. Over the next several days after fracture, the circulation increases and peaks at approximately 2 weeks.[9] Recognize that although there is a relative increase in vascular budding, the dramatic volume of cellular activity creates a state of hypoxia at the fracture that is highly conducive for cartilage formation.[9]

PROCESS OF BONE HEALING

Bone healing can be characterized by the following sequence of events:
■ Fracture occurs.
■ Bleeding occurs, and a hematoma results.
■ Granulation tissue is formed by the hematoma (soft callus formation).

■ Osteoblasts produce new bone, and a bony or hard callus is formed.
■ The callus is gradually reabsorbed, and the anatomic contour of the bone is regained.

As with soft tissue, the immediate inflammatory response lasts 24 to 48 hours and is characterized by the development of granulation tissue, blood clotting, and fibroblast and osteoblast proliferation.[3,13] The repair phase of bone healing signals the development of bone scarring, or callus formation, which is usually detected within the first 2 weeks after injury. The degree of callus formation depends on anatomic alignment of the fragments and the degree and quality of immobilization. If motion occurs through the fracture site during this phase, a soft **bone callus** (primarily of cartilage) bridges the fragments.[3,13] This type of callus also forms if the union between the fragments is poor, even when immobilization prevents motion.

Primary cortical healing (hard callus) forms with anatomic alignment and fragment apposition, immobilization, and appropriately applied progressive stress. The remodeling phase of bone healing is an extraordinarily long process that can take up to several years to complete and is strongly influenced by Wolff's law.[1]

As with ligament healing, protection of the injury site is vital to a successful outcome. There is an exceedingly narrow line to follow with respect to motion after bone injury. In many cases a reducing plan of **immobilization** is used to secure the bone fragments, protect the fracture, and provide needed motion for healing. For example, a rigid cast can be applied for a few weeks (2 to 4 weeks), then a limited-range hinge-brace can be used to protect the healing structures and initiate physiologic motion within set limits. Depending on the severity of the insult, some fractures may require secure immobilization for extended periods to allow for proper healing.

EFFECTS OF IMMOBILIZATION ON BONE TISSUE

A major goal for bone healing to occur is to immobilize the fracture site. However, when bone tissue does not receive physiologic loads (ambulation, vertical loads, and muscle contractions), the normal remodeling processes are negatively affected. The rate of normal bone remodeling changes when immobilization lasts slightly longer than 1 week.[5] The "turnover" or remodeling of bone during immobilization is characterized by a loss of calcium, resulting in localized bone loss. Immobilization leads to a reduction in the hardness of bone related to the duration of immobilization.[5] By 3 months, bone strength is only 55% to 60% of normal.[21] The relationship between soft-tissue structures and bone during periods of immobilization reflects the interdependence of muscular contractions, forces acting

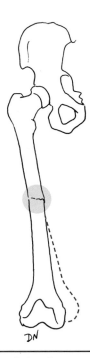

Fig. 10-7 Malunion of the femur. Dotted line indicates normal anatomic alignment.

on joints, compressive loads, circulation (blood flow affecting nutrition), and motion in maintaining bone remodeling equilibrium.

A definite contrast is seen in the care of healing bone tissue. It is necessary to *immobilize* the fracture fragments so healing can occur, yet *minimize the negative effects of* immobilization through the judicious application of progressive motion, exercise, and weight bearing. The length of time needed to regain bone strength after immobilization is considerably longer than the duration of immobilization. Therefore the length of the immobilization is an important component in the overall process of healing bone tissue.

COMPLICATIONS

Occasionally the process of bone healing leads to three distinct complications:
1. Delayed union
2. Nonunion
3. Malunion

In **delayed union,** the dynamic biologic repair processes of bone healing occur at a slower rate than anticipated. Brashear and Raney[3] describe delayed union as clinically detectable when firm callus is not present at 20 weeks (for fractures of the tibia and femur) and at 10 weeks (for fractures of the humerus). An important cause of delayed union is "inadequate or interrupted immobilization."[3] Rehabilitation can significantly affect the healing process either positively or negatively. If therapeutic interventions are begun too soon or too

vigorously, delayed union may occur because of excessive motion occurring at the fracture site. Unfortunately, the trade-off when caring for delayed bone union cases is the need to provide extended periods of immobilization for healing. However, cast braces and walking casts can be used to provide the weight bearing (Wolff's law) necessary to enhance healing.

In **nonunion,** the healing processes have stopped. Nonunion occurs when there is a significant and severe associated soft-tissue trauma, poor blood supply, and infections.

In **malunion,** healing results in a nonanatomic position (Fig. 10-7). Malunion is caused by ineffective immobilization and failure to maintain immobilization for an adequate period of time. For appropriate bone healing to occur, anatomic alignment (apposition) of fragments, adequate fixation (external or internal), and length of time of immobilization must occur in concert. If these factors are not balanced, the chance of complications is increased.

FRACTURE FIXATION: BIOLOGY AND BIOMECHANICS

Rigid anatomic fixation of bone results in primary repair or direct cortical reconstruction. This process generally inhibits periosteal soft tissue bridging callus. The repair process of rigid internal fixation is characterized by haversian remodeling and osteon formation. Creeping substitution is a term used to describe osteoclastic "cutting cones" traversing the cortical fracture fragments, followed by osteoblast formation and revascularization of bone.

The precise application of various internal fixation devices (intermedullary rods, bone plates, and compression screws) to stimulate primary cortical healing are not without inherent risks. The surgical placement of bone plates requires "stripping" the periosteum where the screws and plates are to be fixed. This process obviously devascularizes the periosteal blood supply. In addition, the areas beneath the plate increase the porosity of bone and weaken the mechanical and structural behavior, as well as the architecture of the injured bone. With intramedullary rod application, the medullary canal must be "reamed" to allow for proper anatomic placement of the rod. Again the nutrient arterial system, metaphyseal–diaphyseal system, and medullary circulation are disrupted. During the surgical placement of screws and plates, the surgeon attempts to apply these devices by hand-held screw devices and manual torque wrenches instead of using high-speed drills that might create thermal necrosis of bone and soft tissue, which could contribute to increased bone devitalization.[19,21]

Conversely, nonoperative fracture management involves a complex series of interactions, which stimulate the thermal, chemical, mechanical, and electrical environment of periosteal and cortical bone (Table 10-1).[4,9]

Table 10-1	*Type of Fracture Healing Based on Type of Stabilization*	
Type of Immobilization	**Predominant Type of Healing**	**Comments**
Cast (closed treatments)	Periosteal bridging callus	Enchondral ossification
Compression plate	Primary cortical healing (remodeling)	Cutting cone-type remodeling
Intramedullary nail	Early—periosteal bridging callus	
	Late—medullary callus	Enchondral ossification
External fixator	Dependent on extent of rigidity	
	Less rigid—periosteal bridging callus	
	More rigid—primary cortical healing	
Inadequate	Hypertrophic nonunion	Failed endochondral ossification
		Type II collagen predominates

From Brinker MR, Miller MD: Fundamentals of Orthopaedics. Philadelphia, WB Saunders, 1999.

In cases of nonoperative fracture management, the type of repair is referred to as secondary–periosteal callus. The natural healing sequence on nonoperative diaphyseal fractures include a period of instability (Phase I) in which there is essentially no true biologic support given to the fracture site. The fracture hematoma and proliferative cellular activation provide no mechanical protection of the fragments.

The second phase is the development of the soft callus. Phase II is characterized by the soft-tissue compliance provided the peripheral structures surrounding the fracture fragments. The formation, organization, and gradual maturation of cellular activity in and around the injury site provides for greater stability.[9] As stated by Latta, Sarmiento, and Zych,[9] "peripheral structures supply early vascularization and soft tissue repair. Peripheral soft tissues provide a compliant strength which leads to reduction of acute symptoms long before there is radiographic evidence of healing." Phase III demonstrates a radiographic confirmation of thin "hard callus" (bony ridge).

Generally, hematoma and cartilage are prevalent along with a gradual revascularization of the interfragmentary gap of soft and hard callus formation. Radiographic confirmation of the disappearance of the fracture line is characteristic of Phase IV, the fracture line consolidation phase.

During this stage of nonoperative diaphyseal fracture management, there is a subtle, gradual shrinkage of the central soft callus bone with remodeling, consolidation of the fracture line, and maturation of hard bony callus.

Finally, Phase V structural remodeling is where there is gradual contraction and shrinkage of callus with resultant reorganization and configuration of normal bone anatomy and topography.

EXTERNAL FIXATION AND FRACTURE REPAIR

External fixators are used for a wide variety of clinical situations and allow for modification of stiffness and rigidity of fixation during fracture healing.[3,15]

The geometric composite construct of these elaborate frame configurations usually can be altered by several orders of magnitude. Several factors significantly contribute to the stability, rigidity, stiffness, and compression of the fracture site, as well as the mechanical properties of the frame.[15] The number of pins used; the length, diameter, and type of pin material; the number of side bars set in the spacing between pins; the spacing between side bars and bone surface; pin–bone contact; and proximal–distal pin spacing all contribute to the material characteristics: stability, stiffness, and compression of the fracture site.[4,15]

Fracture healing characteristics using external fixators depend on the rigidity obtained by the device. Overall, the more rigid the fixation, the earlier the radiographic confirmation of bone union. Less rigid fixators create greater periosteal callus formation, whereas rigid fixators characteristically stimulate direct primary cortical fracture healing.[4,15]

As stated, a unique advantage of external fixation is the ability to alter or modify rigidity during various stages of fracture healing. Several models demonstrate the effect of dynamization (mechanisms used to decrease stiffness of the fixation or mechanisms that allow for controlled micromotion between fracture fragments) on blood flow and bone callus formation.[4,9,11,15,20] A 25% increase in fracture site micromotion resulted in a 400% increase in regional blood flow and substantially more callus formation with animals receiving semirigid external fixators compared with rigid external fixation.[15]

BONE FIXATION DEVICES

When caring for patients who have had fractures, the PTA must be aware of various methods used to immobilize or stabilize the fracture so a clear understanding of the extent of trauma can be appreciated. This also allows the PTA to understand the degree of tissue healing necessary before vigorous rehabilitation exercises can be undertaken.

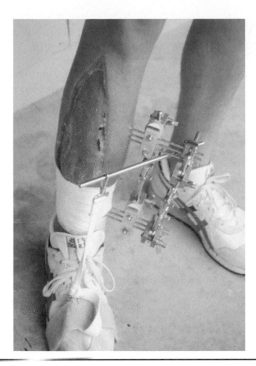

Fig. 10-8 External fixation device (external fixator).

The remarkable sensitivity of bone to normal biologic stress is well known.[1,6,13,18] After fractures, an attempt is made to stabilize the fracture, bring the fragments together by apposition (approximation) and alignment, and remove or minimize forces that may slow the normal healing process. Two general methods of immobilization are used in the treatment of fractures. In one method, the area is immobilized by **external fixation devices.** This method involves the use of casts, traction, splints, and braces and the external fixation devices employed with significant open (compound comminuted) fractures where the risk of infection is present (Fig. 10-8). These ominous-looking devices help fix the fracture site while allowing care of the open wounds with skin grafts, tissue flaps, or débridement. These are classified as external fixation devices because the pins used to immobilize the fracture do not contact the fragments directly, but are used to hold the bone segments in rigid alignment and anatomic apposition. With closed (simple) fractures, various rigid lightweight fiberglass casts, plaster casts, hinged-plaster casts, and adjustable-range hinged braces are used for immobilization.

The second method of immobilization uses **internal fixation devices** and is best for displaced fractures where external fixation does not provide the degree of immobilization necessary to effect healing. (See Box 10-1 for the AO classification system, designed by the Association for the Study of Internal Fixation [ASIF or AO].) Internal fixation is called **open reduction with internal fixation (ORIF)** and involves surgically exposing the fracture site to reduce, approximate, and align the bone fragments. The materials used for ORIF procedures

include metals (stainless steel and metal alloys of cobalt–chromium–molybdenum and titanium) and nonmetals (high-density polyethylene, polymethyl-methacrylate, silicones, and ceramics). Metal internal fixation devices frequently are combinations of screws, staples, pins, nails, tension-band wires, and various plates. The placement of these materials can affect the delivery of certain therapeutic agents, such as ultrasound. Also, a hole or tunnel defect in a bone with or without a screw in it effectively reduces the overall strength of the bone up to 50%.[13] Even after screw removal, the bone will not regain normal strength for up to 1 year.[13]

Metal internal fixation devices occasionally loosen and can "back out," as is the case with screws. If the PTA notes signs of hardware loosening (pain, swelling, or crepitus), he or she must immediately consult with the supervising physical therapist and physician. Many metal fixation devices are designed to be left in place, as with most plates, but these devices should be removed if metal allergy reactions occur. Table 10-2 depicts the various internal fixation devices.

FACTORS INFLUENCING BONE HEALING

Several key factors are implicated in delayed biologic fracture repair. Tobacco smoke, malnutrition, inadequate reduction of the fragments, excessive motion from inadequate immobilization, poor vascular supply, soft-tissue interposition between fracture fragments, and infection significantly limit spontaneous fracture repair.[2,4]

Cigarette smoke is a vasoconstrictor that may reduce blood supply to the injury site. In addition, smoking directly interferes with osteoblast formation.[21] Protein, malnutrition, and calorie deprivation reduce skeletal muscle mass and may contribute to reduced periosteal and cortical bone formation.[4] Poor reduction of the

Table 10-2	Internal Fixation Devices
Type	**Use**
Compression plate	Diaphyseal fractures
Intramedullary rod	Lower extremity diaphyseal fractures (femur, tibia); removed at 1 or 2 years
Reconstruction plate	Used in pelvic and distal humerus fractures
Tension wires	Patella fractures and olecranon fractures
Sliding hip screws	Intertrochanteric hip fractures
Condylar screws	Distal femur fractures
Cannulated screws	Femoral neck fractures

From Miller M: Review of Orthopaedics. Philadelphia, WB Saunders, 1992.

Table 10-3	Biologic and Mechanical Factors Influencing Fracture Healing
Biologic Factors	**Mechanical Factors**
Patient age	Soft-tissue attachments to bone
Comorbid medical conditions	Stability (extent of immobilization)
Functional level	Anatomic location
Nutritional status	Level of energy imparted
Nerve function	Extent of bone loss
Vascular injury	
Hormones	
Growth factors	
Health of the soft-tissue envelope	
Sterility (in open fractures)	
Cigarette smoke	
Local pathologic conditions	
Level of energy imparted	
Type of bone affected	
Extent of bone loss	

From Brinker MR, Miller MD: Fundamentals of Orthopaedics. Philadelphia, WB Saunders, 1999.

fracture fragments and inadequate immobilization create excessive motion and reduced vascular supply to the bone (Table 10-3).[21] Occasionally a sleeve of soft tissue becomes interposed within the fracture site, significantly reducing both primary, cortical, and secondary–periosteal bridging callus, and rendering the fragments devitalized.

Infectious organisms have many deleterious effects on both implants and the host bone environment. Orthopedic implant loosening, bone resorption, bone destruction, and reactive periosteal elevation can occur in the presence of infection.[4]

STIMULATION OF FRACTURE REPAIR

There are several methods available to augment, stimulate, or enhance fracture repair. Bone grafts are used to fill osseous defects and stabilize fractures. Bone autografts are taken from the same individual. Allograft bone tissue is used from the same species. An example of a fresh autograft is harvesting bone from the iliac crest to transpose (heterotopic transportation) to the lumbar spine for fusion.

Conversely, cadaveric bone allografts must be sterilized chemically. This process renders all cells nonviable. In both autografts and allografts, the implanted graft acts as a scaffold to support the growth of host bone tissue. This process is known as passive osteoconduction.[4] Gradually the implant bone tissue becomes revascularized with stimulation and transportation of osteoblasts into the new graft. This process is referred to as osteoinduction.[4] Although the sequence of events is similar (passive osteoconduction, gradual revascularization, and osteoinduction) with both graft materials, allogenic bone requires a longer time for creeping

substitution to take place. Additional materials used for osteoconduction that support vascular ingrowth, growth, attachment, division, and remodeling of bone include ceramics, bioactive glass, and synthetic polymers.[4]

Ceramic bone graft substitutes include hydroxyapatite and tricalcium phosphate. Some of these graft substitutes are formed from marine coral and crystalline hydroxyapatite. These bone substitutes generally have been shown to be as effective as autograft bone.[4]

Two clinically relevant methods of fracture healing augmentation are electromagnetic field application and low-intensity ultrasound. The use of exogenously applied pulsed electromagnetic fields over nonunion fractures is based on the piezoelectric effect in response to load deformation of crystalline–collagen component's of Wolff's law.[4] The use of specific electrical stimulation waveforms to induce bone formations is supported by scientific investigation and clinical observation that electric stimulation affects enchondral bone formation and connective tissue repair.

The use of nonthermal, low-intensity ultrasound (30 mW/cm^2) has very strong biologic value to stimulate chondroblasts, osteoblasts, blood flow, and to enhance greater mechanical and histologic influence on enchondral and periosteal bone healing. Various studies have demonstrated the use of brief low-intensity ultrasound on the order of 20 minutes per day can reduce the time to fracture union by as much as 35%.[4]

CLINICAL APPLICATION OF REHABILITATION TECHNIQUES DURING BONE HEALING

Immobilization after bone injury may not be total. Nonimmobilized structures should be exercised throughout the period of immobilization. For example, a program of lower extremity strengthening and endurance activities (stationary cycle, treadmill, and leg extension) should be instituted for patients with upper extremity fractures. The same principle applies for patients with lower extremity fractures. Endurance activities can be either single-leg stationary cycling or upper body ergometer (UBE) exercises in these cases.

Specific exercises for the injured area frequently involve isometric muscle contractions. Therapeutic exercise programs during bone healing are designed to minimize muscle atrophy while maintaining or improving muscular strength. Muscle contractions provide forces acting to approximate fragments, improve circulation, promote motion to nonimmobilized body parts, and stimulate the piezoelectric effect.

The cast or brace serves as resistance in the initial phases of active range of motion exercises involving the affected limb. Ankle weights can be applied to the cast or brace for added resistance in later stages. It is best to apply the external resistance superior to the injury site at first, such as in ligament injuries. A more distal application of external force may produce excessive, unwanted shearing, or torque through the fracture site.

Occasionally, electrical muscle stimulation (EMS) is used during cast immobilization to help retard atrophy and maintain strength. A small "window" is cut in the cast to allow the application of the electrodes. The patient is instructed to isometrically contract simultaneously with the electrically evoked muscle contraction. The benefits of electrical stimulation on muscle tissue during immobilization are controversial. The piezoelectric effect is enhanced by applying a negatively charged electrode to stimulate osteoblast activity, which is called *direct current* (any current in which electrons flow in one direction). An externally applied electrode with an external power source is called *inductive* coupling.[13]

Continuous passive motion (CPM) devices are used in some cases of intraarticular or extraarticular fractures of the tibia and femur.[7] Although this appears to conflict with the notion of secure immobilization leading to bone healing, Salter[19] has found positive effects of CPM on the development of chondrocytes and the reduction of intraarticular synovial adhesions when judiciously applied to healing intraarticular fractures.

The goals of rehabilitation programs during immobilization of healing fractures are as follows:

■ Improve the overall fitness of the patient
■ Promote motion of unaffected, nonimmobilized joints
■ Minimize muscle atrophy (isometrics and muscle stimulators)
■ Maintain or improve muscular strength
■ Protect the healing structures; avoid unwanted, premature, or excessive motion
■ Teach safe and effective transfers and gait activities (with cumbersome long-leg plaster casts or external fixators)

After immobilization, progressive exercise must be directed cautiously. Motion and circulation can be promoted by using various thermal agents. Strengthening exercises should systematically progress through isometrics, concentric and eccentric resistance, isokinetics, and closed kinetic-chain resistance exercises. Balance, coordination, and proprioceptive exercises are also included during the postimmobilization phases of rehabilitation. Stationary cycle ergometers, upper body ergometers, stair climbers, and treadmills are tools that can enhance cardiorespiratory fitness both during and after immobilization.

❖ ADDITIONAL FEATURES

Bone Injury and Repair of Inflammation: Fracture site hematoma. Granulation tissue forms around fracture site. Osteoblasts and fibroblasts proliferate.

Bone Matrix: Organic components—40% dry weight of bone, collagen, proteoglycans, glycoproteins, and phospholipids.

Bone Types: Normal bone is lamellar. Immature or pathologic bone is woven, not stress oriented. Mature lamellar bone is cortical or cancellous.

Cancellous Bone: Spongy or trabecular. Fractures generally progress at 6 weeks. Examples: calcaneus, vertebral body, radius, pelvis, and tibia.

Cortical Bone: Eighty percent of adult skeleton.

Joint Involvement: If the fracture involves a joint, bone union may be delayed secondary to dilution of fracture hematoma from synovial fluid.

Mobility at Fracture Site: Excessive mobility interferes with vascularization of fractures and hematoma, and it disrupts bridging callus.

Osteoblasts: Form bone. Increased endoplasmic reticulum, increased Golgi apparatus, and increased mitochondria.

Osteoclasts: Resorb bone. Bone resorption generally is more rapid than bone formation.

Osteocytes: Ninety percent of mature skeleton. Former osteoblasts that serve to maintain bone.

Piezoelectric Effect: Compression side of bone is electronegative and stimulates osteoblasts. The tension side of bone is electropositive and stimulates osteoclasts.

Remodeling: Occurs long after the fracture has healed clinically. Woven bone formed during the repair phase is replaced with lamellar bone. Bone remodeling is affected by mechanical function according to Wolff's law. Removal of external stress can lead to significant bone loss. Bone remodels in response to stress and responds to piezoelectric charges.

Repair: Primary callus forms in about 2 weeks. Soft callus involving enchondral ossification occurs if fracture is not in continuity. Amount of callus is indirectly proportional to the degree of immobilization. Primary cortical healing occurs with immobilization and near anatomic reduction.

REFERENCES

1. Bassett C: Effect of force on skeletal tissue. In Downey JA, Darling RC, eds. Physiological Basis of Rehabilitation Medicine. Philadelphia, WB Saunders, 1971.
2. Bostrom MPG, Boskey A, Kaufman JK, et al: Form and function of bone. In Buckwalter JA, Einhorn TA, Simon SR, eds. Orthopaedic Basic Science: Biology and Biomechanics of the Musculoskeletal System. American Academy of Orthopaedic Surgeons, 2000.
3. Brashear RH, Raney RB: Fracture principles, fracture healing. In Handbook of Orthopaedic Surgery. St Louis, Mosby, 1986.
4. Day SM, Ostrum RE, Chao EYS, et al: Bone injury regeneration and repair. In Buckwalter JA, Einhorn TA, Simon SR, eds. Orthopaedic Basic Science: Biology and Biomechanics of the Musculoskeletal System. American Academy of Orthopaedic Surgeons, 2000.
5. Engles M: Tissue Response. In Donatelli R, Wooden MJ, eds. Orthopedic Physical Therapy. New York, Churchill Livingstone, 1989.
6. Guoping L, et al: Radiographic and histologic analyses of stress fracture in rabbit tibias. Am J Sports Med 1985;13:285–294.
7. Hamilton HW: Five year's experience with continuous passive motion. J Bone Joint Surg 1982;64B:259.
8. Kisner C, Colby LA: Therapeutic Exercise: Foundations and Techniques. Philadelphia, FA Davis, 1990.
9. Latta LL, Sarmiento A, Zych GA: Principles of nonoperative fractures. In Brown BD, Jupiter JB, Trafton PG, eds. Skeletal Trauma: Fractures, Dislocations, Ligamentous Injuries, 2nd ed. Philadelphia, WB Saunders, 1998.
10. Lewis CB, Bottomley JM: Geriatric Physical Therapy: A Clinical Approach. New York, Appleton & Lange, 1994.
11. Mazzocca AD, Caputo AE, Brown BD, et al: Principles of internal fixation. In Brown BD, Jupiter JB, Levine AM, et al, eds. Skeletal Trauma: Fractures, Dislocations, and Ligamentous Injuries. Philadelphia, WB Saunders, 1998.
12. McRae R: Practical Fracture Treatment. New York, Churchill Livingstone, 1994.
13. Miller MD: Review of Orthopaedics. Philadelphia, WB Saunders, 1992.
14. Morris JM: Fatigue fractures. Calif Med 1968;108:268–274.
15. Pollak AN, Ziran: Principles of external fixation. In Brown BD, Jupiter JB, Levine AM, et al, eds. Skeletal Trauma: Fractures, Dislocations, Ligamentous Bone Injuries, 2nd ed. Philadelphia, WB Saunders, 1998.
16. Rang M: Children's Fractures. Philadelphia, JB Lippincott, 1974.
17. Rothstein JM, Roy SH, Wolf SL: The Rehabilitation Specialists' Handbook. Philadelphia, FA Davis, 1991.
18. Salter RB: Textbook of Disorders and Injuries of the Musculoskeletal System, 2nd ed. Baltimore, Williams & Wilkins, 1983.
19. Salter RB, et al: Clinical applications of basic research on continuous passive motion for disorders and injuries of synovial joints. A preliminary report of a feasibility study. J Orthop Res 1983; 3:325–342.
20. Shenk RK: Biology of fracture repair. In Brown BD, Jupiter JB, Levine AM, et al, eds. Skeletal Trauma: Fractures, Dislocations, Ligamentous Bone Injuries, 2nd ed. Philadelphia, WB Saunders, 1998.
21. Steinburg FU: The Immobilized Patient: Functional Pathology and Management. New York, Plenum, 1980.

REVIEW QUESTIONS

Multiple Choice

1. Which of the following describe(s) basic objectives in fracture management and healing? (Circle any that apply.)
   A. Muscular hypertrophy
   B. Approximate bone fragments
   C. Maintain alignment of fracture fragments
   D. Preserve and restore function
   E. Enhance aerobic metabolism

2. The adult skeleton is composed of what percent of compact, cortical bone?
   A. 10%
   B. 30%
   C. 80%
   D. 55%

3. Cells that help synthesize bone are called which of the following?
   A. Osteones
   B. Osteoclasts
   C. Osteocytes
   D. Osteoblasts

4. Immobilization and reduced physiologic stress have what effect on healing bone tissue?
   A. Increased callus formation
   B. Stronger bone
   C. Increased osteoblast activity
   D. Decreased osteoblasts and rapid osteoclast activity

5. Normal bone growth, remodeling, and repair are influenced by which of the following?
   A. Motion
   B. Stress (Wolff's law)
   C. Muscular contractions
   D. Piezoelectric effect
   E. All of the above

6. Three complications that can arise from the process of bone healing are which of the following? (Circle any that apply.)
   A. Decreased cardiorespiratory function
   B. Delayed union
   C. Nonunion
   D. Malunion
   E. Hard callus formation

7. Which of the following are descriptive classifications of fractures? (Circle any that apply.)
   A. Injury site
   B. Force of injury
   C. Configuration of injury
   D. Relationship of fracture fragments to the environment
   E. Resultant functional deficits

8. Which of the following are classifications of pediatric fractures?
   A. Smith-Harris
   B. Salter-James
   C. Salter-Harris
   D. Harris-Jones

9. Which is the most common cause of pathologic fractures?
   A. Tumors
   B. Stress fractures
   C. Metastatic bone disease
   D. Osteoporosis

10. Osteoporosis is characterized by which of the following? (Circle any that apply.)
    A. Decreased quality of bone
    B. Increased quantity of bone
    C. Osteoclast activity greater than osteoblast activity
    D. Decreased quantity of bone
    E. Increased tensile strength of bone

11. The most common pathologic fracture related to osteoporosis is which of the following?
    A. Humeral neck fracture

B. Stress fracture
C. Vertebral body compression fracture
D. Colles's fracture

12. Which of the following are methods of external fixation of fractures? (Circle any that apply.)
   A. Traction
   B. Pins
   C. Screws
   D. Cast-braces
   E. Harrington rods

13. The method of open reduction and internal fixation of fractures is known as what type of procedure? (Circle any that apply.)
   A. ORIF
   B. Reduction with fixation
   C. A surgical procedure to internally stabilize a fracture
   D. A surgical procedure used only to stabilize open or compound fractures

14. Which of the following exercises are commonly used for the immobilized area during recovery from fractures?
   A. High-speed isokinetics
   B. Eccentrics
   C. Isometrics
   D. Concentrics

15. When cast-braces are used (protected limited range), the physician and physical therapist occasionally prescribe what type of muscular activity during the early recovery phase of rehabilitation? (Circle any that apply.)
   A. Isometrics
   B. Active range of motion
   C. Isokinetics
   D. Plyometrics
   E. Closed kinetic chain eccentric loading

16. What adjunctive technique is occasionally used to encourage, stimulate, and enhance muscular contractions during periods of cast immobilization for the treatment of fractures?
   A. Ultrasound
   B. Phonophoresis
   C. Biofeedback
   D. TENS
   E. Electrical muscle stimulation (EMS)

17. Exercise is a significant feature of recovery after fractures. Appropriately applied muscular contractions provide which of the following during recovery from fractures?
   A. Improved circulation
   B. Fragment approximation
   C. Promote motion to nonimmobilized parts
   D. Stimulate the piezoelectric effect
   E. All of the above

18. Which of the following are general goals of recovery during the immobilization of fractures?
   A. Improve patient fitness
   B. Minimize muscular atrophy
   C. Protect healing structures
   D. Teach safe and effective gait and transfers
   E. All of the above

Short Answer

19. Name the two general methods used to immobilize fractures.

20. When treating a patient with an ORIF procedure in which a screw was used to stabilize a fracture, the PTA must be cautious of hardware loosening and "backing out." List three clinical signs of hardware loosening.

True/False

21. Compact bone heals faster than cancellous bone.
22. A reduced rate of bone healing (delayed union) can happen when physical therapy interventions are applied too soon or too vigorously.
23. When treating patients recovering from fractures, it is necessary to actively exercise all nonimmobilized joints.

Essay Questions

Answer on a separate sheet of paper.
24. Identify and describe the phases of bone healing.
25. Discuss the objectives that serve as the foundation of fracture management and bone healing
26. Define osteoblasts, osteoclasts, and osteocytes.
27. Define and discuss Wolff's law.
28. Discuss stress deprivation, immobilization, and normal physiologic stress as they apply to fracture healing.
29. Define three complications of bone healing.
30. Outline and describe six areas of descriptive organization of classifying fractures.
31. Describe the five types of pediatric fractures defined by Salter-Harris.
32. Define pathologic fractures and list four types.
33. Discuss how osteoporosis affects fractures.
34. Define osteomalacia.
35. List common methods of fracture fixation, fixation devices, and fracture classifications.
36. Discuss clinical applications of rehabilitation techniques used during bone healing.

Critical Thinking Application

Develop your own "case study" concerning a patient with a distal tibia fracture. Based on your knowledge of the mechanisms of bone healing, recommend the application of specific rehabilitation procedures (immobilization, protected motion, weight bearing, resistance exercise, aerobic conditioning, proprioception and balance training, etc.) that are consistent with the phases of bone healing and remodeling. Identify the influence of Wolff's law on bone remodeling. In developing your rehabilitation program, consider the effects of immobilization of bone and describe clinically significant complications that could occur after fractures. Identify when an ORIF procedure is generally indicated for fracture stabilization. During each phase of recovery in your case study, address the following issues: the overall fitness of the patient, minimization of muscle atrophy, improvement of muscular strength, and protection of the healing structures.

11

Cartilage Healing

LEARNING OBJECTIVES

1. Discuss the composition and function of articular cartilage.
2. Identify common causes of injury to articular cartilage.
3. Describe the sequence of healing and the extent of intrinsic repair of articular cartilage.
4. Define invasive and noninvasive techniques of stimulating articular cartilage repair.
5. Define and describe the composition and function of the meniscus.
6. Identify and discuss common mechanisms of injury to the meniscus.
7. Describe the mechanisms of intrinsic healing of the meniscus.
8. List common rehabilitation techniques used in the treatment of the injured meniscus.

KEY TERMS

Hyaline cartilage
Osteoarthritis
Chondrocytes
Subchondral bone
Inflammatory
 response

Continuous passive
 motion (CPM)
Meniscus injury and repair
Fibroelastic cartilage
Meniscectomy
Zone I

Red-on-red
Zone II
Red-on-white
Zone III
White-on-white
Vascular access channel

CHAPTER OUTLINE

Articular Cartilage
 Composition
  Articular Cartilage Zones
  Collagen in Articular Cartilage
  Vascular Supply of Articular Cartilage
 Function
 Immobilizations and Response to Healing
 Injury
 Healing and Repair
 Techniques of Stimulating Cartilage Repair
  and Therapeutic Applications
 Alternative Management for Articular
  Cartilage Pathology
  Débridement
  Arthroscopic Osteochondral Autografts

 Autologous Chondrocyte
  Transplantation
 Oral Administration of Glucosamine
  and Chondroitin Sulfate
 Viscosupplementation through
  Intraarticular Hyaluronic Acid
  Injection
Meniscus (Fibroelastic Cartilage)
 Composition
  Neuroanatomy
 Function
 Injury
 Healing
 Clinical Application of Rehabilitation
  Techniques after Meniscal Injury

Understanding the mechanisms involved in the healing of articular **(hyaline) cartilage** and fibroelastic cartilage promotes the appropriate application of rehabilitation techniques. Therefore rehabilitation techniques are based on the foundation of intrinsic cartilage repair (chondrogenesis), time necessary for healing, and extrinsic reparative interventions. **Osteoarthritis** (degenerative joint disease), chondromalacia (softening of hyaline cartilage), meniscal lesions, and many other articular and meniscal pathologic processes are common problems the physical therapist assistant (PTA) sees clinically. Therefore understanding injury and repair of articular cartilage defects and meniscal lesions helps the PTA to understand the rationale for appropriate rehabilitation techniques.

ARTICULAR CARTILAGE
Composition

Articular cartilage covers the ends of bones with synovial joints. It is composed primarily of water (approximately 65% to 80%),[6,9] which provides for load deformation of the cartilage surface.[12] The tensile strength of articular cartilage depends on type II collagen, which is approximately 20% of the total composition of hyaline cartilage.[15] Proteoglycans contribute 10% to 15% of the structure of articular cartilage. These proteoglycans are made up of glycosaminoglycans, which are in part responsible for bearing the compressive strength of articular cartilage. Finally, **chondrocytes** (mature cartilage cells) make up 5% of the articular cartilage.[12,15]

Articular Cartilage Zones

Articular cartilage is an extremely nonhomogeneous tissue. The composition of articular cartilage varies considerably among four distinct zones. The superficial zone of articular cartilage is composed of water and parallel, highly organized collagen fibrils with very limited concentration of proteoglycans.[10] The middle or transitional zone of articular cartilage demonstrates randomly arranged, large diameter collagen and rounded chondrocytes.[10] The deep zone is rich in proteoglycans and lowest in water concentration. Collagen is large with a more organized structure arranged vertically.[10]

The zone of calcified cartilage is the deepest zone that separates cartilage tissue from subchondral bone. This small distinct layer is composed mainly of cells, cartilage, matrix, and inorganic salts (Fig. 11-1 and Table 11-1).

Collagen in Articular Cartilage

Articular cartilage is an extremely unique biologic tissue with both durable and permeable characteristics. Collagen represents more than 50% of the entire dry weight of articular cartilage.[10] The vast majority of collagen in articular cartilage is type II. However, the extracellular matrix also contains types V, VI, IV, X, and XL.

Clinicians must recognize the composition of various collagen types to fully appreciate the remarkable resilience of articular cartilage tissue. Collagen in general contains various amounts of proline, hydroxyproline, and hydroxylysine. The proline content of collagen provides a structure that is highly resistant to tensile

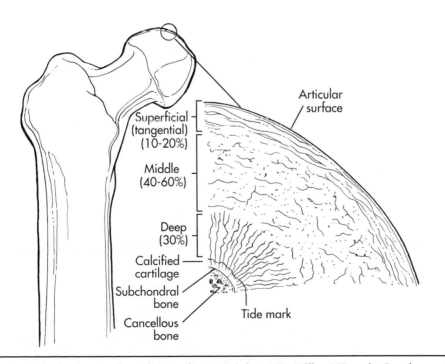

Fig. 11-1 Articular cartilage layers. (From Brinker MR, Miller MD, eds: Fundamentals of Orthopaedics. Philadelphia, WB Saunders, 1999.)

Table 11-1	*Articular Cartilage Layers*			
Layer	**Width (μm)**	**Characteristic**	**Orientation**	**Function**
Gliding zone (superficial)	40	↓ Metabolic activity	Tangential	vs. Shear
Transitional zone (middle)	500	↑ Metabolic activity	Oblique	vs. Compression
Radial zone (deep)	1000	↑ Collagen size	Vertical	vs. Compression
Tidemark	5	Undulation barrier	Tangential	vs. Shear
Calcified zone	300	Hydroxyapatite crystals		Anchor

↑, increased; ↓, decreased

From Brinker MR, Miller MD: Fundamentals of Orthopaedics. Philadelphia, WB Saunders, 1999.

Table 11-2	*Overview of Collagen Types*
Type	**Location**
I	Bone
	Tendon
	Meniscus
	Annulus of intervertebral disk
	Skin
II	Articular cartilage
	Nucleus pulposus of intervertebral disk
III	Skin
	Blood vessels
IV	Basement membrane
V	Articular cartilage (in small amounts)
VI	Articular cartilage (in small amounts)
VII	Basement membrane
VIII	Basement membrane
IX	Articular cartilage (in small amounts)
X	Hypertrophic cartilage
	Associated with calcification of cartilage (matrix mineralization)
XI	Articular cartilage (in small amounts)
XII	Tendon
XIII	Endothelial cells

From Brinker MR, Miller MD: Fundamentals of Orthopaedics. Philadelphia, WB Saunders, 1999.

forces. Conversely, hydroxyproline composition of collagen provides for compressive stability of articular cartilage. Therefore articular cartilage is composed of collagen types that are distinct in organization, structure, and fiber arrangement and that are consistent with the zones of cartilage and their unique physiologic requirements of compression, tension, stiffness, strength, and durability (Table 11-2).[10]

Vascular Supply of Articular Cartilage

Vascularized tissues heal in an organized, predictable fashion. Trauma to vascular tissue incites an intense cascade of events characterized by hemorrhage, inflammation, and fibrin clot formation. Angiogenesis, or neovascularization, is the hallmark of intrinsic repair through mobilization of repair molecules and undifferentiated cells capable of synthesizing matrix and new tissue.[10]

Articular cartilage is a nonhomogeneous avascular structure with a dramatic inability to stimulate, regulate, or organize intrinsic repair. Without an intense vascular response to injury, articular cartilage cannot form a fibrin scaffold or mobilize cells to repair the defect. Chondrocytes are incapable of traveling to the damaged site via a vascular access channel and because these necessary cells are essentially trapped within dense extracellular matrix, they cannot migrate to the injury site.[10]

Therefore spontaneous healing of superficial wounds to articular cartilage is not possible. Rather, weak, fragile proteoglycans surround the injury, whereas chondrocytes do not fill the defect. Deep injury that communicates below the deep, calcified zone into subchondral bone produces a vascular inflammatory response to a limited extent. As expected, a fibrin clot forms a repair-like tissue but ultimately demonstrates biochemical and mechanically inferior weak scar.

Function

The viscoelastic structure of articular cartilage, by virtue of its component parts of collagen, water, and proteoglycans, makes hyaline cartilage incredibly durable.[12,15] Generally, articular cartilage is only 2 to 4 mm thick, yet it is capable of bearing compressive loads many times greater than body weight.[21] Articular cartilage is resistant to wear; almost entirely frictionless; and responsible for influencing and dissipating compression, shear, and tension forces within diarthrodial synovial joints.[12,15,21]

Articular cartilage is also permeable. The chondrocytes within the cartilage must receive nutrition to remain viable. The synovial fluid surrounding the articular cartilage provides the necessary nutrients through joint motion and normal physiologic weight bearing by diffusion, convection, or both.[15] Therefore normal joint motion is needed to maintain the cartilage integrity, fluid movement (lubrication between articulating surfaces), and nutrition of hyaline cartilage.[15]

Table 11-3	*Biochemical Changes of Articular Cartilage*	
	Aging	**Osteoarthritis (OA)**
Water content (hydration; permeability)	↓	↑
Collagen	Content remains relatively unchanged	Becomes disorderly (breakdown of matrix framework) Content ↓ in severe OA Relative concentration ↑ (because of loss of proteoglycans)
Proteoglycan content (concentration)	↓ (Also the length of the protein core and GAG chains decreases)	↓
Proteoglycan synthesis	↓	↑
Proteoglycan degradation	↓	↑↑↑
Chondroitin sulfate concentration (includes both chondroitin 4- and 6-sulfate)	↓	↑
Chondroitin 4-sulfate concentration	↓	↑
Keratin sulfate concentration	↑	↓
Chondrocyte size	↑	
Chondrocyte number	↓	
Modulus of elasticity	↑	↓

From Brinker MR, Miller MD: Fundamentals of Orthopaedics. Philadelphia, WB Saunders, 1999.

Immobilization and Response to Healing

Articular cartilage requires physiologic stress (e.g., cyclical compression) to maintain its unique environment as a strong, tough, fatigue-resistant, permeable, and frictionless tissue.[10,11] The biochemical components of proteoglycans (glycosaminoglycans) chondrocytes, matrix-molecules, and collagen significantly contribute to its structure, composition, and mechanical properties.[10,11]

Just as collagen is varied and distinct among the zones of articular cartilage, so are proteoglycans distributed in different concentrations between zones. Because these proteoglycan molecules—including chondroitin sulfate, keratan sulfate, and dermatan sulfate—bind and attract water (hydrophilic), their concentration and distribution among zones influence the various mechanical wear characteristics of articular cartilage.[10,11]

The removal of normal physiologic loading, unloading, and joint motion have profoundly negative effects on the biochemical and mechanical characteristics of articular cartilage.[10,11]

The significance of articular cartilage atrophy and degeneration is related to the magnitude and duration of immobilization. Joint contact surfaces suffer greater degenerative changes than noncontact areas of articular cartilage (Table 11-3).[10,11]

Chondrocyte necrosis and subchondral bone degenerative lesions occur with prolonged rigid immobilization. Generally, immobilization and lack of physiologic stress cause a reduction in the synthesis and concentration of proteoglycans, which ultimately leads to surface fibrillation, fissures, and ulceration of the various zones of articular cartilage.[10,11]

Injury

Articular cartilage can be damaged in many ways.[15,21] Erosion of the articular surface and degeneration can be seen clinically in patients ranging from young athletes to elderly people. Causes of degenerative joint disease include related joint instability, blunt trauma, repetitive overloading, and immobilization.[21] Articular cartilage degeneration is generally characterized by three progressively overlapping degenerative events (Fig. 11-2).[21] Initially the hyaline cartilage begins to fray or fibrillate. Progressive destruction leads to blistering of the articular surface. Further joint deterioration leads to splitting or clefting (fissuring) of the surface, which affects the deeper layers of cartilage and eventually progresses to denuded bone.[21] Although blunt trauma, progressive friction abrasion, and a sharp concentration of weight bearing forces mechanically erode articular cartilage, causing various degrees of wear, joint immobilization does not cause mechanical changes. However, joint immobilization may lead to loss of the load bearing structural compression-resistant component proteoglycans (glycosaminoglycans).[15] Such loss is related to decreased normal joint loading (which is needed for cartilage nutrition) and physiologic motion.

Hyaline cartilage erosion can occur after trauma, penetrating injury, infection or compressive loads, joint

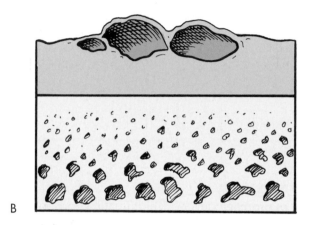

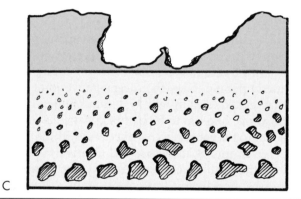

Fig. 11-2 Articular cartilage degeneration generally is characterized by three progressive overlapping stages: **A,** Fibrillation or fraying of articular cartilage. **B,** Blistering of articular surface. **C,** Splitting, clefting, or fissuring of articular surface.

immobilization, and reduction of normal joint mechanics. The therapeutic application of exercise and functional activities must be adjusted and modified to minimize the progressive destruction of tissue in patients who have a range of osteoarthritic changes to articular cartilage changes caused by long-term immobilization.

Healing and Repair

Articular cartilage defects heal differently, depending on the extent or depth of the injury.[12,15,21] Less serious, more superficial lesions of articular cartilage do not remodel or heal as well as deeper or full-thickness injuries. Healing of these superficial layers occurs through proteoglycans and chondrocyte proliferation, but the strength, composition, and durability of this healing tissue are exceedingly weak and inferior to those of normal articular cartilage.[15]

The reason superficial articular cartilage defects do not heal as well as deeper injuries is that these injuries do not stimulate an inflammatory reaction.[15] The thickness of the articular cartilage (2 to 4 mm) forms a barrier between the superficial layers of the cartilage and subchondral blood vessels, effectively eliminating any contact among fibrin, fibroblasts, and inflammatory response cells (neutrophils, macrophages). In effect, the chondrocytes do not adhere to the defect and do not fill the injury site with new tissue.

Deeper wounds or full-thickness injuries expose **subchondral bone** blood vessels to the defect site, which stimulates the acute **inflammatory response.** Full-thickness cartilage injuries heal spontaneously with large amounts of type I collagen. (Articular cartilage is primarily composed of type II collagen.) In fact, 1 year after injury, approximately 20% of the repaired defect remains type I collagen.[15] Although full-thickness injuries heal considerably better than superficial wounds, the quality of the scar formed within the defect remains inferior to normal articular cartilage, and the healed scar does not maintain its integrity over time.[15]

Techniques of Stimulating Cartilage Repair and Therapeutic Applications

When treating patients recovering from injury, immobilization, or disease of the articular cartilage, appropriate physical therapy measures are those that stimulate cartilage repair.

Arthroscopic surgical shaving of articular cartilage is a common practice in patients with femoral and patellar articular cartilage disease.[5,9] The procedure is designed to remove the loose fibrillated tissue and smooth the articular surface contours. Ideally removing the irritated tissue lessens the symptoms of pain and dysfunction. Articular cartilage repair is promoted when the injury site can go through the inflammatory process and when factors lead to chondrocyte proliferation. Therefore with some cartilage defects, surgically abrading or drilling multiple small holes (perforating) through the cartilage layers down to bone stimulates bleeding and initiates the healing process.

Noninvasive therapeutic measures also are beneficial in the treatment of articular cartilage injury. Limited weight bearing activities can arrest symptoms of pain

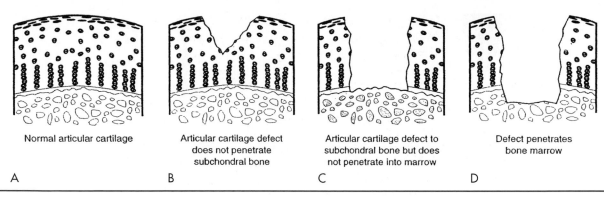

Normal articular cartilage	Articular cartilage defect does not penetrate subchondral bone	Articular cartilage defect to subchondral bone but does not penetrate into marrow	Defect penetrates bone marrow
A	B	C	D

Fig. 11-3   The various types and depths of articular cartilage defects or lesions that can be created in animal models to evaluate repair processes in articular cartilage. **A,** Normal articular cartilage is typically organized histologically into zones. **B,** A partial-thickness (superficial or shallow) defect penetrating to the middle zone is isolated from the blood supply and marrow space. Such a defect typically does not elicit or demonstrate a repair response. **C,** A lesion that penetrates to the subchondral bone but does not penetrate into the marrow space, if truly isolated from the marrow, will not repair. However, even a very small communication of the lesion with the marrow blood supply will elicit a repair response. Full-thickness lesions usually are in this category. **D,** A defect that penetrates through all zones of the articular cartilage and penetrates into the marrow space typically demonstrates a repair response that results in fibrocartilaginous tissue. (From Jackson DW, et al: Cartilage substitutes: overview of basic science and treatment options. *J Am Acad Orthop Surg* 2001;9:42.)

and swelling in some cases of articular cartilage injury. Reducing vertical compressive loads (stair climbing, squats, and walking) is a critical first step in the care of tibiofemoral articular cartilage defects. Patients can maintain strength with isometric exercise or limited open kinetic-chain progressive–resistive exercise.

In cases of patellofemoral articular cartilage disease, vertical compressive loads generally do not negatively affect function. However, full range of motion (ROM) knee extension exercises may produce symptoms of pain, swelling, and crepitus (noise, grinding, and cracking). Limited ROM exercises that do not produce pain and crepitus, along with isometric exercises, are most appropriate with patellofemoral disease.

As mentioned in Chapter 9, **continuous passive motion (CPM)** is used in the care of articular cartilage injury. Again, the benefits from the use of CPM are limited to full-thickness hyaline cartilage defects.[17,18] Salter and colleagues[17,18] demonstrated that CPM used on full-thickness cartilage injury in rabbits showed healing of the defect with tissue resembling hyaline cartilage. Salter and associates,[16–18] who believe that CPM can help stimulate chondrocyte formation, also found that using CPM with full-thickness hyaline cartilage injuries improves articular cartilage nutrition by enhancing fluid mechanics, inhibiting adhesions, and clearing the joint of noxious material.

Maintaining near-normal joint motion through modified exercise regimens and weight bearing activities (depending on the location and severity of the articular defect) are necessary both for healing of cartilage injuries and maintenance of hyaline cartilage nutrition.

Alternative Management for Articular Cartilage Pathology

Various surgical interventions are at the disposal of the surgeon that are designed to stimulate an intense inflammatory response or to débride–irrigate (lavage) cartilage debris from within the joint (Fig. 11-3).

Operative repair or stimulation procedures generally are described as drilling, abrasion, chondroplasty, or microfracture techniques, all of which are used to create a vascularized ingrowth of chondrocyte cells and collagen that migrate to the injury site.[5]

The typical outcome of these "penetrating" techniques is the partial development of fibrocartilage consisting of type I collagen, which attempts to fill the defect. Normal hyaline cartilage contains predominantly type II collagen; therefore the repair tissue that forms from surgical stimulation techniques is histochemically and biochemically fragile and weak when compared with structurally intact articular cartilage. It should be remembered that normal cartilage is a nonhomogeneous tissue with anatomically distinct layers of differing collagen types with various orientations and biochemical contributions to compression, shear, and tensile loads.

The long-term outcome of these various surgical interventions is highly unpredictable without consistent alleviation of symptoms or increased function (Fig. 11-4).

Débridement

Short-term temporary relief of symptomatic articular cartilage lesions can be achieved with arthroscopic lavage or débridement of cartilaginous debris. Essentially, arthroscopic débridement removes particles of

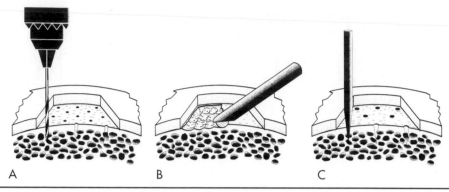

Fig. 11-4 Various methodologies currently used to elicit repair tissue in articular cartilage defects. **A,** Current methods involve penetrating the underlying bone endplate by drilling, as proposed in the Pridie procedure. Variations include, **B,** abrasion and, **C,** microfracture. All these techniques penetrate the subchondral bond to open communication with a zone of vascularization to initiate fibrin clot formation and obtain the potential benefit of vascular ingrowth or migration of more primitive mesenchymal cells from the bone marrow. These communications open the defect to the migration of many types of cells, including fibroblasts and inflammatory cells. These cells may compete with a limited number of the primitive mesenchymal cells to occupy the fibrin matrix, contributing to a variety of repair scenarios. These methods penetrate the subchondral bone plate and tidemark, but the intent is not to disrupt the integrity of the subchondral bone. Large disruption or removal of the subchondral bone end plate may result in detrimental mechanical, structural, and biologic changes. (From Jackson DW, et al: Cartilage substitutes: overview of basic science and treatment options. *J Am Acad Orthop Surg* 2001;9:45.)

cartilage, degradative enzymes (matrix metalloproteinases [MMPs]), and proinflammatory cytokines, all of which contribute to the painful disability of articular cartilage osteoarthritic lesions. Therefore the benefit of arthroscopic débridement is temporary with no true inflammatory response or cellular proliferation. Joint lavage (irrigation) with saline inflow provides a substantial isolated benefit by removing tissue debris and inflammatory cells even without surgical intervention of articular shavers with suction.[5]

Arthroscopic Osteochondral Autografts

Full-thickness articular lesions (osteochondral) can be surgically "filled with transplanted plugs" of intact bone and articular cartilage using the technique of mosaicplasty or osteochondral autograft transplantation system (OATS) (Fig. 11-5).

The surgeon prepares the lesion by removing all nonviable surrounding tissue from the crater, thereby creating precise borders or "edges and floors" of the lesion. Multiple full-thickness bone plugs are surgically harvested from a relative non–load-bearing surface of the femur, usually the superior lateral femoral condyle or, less often, the inferior condylar notch. Actually, harvest site morbidity is a concern because full-knee ROM provides significant contact pressure of the mentioned harvest sites.[5] These cylindrical osteochondral plugs become revascularized (incorporated) into

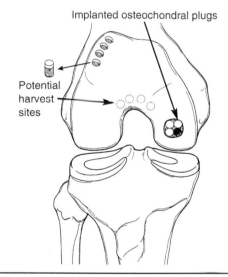

Fig. 11-5 Osteochondral plug transplantation technique. The lesion site is prepared by débriding any loose articular cartilage, and the number and size of the plugs to be used for repair are determined. The holes to receive the plugs are drilled in the floor of the lesion. With use of specialized harvesting instrumentation, the osteochondral plugs are procured from suitable sites so as to approximate the surface geometry of the lesion site. The plugs are then implanted to the appropriate depth into the holes placed in the lesion base. (From Jackson DW, et al: Cartilage substitutes: overview of basic science and treatment options. *J Am Acad Orthop Surg* 2001;9:48.)

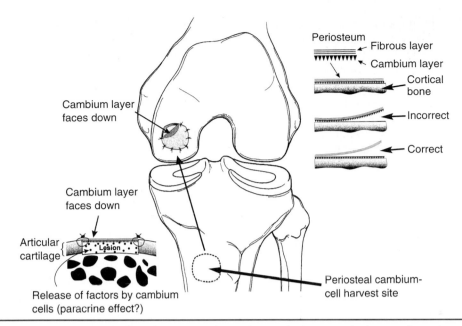

Periosteum
← Fibrous layer
← Cambium layer
Cortical bone
← Incorrect
← Correct

Cambium layer faces down

Cambium layer faces down

Articular cartilage

Lesion

Release of factors by cambium cells (paracrine effect?)

Periosteal cambium-cell harvest site

Fig. 11-6 Autologous chondrocyte implantation technique. Articular cartilage is procured, and its chondrocytes are enzymatically released and expanded in cell culture. When a sufficient number of cells are obtained, a second operation is performed for implantation of the cultured cells. A periosteal flap with matching geometry is harvested and sutured in place with the cambium cell layer facing the defect (down). Care must be taken to ensure that the cambium cells remain attached to the periosteal fibrous layer *(inset)*. (From Jackson DW, et al: Cartilage substitutes: overview of basic science and treatment options. *J Am Acad Orthop Surg* 2001;9:46.)

the lesion. These "press-fit" plugs contain viable hyaline cartilage, which tends to "survive" over time and remains structurally stable.[5]

Several key factors may compromise the outcome of the OATS technique. The convex geometry of the femoral condyles contributes to a relative joint incongruence because the shape of the plugs may not match the surrounding surface with anatomic precision. In addition, the depth placement of the chondral plugs is critical because the donor plugs may collapse or "settle" over time or may be inserted with too much "pride" (the surface of the plugs may sit too high above the horizon of the chondral plate).[5]

Autologous Chondrocyte Transplantation

Because of substantial variations in collagen types, orientation, proteoglycan content, extracellular matrix composition, and avascularity of the four anatomically distinct zones of articular cartilage, a tissue transplantation procedure is available to "generate" a biologic substitute tissue.[5]

The autologous chondrocyte transplantation procedure calls for two separate surgical interventions. First the surgeon "harvests" articular cartilage from a "minor" load bearing surface of the superior medial or lateral femoral condyle. The harvested tissue is peeled off in several strips 5 mm wide and 15 mm long and

placed in sterile vials. This harvested tissue is sent to a specific laboratory, where the chondrocytes are enzymatically separated from the extracellular matrix. The chondrocyte cells are cultured and multiplied for 4 to 6 weeks. The second procedure prepares the chondral defect through débridement. A separate small incision is made over the proximal anteromedial aspect of the tibia to harvest a "periosteal patch" 1 to 2 mm larger than the femoral condyle defect. This layer of periosteum is secured with fibrin glue and sutures. The cultured chondrocytes are injected under the patch to fill the defect with biologically active viable chondrocytes (Fig. 11-6).

Oral Administration of Glucosamine and Chondroitin Sulfate

Articular cartilage is composed of various collagen types and an extensive extracellular matrix (ECM) of glycosaminoglycans (GAGs) and proteoglycans. Major GAGs in human connective tissue are keratan sulfate, dermatan sulfate, heparin sulfate, chondroitin sulfate, and hyaluronic sulfate.

Degenerative articular cartilage disease processes generally demonstrate an imbalance between production synthesis of proteoglycans and degradation of GAGs.

It should be recognized that proteoglycans and GAGs are extremely hydrophilic because of large negatively charged macromolecules referred to as *aggregates*. The binding and attraction for water contributes significant and important biochemical properties to articular cartilage to resist and influence compression and shear forces.

Catabolic processes involved with osteoarthritis (MMPs, cytokines, and growth factors) create an imbalance between GAGs and proteoglycan synthesis and degradation. With reduction in proteoglycan content of articular cartilage (keratin sulfate, dermatan sulfate, heparin sulfate, hyaluronic acid, and predominantly chondroitin sulfate), the fluid-binding capacity of the large aggregate GAGs is lost. The result is a biochemically weaker structure that is increasingly vulnerable to compression, shear, and tensile loads, further stimulating the degradative processes of osteoarthritis.

The exogenous oral administration of two key constituents of articular cartilage proteoglycans and GAGs (glucosamine and chondroitin sulfate) may contribute to the reestablishment of fluid attraction, thereby reducing degenerative effects or preventing further erosion.

Generally, glucosamine is an amino saccharide that participates in the synthesis of GAGs and proteoglycans by chondrocytes.[3] Glucosamine is also an active substrate for the production of chondroitin sulfate, hyaluronic acid, and other proteoglycans in the articular cartilage matrix.[3]

Chondroitin sulfate is a GAG and significant constituent of large molecular mass proteoglycans referred to as *aggrecan*. The oral administration of glucosamine or chondroitin sulfate proposes a gradual "chondroprotective" role by reestablishing the water-binding nature of the articular cartilage matrix.

Clinical trials and commercial products recommend daily doses of 500 mg three times daily as an effective regimen.[3] Glucosamine sulfate generally appears to have a more rapid onset of effects (4 to 8 weeks), as compared with chondroitin sulfate (3 to 6 months).[3] Overall, Brief and associates describe the clinical efficacy of these agents as follows:

> . . . a progressive and gradual decline of joint pain and tenderness, improved mobility, and sustained improvement after drug withdrawal. In addition, there are fewer side effects when compared with other drugs used to treat the symptoms of osteoarthritis, as well as a lack of toxicity associated with short-term use of these agents.[3]

Viscosupplementation through Intraarticular Hyaluronic Acid Injection

Hyaluronic acid is a proteoglycan constituent of articular cartilage matrix and synovial fluid. Both fibroblasts and synoviocytes synthesize hyaluronic acid into the joint space of the knee.[24]

The normal, nonpathologic human adult knee contains approximately 2 mL of synovial fluid with a hyaluronic acid concentration of 2.5 to 4.0 mg per mL.[24]

Osteoarthritis creates a deficit in volume and molecular mass of hyaluronic acid.[24] This reduction in hyaluronic acid causes lower viscosity, high stress concentration, and lowered elastic properties of the synovium and articular cartilage matrix.[24]

Injecting hyaluronic acid proposes to benefit the osteoarthritic knee by reducing pain and inflammation, replenishing decreased volume of hyaluronic acid, and stimulating intrinsic synovial synthesis of hyaluronic acid.[24] Hyaluronic acid is manufactured from purified and isolated noninflammatory hyaluronate from rooster combs.[24] Therefore patients with known hypersensitive allergic reaction to avian products should be carefully identified. Hyaluronic acid injections are shown to reduce inflammation by limiting prostaglandins, reducing circulating proinflammatory cytokine, and decreasing the release of arachidonic acid from synovial fibroblasts.[24]

Typically, commercially available hyaluronic acid preparations are injected into the affected knee joint once a week for a total of 3 weeks. At present, there is no consensus about the clinical efficacy of hyaluronic acid intraarticular injections. Several clinical trials have demonstrated no increased joint function or pain relief when compared with traditional nonsteroid antiinflammatory agents or intraarticular steroidal preparations. However, clinical trials of hyaluronic acid injections versus placebo favor its use. The rate of side effects is approximately 1% per injection. Local site reaction of pain, warmth, and swelling are most common and last 1 to 2 days.[24]

MENISCUS (FIBROELASTIC CARTILAGE)

Understanding **meniscus injury and repair** is a necessary foundation for the appropriate delivery of rehabilitation programs. The PTA also must be aware of the differences in healing between articular cartilage and **fibroelastic** (meniscus) **cartilage.**

Composition

Fibroelastic cartilage is found within the synovial joints of the acromioclavicular joint, sternoclavicular joint, glenohumeral joint, hip, and knee. A large percentage of fibroelastic cartilage is water,[8] whereas a major constituent of meniscal tissue is collagen. Meniscal tissue contains four types of collagen:[1] type I collagen comprises about 90%, whereas types II, V, and VI account for 1% to 2% each in the total collagen in the meniscus. Proteoglycans and elastin (0.6%) complete the components of fibroelastic cartilage.[1]

Neuroanatomy

Once considered aneural, the meniscus of the knee is now recognized to contribute to joint stability by virtue of mechanoreceptors located within the anterior and posterior horns. Three distinct types of afferent mechanoreceptors in the meniscus are Golgi tendon organs, Ruffini endings, and Pacinian corpuscles.[1,2] These highly specific organs provide a protective–reactive afferent feedback mechanism to guard against hyperextension and hyperflexion motions in the knee. The specific location of these mechanoreceptors (the posterior horns more richly innervated than the anterior horns) is indicative of the protective stimulation created by compression and tension of the meniscal horns during extremes of flexion and extension.

Function

The menisci of the knee are semilunar (C-shaped) fibroelastic tissues that have several functions. Generally the meniscus dissipates extreme compressive (vertical) loads. By virtue of its anatomic position within the knee and its collagen makeup, the meniscus acts as a mechanical buffer between the load bearing surfaces of the tibia and the femur. The meniscus of the knee also functions as a shock absorber.[1] Studies have shown that a knee without a meniscus has 20% less shock-absorbing capacity than normal knees.[23] Total **meniscectomy** (complete removal), subtotal meniscectomy (partial removal), and repair (suturing of torn parts) are discussed elsewhere in this chapter. The concept of partial removal and repair of the meniscus is in part founded on maintaining as much viable tissue as possible to serve in load bearing, shock absorption, joint stability, and lubrication.

The meniscus functions as a secondary restraint in joint stability. Several factors influence its effect, including ligament stability, joint surface congruency, and joint compression loads.[1] Significant joint instability does not occur with an isolated, total meniscectomy. However, a meniscectomy combined with anterior cruciate ligament injuries produces profound joint instability.[20]

The meniscus also limits knee hyperextension as a passive restraint and functions in joint lubrication and nutrition.[8] Normal physiologic joint motion promotes the lubricating effects of a thin layer of fluid between the joint surfaces. The meniscus may spread this lubrication medium during motion.[14]

Injury

Injuries to the meniscus can be traumatic or degenerative. Traumatic intraarticular fibrocartilage tears usually occur in a younger population (<40) and generally result from a combination of compression, torque, acceleration, or deceleration. These events usually occur during running, jumping, twisting, and dynamic change-of-direction activities.

Degenerative meniscal tears typically occur in an older population (>40). These injuries do not present with a history of sudden trauma, but rather with a minor event that precipitates complaints of pain and dysfunction.[1]

Healing

The vascular anatomy of the meniscus profoundly influences the type of healing that occurs and the degree of remodeling, such as with articular cartilage. The peripheral borders of the medial and lateral meniscus of the knee are vascularized between 10% and 30% of the width of the tissue.[1] If an injury occurs within a nonvascular region of the meniscus, spontaneous, intrinsic repair is not possible because no vascular supply communicates with the injury site. However, if the injury extends to the periphery where the cartilage is vascularized, then healing is possible through the inflammatory–response mechanism.

Surgical repair or excision of meniscal tissue is based on the extent of the injury and whether the injury is located within a vascularized area. If the tear is within the vascularized peripheral border (only 15% to 20% of all meniscal injuries occur within the vascularized bed of the meniscus), arthroscopic repair can be done by placing sutures in the meniscus to approximate the torn tissue.[1] Surgeons refer to the following zone system of evaluating meniscal injuries:[4]

Zone I   Both portions of the meniscus are torn within the vascularized periphery; **"red-on-red"**

Zone II   One portion of the meniscus is torn within the vascularized periphery, whereas the other portion is in the avascular region; **"red-on-white"**

Zone III   No blood supply on either side of the injury; **"white-on-white"**

Both red-on-red and red-on-white zones are considered reparable. However, in animal studies,[2] if an injury is present within the white-on-white nonvascularized Zone III area of the meniscus, researchers surgically create a **"vascular access channel"** to connect the blood supply of the periphery to the area of injury without circulation.[1,3] This study shows that the blood vessels migrated to the injury site and provided an avenue for repair.

When injuries occur in an avascular portion of the meniscus, the surgeon must perform either a subtotal (partial removal) or total meniscectomy. After either of these procedures, some studies have shown partial or complete regeneration of fibrocartilaginous tissue.[1] However, for the regeneration of tissue to occur after a meniscectomy, the tissue must be removed to expose the vascular synovium.[1]

Arnoczky and colleagues[1] state:

Thus it appears that the synovial and peripheral meniscal vasculatures are capable of generating a connective tissue replacement for the removed meniscus. It should be noted, however, that this regeneration is not always complete and does not occur in all cases.

Clinical Application of Rehabilitation Techniques after Meniscal Injury

The mechanics of meniscal injury, surgical repairs, meniscectomies, and criteria-based programs are covered in Chapter 19. However, an understanding of how and why fibroelastic cartilage responds to a repair procedure versus a meniscectomy and how these procedures affect the course of rehabilitation is clinically relevant to the PTA.

In general terms, after a subtotal or total meniscectomy, treatment focuses on pain management, reduction in swelling, improved ROM, normalized gait, increased strength, increased girth of the thigh musculature, development of aerobic fitness, and improved proprioception. With a meniscectomy patient, ROM exercises (active and active assistive) can be instituted immediately and progressed according to the patient's tolerance. Weight bearing should progress in the same manner.[19] Usually full weight bearing is used within 10 days of surgery.[19] Stationary cycling, isometric exercise progressing to concentric and eccentric resistance exercise, and progressive closed kinetic-chain exercises can be initiated when pain, swelling, and strength allow. Gaining full ROM and progressive weight bearing does not alter or inhibit the healing processes after a meniscectomy and depends on whether or not there is any associated articular cartilage defect.

The rehabilitation program after meniscal repair has the same long-range goals (reduced pain and swelling, progressive motion, strength, and progressive weight bearing) as for a meniscectomy patient, but its implementation must be altered, taking into account the initiation of weight bearing and ROM exercises in relation to the healing process of a repaired meniscus.[3,15] In a surgically repaired meniscus, if full or even partial weight bearing is progressed too soon, the compressive forces and load bearing mechanics during gait disrupt the healing processes.[2,4] Full weight bearing generally is not allowed until 4 to 6 weeks after surgery.[19] However, toe-touch weight bearing may be allowed at 3 weeks and progressive partial weight bearing 4 to 5 weeks after surgery.

ROM also can influence the healing of a repaired meniscus. If full flexion is allowed too early, the motion created within the knee may place "undue stress upon the sutures and the repair site."[4] Therefore ROM activities must progress cautiously until secure healing of the sutured meniscus has occurred.

The contrasts in rehabilitation programs between those used for meniscectomies and repaired (sutured) meniscus are founded on the nature and disposition of healing mechanics related to forces acting on the meniscus (weight bearing and ROM), time, and the vascular supply supporting the healing tissues. Strengthening exercises can be initiated if they progress gradually from isometrics, to multiangle isometrics, to open kinetic-chain exercises, to isokinetics, and finally, to closed-chain resistance exercises.

Many rehabilitation programs are organized in phases (maximum protection phase, moderate protection phase, and minimum protection phase), which are developed in part to minimize unwanted forces on healing tissues.[22] For meniscal injuries, phased programs allow for continued clinical assessment of a patient's progress while restraining unnecessary motion and weight bearing and allowing for proper, secure healing.

❖ ADDITIONAL FEATURES

Articular Cartilage: Concentration of collagen, proteoglycans, and water influences tensile forces, compression, shear, and permeability.

Articular Cartilage Composition: Chondrocytes, matrix, type II collagen, proteoglycans, and noncollagenous proteins.

Articular Cartilage Injury and Repair: Intrinsic repair depends on the nature and extent of the injury. Trauma that penetrates cartilage but not subchondral bone leaves a defect that does not heal. Penetration of subchondral bone stimulates intense vascular response that allows weak fibrous tissue to fill the defect.

Deep Zone: Largest part of the articular cartilage. Contains the largest collagen fibrils and has the highest proteoglycan content and lowest water content.

Injuries in Vascular Zones of the Meniscus: Intrinsic repair is possible if the lesion communicates with a blood supply. Stimulates inflammatory response. If an injury occurs in the vascular zones, a fibrin clot forms that acts as a scaffold for ingrowth of vessels.

Meniscus Gross Anatomy: Extension of the tibia; peripheral border is thick, convex, and attached to the capsule; the opposite border tapers to a thin free edge. Medial meniscus is semicircular; lateral meniscus is nearly circular. Tibial portion of capsular attachment of medial meniscus is referred to as the coronary ligament.

Meniscus Neuroanatomy: Horns of the meniscus are innervated; there is less innervation of the bodies of the meniscus. The central third of the meniscus is aneural. The sensory afferent arc may provide proprioception information concerning joint position.

Meniscus Vascular Anatomy: Blood supply from the lateral and medial genicular arteries. Vessels penetrate 10% to 30% of the periphery of the medial meniscus and 10% to 25% of the lateral meniscus.

Structure and Function of Articular Cartilage: Proteoglycans and water provide stiffness to compression; proteoglycans contribute resiliency and durability. Articular cartilage is a nonhomogeneous tissue. Elaborate organization of cells and matrix that varies considerably in depth.

Transition Zone of Articular Cartilage: Several times the volume of the superficial zone. Contains large collagen fibrils.

Vascular Zone I of Meniscus: "Red-on-red." The location of the tear is vascular on both sides. Reparable intrinsic healing is possible.

Vascular Zone II of Meniscus: "Red-on-white." The location of the tear is vascular on one side. Reparable intrinsic healing is possible.

Vascular Zone III of the Meniscus: "White-on-white." The location of the tear is avascular on both sides. There is no intrinsic repair.

Zones of Articular Cartilage: Superficial zone is the thinnest zone. Gliding surface of joint is covered with a thin, clear liquid that is almost entirely frictionless.

Zone of Calcified Cartilage: Separates softer cartilage from subchondral bone. Forms anchor for hyaline cartilage to attach to bone.

REFERENCES

1. Arnoczky SP, et al: Meniscus. In Buschbacher JA, Woo SL-Y, eds. Injury and Repair of the Musculoskeletal Soft Tissues. Rosemont, IL, American Academy of Orthopaedic Surgeons, 1988.
2. Arnoczky SP, Warren RF: The microvasculature of the meniscus and it's response to injury: an experimental study in the dog. *Am J Sports Med* 1983;11:131–141.
3. Brief AA, et al: Use of glucosamine and chondroitin sulfate in the management of osteoarthritis. *J Am Acad Orthop Surg* 2001; 9:71–78.
4. Hammesfahr JR: Surgery of the knee. In Donatelli R, Wooden MJ, eds. Orthopaedic Physical Therapy. New York, Churchill Livingstone, 1989.
5. Jackson DW, et al: Cartilage substitutes: overview of basic science and treatment options. *J Am Acad Orthop Surg* 2001;9:37–52.
6. Jaffe FF, et al: Water binding in the articular cartilage of rabbits. *J Bone Joint Surg* 1974;56A: 1031–1039.
7. Johnson LL: Diagnostic and Surgical Arthroscopy. St Louis, Mosby, 1980.
8. MacConaill MA: The function of intraarticular fibrocartilages, with special reference to the knee and inferior radio-ulnar joints. *J Anat* 1932;66:210–227.
9. Mankin HJ: The water of articular cartilage. In Simon WH, ed. The human joint in health and disease. Philadelphia, University of Pennsylvania Press, 1978.
10. Mankin HJ, et al: Articular cartilage structure, composition, and function. In Buckwalter JA, Einhorn TA, Simon SR, eds. Orthopaedic Basic Science, Biology, and Biomechanics, 2nd ed. Rosemont, IL, American Academy of Orthopaedic Surgeons, 2000.
11. Mankin JH, et al: Articular cartilage repair and osteoarthritis. In Buckwalter JA, Einhorn TA, Simon SR, eds. Orthopaedic Basic Science, Biology, and Biomechanics, 2nd ed. Rosemont, IL, American Academy of Orthopaedic Surgeons, 2000.
12. Miller MD: Review of Orthopaedics. Philadelphia, WB Saunders, 1992.
13. O'Donoghue DH: Treatment of chondral damage to the patella. *Am J Sports Med* 1981;9:10–12.
14. Radin EL, Bryan RS: The effect of weight bearing on regrowth of the medial meniscus after meniscectomy. *J Trauma* 1970;12:169.
15. Rosenberg L, et al: Articular cartilage. In Woo SL-Y, Buckwalter JA, editors: Injury and Repair of the Musculoskeletal Soft Tissues. Rosemont, IL, American Academy of Orthopaedic Surgeons, 1988.
16. Salter RB, et al: Clinical applications of basic research on continuous passive motion for disorders and injuries of synovial joints: a preliminary report of a feasibility study. *J Orthop Res* 1983;3:325–342.
17. Salter RB, et al: Continuous passive motion and the repair of full-thickness articular cartilage defects: a one year follow-up. *Trans Orthop Res Soc* 1982;7:167.
18. Salter RB, et al: The biological effect of continuous passive motion on healing of full-thickness defects in articular cartilage: an experimental study in the rabbit. *J Bone Joint Surg* 1980; 62A:1232–1251.
19. Seto JL, Brewster CE: Rehabilitation of meniscal injuries. In Greenfield BH, ed. Rehabilitation of the Knee: A Problem-Solving Approach. Philadelphia, FA Davis, 1993.
20. Shoemaker SC, Markolf KL: The role of the meniscus in the anterior-posterior cruciate-deficient knee. *J Bone Joint Surg* 1986; 68A:71–79.
21. Threlkeld JA: Electrical stimulation of articular cartilage. In Currier DP, Nelson RM, eds. Dynamics of Human Biologic Tissues. Philadelphia, FA Davis, 1992.
22. Timm KE: Knee. In Richardson JK, Iglarsch ZA, eds. Clinical Orthopaedic Physical Therapy. Philadelphia, WB Saunders, 1994.
23. Voloshin AS, Wosk J: Shock absorption of meniscectomized and painful knees: a comparative in vivo study. *J Biomed Eng* 1983;5:157–161.
24. Watterson JR, Esdaile JM: Viscosupplementation: therapeutic mechanisms and clinical potential in osteoarthritis in the knee. *J Am Acad Orthop Surg* 2000;8:277–284.

REVIEW QUESTIONS

Multiple Choice

1. What percent of articular cartilage is water?
   A. 10% to 20%
   B. 65% to 80%
   C. 35% to 50%
   D. 15% to 40%
2. Which of the following characterizes articular cartilage?
   A. Frictionless
   B. 2 to 4 mm thick (generally)
   C. Quite durable—resistant to wear
   D. Able to dissipate compressive loads many times greater than body weight
   E. All of the above
3. Which of the following describe(s) how articular cartilage can become damaged? (Circle any that apply.)
   A. Joint instability
   B. Immobilization
   C. Fever
   D. Repetitive overload
   E. Non–weight-bearing and reduced physiologic loading
4. Which of the following describe(s) how joint immobilization affects articular cartilage? (Circle any that apply.)
   A. Increased articular wear
   B. Increased friction abrasion
   C. Loss of proteoglycans
   D. Reduced mechanical loading leading to degeneration
   E. Improved healing of superficial wounds
5. Which of the following characterize(s) how significant articular cartilage lesions heal? (Circle any that apply.)
   A. Reduced blood supply to deep lesion
   B. Reduced inflammatory response
   C. Increased vascular supply to lesion
   D. Chondrocytes communicate with the wound
   E. Reduced chondrocytes in deep wounds
6. Femoral and retropatellar arthroscopic abrasion is designed to do which of the following? (Circle any that apply.)
   A. Promote articular cartilage repair with deep, significant wounds.
   B. Smooth the articular surface.
   C. Stimulate the inflammatory process.
   D. Elicit repair via subchondral bone bleeding.
   E. Improve patellofemoral joint stability.

7. Which of the following describes the functions of the meniscus?
   A. Dissipation of compressive loads
   B. Joint lubrication
   C. Load bearing
   D. Joint stability
   E. All of the above

8. Degenerative tears of the meniscus occur typically to people of which age?
   A. Younger than 30 years old
   B. Older than 40 years old
   C. Between 30 and 40 years old
   D. Between 70 and 80 years old

9. Which of the following describes the mechanism of injury of an intraarticular fibrocartilage tear?
   A. Twisting
   B. Torque
   C. Deceleration
   D. Compression
   E. All of the above

10. What percentage of the periphery is vascular in the medial and lateral meniscus?
    A. 5% to 10%
    B. 40% to 50%
    C. 10% to 30%
    D. 20% to 40%

11. What percentage of meniscal tears occurs in the vascular border of the meniscus?
    A. 5%
    B. 40%
    C. 15% to 20%
    D. 10%

12. If an injury occurs to an area of the meniscus where the tear is vascular on both sides, it is called which of the following? (Circle any that apply.)
    A. Reparable
    B. Red-on-white
    C. Red-on-red
    D. Nonreparable
    E. Zone III

13. Which zones of injury are considered reparable? (Circle any that apply.)
    A. Red-on-white
    B. White-on-white
    C. Red-on-red
    D. Zone II
    E. Zone I

14. Identify the characteristics of rehabilitation after an isolated meniscal repair as compared with total or subtotal meniscectomy. (Circle any that apply.)
    A. Long-term goals are basically the same.
    B. Weight bearing and full range of motion should be deferred until secure healing has occurred.
    C. Closed-chain exercises begin 2 weeks after repair.
    D. Full weight bearing is allowed as soon as pain allows.
    E. Full knee flexion is allowed 1 week postoperatively.

Short Answer

15. Name the three classic surgical procedures used to correct tears of the meniscus.

16. The meniscus of the knee can be injured in two distinct ways. Name the two classifications of meniscal injuries.

True/False

17. If an injury were to occur to the central nonvascular portion of the meniscus, spontaneous intrinsic repair is not possible.

18. Normal joint motion and compressive loads are necessary for hyaline (articular) cartilage to remain viable.

19. The deeper and more extensive the damage to articular cartilage, the less "healing" occurs.

20. Superficial articular cartilage lesions heal much quicker and to a greater degree than significant wounds.

21. CPM is used to help stimulate cartilage nutrition in partial-thickness articular cartilage lesions.

22. The meniscus of the knee serves as a primary joint restraint.

23. The central portion of the medial and lateral meniscus is essentially avascular.

Essay Questions

Answer on a separate sheet of paper.

24. Discuss the composition and function of articular cartilage.

25. Identify common causes of injury to articular cartilage.

26. Describe the sequence of healing and the extent of intrinsic repair of articular cartilage.

27. Define invasive and noninvasive techniques of stimulating articular cartilage repair.

28. Define and describe the composition and function of the meniscus.

29. Identify and discuss common mechanisms of injury to the meniscus.

30. Describe the mechanisms of intrinsic healing of the meniscus.

31. List common rehabilitation techniques used in the treatment of the injured meniscus.

Critical Thinking Application

Develop your own "case study" concerning a patient with superficial articular cartilage degeneration of the patellofemoral joint. Based on your knowledge of the mechanisms of articular cartilage healing, recommend the application of rehabilitation techniques (e.g., immobilization, protected motion, CPM, ROM, resistance exercise, closed kinetic-chain exercises, aerobic conditioning, proprioception, and balance training) that are consistent with the stages of articular cartilage repair. Make specific reference to modification in exercise and functional activities based on your knowledge of patellofemoral compressive forces during the performance of various open- and closed-chain activities. In developing your program, ask these questions: How do more significant articular cartilage defects heal in comparison to superficial wounds? Is physiologic motion necessary for the nutrition of articular cartilage? List invasive surgical techniques used to stimulate subchondral bone bleeding in cases of femoral and patellar articular cartilage disease. In terms of a meniscal injury, develop a list of reasons related to motion, weight bearing, and closed-chain functional activities that contrast the rationale for alteration in rehabilitation between meniscal repairs and subtotal meniscectomy.

12

Muscle and Tendon Healing

LEARNING OBJECTIVES

1. Define and contrast the terms sprain and strain.
2. Discuss direct and indirect muscle injuries.
3. Define and describe complete and incomplete muscle injuries.
4. Identify and describe the sequence of muscle injury repair.
5. List the effects of immobilization of muscle tissue.
6. Describe clinically relevant rehabilitation techniques used during periods of muscle injury, repair, and immobilization.
7. Define and describe the organized stages of tendon healing.
8. Contrast intrinsic and extrinsic capacity of tendon tissue to heal.
9. Outline and describe the effects of motion and immobilization on tendons.
10. Discuss clinical applications of rehabilitation techniques during tendon healing.

KEY TERMS

Sprain

Strain

Microtrauma

Overuse

Indirect muscle injury

Direct muscle injury

Contusion

Incomplete muscle tears

Complete muscle tears

Immobilization

Atrophy

Tendinitis

Tenocytes

Protected motion

CHAPTER OUTLINE

Muscle
  Definitions
    Structure of Muscle
    Muscle Bioenergetics
  Injury and Healing
    Muscle Injury
    Classification of Muscle Injury
  Muscular Adaptation to Resistance
      Exercise
  Neural Adaptations to Resistance Exercise
    Polymorphism
  Effects of Immobilization
  Clinical Applications of Rehabilitation
      Techniques on Skeletal Muscle during
      Recovery and Immobilization

Tendon
  Anatomy
    Connective Tissue in Tendon
    Vascular Supply of Tendon
    Innervation of Tendon
  Response to Injury
    Injury and Repair of Tendon
    Effects, Remobilization, and Exercise
  Effects of Motion and Immobilization
  Clinical Applications of Rehabilitation
      Techniques during Tendon Healing

Injuries to muscle and tendon are common, clinically significant conditions treated with physical therapy procedures. The physical therapist assistant (PTA) must recognize the different types of injuries that occur to muscle, tendon, and the musculotendinous junction, and must appreciate how these specific tissues respond to injury and immobilization. A general understanding of injury, healing response mechanisms, and the effects of muscle position during immobilization guide the choice of therapeutic interventions to enhance recovery and minimize the deleterious effects of immobilization.

MUSCLE
Definitions

When treating patients recovering from injury to muscle, it is wise to clarify the exact nature of the original injury. The mechanisms of injury, specific tissue response to the insult, and the rationale for rehabilitation become focused, and the purpose of rehabilitation techniques is clarified.

Previously a **sprain** was defined as an injury to ligament tissue. A **strain** refers to an injury involving muscle and tendon tissue. It also may be referred to as a pulled muscle or a muscle tear.[13] **Microtrauma** injuries resulting in pain and dysfunction are called **overuse** injuries.[21] Although not entirely related to just muscle and tendon tissue, *overuse* is a term frequently used to describe repetitive microtrauma injury to muscle and tendon.

In an **indirect muscle injury** the muscle or, more commonly, the musculotendinous junction[15] becomes injured by a sudden stretch or concentric or eccentric muscle contraction. Also included in the definition of indirect muscle injury is delayed onset muscle soreness (DOMS) (see Chapter 5). Indirect strains are classified as either complete or incomplete tears.[13] **Direct muscle injury** refers to lacerations, surgical incisions, contusions, or blunt trauma. Clinically both direct and indirect musculotendinous injuries are seen. Occasionally severe contusions to muscle result in bone deposits within the muscle tissue, producing myositis ossificans. If the injury extends deeply enough to contuse bone, periosteal or heterotopic bone (bone tissue separate from the underlying contused bone) can form within the muscle.[13]

Structure of Muscle
The multinucleated cellular unit of human muscle is the myofiber. Multiple myofibers combine to form "fascicles," which cluster to create entire or whole muscle.

Single muscle fibers are surrounded by the sarcolemma or plasma membrane. An external adjacent connective tissue basement membrane that connects with extracellular matrix (ECM) is composed of collagen, laminin, fibronectin, chondroitin sulfate, hyaluronic acid, and heparin sulfate. General functions of the basement membrane are to I-serve as a termination point for synaptic transmission; II-serve as an attachment for myofibers, connective tissue, motor–nerve, and muscle–tendon junction; III-serve as confinement structures for satellite cell regeneration; and IV-regulate neuromuscular junction (Fig. 12-1).[2,14]

The sarcolemma is synonymous with the cytoplasm of the other cell types and as such contains various important cellular organelles. Mitochondria, Golgi apparatus, and a complex ECM of collagen, glycoproteins, and specific link proteins referred to as integrins comprise the chemical milieu of sarcolemma.[2,14]

Sarcoplasmic Reticulum
A complex muscle membrane system exists to facilitate and communicate electrical impulse signals to trigger calcium release that stimulates specific muscle contractile proteins to generate tension and force production.[2,14]

The sarcoplasmic reticulum is an elaborate system of chemical membranes that are arranged longitudinally along the myofibrils.[2,14] An intercommunicating system of tubules (transverse system or T-tubes) runs perpendicular to the long axis of the myofibrils and interdigitates with the sarcoplasmic reticulum (SR). Specifically, the SR stores and releases calcium in response to motor nerve impulse signals to invoke synchronous muscle contractions.

Connective Tissue
The histologic organization of muscle is arranged in an orderly hierarchy of connective tissue compartments. Each myofiber is surrounded by a sheath of connective tissue called the endomysium. The major constituents of connective tissue are collagen with small relative contributions from elastin. Multiple muscle fibers are bound into groups of fascicles. The muscle fascicles are surrounded by noncontractile tissue. McComas[23] eloquently describes several key functions of noncontractile connective tissue:

I. In development the connective tissue serves as a scaffolding upon which the muscle fibers can form. When the muscle development is complete, the connective tissue continues to hold the muscle fibers together and largely determines the gross structure of the muscle belly. II. The loose connective tissue of the perimysium provides a conduit for the blood vessels and nerves that supply the muscle fibers, III. The connective tissue tends to resist passive stretching of the muscle and ensures that the forces are distributed in such a way as to minimize damage to the muscle fibers and the wavy collagen bundles enable the muscle belly to regain its shape when the passive forces are removed, and IV. The endomysium through lateral connections to the muscle fiber conveys part of the contractile force to the tendon.[23]

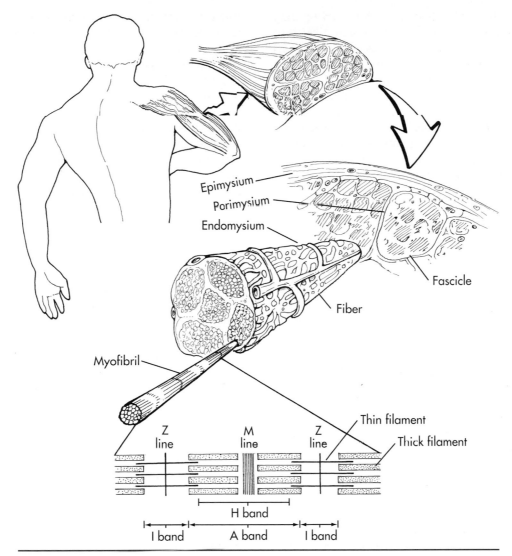

Fig. 12-1 Skeletal muscle architecture. (From Brinker MR, Miller MD: Fundamentals of Orthopaedics. Philadelphia, WB Saunders, 1999.)

Contractile Proteins

The highly organized sequential structure of the myofibril is the cellular-contractile unit called the sarcomere. Electron microscopy survey of a sarcomere reveals alternating light and dark successive bands that give "voluntary" muscle its characteristic "striped" appearance. The dark band structure is referred to as the A-band. The A-band is composed of quite thick, dark protein filaments called myosin. Two large isoforms called heavy chain (myosin heavy chain [MHC]) also are present. A very large longitudinal stabilized protein called titin contributes to the organization, arrangement, stability, and elasticity of the myosin filament.[14]

The light bands of the sarcomere are called I-bands. I-bands are composed of thin protein filaments called actin. Actin filaments contain a few strengthening and regulatory proteins called troponin, tropomyosin, and nebulin.[14] Components assist with organization support of actin filaments. Actin filaments are in part given positional arrangement from protein tropomyosin and from the Z-line or Z-disk within the center of each I-band.[2,14] Troponin and tropomyosin are calcium-sensitive regulatory proteins involved with actin filaments and are essential for sarcoplasmic calcium binding, allowing for resultant muscle contraction and force production.

Muscle Fiber Types

Descriptions of muscle fiber types vary according to physiologic categories and numerous identifying techniques.

Generally, two categories of muscle fiber types are identified:[1,2] fast twitch and slow twitch. Based on cellular characteristics, metabolic (glycolytic and oxidative) demands, neuromuscular responses, and MHC isoform content, subclassifications of muscle fiber types are used to more accurately describe unique forms and distribution of specific fiber types. Fast-twitch muscle can be subdivided (via glycolytic and oxidative capabilities) into fast oxidative-glycolytic (FOG) and fast glycolytic (FG) fibers. FOG fibers generally have a higher capacity for cellular oxidation and glycolysis when compared with other muscle fiber types. FG fibers demonstrate low oxidation and a high glycolytic capacity. Specifically, FG fibers produce the greatest tension and generate the quickest contractile velocity among all fiber types. However, FG fibers also fatigue the fastest.

Conversely, slow-twitch muscle fibers demonstrate slow oxidative qualities with slow velocity of contraction and low tension development, and they are very fatigue resistant.

Type I fibers are slow-twitch, oxidative fibers with the least glycogen and glycolytic enzyme content. Type I muscle fibers demonstrate the slowest contraction velocity with the greatest resistance to fatigue. Type I fibers have the highest myoglobin and mitochondria content among all muscle fiber types. Therefore these fibers possess the greatest oxidative capacity. These fibers are also described as red fibers because of their rich oxidative enzyme content. It may be helpful to remember "slow red ox" as a useful means of identifying the characteristics of type I muscle fiber.

Type IIa fibers are fast-twitch oxidative fibers. Type IIa muscle fibers possess relatively high myoglobin and mitochondria content as compared with type IIb muscle fibers. Generally, type IIa fibers demonstrate more rapid contraction than type I fibers. Overall, type IIa fibers are more fatigue resistant than type IIb fibers because of their higher oxidative enzyme content. The MHC isoforms of type IIa fibers are defined as fast red or FOG fibers. The MHC of type IIb fibers is referred to as fast white.

The type IIc fiber is termed an intermediate fiber because of the presence of both MHC isoforms.

The type IIm is a unique super fast fiber type with a genetically distinct myosin. Type IIm fibers are most commonly expressed in the masseter muscle of the jaw.

Neuromuscular Junction

A single nerve axon with each muscle fiber it innervates is called a motor unit. Individual nerve terminals that contact a single muscle fiber are referred to as motor end plates. Numerous cellular components are observed within the motor end plate, including mitochondria, endoplasmic reticulum, and glycogen. Unique structures called vesicles are the storage clusters of the neurotransmitter acetylcholine (ACH). The storage vesicles are found at the presynaptic nerve terminal. In addition to ACH, adenosine triphosphate (ATP) and proteoglycans are also found at the presynaptic nerve terminals.[2,9,14] The deactivating enzyme that affects ACH is acetylcholinesterase (ACHE).

Generally, three types of motor neurons are described in human muscle tissue.[2,9,14] I. Alpha-motor neurons innervate extra fusal (striated muscle outside the muscle spindle) muscle fiber. II. Beta-motor neurons innervate both extrafusal and intrafusal (striated muscle within the muscle spindle) muscle fiber. III. Gamma-motor neurons innervate intrafusal muscle fibers exclusively. Muscle spindles are sensory receptor structures that regulate tension in muscle tissue.

A highly structured and specific sequence of orderly electrochemical events are involved with neuromuscular stimulation. Initially, an electric impulse travels from an axon to its anatomically precise motor end plate. Calcium (CA^{2+}) channels located throughout the nerve terminal membrane are stimulated to "open." This action creates a release of CA^{2+} from the sarcoplasmic reticulum, which initiates the presynaptic release of ACH from the vesicles.

A tenfold increase in CA^{2+} intracellular concentration initiates the contraction phase of the excitation-contraction process.[2,9,14] Once CA^{2+} is liberated from the sarcoplasmic reticulum, muscle contraction between CA^{2+} and sensitive regulating proteins troponin and tropomyosin stimulates contractile filaments.[2,9,14]

Muscle Bioenergetics

Generally, metabolic pathways are described as either anabolic (synthesis) or catabolic (degradative). Anabolic energy metabolism requires ATP hydrolysis for energy by way of synthesizing complex molecules from reduced or simple precursors.[2,14]

Catabolic energy metabolism, by contrast, degrades complex molecular structures to simple forms to liberate energy as ATP.[2,14]

Glycolysis is a degradative pathway for carbohydrate metabolism. Generally, glycolysis breaks down glucose to liberate energy and form ATP. Anabolic glycolysis processes occur in the cytosol of cells. The end stage product of anaerobic glycolysis is lactate, which ultimately creates an acidic (acidosis via the toxic substance lactic acid) environment, leading to muscle fatigue. The major catalytic regulatory enzyme involved with anabolic glycolysis is phosphofructokinase.

Glucose is stored as glycogen in the liver and muscle tissue. Glycogenolysis is the catabolism of glycogen (which occurs in the cytosol of cells) to glucose and ATP for energy use.

The aerobic oxidative energy pathway is the tricarboxylic acid cycle (citric acid, Krebs' cycle), which leads to oxidative phosphorylation and degradation of fatty acids, carbohydrates, and amino acids. This aerobic energy pathway occurs in the mitochondria of cells. Generally, in aerobic metabolism, oxygen is combined with hydrogen to produce water and ultimately ATP for energy use.

Injury and Healing

Muscle tissue heals by acute, intense inflammatory response. The highly vascular and innervated nature of muscle is very conducive to repair and healing. In addition, with most muscle injuries, the speed at which the tissue is repaired is directly related to the degree of vascularity within the injury site during the repair phase of healing.[21] When a blunt trauma to a muscle **(contusion)** occurs, an acute inflammatory response creates connective tissue scarring; strength loss and dysfunction result.[6] When muscle lacerations and surgical incisions occur, muscle tissue tends to heal with dense connective scar tissue.[15] To minimize this scar tissue and achieve more normal functioning, the muscle tissue must be in near-anatomic approximation.

Incomplete muscle tears are clinically much more common than **complete muscle tears.**[13] Sudden stretching, rapid and eccentric muscle loading, running, jumping, and dynamic change-of-direction activities can lead to various muscular strains.

Animal studies have shown that after an incomplete muscle tear, hemorrhage, edema, fibroblasts, and granulation tissue are present within 4 days.[23] Scar tissue forms at 1 week with a resultant decrease in the muscle's ability to generate active force during the initial stages of healing.

Clinically the musculotendinous junction appears to be much more susceptible to indirect, incomplete muscle strain than is the muscle belly.[13] In addition, eccentric muscle contractions are a frequent cause of indirect muscle strains.

Muscle Injury

Muscle tissue is unique because it possesses the ability to regenerate (replace with biochemical, biomechanical, histologic, and immunologic similar tissue) and repair (replace with fibrous scar tissue) after direct or indirect muscle injury.

The biologic characteristics of the reparative process of mammalian striated muscle are a complex series of molecular, cellular, vascular, neurologic, and immunohistochemical events either directly or indirectly under genetic embryologic control with specific cell-signaling actions from various cytokines and growth factors.[14] The following sections review the essential elements of vascular endothelial repair or neovascularization, reinnervation, and molecular–cellular driven repair processes involving growth factors, cytokines, and synthetic degradative tissue homeostasis that include matrix metalloproteinases (MMPs), a family of degradative enzymes.

Angiogenesis

Vascular supply is a critical and essential component of muscle tissue repair. A direct or indirect injury to striated skeletal muscle involves disruption of the intimate blood supply of the damaged muscle tissue to varying degrees. The creation of new vascular tissue is called angiogenesis or neovascularization.[14] Basic arterial anatomy describes three fundamental layers of endothelial cells, connective tissues, and smooth muscle. The innermost layer is the tunica intima, consisting of endothelial cells, basement membrane, and connective tissue. The middle layer is the tunica media, with its primary constituents being connective tissue and smooth muscle cells. The outermost layer is the tunica adventitia, which is composed mainly of connective tissue. Arterial walls also contain a complex distribution of sympathetic innervation.[14]

The extracellular matrix composition of the vascular system is a complex array of collagen, elastin, glycosaminoglycans (chondroitin, heparin, dermatan, and hyaluronic acid), and glycoproteins (laminin and fibronectin).

In general, with muscle injury of any significance, intrinsic vascular regeneration requires the intricate interplay of endothelial cell migration and proliferation, connective tissue reorganization, and the synthesis, degradation, and deposition of matrix constituents (glycosaminoglycan [GAGs], glycoproteins, and collagen) to assist with basement membrane (basal lamina) formation and smooth muscle cell repopulation to reorganize damaged vascular tissues that supply the injured muscle fibers with oxygen, water, and reparative growth factors.

Degradative Enzymes

The reparative process of vascular muscle tissue is a finely tuned balance between proliferation and degradation. Damaged vascular tissues are enzymatically degraded to allow for removal by the inflammatory cellular molecular response cascade described in the preceding sections.

A family of zinc-bound enzymes called MMPs are secreted by various and specific regulatory cytokines and growth factors that have been stimulated by the inflammatory products of the arachidonic acid metabolic pathways. These degradative enzymes are classified according to the specific tissue they degrade. For example, interstitial collagenases degrade types I, II, III, VII, VIII, and X collagen. Stromelysins degrade type IV collagen, fibronectin, and proteoglycans. Therefore gelatinases degrade gelatin and elastin.[14]

Because the connective tissue and extracellular matrix composition of vascular tissue is composed of various collagen types, MMPs are essential regulators of efficient and effective decomposition of damaged matrix and collagen constituents, proteins, glycoproteins, and GAGs.[14]

Revascularization of damaged muscle tissue depends on several factors that are in turn regulated by stimulation, deposition, and proliferation of collagenous scar tissue. The function of MMPs must be kept in check by tissue inhibitors of metalloproteinases (TIMPs). Generally, TIMPs function to regulate the overproduction of MMPs, which create an overzealous cascade of degradation versus stimulation and proliferative repair processes.[14]

Cytokines and Growth Factors

Various soluble peptide cell-signaling molecules, which are produced by numerous cells, have direct mechanisms of tissue repair.[26]

Angiogenic growth factors serve as molecular stimulants to propagate the synthesis, proliferation, and deposition of cells involved in healing (repair and regeneration) of all musculoskeletal tissues.[26] Fibroblast growth factor (FGF) is an angiogenic factor that acts to stimulate neovascularization of damaged tissue.

Platelet-derived growth factor (PDGF) is a strong mitogen that is present in high concentration in vascular endothelial cells. Transforming growth factor (TGF) and epidermal growth factor (EGF) are both stimulants to endothelial cell proliferation and angiogenesis.[26] Vascular endothelial cell growth factor (VEGF) is a direct neovascular growth factor stimulant found in endothelial cells.

Generally the complex cascade of proinflammatory cells after injury signal the stimulation of various growth factors and cytokines, which further directs the appropriate organization, proliferation, and degradation of specific cells to assist in repopulation of endothelial cells, connective tissue, and smooth muscle.

The reorganization of the lumen in neovascular tissue may be partially or completely occluded from the repair process and eventual scar formation after muscle injury.

It should be recognized that the highly structured process of cell stimulation, migration, synthesis, proliferation, organization, deposition, degradation, and ultimate tissue homeostasis and regeneration is rarely complete. The repair process eventually outbalances the regenerative abilities of neuromuscular and vascular tissue, leaving a partially repaired organ system. Naturally the severity and complexity of the initial trauma directs or "drives" the degree of tissue healing.

Depending on the nature of musculovascular injury, the regenerative and repair process of angiogenesis usually results in functionally insignificant scarring of the lumen.[26]

Reinnervation

The repair and regenerative abilities of various orthopedic tissues are quite characteristic of peripheral nerves. The relative severity and complexity of muscle tissue injury makes functional regeneration of motor and sensory cutaneous nerve highly unpredictable.

Minor grades of muscle trauma that do not disrupt the organization of the connective tissue mix, vessels, and nerve usually result in myotube and myofiber reorganization and spontaneous restoration of the "three

Cs": I-color, II-consistency, and III-contractibility of the damaged muscle fibers. However, with muscle injury that disrupts the continuity of the muscle's connective tissue, blood supply, and nerve supply, the functional restoration of peripheral motor nerve depends largely on the degree of distal target site reinnervation of the axon reconnecting across the injury site.

The remarkable intimate and complex blood supply of peripheral nerve tissue is directly related to repair and regeneration. Transient compression–conduction blocks of peripheral nerve can occur with tourniquet application during surgical procedures. Retraction of peripheral blood flow to allow for improved vision of the surgical field is necessary. However, compression also reduces oxygen and nutrients, which maintain function of peripheral nerves.

Reorganization of antegrade axon transmission across the injury site (e.g., compression blunt trauma and sharp dissection) ultimately depends on the reconstruction of appropriate blood supply to the nerve (necessary to transport oxygen, cytokines, growth factors, MMPs, inflammatory cells, repair molecules, and connective tissue matrix constituents) synthesis and deposition of collagen, fibroblasts, laminin, and glycoproteins to reorganize the connective tissue matrix (epineurium, endoneurium, and perineurium) and anatomically precise reconnection with target sites.

Satellite Cells

Muscle tissue damage may incite the activation of myosatellite cells that propagate to form (precursors of) myoblasts. Satellite cells are undistinguished spindle-shaped cells located between the sarcolemma and basal lamina of individual muscle fibers.[2] Satellite cells are dormant nonactivated cells with very limited organelle number and function. However, when muscle tissue is damaged, exposing the satellite cells to the sarcoplasm (cytoplasm in general cell types), the dormant satellite cells differentiate to myoblasts, which help form myotubes as direct precursors to new muscle fibers.

Classification of Muscle Injury

To effectively predict the degree of intrinsic muscle regeneration and repair, Buckwalter[6] has classified muscle tissue injury into three categories. A type I muscle injury is described as either direct or indirect and damages muscle fiber substance but does not affect the extracellular matrix, blood supply, or innervation of the injured muscle. Examples of a type I muscle injury are blunt trauma, mild stretching, or contraction injury (concentric or eccentric), minimally invasive surgical procedures, and temporary ischemia. Because of muscles' highly neurovascular composition, these injuries heal spontaneously through intrinsic fiber regeneration (myoblasts) composition, organization, and function because the blood and nerve supply remain intact. In a type I injury, the damaged area appears as functional regenerated muscle fiber and not weak, fragile, or immature collagenous scar tissue.

In type II injury, there is injury to muscle tissue and nerve supply, but not the extracellular matrix (noncontractile, connective tissue elements) or vascular supply. Examples are peripheral isolated nerve neuropraxia (stretch), blunt trauma, and neuromuscular stretching injuries. The potential for functional recovery exists in these cases because the connective tissue maintains order and structure of the muscle, and the blood supply is not compromised when regenerating nerve tissue contacts an intact neuromuscular junction.

Conversely, with type III muscle injury, muscle fiber, matrix, and nerve and vascular supply are damaged. Usually highly differentiated myoblasts can either survive the trauma or are capable of migrating to the injury site. However, because the matrix is damaged, the order, structure, and composition of regenerating myoblasts cannot form functional contracting muscle tissue. Generally with type III muscle injury, there appears a predominant composition of collagenous–fibrous scar formation rather than functional regenerating muscle tissue.

Heterotopic Bone Formation

Occasionally, severe blunt injury, deep contusion, surgical exposures, and certain fractures (femoral head fracture, elbow fracture, proximal humerus) result in heterotopic bone formation (ectopic bone formation).

Myositis ossificans is the specific term used to describe heterotopic bone formation after blunt trauma to muscle. Generally, if the contusion is severe (deep versus superficial), there is a periosteal reaction in which undifferentiated mesenchymal cells proliferate during the first 3 to 4 days. During the following 5 to 8 days, cartilage develops with gradual calcification and neovascularization with subsequent bone deposition.

Deep tissue stimulation of massage, thermal agents (ultrasound, hot packs, and whirlpool), aggressive exercise, and passive stretching are to be avoided. In cases of predictable ectopic bone formation after specific fractures and subsequent surgical exposures (e.g., humerus fractures, fracture dislocation of the elbow, femoral head fractures, pelvis and acetabular fractures), oral ingestion of a specific nonsteroidal antiinflammatory drug (NSAID) indomethacin and low-dose radiation has proved effective at preventing nearly all heterotopic bone formation.

Muscular Adaptation to Resistance Exercise

As described by Alway,[2] muscular response to resistance training is an extremely complex and interrelated series of intrinsic neural biochemical, hormonal, and endocrine activity directly under genetic control. Alway[2] proposes a four-step model for muscular adaptation in response to resistance stimuli.

Step I requires a stimulus of resistance or muscular contraction against an applied load, either concentric or eccentric, with adequate intensity and frequency of load. This stimulus initiates a series of complex cellular and molecular changes that are regulated by transcription of DNA to RNA, then to translation of messenger RNA (mRNA) to the synthesis of protein (Fig. 12-2).[2]

The cellular events involved with signal activation of DNA and RNA require production of muscle force, which leads to myosin cross-bridges and subsequent binding to actin. The conversion of the contraction stimulus to protein synthesis is regulated by the biochemical signals initiating DNA and RNA activity.[2] Two cell nuclei are identified in muscle tissue. Myonuclei are postmitotic and are genetically consistently "fixed" in terms of volume. Satellite cells can divide, propagate, and increase protein synthesis when activated (Figs. 12-3 to 12-5).[2]

Step 2, as outlined by Alway,[2] generally involves genetic control of mRNA levels that stimulates a greater degree of mRNA efficiency and increased contractile proteins per nuclei (Figs. 12-6 to 12-8).

Steps 3 and 4 of Alway's description of muscular adaptation to resistance exercise involves increased mRNA transcription capacity and modification of gene transcription. The increase of both mRNA efficiency and capacity leads to the activation of dormant satellite cells with cell differentiation and increases volume of myonuclei (Figs. 12-9 to 12-12).

This intricate and complex interaction between resistance exercise and signal activation of mRNA ultimately leads to an increase in protein synthesis and more myosin cross-bridges, creating potential for increase in strength and power.[2]

Neural Adaptations to Resistance Exercise

Sequential motor unit recruitment is referred to as the "size principle" in which small motor units, or slow-twitch or type I muscle fibers, are activated before large

---

Muscular Adaptations:
Step 1: RNA activity

• Onset of resistance training = ↑ RNA activity

  • Translation capacity and/or efficiency for same amount of mRNA ↑
  • Ribosomal (rRNA) ↑ for capacity for protein synthesis ↑
  • Protein synthesis ↑ (but not measurable at the muscle fiber level)

Fig. 12-2 Molecular and muscular adaptations: Step 1: RNA activity. (From Alway S: Cellular and molecular regulation of muscle hypertrophy. NSCA Conference, 2000.)

Muscular Adaptations:
Step 1: RNA activity (translational)

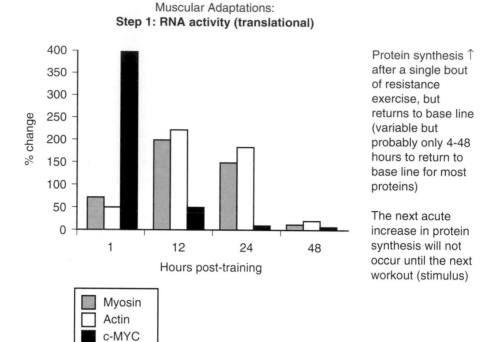

Protein synthesis ↑ after a single bout of resistance exercise, but returns to base line (variable but probably only 4-48 hours to return to base line for most proteins)

The next acute increase in protein synthesis will not occur until the next workout (stimulus)

Fig. 12-3 Molecular and muscular adaptations: Step 1 (translating). (From Alway S: Cellular and molecular regulation of muscle hypertrophy. NSCA Conference, 2000.)

Myonuclei and Satellite Cells

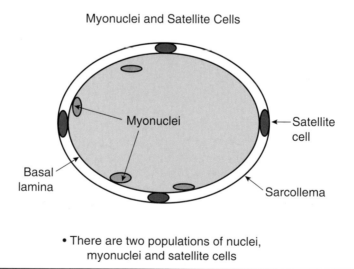

• There are two populations of nuclei, myonuclei and satellite cells

Fig. 12-4 Satellite cells and myonuclei. (From Alway S: Cellular and molecular regulation of muscle hypertrophy. NSCA Conference, 2000.)

Muscular Adaptations
Step 1: RNA Activity (translational)

• All initial protein synthesis and RNA activity changes occur in the myonuclei

• Satellite cells are normally dormant at rest and in step 1 of adaptations to resistance training-induced muscle hypertrophy

Fig. 12-5 Protein synthesis: Molecular adaptations: Step 1. (From Alway S: Cellular and molecular regulation of muscle hypertrophy. NSCA Conference, 2000.)

Muscular Adaptations
Step 2: Increase mRNA Levels

• After initial "lag" mRNA for contractile proteins ↑
  • transcriptional efficiency ↑
  • mRNA stability ↑
  • transcriptional capacity ↑
  • transcriptional factors ↑

Fig. 12-6 Muscular and molecular adaptations: Step 2. (From Alway S: Cellular and molecular regulation of muscle hypertrophy. NSCA Conference, 2000.)

Muscular Adaptations
Step 2: Increase mRNA Levels

• When translational capacity is reached, continued hypertrophy can no longer be maintained

• mRNA synthesis is controlled by transcription rate of the muscle gene

• mRNA for contractile proteins must ↑ if hypertrophy is to occur

Fig. 12-7 Muscular and molecular adaptations: mRNA increase: Step 2. (From Alway S: Cellular and molecular regulation of muscle hypertrophy. NSCA Conference, 2000.)

Muscular Adaptations
Step 2: Increase mRNA levels

  • mRNA for muscle proteins

  • mRNA for transcriptional factors

Muscular Adaptations
Step 2: Increase mRNA levels/transcriptional efficiency

  • mRNA for contractile proteins ↑ per nuclei

Fig. 12-8 Muscular and molecular adaptations: Step 2. (From Alway S: Cellular and molecular regulation of muscle hypertrophy. NSCA Conference, 2000.)

Muscular Adaptations:
Step 3: Increase mRNA transcriptional capacity

  • After a limited fiber size increase threshold for nuclear control (transcription and translation) is exceeded (protein degradation has not stopped)

  • mRNA for contractile proteins must ↑ even more if hypertrophy is to continue and not plateau

  • Problem – limited capacity for transcription/nuclear domains because limited myonuclei and nuclei/cytoplasm domain is ~ constant

Fig. 12-9 Satellite cells and myonuclei. (From Alway S: Cellular and molecular regulation of muscle hypertrophy. NSCA Conference, 2000.)

Nuclei have Fixed Central Domains

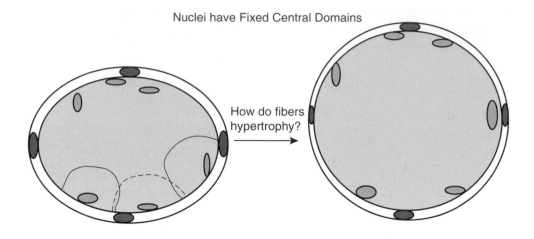

How do fibers hypertrophy?

Myonuclei are post mitotic

Satellite cells – dormant; but can divide if activated

Fig. 12-10 Step 3: Increase mRNA capacity. (From Alway S: Cellular and molecular regulation of muscle hypertrophy. NSCA Conference, 2000.)

Satellite Cells Proliferate

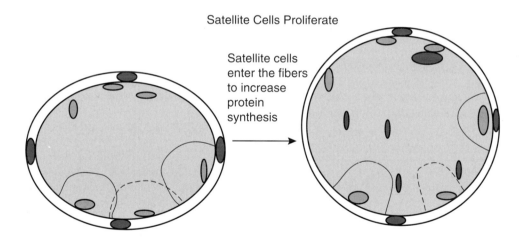

Satellite cells enter the fibers to increase protein synthesis

Satellite cells – divide – some enter the fiber to increase transcriptional capacity (mRNA); some may start new fibers

Fig. 12-11 Satellite cell activation and proliferation. (From Alway S: Cellular and molecular regulation of muscle hypertrophy. NSCA Conference, 2000.)

motor units, or fast-twitch type IIa or type IIb muscle fibers. The "motor unit" is defined as a single alpha motoneuron and the muscle fibers that it innervates. The three major fiber types identified in humans (types I, II, and IIIb) correspond to three distinct isoforms of MHCs, a marker of a muscle's oxidative and glycolytic capacity. The content or composition for MHC within the three human muscle fiber types determine the rate

of cross-bridging and the contractile velocity of the expressed fiber type.[2,9]

Polymorphism

Human muscle biologic plasticity enables a relative interconversion of fiber types, depending on the specific mode of exercise employed. Changes in fiber types distribution is referred to as polymorphism. The expres-

---

Increased muscle hypertrophy

- Increased transcriptional efficiency
  - Increased transcription per muscle nuclei
- Increased translational capacity
- Increase transcriptional capacity
  - Satellite cell activation
  - Increased myonuclei number
  - Satellite cell differentiation
- Increased mRNA stability
- Increased protein

Fig. 12-12 Cellular molecular hypertrophy. (From Alway S: Cellular and molecular regulation of muscle hypertrophy. NSCA Conference, 2000.)

BOX 12-1

Effects of Immobilization on Skeletal Muscle Tissue (Shortened)

Muscle atrophy (type I)
Sarcomeres decreased
Increased protein breakdown
Decreased muscle extensibility after immobilization
Decreased muscle weight
Decreased force generating capacity
Increase in connective tissue
Decreased anaerobic glycolytic enzymes
Decreased aerobic oxidative enzymes

---

sion "specificity of exercise" is best characterized by neuromuscular characteristics of muscle fiber types being able to convert (relative percentage increase) to a greater percentage of another fiber type, depending on the precise application of training variables of frequency, intensity, rate, velocity, and duration.

There is general consensus that endurance training of muscle increases the relative percentage of type IIa fibers "at the expense of type IIb fibers."[2,3,23] Also, specific strength development without the use of aerobic exercise preferentially increases the percentage of type IIb fibers. It appears that interconversion between type II fibers is greater than changes between fiber types I and II.

There is some evidence that the reverse size principle is employed with intense eccentric force that preferentially activates fast motor unit fibers while inhibiting slow motor unit fibers.

Effects of Immobilization

Perhaps the most profound change in human skeletal muscle during **immobilization** is **atrophy.** The degree of atrophy depends on both the duration of immobilization and the position or stretch imposed on the muscle.[6,12,13] When a muscle is immobilized in a shortened position, it may atrophy more than muscle casted in a lengthened position. Sarcomeres decrease up to 40% in muscles immobilized in a shortened position.[28] However, sarcomere numbers are replaced when immobilization is ended.[28] Muscles that are immobilized in a shortened position are also less extensible after cast removal than muscles immobilized in a stretched position. Finally, muscles immobilized in a shortened position undergo far greater rates of protein degradation than muscle casted in a passive tension, or stretched, position.[17]

Muscle fiber types are also affected by position during immobilization. When muscles are immobilized in a shortened position, type I muscle fibers (slow-twitch [red] oxidative) atrophy (decrease in both number of fibers and fiber diameter) far more than type II fibers (fast-twitch [white] glycolytic).[20] When a large percentage of type I muscle fibers atrophy during periods of immobilization, the relative number of type II fibers increases.[2,5,27,29]

Conversely, muscles immobilized in a lengthened position demonstrate an increase in sarcomere numbers up to 20% after 4 weeks of immobilization.[28] Protein synthesis also increases. Generally, muscles immobilized in a shortened position experience accelerated atrophy (type I fibers), decreased numbers of sarcomeres, reduced protein synthesis, and decreased oxidative and anaerobic enzyme levels.

Muscle atrophy also results in a decrease in muscle weight.[2,5,10,27] Muscle that has atrophied and lost weight also loses its ability to generate force and tension.[10] The greatest amount of atrophy occurs within 1 week of immobilization, and muscle fiber size decreases by approximately 17% within 3 days of immobilization.[4] Box 12-1 depicts the various physiologic changes that occur in skeletal muscle during immobilization.

Clinical Applications of Rehabilitation Techniques on Skeletal Muscle during Recovery and Immobilization

The healing response of muscle is far greater than bone, ligament, or tendon tissue because of the highly vascular makeup of human skeletal muscle.[10] Specific rehabilitation programs directed at maintaining muscular strength and minimizing atrophy during prolonged periods of immobilization attempt to enhance and magnify intrinsic muscular repair.

Typically, isometric muscle contractions are initiated during immobilization. However, Gould and colleagues[19] described a protocol involving 400 maximal isometric contractions with normal healthy subjects casted for

2 weeks. The results of their program showed no attenuating effect on loss of strength. Other studies have shown beneficial effects of isometrics on reducing strength loss during immobilization.[26] In a later study, Gould and colleagues[19] demonstrated that a protocol of electrical muscle stimulation for 16 hours per day during immobilization reduced the negative effects of atrophy and loss of strength in patients after open meniscectomy.

Combination protocols involving maximal voluntary isometric muscle contractions, with electrically evoked muscle stimulation, appear to provide more consistent results than either isometrics or muscle stimulation alone.[3,11] The effects of electrical muscle stimulation and isometric contractions during immobilization may retard disuse atrophy, reduce strength losses, and minimize the loss of aerobic oxidative enzymes (succinic dehydrogenase).[3,18,19,26]

Concentric and eccentric dynamic muscle contractions also can be used during immobilization provided a range-limiting hinged cast-brace is used. As stated, muscles that are immobilized in a lengthened position increase in muscle weight and protein synthesis. Therefore stretching immobilized muscle along with using hinged cast-braces, combined isometric muscle contractions, and electrically evoked muscle contractions may promote strength while minimizing atrophy during immobilization.[3]

Recovery from muscle injury (direct or indirect) not related to immobilization is directed at reducing pain (oral analgesics), eliminating swelling (NSAIDs, ice, elevation, and elastic wraps), and improving function. Once the acute inflammatory phase is controlled, ice packs, elastic compression bandages, elevation, and gentle isometric muscle contractions are applied. Depending on the severity of injury, gentle active range-of-motion (ROM) activities can be initiated during the early repair phase of healing. With severe muscle contusions, it is wise to avoid progressive motion, massage, heat, or exercise early in the rehabilitation program. Myositis ossificans may develop with vigorous activity. In these cases, rest, ice, elevation, medication, and the delayed judicious use of motion, exercise, and thermal agents are recommended.

Progressive isometric muscle contractions (e.g., weighted straight-leg raises) or isometric static holds with resistance can be initiated soon after many direct and indirect muscle strains. Once pain and motion improve, concentric and eccentric resistance exercise and isokinetics can begin. With most unilateral muscle injuries, the patient is instructed in general aerobic, strength, and flexibility programs that do not compromise the healing processes of the injured structures.

With all direct and indirect muscle strains, the timing for applying motion and resistance exercise, and the intensity of effort, must be specific to each patient. The degree of injury, which structures are involved, repair (intrinsic regeneration, scar formation, or surgical repair), and pain tolerance strongly influence the rehabilitation protocol. Relatively minor muscle strains heal spontaneously with conservative treatment consisting of ice, compression wraps, elevation, gentle active motion, isometrics progressing to isotonic and isokinetic exercise, and closed-chain functional activities.

More severe muscle injuries may require longer periods of rest, ice, compression, and elevation along with delayed yet progressive motion, exercise, gait, and functional activities. Box 12-2 describes various therapeutic techniques used for immobilization and healing skeletal muscle injuries.

BOX 12-2

Therapeutic Interventions during Immobilization and Healing of Skeletal Muscle

IMMOBILIZATION
Treatment
Isometric muscle contractions (10-second hold) in combination with electrically evoked muscle contractions. Stretch immobilized muscle if possible. Aerobic, strength, and flexibility programs for general fitness. Perform concentric–eccentric muscle contractions with hinged cast-braces if possible. Weight bearing as tolerated.

INDIRECT MUSCLE STRAINS, MUSCLE PULLS, OR TEARS
Treatment
Rest, ice, compression, elevation (RICE). Gentle, active ROM, progressive exercise. Isometrics, isotonics, isokinetics. Stationary cycle. Weight bearing as tolerated. NSAIDs. Do not overstretch muscles too soon after injury. Allow for scar formation and regeneration of muscle tissue. General fitness program.

DIRECT MUSCLE INJURY, LACERATIONS, AND BLUNT TRAUMA INCISIONS
Treatment
RICE. Weight bearing as tolerated. Gentle isometrics. Active ROM. General fitness programs. NSAIDs. *Caution:* Progress very gradually with severe muscle contusions. Progressive–resistive exercise. Concentric–eccentric isotonic and isokinetic exercise. Allow for scar formation. No vigorous motion during acute phase or early repair phase.

TENDON

Because tendon attaches to bone via muscle, the two structures are interrelated and are frequently injured together (e.g., musculotendinous junction muscle strains). However, a number of injuries seen clinically involve isolated tendon pathologic processes (**tendinitis** or Achilles tendon ruptures).

Tendon receives its blood supply generally from the musculotendinous junction, synovium, periosteal attachments, and the length of the tendon itself.[8,22] The tendon–bone interface and musculotendinous junction provide nutrition to the distal third of the tendon.[6] The midportion of the tendon receives its blood supply primarily from the synovial sheath, or paratenon.[8]

Anatomy

The primary cellular component of tendon is the fibroblast.[31] Fibroblasts are called tenoblasts and tenocytes specifically in tendon tissue. The metabolically active tenoblasts have large endoplasmic reticulum, well-developed Golgi apparatus, and greater volume of mitochondria than the less metabolically active tenocyte. Chondrocytes are found at pressure sites and insertion attachments. Microscopic examination of osseotendinous junctions by way of Sharpey's fibers reveal gradual histochemical changes of tissues from tendon to fibrocartilage to mineralized fibrocartilage and finally to bone. Collagen and elastin composition in human tendon represent 75% and 2% of the dry mass of tendon, respectively.[31] Collagen composition is mostly type I, with representative smaller amounts of type II and V collagen.[31] The extracellular matrix of tendon is composed of proteoglycans, GAGs, and matrix glycoproteins. Chondroitin sulfate and dermatan sulfate are the major GAG constituents of tendon. Macromolecule glycoproteins, fibronectin, and thrombospondin have been identified in human tendon and act to bind (adhesive-glycoprotein) other glycoproteins and cells together within the cellular matrix. Universally, tendons appear as hypovascular, shiny, white, dense, and fibroelastic tissue macroscopically.

Connective Tissue in Tendon

Although there are specific anatomic variations of tendons, most human tendons have a hierarchic network of connective tissue that surrounds the tendon proper and the primary, secondary, and tertiary bundles of tendon fiber. The paratenon is loose areolar connective tissue composed mainly of types I and III collagen, elastin, and synovial cells. The paratenon surrounds the tendon and functions as an "elastic sleeve" to provide reduced friction, free movement, and orientation of tendons against surrounding tissues.[31] The epitenon is directly under the paratenon. The epitenon is a fine sheath of connective tissue that envelops the entire tendon. Deep within the tendon, the endotenon forms a network of connective tissue around the subfascicle, fascicle, and fiber bundles of tendon tissue. The endotenon organizes, orients, and provides gliding surfaces for the tendon fibers and carries nerves and vessels to portions of the tendon (Fig. 12-13).

Vascular Supply of Tendon

Generally, tendons are extracellular tissues with relatively low metabolic demands because of tenuous blood supply when compared directly with many other tissues.[31] Basically, tendon receives blood supply from three sources.[31] The osteotendinous junction, musculotendinous junction, paratenon, and intratendinous network supply varying amounts of blood to tendon. The osteotendinous junction typically supplies the lower or distal one third of tendon.[31] Because there is a mineralized fibrocartilaginous barrier between bone and tendon tissue, there is no circulation to the body of the tendon through the osteotendinous junction. Tendons receive vascular supply at their proximal third by way of vessels from muscle tissue at the musculotendinous junction. It is apparent that there is a sudden and relatively dynamic change from the rich vascularity of muscle to the sparse network of vessels at the proximal third of tendon at the musculotendinous junction.[31] Generally the body of tendon tissue receives circulation from the thin network of arteries, capillaries, and vessels within the intratendinous connective tissue, paratenon, and endotenon.[31]

Innervation of Tendon

Tendons are innervated at the musculotendinous junction with relatively little contribution within the intratendinous substance.

Sensory (afferent) mechanoreceptors type I Ruffini corpuscles are pressure- and stretch-sensitive with a relatively slow rate of response. Type II Pacinian corpuscles are rapid reactors to pressure, acceleration, and deceleration movements. Type III Golgi tendon organs are tension receptors that give input on position, active muscle contraction, and passive stretch. Type IV free nerve endings are responsive to pain and are found primarily within peritendinous tissue.[31]

Response to Injury

Tendons heal through three organized stages: inflammation, repair, and remodeling.[16] Inflammation occurs within 72 hours after injury, whereas collagen synthesis and fibroblasts are arranged in a random, disorganized fashion within 1 to 4 weeks after injury.[15]

Curwin and Stanish[8] cite Chavapil[7] for further classification and organization of tendon healing into four stages:
1. Cell mobilization
2. Ground substance proliferation

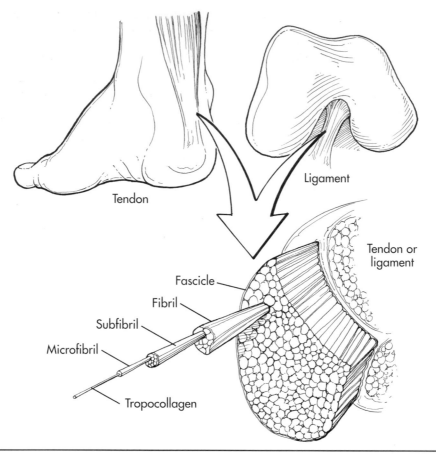

Fig. 12-13 Tendon and ligament architecture. (From Brinker MR, Miller DS, eds: Fundamentals of Orthopaedics. Philadelphia, WB Saunders, 1999.)

3. Collagen protein formation
4. Final organization

Tendons have both an intrinsic and extrinsic capacity to heal.[16] Therefore tendons can heal spontaneously from the formation of **tenocytes** (tendon cells) and from fibroblasts and vascular–inflammatory response mechanisms from adjacent tissues.[16]

When tendons are injured to the degree that a gap disrupts the normal anatomic continuity, collagen, granulation tissue, and fibroblasts migrate to the gap and fill it with scar tissue. The process of tendon healing depends largely on the degree of injury, the degree or contribution of vascular–inflammatory response from other structures, the amount of mobilization or immobilization after injury, and the need for surgical repair to approximate the torn tissue to obliterate the gap.

Tendon healing is a slow process requiring periods of rest and limited, controlled stress to develop strength. Gelbermann and colleagues[16] report that fibroblasts vigorously reorient along the long axis of the tendon to form dense connective tissue within 21 to 42 days after injury. Complete maturation of tendon scar appears 112 days after injury.[16]

Although tendons possess the capacity to heal, ultimately healed tendon is not strong enough to keep the torn tissue together.[13] Thus although minor tendon strains (incomplete) may be able to heal nicely, more severe tendon injury (Achilles tendon rupture) may require surgical repair for increased strength.

The fundamental concept behind suture repair of torn tendon is to minimize scar formation by using sutures to close or repair the gap. In response to surgical repair of the tendon, Miller[24] reports, "Tendon repairs are weakest at 7 to 10 days, they regain a majority of their original strength at 21 to 28 days, and achieve maximal strength in 6 months."

Injury and Repair of Tendon

Three distinct phases of healing characterize the repair process after injury or surgical repair of tendon. As with other vascular structures, initial response to injury is representative of the acute inflammatory cascade. Trauma incites a complex series of chemical events that mobilize cells and chemotactic agents to the injury site to stimulate coagulation, control hemorrhage, and initiate a fibrocollagenous fragile mesh of the phospholipids fibrin and fibronectin that connects with collagen to form a tenuous scaffold or plug.

Necrotic cellular debris is removed from the wound site and secondary tissues via the process of phagocytosis. Polymorphonuclear leukocytes, lymphocytes, and macrophages migrate into the site in response to histamine, fibronectin, and bradykinin to stimulate vascular permeability, vasodilation, and the release of prostaglandins.

As with other tissues, there is no clear precise delineation between the distinct phases of injury repair. With the gradual removal of cellular waste from the injury site, an accumulation of fibroblasts and myofibroblasts signal the initiation of the proliferative Phase II of healing. Neoangiogenesis or capillary budding is characteristic of this phase of injury repair. Extracellular matrix collagen (type III collagen: weak, fragile, and immature with deficient crosslinks) and glycosaminoglycans are produced by the fibroblasts. Tenacious adherence of the fibroblasts and myofibroblasts is increased by the presence of fibronectin during the proliferative phase. Rapid synthesis of and increases in fibroblasts, myofibroblasts, fibronectin, type III collagen, extracellular matrix proteins, and glycosaminoglycans are the hallmark of the proliferative phase. In the latter stages of the proliferative phase, there is a subtle and gradual shift in which fibroblasts synthesize type I rather than type III collagen, which is devoid of cross-links.

The final phase of healing is referred to as the maturation or remodeling phase. There is a characteristically slow decline in synthetic activity of fibroblasts, myofibroblasts, and extracellular matrix glycoproteins. The density of tendon collagen reverts to almost exclusively type I collagen. Collagen fibrillar alignment is influenced by compression and tension stress, whereas the fibers reorient along lines of protected gradual contraction and stretching. This final phase may last 1 year or more, depending on the extent of initial injury.

Relevant therapeutic application of exercise and functional activities after tendon injury and repair must be tempered by the fact that ultimate tensile strength of damaged tendon may be reduced by as much as 30% permanently.[31]

Effects, Remobilization, and Exercise

Generally the destructive effects of prolonged inactivity to tendon are reversible. Clearly, early protected motion and appropriately applied stress result in an acceleration of collagen synthesis, fiber orientation and alignment, vascular proliferation, and afferent stimulation. However, as with other tissues of limited intrinsic vascular supply, the quality of collagen deposition reflects reduced ultimate load to failure and tensile strength when compared with noninjured tendon. Repaired and remodeled tendon demonstrates a disproportionate amount of weak, fragile type III collagen

in contrast to nonpathologic tendon composition of type I collagen.[31]

Ultimately, the biochemical, biomechanical, and tensile strength of remobilized tendon does not regain normalized physiologic composition, orientation, quality, and quantity of noninjured tendon tissue.

Effects of Motion and Immobilization

As with other musculoskeletal tissues, long-term negative effects occur with immobilization of the tendon. Overall tensile strength is decreased, proteoglycans (glycosaminoglycans) are significantly reduced, and water content of tendon is severely compromised.[1,30] Conversely, stress and exercise produce increased tensile strength, stiffness, and increased collagen size.[30]

Historically it was felt that early motion after tendon injury and repair produced gap formation, accelerated adhesion formation, delayed collagen maturation, increased scar size, and disorganized collagen and fibroblast formation.[16] Miller[24] suggests that early motion provides increased motion but decreased tendon strength. Conversely, immobilization creates improved strength of the tendon but with less motion. Periods of immobilization also reduce tendon–bone junction strength.[24]

Early and limited **protected motion** appears to provide greater tensile strength, less adhesion formation, and earlier organization, orientation, and remodeling of collagen, and it does not contribute significantly to gap formation.[16] The degree of motion (excursion within the tendon sheath) after injury and repair must be slight with protection from excessive stress, which would be detrimental to healing.

Clinical Applications of Rehabilitation Techniques during Tendon Healing

Rehabilitation protocols during tendon healing reflect the extent of injury and indicate whether or not surgical repair and immobilization were used. Tendinitis is a common clinical pathologic process; generally treatment focuses on pain management and reduction of swelling and involves RICE (rest, ice, compression, and elevation), NSAID medications, and physical therapy. Gradually a course of gentle stretching with resistive exercise emphasizing eccentric muscle contractions is used.[8] Some type of limited protection may be needed to avoid excessive, unwanted motion, and factors that exacerbate the pain are removed. For example, with patellar tendinitis (jumper's knee) it may be necessary to limit running and jumping activities; with bicipital tendinitis, it may be necessary to avoid overhead motions; and with tennis elbow (lateral epicondylitis), it may be wise to avoid using hand tools, playing tennis, or generally engaging in excessive wrist flexion, extension, pronation, and supination. Surgery and subsequent immobilization are rare treatments. Naturally, modifications in activities are necessary to reduce pain, but total cessation of activity usually is not needed. Many activities that cause pain can be removed and supplemented with other activities that do not cause pain. Specific tendon pathologies and comprehensive rehabilitation programs are covered in detail in later chapters.

More severe tendon injuries that necessitate surgical repair (although ruptured Achilles tendons may be casted instead of surgically repaired in some cases) and subsequent periods of limited immobilization require judicious application of stress, exercise, weight bearing, and pain and swelling management. If stress (stretching and exercise) is added too soon or too vigorously after surgical repair or long periods of immobilization, stretching out of the repair and reinjury may occur.

✤ ADDITIONAL FEATURES

Age Influence on Tendon: Tensile strength and strain increase with age.

Controlled Motion: Proper environmental factors contribute to the quality, quantity, and histologic appearance of healing tendon. With protected motion, greater orientation and concentrations of collagen and proteoglycans predominate.

Exercise of Tendons: Tendons can be influenced significantly with exercise. Exercise may enhance collagen synthesis, increase collagen fiber diameter, and increase tensile strength. Cross section of tendon increases with age. The ultimate tensile strength of mature and old tendon is significantly higher than immature tendon.

Immobilization of Muscle: Disuse or immobilization leads to atrophy, loss of strength, decreased force production, fatigability, decreased protein synthesis, and decreased insulin sensitivity, which results in reduced glucose use by muscle. Loss of mass and force production are significantly more prominent with muscles immobilized with no tension than those muscles immobilized under some tension.

Loading Tendons during Healing: With controlled loading (e.g., stress), collagen production sharply decreases, slowing the remodeling process.

Muscle Contusion: Nonpenetrating blunt trauma. Speed of recovery is related directly to vascular ingrowth during the repair phase.

Severe Blunt Trauma: Deep nonpenetrating blunt injury to muscle that contacts periosteum and bone. May develop heterotopic bone formation within the muscle called myositis ossificans.

Tendon: When tension and force production of the muscle–tendon–bone complex exceeds the resistance of this structure, failure occurs at the weakest point. Tendons receive their blood supply from the perimysium, periosteal insertion, and paratenon. May also receive blood supply by synovial diffusion at vascular areas of tendon.

Tendon Healing: Intrinsic healing of injured or surgically repaired tendon varies histochemically and biomechanically among different tendons at different anatomic locations. Generally as healing progresses during the repair and maturation phases, at 5 to 6 months, there are minimal differences in cellularity and vascularity between healing and normal tendon.

REFERENCES

1. Akeson WH: An experimental study of joint stiffness. *J Bone Joint Surg* 1961;43A:1022–1034.
2. Alway SE: Cellular and molecular regulation of muscle hypertrophy. NSCA Conference, 2000.
3. Behm D: Debilitation to adaptation. *J Strength Cond Res* 1993; 7:25–75.
4. Booth FW, Seider MJ: Recovery of skeletal muscle after three months of hindlimb immobilization in rats. *J Appl Physiol* 1979; 47:435–439.
5. Caplan A, et al: Skeletal muscle. In Woo SL-Y, Buckwalter JA, eds. Injury and Repair of the Musculoskeletal Soft Tissues. Rosemont, IL, American Academy of Orthopaedic Surgeons, 1988.
6. Buckwalter JA: Musculoskeletal soft tissues. In Baratz ME, Watson AD, Impriglia JE, eds. Orthopaedic Surgery, the Essentials, 2nd ed. New York, Thieme, 1999.
7. Chavapil M: Physiology of Connective Tissue. Newton, MA, Butterworth, 1967.
8. Curwin S, Stanish WD: Tendinitis: Its Etiology and Treatment. Lexington, MA, Collamore Press, DC Heath, 1984.
9. Deschenes MR, et al: The neuromuscular junction: Structure, function, and its role in the excitation of muscle. *J Strength Cond Res* 1994;103–109.
10. Engles M: Tissue response. In Donatelli R, Wooden MJ, eds. Orthopaedic Physical Therapy. New York, Churchill Livingstone, 1989.
11. Eriksson E, Haggmark T: Comparison of isometric muscle training and electrical stimulation supplementing isometric muscle training in the recovery after major knee ligament surgery. *Am J Sports Med* 1979;7:369–171.
12. Fitts RH, Brimmer CJ: Recovery in skeletal muscle contractile function after prolonged hind limb immobilization. *J Appl Physiol* 1985;59:916–923.
13. Garrett W, Tidball J: Myotendinous junction: structure function, and failure. In Woo SL-Y, Buckwalter JA, eds. Injury and Repair of the Musculoskeletal Soft Tissues. Rosemont, IL, American Academy of Orthopaedic Surgeons, 1988.
14. Garrett WE, Best TM: Anatomy, physiology, and mechanics of skeletal muscle. In Buckwalter JA, Einhorn TA, Simon SR, eds. Orthopaedic Basic Science, Biology and Biomechanics of the Musculoskeletal System, 2nd ed. Rosemont, IL, American Academy of Orthopaedic Surgeons, 2000.
15. Garrett WE, et al: Recovery of skeletal muscle after laceration and repair. *J Hand Surg* 1984;9A:683–692.
16. Gelbermann R, et al: Tendon. In Woo SL-Y, Buckwalter JA, eds. Injury and Repair of the Musculoskeletal Soft Tissues. Rosemont, IL, American Academy of Orthopaedic Surgeons, 1988.
17. Goldspink DF: The influence of immobilization and stretch on protein turnover of rat skeletal muscle. *J Physiol* 1977;264:267–282.
18. Gould N, et al: Transcutaneous muscle stimulation to retard disuse atrophy after open meniscectomy. *Clin Orthop* 1983;178:190–197.
19. Gould N, et al: Transcutaneous muscle stimulation as a method to retard disuse atrophy. *Clin Ortho Rel Res* 1982;164:215–220.
20. Halkjaer-Kristensen J, Ingemann-Hansen T: Wasting of the human quadriceps muscle after knee ligament injuries: II muscle fibre morphology. *Scand J Rehab Med* 1985;13:12–20.
21 Järvinen M: Healing of a crush injury in rat striated muscle. *Acta Pathol Microbiol Scand* 1976;142:47–56.
22. Johanson MA, Donatelli R, Greenfield BH: Rehabilitation of microtrauma injuries. In Greenfield BH, ed: Rehabilitation of the Knee: A Problem-Solving Approach. Philadelphia, FA Davis, 1993.
23. McComas AJ: Skeletal muscle, form and function. Champaign, IL, Hum Kinet, 1996.
24. Miller MD: Review of Orthopaedics. Philadelphia, WB Saunders, 1991.
25. Nikolaou PK, et al: Biomechanical and histological evaluation of muscle after controlled strain injury. *Am J Sports Med* 1987;15:9–14.

26. Rosier RN, et al: Molecular and cell biology in orthopaedics. In Buckwalter JA, Einhorn TH, Simon PR, eds. Basic Science, Biology and the Biomechanics of the Musculoskeletal System. Rosemont, IL, American Academy of Orthopaedic Surgeons, 2000.

27. Rozier CK, Elder JD, Brown M: Prevention of atrophy by isometric exercise of a casted leg. *J Sports Med Phys Fit* 1979;19:191–194.

28. Tabary JC, et al: Physiological and structural changes in the cat's soleus muscle due to immobilization at different lengths by plaster casts. *J Physiol* 1972;224:231–244.

29. Tomanck RJ, Lund DD: Degeneration of different types of skeletal muscle fibers: II. Immobilization. *J Anat* 1974;118:531–541.

30. Woo SL-Y, et al: Mechanical properties of tendons and ligaments: II. The relationships of immobilization and exercise on tissue remodeling. *Biorheology* 1982;19:397–408.

31. Wool SL-Y, et al: Anatomy, biology, and biomechanics of tendon and ligament. In Buckwalter JA, Einhorn TA, Simon SR, eds. Orthopaedic Basic Science, Biology and Biomechanics of the Musculoskeletal System, 2nd ed. Rosemont, IL, American Academy of Orthopaedic Surgeons, 2000.

REVIEW QUESTIONS

Multiple Choice

1. Which of the following is most susceptible to indirect, incomplete muscle strains?
   A. Muscle belly
   B. Biceps
   C. Quadriceps
   D. Musculotendinous junction

2. Which type of muscle contraction is a frequent cause of indirect muscle strain? (Circle any that apply.)
   A. Isometric
   B. Isokinetic
   C. Concentric
   D. Eccentric
   E. Isotonic

3. The most profound change in human skeletal muscle during immobilization is atrophy. The degree of muscle atrophy depends on which of the following?
   A. The significance of the injury
   B. The type of surgical procedure
   C. The duration of immobilization and the position or stretch imposed on the limb during immobilization
   D. The amount of bleeding

4. Which type of muscle fiber atrophies to a great degree when muscle is immobilized in a shortened position?
   A. Type I—slow-twitch
   B. Type II—fast-twitch
   C. Fast-twitch—A
   D. Fast-twitch—AB
   E. Fast-twitch—B

5. An increase in sarcomeres up to 20% and protein synthesis is seen when muscle is which of the following?
   A. Immobilized for 6 weeks or longer
   B. Immobilized in a lengthened position
   C. Immobilized in a shortened position
   D. Not severely damaged

6. The healing response of muscle is which of the following?
   A. The same as bone
   B. Less than ligaments
   C. Similar to cartilage
   D. Greater than bone, ligament, or cartilage

7. The use of electrically evoked muscle stimulation in conjunction with isometric muscle contractions during periods of immobilization may do which of the following? (Circle any that apply.)
   A. Retard disuse atrophy.
   B. Minimize strength loss.
   C. Reduce the loss of succinic dehydrogenase.
   D. Enhance cardiovascular fitness.
   E. Greatly enhance eccentric strength.

8. When a severe, deep muscle contusion occurs, it is wise to avoid heat, early progressive motion, or massage because of which of the following?
   A. These treatments are too painful.
   B. These treatments are ineffective for pain and swelling relief.
   C. These treatments may promote myositis ossificans (MOT).
   D. Motion can effectively eliminate a hematoma by itself.

9. Tendons heal by way of three organized stages of inflammation, repair, and remodeling. However, tendons have the capacity to heal by which of the following?
   A. Inflammatory response only
   B. Intrinsic repair only
   C. Extrinsic repair only
   D. Both intrinsic and extrinsic repair

10. A tendon generally receives its blood supply from which of the following? (Circle any that apply.)
    A. The muscle belly
    B. Bone
    C. Synovium
    D. Musculotendinous junction
    E. Articular surfaces

11. Which of the following describes the effects of early, limited, and protective motion during tendon healing?
    A. Decreased tendon strength
    B. Reduced bone strength
    C. Less adhesion formation
    D. Increased gap formation

12. Which of the following describes a common course of rehabilitation for cases of tendinitis?
    A. Surgery and immobilization–rehabilitation
    B. RICE, protection, and progressive exercise
    C. Full ROM and active exercise
    D. Rigid immobilization

13. Tendon injuries that require surgical repair are best treated with which of the following?
    A. Nonrestrictive full ROM exercises after immobilization
    B. Temporary rigid immobilization followed by closed-chain resistance exercise
    C. Limited immobilization, gentle protected ROM, and appropriate exercise
    D. Rigid, long-term immobilization, non–weight bearing, followed by unlimited exercise

Short Answer

14. A muscle injury that occurs as a result of sudden stretch (concentric or eccentric muscle contraction) is referred to as

    _____ .

15. A muscle injury that occurs as a result of a contusion, laceration, or surgical incision is called _____ .

True/False

16. Generally, muscle tissue heals by way of intense, acute inflammatory response.
17. Indirect, incomplete muscle strains are more common than complete muscle strains.
18. If a muscle is immobilized in a shortened position, it will atrophy more than if the muscle were placed in a lengthened or stretched position.
19. Concentric and eccentric muscle contractions can be used in selected cases with range-limiting hinged cast-braces.
20. Controlled motion, limited stress, and appropriately applied exercise are necessary adjuncts during periods of tendon healing.
21. Tendinitis is best treated with surgical excision and periods of immobilization.

Essay Questions

Answer on a separate sheet of paper.

22. Define and contrast the terms *sprain* and *strain*.
23. Discuss direct and indirect muscle injuries.
24. Define and describe complete and incomplete muscle injuries.
25. Identify and describe the sequence of muscle injury repair.
26. List the effects of immobilization of muscle tissue.
27. Describe clinically relevant rehabilitation techniques used during periods of muscle injury, repair, and immobilization.
28. Define and describe the organized stages of tendon healing.
29. Contrast the intrinsic and extrinsic capacity of tendon tissue to heal.
30. Outline and describe the effects of motion and immobilization on tendons.
31. Discuss the clinical applications of rehabilitation techniques during tendon healing.

Critical Thinking Application

Based on your understanding of the mechanisms of muscle injury and repair, develop a list of rehabilitation techniques you would recommend after immobilization, indirect muscle strain, and direct muscle injury. Organize and construct a working rehabilitation plan that focuses attention on the restoration of motion, soft-tissue extensibility, strength, power, neuromuscular endurance, cardiovascular fitness, proprioception and balance, and functional closed kinetic-chain exercises. Be certain to categorize your therapeutic interventions so that they are consistent with the stages of muscle tissue healing and time constraints. What adjunctive techniques would you recommend to stimulate muscle reeducation? Which thermal agents would you encourage during each phase of muscle healing? Are there any contraindications for employing massage, heat, and passive motion after a muscle injury? Explain. Describe in detail the specific application of isometric, concentric, and eccentric muscle contractions during each phase of intrinsic muscle repair. Describe the clinical rationale for use of early protected motion versus immobilization after tendon injury or surgical repair.

13 Neurovascular Healing and Thromboembolic Disease

LEARNING OBJECTIVES

1. Identify neural anatomy.
2. Discuss the vascular supply to nerve tissue.
3. Understand the mechanical behavior of nerve tissue.
4. Identify the causes and classification of nerve injury.
5. Discuss intrinsic nerve healing.
6. Describe methods of surgical repair of nerve injury.
7. Identify structure and composition of vascular tissue.
8. Discuss the vascular response to injury.
9. Explain the various signs and symptoms of vascular injury.
10. Discuss the pathophysiology of thromboembolic disease.
11. Recognize risk factors of deep vein thrombosis and pulmonary emboli.

KEY TERMS

Peripheral nervous system (PNS)
Epineurium
Perineurium
Endoneurium
Creep
Neurapraxia
Axonotmesis
Neurotmesis
Compression neuropathy
Traction neuropathy
Ischemia
Meralgia paresthetica
Anoxia

Double crush syndrome
Neurorrhaphy
Endothelial cells
Smooth muscle
Lumen
Tunica intima
Tunica media
Tunica adventitia
Vein
Artery
Intimal hyperplasia
"Hard" signs
"Soft" signs
Thromboembolic disease

Deep vein thrombosis (DVT)
Pulmonary embolism (PE)
Virchow's triad
Homans' sign
Pleuritic pain
Dyspnea
Tachypnea
Warfarin (Coumadin)
Low-molecular-weight heparin
Intermittent pneumatic compression

CHAPTER OUTLINE

Peripheral Nerve Injury
  Vascular Supply
  Mechanical Behavior of Nerve
  Causes and Classification of Nerve Injury
  Compression and Traction Neuropathy
  Methods of Peripheral Nerve Repair
  Recovery after Peripheral Nerve Injury
  Assessment of Peripheral Nerve Functional
    Recovery
Vascular Injury
  Structure and Composition
  Vascular Response to Injury
  Mechanisms of Injury
  Signs and Symptoms of Vascular Injury
  Diagnostic Studies
  Methods of Vascular Repair
Thromboembolic Disease
  Pathophysiology of Thromboembolism
  Virchow's Triad
  Risk Factors
  Signs and Symptoms of Deep Vein Thrombosis
  Diagnostic Studies
  Pulmonary Emboli
    Signs and Symptoms
  Pharmacologic Treatment of Thromboembolic
    Disease

PERIPHERAL NERVE INJURY

In general terms, peripheral nerve can be traumatized by a number of causative factors: mechanical, thermal, chemical, and ischemic. As an organ system, the **peripheral nervous system (PNS)** is highly vascularized. As such, a mechanical insult to nerve (e.g., compression, stretch, or severance) stimulates an intense inflammatory reaction (Fig. 13-1).

Vascular Supply

Peripheral nerve has a complex and extensive blood supply. The PNS requires an ongoing nutritive energy supply for maintenance of nerve conduction. Longitudinal extrinsic vessels connect with regional feeding vessels that form a plexus of vessels within the **epineurium, perineurium,** and **endoneurium** connective tissue network within the nerve fiber (Fig. 13-2).[1,3]

The initial response to trauma once again is predictable with vascular tissue. There is an increase in vascular permeability with release of the potent chemical mediators histamine and serotonin. The end result is an increase in edema within the defined connective tissue barriers (epineurium, perineurium, and endoneurium) of the nerve fiber. The dramatic change in fluid pressure

and tissue edema adversely affect oxygen transport, nutrition, ion content, and nerve conductivity of the traumatized nerve fiber.[1,3]

Mechanical Behavior of Nerve

Nerve tissue is highly deformable, expressing relatively similar viscoelastic mechanical behavior as other soft tissues. Essentially, two load deformation terms are used to quantify a tissue's ability to structurally and mechanically adapt to time-dependent forces. **Creep** is a term used to describe a tissue's ability to change or "creep" to a new length in response to a rapidly applied load.[1,3] Stress relaxation describes a deforming force applied to soft tissue and held constant. As the force remains constant, the load absorbed by the tissue slowly reduces.[1,3]

Peripheral nerve tissue responds to these two viscoelastic properties by demonstrating ultimate load-to-failure values of 20% to 60%. Although peripheral nerve tissue may tear at strain rates approaching 20%, ischemic changes, which profoundly affect nerve function, may occur at strain rates of 15% or less.[1,3]

Causes and Classification of Nerve Injury

As stated, trauma to peripheral nerve can come from many sources such as mechanical, thermal, chemical, and ischemic sources. Mechanical sources of trauma are contusion, concussion, stretch, compression, laceration, and division.[1,3] Three distinct categories of nerve injury are neurapraxia, axonotmesis, and neurotmesis.[1,3]

Type I or first-degree nerve injuries are referred to as **neurapraxia.** As a general rule, neurapraxia is a reduction in nerve conduction at the specific site of injury. There are a few commonalities with first-degree neurapraxia. The lesion is local, the anatomic continuity of the axon is maintained, and all pathologic changes associated with neurapraxia generally are reversible if the cause of the compression is removed.[1,3]

In a very broad sense, motor nerve is at greater risk for injury than sensory nerve.[1,3] Grossly predictable, motor and sensory nerve may fail in the following order: motor, proprioceptor, touch, temperature, and pain, with recovery occurring in the reverse order.[1,3]

A type II nerve injury is defined as **axonotmesis.** In this injury, all neural connective tissue (epineurium, perineurium, and endoneurium) remain intact with physiologic disruption of the axon. Because the connective tissue sheaths remain unaltered, regeneration of axon distribution to target sites are directed within the confines of the connective tissue.[1,3] Therefore the expected functional recovery should be complete.[1,3]

A type III axonotmesis is defined as axonal injury, as well as anatomic disruption of endoneurium connective tissue. The epineurium and perineurium remain intact. Healing and functional recovery are highly unpredictable and mostly incomplete. Without direc-

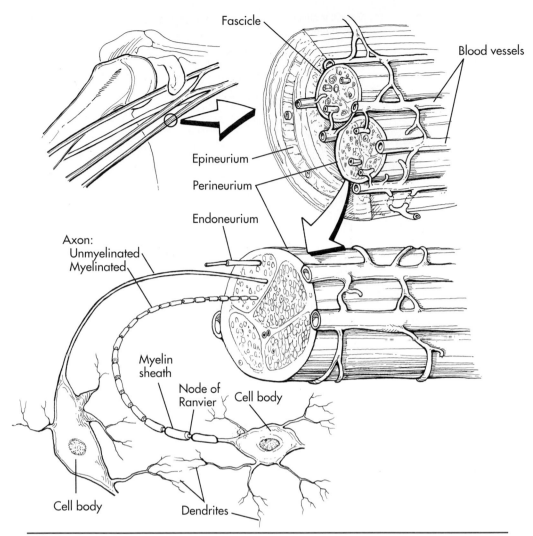

Fig. 13-1 Nerve architecture. (From Brinker MR, Miller MD: Review of Orthopaedics, 2nd ed. Philadelphia, WB Saunders, 1999.)

tional support of the endoneurium, intrafascicular fibrosis occurs, which limits axon regeneration.[1,3]

Type IV axonotmesis is defined as a loss of continuity of the axon with disruption of the endoneurium and perineurium. The epineurium remains intact. In this injury scenario, fibrosis within the nerve fiber is magnified with significant neuronal damage. Expectations are bleak for function and recovery.[1,3] Surgical excision of damaged nerve segments with repair, reconstruction, or grafting of the nerve are necessary.[1,3]

The final classification of peripheral injury is a type V **neurotmesis,** complete severance, and total loss of nerve trunk continuity. Surgical grafting and reconstruction are essential.[1,3]

Compression and Traction Neuropathy

Two general types of compression nerve injury are acute and chronic in origin. In either case, the physiologic consequence of compression or traction on peripheral

nerve tissue is mechanical disruption of nerve fiber and **ischemia** (Fig. 13-3). Anatomically, certain peripheral nerves are at risk for compression because of the surrounding soft tissue and bone, which limits three-dimensional motion of the nerve. Specifically at risk are the common peroneal nerve behind the fibular head and the radial nerve within the spinal groove of the humerus, as well as the median nerve within the soft tissue confines of the arch of the carpal tunnel and the lateral femoral cutaneous nerve within the inguinal ligament **(meralgia paresthetica).**

It is interesting to note that spinal nerve roots are more susceptible to compression injury than peripheral nerves because of the anatomic variant that spinal nerve roots demonstrate no epineurium or perineurium connective tissue.[1,3]

The biologic responses of the PNS to acute and chronic compression include obstruction of intraneural blood vessels, **anoxia,** local ischemia, nerve fiber deformation,

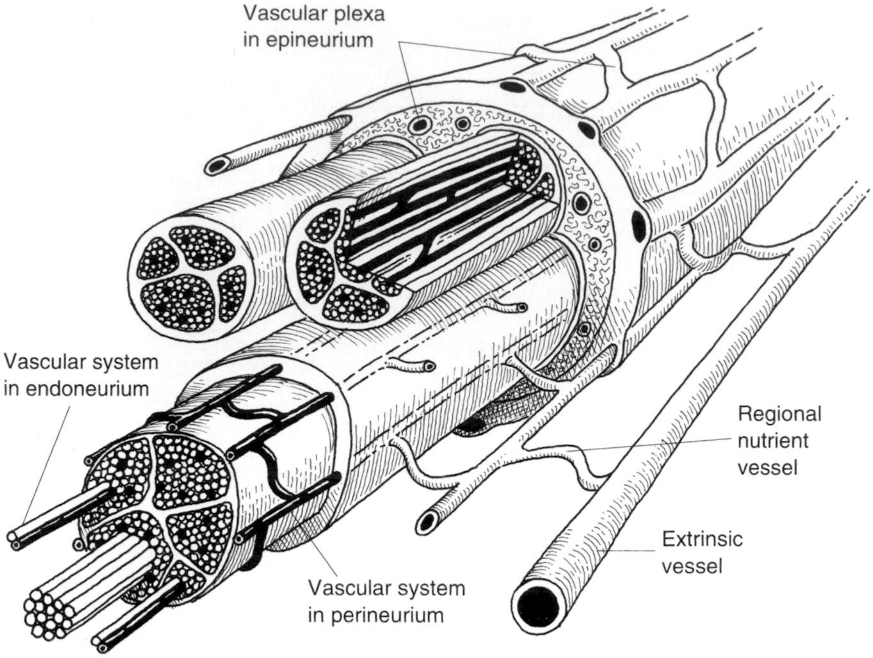

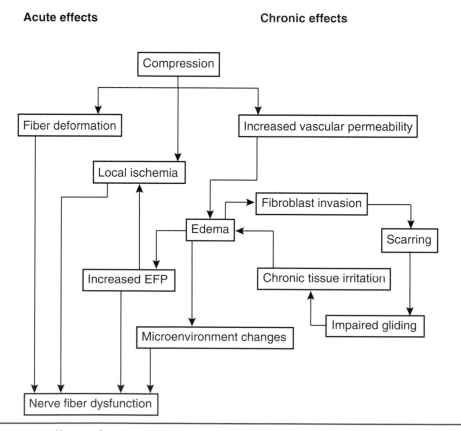

Fig. 13-2 Blood supply of a peripheral nerve. (Adapted with permission from Lundborg G: Nerve Injury and Repair. New York, Churchill Livingstone, 1988.)

Acute effects   **Chronic effects**

Fig. 13-3 Effects of compression on intraneural tissue. (Adapted with permission from Lundborg G: Nerve Injury and Repair. New York, Churchill Livingstone, 1988.)

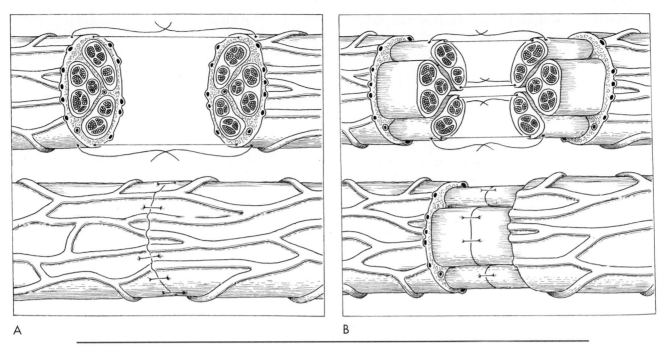

Fig. 13-4   A, Epineurial neurorrhaphy; **B,** Group fascicular neurorrhaphy. (Adapted with permission from Lundborg G: Nerve Injury and Repair. New York, Churchill Livingstone, 1988.)

increased vascular permeability, intraneural edema, and fibroblastic proliferation with resultant diminished nerve gliding.

Traction or stretch neuropathy is classified as acute or chronic with the magnitude of injury following the various grades of neurapraxia, axonotmesis, and neurotmesis, as outlined and described.

A practical and common description of acute traction neurapraxia is the term "burner" or "stinger" experienced by athletes, in which the shoulder is depressed with concomitant contralateral head and neck flexion that creates a brachial plexus stretch.

Occasionally with lengthy surgical procedures, prolonged wide exposure of the visual field inadvertently may stretch surrounding peripheral nerve tissue. Surgical procedures also may require prolonged tourniquet application, with cuff pressures occluding extrinsic neural blood supply.[1,3]

The application of physical therapy (range of motion [ROM]) interventions after prolonged joint immobilization may increase premature and intensive stretch that may elicit traction neurapraxia.[1,3] Appropriate slow, controlled stress devoid of high velocity or forcible motion during the maximum protection phase of postoperative care or prolonged joint immobilization protects peripheral nerve from unwanted injury.

Some patients may experience symptoms of peripheral nerve compression or entrapment at more than one level of the same nerve. The term **double crush syndrome** is used to describe symptoms of carpal tunnel median nerve compression neuropathy and cervical nerve root

injury. This syndrome is not exclusive to the example given and also may include ulnar nerve entrapment neuropathy of the elbow. An explanation for this phenomenon is that a compressive lesion at one level of the nerve may make a distal segment of the same nerve more susceptible to injury.[1,3]

It is suggested that compression reduces nerve conduction, blood supply, and plasma membrane proteins that decrease the quality of distal nerve segments, making the nerve highly sensitive to mechanical or compressive deforming forces.[1,3]

Methods of Peripheral Nerve Repair

The term **neurorrhaphy** is synonymous with direct coaptation or surgical apposition of corresponding nerve stumps.[1,3] This specific surgical intervention is reserved for neurotmeses with complete severance of nerve trunk continuity. Two basic objectives for direct fascicular repair (neurorrhaphy) are to maximize the number of axons that regenerate across the impaired area and the accuracy with which the axons reinnervate distal target sites (Fig. 13-4).[1-3]

Skeletal stability is essential for direct coaptation surgical repair to be effective. There must also be a well-vascularized tissue bed. The procedure itself requires that appropriate tension be applied to the injury site.[1,3] Animal studies demonstrate that minimal tension on the repair produces better results than do tension-free repairs. Overall, there are four identified steps in the direct coaptation repair of denervated tissue. First, there must be clean preparation of the traumatized nerve stumps. Second, there must be manual approximation of the tissue stumps with correct tension produced at the repair site. Third, there must be direct connection among nerve stumps fascicle to fascicular group. Fourth, the coaptation must be maintained with sutures, fibrin glue, or interstitial clot.[1,3] Denervated tissue undergoes dynamic pathologic changes without reinnervation of peripheral nerve neurotmesis. Distal site denervated bone becomes osteoporotic, joint capsules and periarticular soft tissues become fibrotic, and muscle atrophies with decreased muscle fiber volume. There is muscle fiber weight loss of 30% the first month and approximately 60% the second month after denervation.[1,3]

Autografts are used in addition to direct coaptation of nerve. Autografts are selected whenever direct repair is not possible because of poor tension at the repair site. The most common autograft for peripheral nerve repair is the sural nerve.[1,3] Other sources are the anterior branch of the medial antebrachial cutaneous nerve, the lateral femoral cutaneous nerve, and the superficial radial sensory nerve.[1,3]

Currently, good to excellent results can be expected in approximately 50% of surgically repaired peripheral nerves. A few generalizations can be made concerning surgical reconstruction of peripheral nerves. Younger patients normally do better than older patients. Patients with prompt surgical repairs do better than those with late repairs. Patients with distal repairs do better than those with proximal repairs. Patients with short nerve grafts do better than those with long nerve grafts.[1,3]

Recovery after Peripheral Nerve Injury

Protection of the repair site is the most important factor after surgical coaptation or autograft of peripheral nerve. Overzealous ROM exercise during early recovery of a graft or neurorrhaphy can easily disrupt fragile healing of fascicle sutures and axonal regeneration. Typically, postoperative splinting is used to maintain appropriate tension and mechanical properties of the repaired nerve.[1,3] Compressive dressings are used to decrease venous congestion and edema. ROM exercises are employed cautiously to encourage venous return, muscle activation, and lymphatic flow, and to reduce the potential for adhesions of muscle and connective tissue.[1,3] Vascular supply to the healing and repaired nerve tissue must be continuously enhanced to influence axonal regeneration. Superficial heat application may encourage peripheral vascular blood flow to the healing tissues. Electrical stimulation may be of some benefit to initiate muscle contraction, increase blood flow, and stimulate removal of cellular debris.[1,3] Neuromuscular and sensory reeducation exercise are initiated early and progressed continuously during all phases of peripheral nerve injury and repair. Continuous stimula-tion of distal target sites of reinnervation is essential to redirect axonal regeneration and to facilitate motor reeducation. Various sensory stimulation tactics are used to decrease hypersensitivity. Light touch, pressure, vibration, thermal stimuli, texture, and stimulation of the afferent mechanoreceptor system (proprioception and kinesthesia) are critical components of functional recovery of nerve injury or repair.

Assessment of Peripheral Nerve Functional Recovery

To document the quality and quantity of motor and sensory nerve recovery after injury or surgical repair, an objective grading system is used to determine the level of functional recovery. The Mechanical Research Council Grading System is used for continued assessment of both motor and sensory recovery.[1,3] Motor recovery is graded M0 through M5 and sensory recovery S0 through S4. A parallel analogy is manual muscle strength testing: trace, 1; poor, 2; fair, 3; good, 4; and normal, 5.

With an excellent result after nerve repair, a grade of M5, S4 is used to describe full motor reinnervation and complete sensory recovery. A good result is described as M3, S3; a fair result is M2, S2; and a poor result is M0 to M1, S0 to S1.

By establishing objective documentation relating to functional motor and sensory nerve recovery after injury or surgical repair, appropriate physical therapy interventions can be explored to stimulate, regulate, or enhance specific motor or sensory functions.

VASCULAR INJURY

The peripheral vascular system frequently is damaged with orthopedic trauma, surgery, or disease. The importance of revascularization of bone and soft tissues after injury is well documented and firmly established. Without a continuous supply of oxygen, red blood cells (RBCs), water, gases, growth factors, proliferative cells, bone, and soft tissues become anoxic and necrotic, and eventually cease to function properly.

The complex relationship among musculoskeletal injury, surgical procedures, and diseases and the vascular response to injury are profoundly important for restoration of function.

Structure and Composition

Grossly, vessels consist of three basic components: **endothelial cells, smooth muscle,** and connective tissue.[1-3] Arteries and veins consist of three identifiable concentric layers (lamina) that form the **lumen** or "walls" of this elastic tissue. The innermost layer is referred to as the **tunica intima,** which consists of connective tissue, endothelial cells, and a basement membrane. The middle or intermediate layer is the **tunica media,** which is composed of smooth muscle cells and connective tissue. The outermost layer is the **tunica adventitia,** with connective tissue and fibroblasts that blend with loose surrounding connective tissue.[2] Between the tunica media and adventitia is an external elastic membrane (elastica externa). Between the tunica intima and tunica media is an internal elastic lamina (elastica interna).

It is interesting to note that the outermost walls of large vessels contain their own microvascular system. The arterial tunicae are innervated with sympathetic nerves. Although **veins** contain the same three layers of tunicae, the relative percentage of smooth muscle and elastic components are less than that of **arteries.**[2] Also, the contribution of connective tissue in veins is much greater than that of arteries. These anatomic distinctions obviously contribute to the vasomechanical differences noted between highly elastic muscular arteries and relatively less elastic veins. There is great variation in biochemical composition within the vascular system, depending on regional anatomic requirements. Generally, peripheral vascular histochemical composition includes extracellular matrix, collagens, elastin, proteoglycans, laminin, fibronectin, squamous epithelial (endothelial) cells, and smooth muscle cells.[2]

Vascular Response to Injury

As with other types of soft tissue, specific injuries to vessels incite an organized, predictable inflammatory response with distinct overlapping sequential phases of events: coagulation, inflammation, fibroplasia, and remodeling and maturation.[1-4]

Depending on the nature and severity of vascular injury, the proliferative cellular healing of damaged lumen may actually thicken vessel walls, reducing blood flow. The most significant histochemical event of the healing process is referred to as **intimal hyperplasia.**[2] This process is defined as smooth muscle cell proliferation after arterial injury.

Mechanisms of Injury

Vascular injury from traction, avulsion, compression, or penetration can occur with blunt orthopedic trauma or elective or emergency surgical procedures (Table 13-1).[2] Identifiable arterial injury can occur with specific shoulder dislocation and humeral neck fractures, which result in associated injury to the axillary artery. Supracondylar humerus fractures and elbow dislocation can produce associated brachial artery injury.[2] Posterior dislocation of the knee and supracondylar fracture of the femur in the lower extremity can result in popliteal artery injury (Table 13-2). Total hip arthroplasty can involve injury to the common or external iliac artery. Total knee arthroplasty poses a risk to the popliteal artery as well.

Signs and Symptoms of Vascular Injury

General signs and symptoms of peripheral arterial injury are defined as either "hard" or "soft."[2]

"Hard" signs include the traditional occlusive signs of pulselessness, pallor, paresthesias, pain, and paralysis.[2] In addition, overt signs of massive bleeding and a rapidly expanding hematoma are classic examples of arterial occlusion.[2]

"Soft" signs include a history of arterial bleeding, hematoma over a peripheral artery, and a neurologic deficit of a nerve parallel to an anatomically identified artery.[2] After specific fractures, dislocations, and selected surgical procedures (e.g., posterior knee dislocation, total knee arthroplasty, or glenohumeral dislocation), continuous reassessment of peripheral pulses (dorsalis pedis or radial) is essential to identify potential vascular injury. In addition, skin color, temperature, edema, and digital capillary refill are routinely assessed in all suspected peripheral vascular injuries.

Table 13-1	*Arterial Injuries Associated with Orthopedic Operative Procedures*
Orthopaedic Procedure	**Artery Injured**
UPPER EXTREMITY	
Clavicular compression plate	Subclavian artery
Modified Bristow procedure	Axillary artery
Closed reduction humeral fracture	Brachial artery
LOWER EXTREMITY	
Total hip arthroplasty	Common or external iliac artery
Internal fixation of acetabular fracture	External iliac artery or superficial femoral artery
Nail-plate fixation of intertrochanteric or subtrochanteric hip fracture	Profunda femoris artery
Subtrochanteric osteotomy	Profunda femoris artery
Total knee arthroplasty	Popliteal artery
Meniscectomy	Popliteal artery
External fixator pin or locking screw	Superficial femoral, profunda femoris, or tibial arteries
SPINE	
Anterior spinal fusion	Abdominal aorta
Resection of nucleus pulposus	Right common iliac artery and vein, inferior vena cava

From Browner BD, Jupiter J, Levine A, et al: Skeletal Trauma, 2nd ed. Philadelphia, WB Saunders, 1998.

Table 13-2	Arterial Injuries Associated with Fractures and Dislocations	
Fracture or Dislocation	**Artery Injured**
UPPER EXTREMITY	
Fracture of clavicle or first rib	Subclavian artery
Anterior dislocation of shoulder	Axillary artery
Fracture of neck of humerus	Axillary artery
Fracture of supracondylar area of humerus	Brachial artery
Dislocation of elbow	Brachial artery
LOWER EXTREMITY	
Fracture of shaft of femur	Superficial femoral artery
Fracture of supracondylar area of femur	Popliteal artery
Posterior dislocation of the knee	Popliteal artery
Fracture of proximal tibia or fibula	Popliteal artery, tibioperoneal trunk, tibial artery, or peroneal artery
Fracture of distal tibia or fibula	Tibial or peroneal artery

From Browner BD, Jupiter J, Levine A, et al: Skeletal Trauma, 2nd ed. Philadelphia, WB Saunders, 1998.

Diagnostic Studies

Noninvasive diagnosis of vascular occlusion is made with Doppler flow detection or duplex ultrasonography.[2] With Doppler flow, a comparison is made with the noninvolved extremity. In this way, an arterial pressure index (API) is calculated by dividing the Doppler systolic pressure of the involved extremity with that of the uninvolved extremity.[2]

Research has shown a high predictability of approximately 97% in assessing arterial injury with an API of 0.90 or lower.[2] Duplex ultrasonography is the combination of ultrasound imaging and pulsed Doppler flow detection.

Percutaneous arteriography is the gold standard invasive technique for diagnostic elucidation of suspected vascular injury. This technique requires that dye proximal (antegrade) or distal (retrograde) is injected to the suspected injury, then multiple sequential plain film radiographs are taken of the area.[2]

Methods of Vascular Repair

A general analogy of repair techniques can be drawn from peripheral nerve repair. Generally, direct repair of vascular defects, including arteriorrhaphy or anastomosis, involves direct suturing of traumatized vessel. Autografting techniques or synthetic graft material (polytetrafluoroethylene [PTFE]) or Dacron are used for interposition grafting.[2,3]

THROMBOEMBOLIC DISEASE*[4]

Thromboembolic disease, deep vein thrombosis (DVT) that propagates to **pulmonary embolism (PE),** is among the most common causes of mortality and morbidity in hospitalized patients.

Hip and knee arthroplasty place patients at very high risk of developing thromboembolic disease without any other known risk factors. Generally, most high-risk orthopedic patients have a 40% to 70% chance of developing DVT.

Pathophysiology of Thromboembolism

Most thrombi are initiated in the valve cusps of deep veins in the lower leg. Thromboplastin, thrombin, and fibrin are part of the coagulation cascade of events that stimulate the adherence of platelets to vessel walls. Platelet adherence at valves creates build-up of blood cells that coagulate into a thrombus.

A dislodged clot from the thrombus is referred to as an *embolus.* Pulmonary embolism is a life-threatening consequence in which the lower lobes of the lungs are involved four times more often than the upper lobes.

Virchow's Triad

Three classic factors generally lead to the development of DVT. Categorically referred to as **Virchow's triad,** the factors include hypercoagulability, venous stasis, and endothelial vessel wall injury. These factors contribute to the pathogenesis of thrombus and emboli. Hypercoagulation is the result of tissue trauma (surgery or injury) that initiates and propagates an imbalance between fibrinolysis and coagulation. Trauma exposes collagen fragments, thromboplastin, and fibrinogen, which in turn stimulates platelet activity and volume. The initial trauma of surgery shifts the balance more toward coagulation than fibrinolysis and ultimately the formation of DVT.

Vessel wall injury and venous stasis are directly related to various orthopedic surgical procedures, such as total joint arthroplasty, pelvic fractures, and femur fractures.

Deep vein thrombosis progresses in one of three ways: The thrombus undergoes partial or complete lysis, with complete or near-complete recannulization of the thrombosed blood vessel; the thrombus becomes more organized, resulting in further occlusion of the vessel; or the thrombus becomes dislodged in whole or in part and escapes to a proximal site in the vascular system as an embolism.

Risk Factors

Several intrinsic and extrinsic risk factors are identified as additive factors in the potential development of

---

*This section, "Thromboembolic Disease," is reproduced with written permission from Orthopedic Practice, vol 13, LaCrosse, Wisc, March 2001, Orthopedic Section, APTA.

thromboembolic disease. Surgery, trauma, obesity, malignancy, age over 40 years, oral contraceptives, and immobility are well-known causative factors in the development of DVT. In addition, smoking, heredity, congestive heart failure, prior history of DVT, and varicose veins contribute as risk factors for the development of thromboembolic disease.

Signs and Symptoms of Deep Vein Thrombosis

Very high levels of suspicion must accompany all complaints of proximal thigh pain, inguinal and lower leg pain after postoperative joint arthroplasty, pelvic fractures, femur fractures, spinal surgery, and general trauma.

Symptoms are nonspecific, with generally diffuse complaints of leg pain and tenderness after surgery. Signs include edema, palpable warmth, skin discoloration, prominent superficial veins, and the presence of **Homans' sign.**

Approximately 50% of cases of DVT are asymptomatic. Symptoms generally arise locally from relatively large thrombi (including or excluding) inguinal and proximal thigh veins.

Diagnostic Studies

Testing or diagnostic procedures must be sensitive, accurate, specific, reliable, and reproducible to convey the precise anatomic status of the patient's pathology. Duplex ultrasonography is the current gold standard, noninvasive diagnostic study for suspected DVT. This test combines Doppler assessment and ultrasound examination of the venous system with manual compression. Veins that do not easily compress with normal pressure on the transducer may be considered positive for DVT.

Clinical probability estimates of physical examination alone of Homans' sign, edema, and palpable firmness are approximately 50% reliable for positive DVT. Generally, proximal thrombi of the inguinal area, deep proximal thigh, and popliteal are considered more dangerous than deep calf vein thrombi because distal clots are smaller and less frequently associated with major complications.

Pulmonary Emboli

Pulmonary emboli are a result and complication of DVT. A dislodged deep vein thrombus may travel to the pulmonary artery or obstruct the pulmonary blood supply. The result is hypoxia from constriction of the bronchioles, mediated by vasoconstrictive substances such as serotonin, histamine, and prostaglandins. The net effect is pulmonary infarction, shock, and congestive heart failure.

Signs and Symptoms

Generally, patients with symptomatic pleuritic PE may complain of **pleuritic pain, dyspnea,** or **tachypnea.** These signs and symptoms of PE are related to the size of the embolus and cardiopulmonary status of the patient.

Pharmacologic Treatment of Thromboembolic Disease

High-risk orthopedic patients undergoing total joint arthroplasty are treated with **warfarin (Coumadin),** heparin, or **low-molecular-weight heparin** (LMWH; Enoxaparin). The judicious use of LMWH has proved to be both safe and effective in the prevention and treatment of DVT in orthopedics. The use of LMWH is more predictable than heparin, with 92% bioavailability compared with 29% bioavailability of heparin.

Therapeutic administration of anticoagulation begins 12 to 24 hours postoperatively. Optimal therapeutic effect of warfarin takes 4 to 7 days. The method of delivery for Enoxaparin is through subcutaneous injection (not muscular injection). Coumadin is indicated for prophylaxis and treatment of DVT or PE, and the duration of therapy may take 3 or 4 months. Coumadin is administered either intravenously or subcutaneously.

Nonpharmacologic treatment of DVT generally includes antiembolism stockings or **intermittent pneumatic compression.** Contraindications for the use of pneumatic compression devices include local ulceration, cellulitis, and arterial insufficiency.

❖ ADDITIONAL FEATURES

Axonotmesis: Type II peripheral nerve injury. Two subclasses, III and IV. Generally, loss of continuity of axons, with varying degrees of connective tissue function.

Blood Supply to Peripheral Nerve: Complex arrangement of superficial longitudinal and segmental longitudinal arterial systems.

Clinical Probability Estimate of Suspected Pulmonary Emboli: A high clinical probability of 80% to 100% of PE exists with unexplained dyspnea, tachypnea, or pleuritic pain.

Cold Ischemia: Cold, pulseless hand or foot with little or no capillary refill.

Common Arterial Injuries in Orthopedics: Fracture or dislocation of the upper extremity—subclavian artery, axillary artery, brachial artery. Fracture or dislocation of the lower extremity—femoral, popliteal, tibial, and peroneal arteries.

Connective Tissue Components of Peripheral Nerve: Epineurium, perineurium, and endoneurium.

Denervation: Distal tissues undergo physiologic changes; bone—osteoporosis, joint fibrosis, or muscle atrophy.

Direct Surgical Repair: Neurorrhaphy—primary repair, skeletal stability is essential. Too much tension on the repair decreases results, as does no tension. Moderate tension improves outcomes.

"Hard" Signs of Arterial Injury: Pulselessness, pallor, paresthesia, pain, paralysis, and poikilothermia.

Neurotmesis: Type V injury—complete physiologic disruption of nerve.

Peripheral Nerve Injury Classification: Neurapraxia type I—axon maintains continuity, no distal degeneration, usually because of compression.

Rehabilitation After Peripheral Nerve Injury: Splinting for protection of healing tissue, warm to propagate blood flow, ROM to prevent adhesion, motor and sensory stimulation to facilitate reeducation.

Risk Factors for DVT: Age over 40 years; prior history of DVT, malignancy, trauma, immobility, surgical procedures, low cardiac output, varicosity, and obesity.

Signs and Symptoms of DVT: Peripheral edema, warmth, skin discoloration, prominent superficial veins, Homans' sign, leg pain, and tenderness.

"Soft" Tissue Signs of Arterial Injury: Questionable history of bleeding, location of a penetrating wound or blunt trauma to an artery, and neurologic deficit at a nerve directly next to a known artery.

Virchow's Triad: Stasis, prolonged immobility, vessel wall injury, trauma, fractures, surgical procedures, and a hypercoagulable state.

REFERENCES

1. Bodine SC, Lieber RL: Peripheral nerve physiology, anatomy, and pathology. In Buckwalter JA, Einhorn TA, Simon SR, eds. Orthopaedic Basic Science, Biology, and Biomechanics of the Musculoskeletal System, 2nd ed. Rosemont, IL, American Academy of Orthopaedic Surgeons, 2000.
2. Feliciano DV: Evaluation and treatment of vascular injuries. In Browner BC, Jupiter JB, Levin AM, et al, eds. Skeletal Trauma, Fractures, Dislocations, Ligamentous Injuries, 2nd ed. Philadelphia, WB Saunders, 1998.
3. Lee SK, Wolfe SW: Peripheral nerve injury and repair. *J Am Acad Orthop Surg* 2000;8:243–252.
4. Shankman G: Thromboembolic disease, anticoagulation therapy. *Orthopedic Practice* Vol 13, March 2001, APTA.

REVIEW QUESTIONS

Multiple Choice

1. Connective tissue barriers of peripheral nerve tissue include which of the following? (Circle all that apply.)
   A. Endoneurium
   B. Myosin
   C. Perineurium
   D. Epineurium

2. As an organ system, the peripheral nervous system can be described as which of the following?
   A. Moderately vascularized
   B. Minimally vascularized
   C. Highly vascularized
   D. Avascular

3. Peripheral nerve tissue demonstrates ultimate load-to-failure values of how much?
   A. 10% to 30%
   B. 20% to 60%
   C. 25% to 45%
   D. 70% to 90%

4. When a peripheral nerve lesion is local, the anatomic continuity of the axon is maintained and all pathologic changes generally are reversible. This is called which of the following?
   A. Axonotmesis
   B. Neurapraxia
   C. Neurotmesis
   D. Neuralgia

5. The biologic response of the peripheral nervous system to acute or chronic compression or traction is which of the following? (Circle all that apply.)
   A. Epineurial deformation
   B. Anoxia
   C. Decreased vascular permeability
   D. Intraneural edema

6. "Burner" or "stinger" is a term used to describe which classification of nerve pathology?
   A. Axonotmesis
   B. Neurapraxia
   C. Neurotmesis
   D. Neuropathy

7. The innermost layer of the lamina of vessels is referred to as which of the following?
   A. Tunica media
   B. Tunica adventitia
   C. Tunica intima
   D. Elastica interna

8. Gross anatomic components of vessels consist of which of the following? (Circle all that apply.)
   A. Skeletal muscle
   B. Endothelial cells
   C. Macrophages
   D. Connective tissue

9. Intimal hyperplasia refers to which of the following?
   A. Decreased perfusion
   B. Connective tissue proliferation
   C. Smooth muscle cell proliferation
   D. Reduced epithelial cells

10. Supracondylar humerus fractures and elbow dislocations may result in which vascular injury?
    A. Ulnar artery
    B. Axillary artery
    C. Brachial artery
    D. Subclavian artery

11. Which of the following examples are "hard" signs of vascular injury? (Circle all that apply.)
    A. Pain
    B. Pallor
    C. Pulselessness
    D. All of the above

12. Risk factors for developing thromboembolic disease include which of the following?
    A. Total hip replacement
    B. Total knee arthroplasty
    C. Immobility
    D. All of the above

13. High-risk orthopedic patients demonstrate a risk of which percent for developing deep vein thrombosis (DVT)?
    A. 10% to 20%
    B. 70% to 90%
    C. 40% to 70%
    D. 5% to 15%

14. Which of the following describe Virchow's triad? (Circle all that apply.)
    A. Venous stasis
    B. Hypertension
    C. Endothelial cell wall injury
    D. Hypercoagulability

15. Signs of DVT after trauma or surgery include which of the following? (Circle all that apply.)

A. Presence of Homans' sign
B. Cool skin
C. Edema
D. Skin discoloration

16. Approximately what percent of patients with DVT are asymptomatic?
    A. 10%
    B. 50%
    C. 20%
    D. 15%

17. What is the chance that a patient with a positive Homans' sign, edema, and palpable tissue firmness has DVT?
    A. 30%
    B. 20%
    C. 10%
    D. 50%

Short Answer

18. Describe the gross anatomic connective tissue barriers of peripheral nerve tissue.

19. Outline and describe three classifications of peripheral nerve injury.

20. Certain peripheral nerves are a risk for compression because of surrounding soft tissue and bone that limit three-dimensional motion of nerves. Name four nerves.

21. Acute traction neurapraxia is also referred to as a _____

    or _____ .

22. A compressive nerve lesion at the proximal location may involve the distal segment of the same nerve. Name this syndrome.

23. Name the three layers of vessel gross anatomy from deep to superficial.

24. Total arthroplasty of the hip and knee poses a risk to which arteries?

25. Describe "hard" signs of vascular injury.

26. Name the components of Virchow's triad.

27. List the risk factors for developing DVT.

28. Describe the signs of DVT.

True/False

29. Peripheral nerve tissue is avascular.
30. Peripheral nerve tissue is highly deformable, with viscoelastic properties similar to other soft tissue.
31. Peripheral nerve tissue healing is highly predictable.
32. Type I axonotmesis nerve injury results in disruption of the epineurium, perineurium, and endoneurium.

33. Meralgia paresthetica is compression of L4 to L5 nerve roots.
34. Neurotmesis nerve injury results in total severance and loss of nerve trunk continuity.
35. Spinal nerve roots are more susceptible to compression injury than peripheral nerve tissue because of the anatomic variation that spinal nerve roots demonstrate no epineurium or perineurium connective tissue.
36. Proximal nerve compression reduces conductivity, blood supply, and a reduction in plasma membrane proteins that decrease the quality of the distal nerve segments, making the nerve less sensitive to mechanical or compressive deforming forces.
37. Animal studies demonstrate that tension-free surgical repairs are essential for complete healing.
38. Anatomically, veins demonstrate more connective tissue than arteries, rendering veins less "elastic" than arteries.
39. Pulselessness, pallor, paresthesias, pain, and paralysis are examples of "soft" vascular signs of injury.
40. Approximately 10% of patients have asymptomatic DVT.
41. The presence of Homans' sign, edema, and palpable soft tissue firmness is only 50% reliable for positive DVT.

Essay Questions

Answer on a separate sheet of paper.
42. Discuss the general vascular supply of peripheral nerve tissue and outline the consequences of the intense inflammatory response to injury.
43. Name the classifications of peripheral nerve injury.
44. Discuss the gross anatomic structures and composition of vessels.
45. Name and discuss a significant event or consequence of proliferative cellular healing involving damaged lumen.
46. Name and discuss three factors that contribute to the pathogenesis of DVT.
47. Discuss signs and symptoms of DVT.

Critical Thinking Application

The patient you are treating in the hospital is 2 days postoperative, total knee arthroplasty. Chart review reveals a 40-year history of smoking, obesity, and congestive heart failure. Your patient is 78 years old. The patient reports "groin pain" and a swollen foot. The patient also states that his lower leg below the operated knee and his foot feels cold. The patient is demonstrating profound difficulty dorsiflexing his foot on the operative leg.

In groups, using your knowledge and understanding of neurovascular gross anatomy, composition, function, and response to overt injury, discuss the neurologic and vascular signs and symptoms your patient is experiencing. Sequentially cite specific peripheral nerve pathology that may explain your patient's symptoms. How and why would a total knee arthroplasty contribute to a loss of dorsiflexion? Discuss and define specific arterial and venous supply to the knee, lower leg, and foot, and explain causative factors that contribute to reports of paresthesia involving the leg and foot. Does clinical probability demonstrate the existence of DVT in this patient? How certain are you that DVT is confirmed with clinical examination alone? Demonstrate on each person in your group the performance of Homans' sign and palpate specifically the inguinal area, proximal thigh, popliteal fossa, medial thigh, gastrocnemius, and anterior lower leg. Palpate the dorsalis pedis artery. Explain and describe acute compression neurapraxia with specific anatomic reference to this patient. Discuss the complex interrelationship of musculoskeletal (muscle, tendon, ligament, cartilage, and bone) and neurovascular repair after total knee arthroplasty.

PART III

COMMON MEDICATIONS IN ORTHOPEDICS

This section establishes an awareness of key elements, terms, and definitions involving antiinflammatory and antibiotic agents that provide the student physical therapist assistant (PTA) and practicing clinician with a cursory introduction to the basics of orthopedic pharmacology.

Orthopedic physical therapy interventions involving the PTA do not divest interest in or responsibility for the care of the whole patient. Knowledge concerning neurovascular anatomy and healing of various organ systems of the body play essential roles in the delivery of physical therapy procedures. Therefore an appreciation of antibacterial medications and antiinflammatory agents aids the PTA in understanding the complexity and interdependence of medications and orthopedic health care.

This section is presented as a means of broadening the focus of specific PTA education; to expose the student to concepts of prophylactic antibacterial medications; bacterial adherence to orthopedic internal fixation devices; infections involving total joint arthroplasty and various fractures; classifications of antibiotic medications and related offending organisms; nonsteroidal antiinflammatory drugs (NSAIDs); and corticosteroids related to acute and chronic pain and inflammation.

In the day-to-day delivery of physical therapy, the PTA encounters many orthopedic afflictions requiring medications to target specific bacterial organisms, as well as antiinflammatory agents to control pain and swelling.

A basic understanding of drug administration routes, bioavailability, and rationale for use of single or multiple antibiotics with both bactericidal and bacteriostatic actions, as well as the use of NSAIDs versus the use of corticosteroids, allows the student and clinician to more efficiently and effectively enhance patient care.

14 Concepts of Orthopedic Pharmacology

LEARNING OBJECTIVES

1. Define components of pharmacokinetics.
2. Discuss the drug "schedule" classification.
3. Identify five mechanisms of antibiotic activity.
4. Discuss the difference between bactericidal and bacteriostatic activity.
5. Identify six classifications of antibiotics.
6. Explain the rationale of preoperative antibiotics.
7. Discuss the mechanisms of bacterial adherence to orthopedic implants.
8. Explain the antiinflammatory effects of corticosteroids.
9. Discuss the effects of nonsteroidal antiinflammatory drugs.
10. Explain the difference between COX-1 and COX-2 inhibition.

KEY TERMS

Pharmacokinetics
Absorption
Bioavailability
First-pass effect
Metabolism
Pharmacodynamics
Bactericidal
Bacteriostatic
Antibiotics
Penicillins
Cephalosporins

Aminoglycosides
Tetracyclines
Macrolide antibiotic
Lincosamide antibiotic
Fluoroquinolones
Quinolones
Infection
Glycocalyx
Corticosteroids
Arachidonic acid
Cyclooxygenase

Lipoxygenase
Nonsteroidal antiinflammatory drugs (NSAIDs)
Prostaglandins
COX-1
COX-2
Inflammation
Thromboxanes
Leukotrienes

CHAPTER OUTLINE

Pharmacology: Definitions
Classification of Drugs
Antibiotics
  Penicillins
  Cephalosporins
  Aminoglycosides
  Tetracyclines
  Macrolide and Lincosamide Antibiotics
  Fluoroquinolones in Quinolones
  Miscellaneous Antibiotics
Infections and Orthopedics
  Preoperative Prophylaxis
  Fractures
  Bacterial Adherence to Orthopedic Implants

Severe Open Fractures
Infection in Total Joint Arthroplasty
Corticosteroids
  Intraarticular and Paraarticular Corticosteroid Injections
Nonsteroidal Antiinflammatory Drugs (NSAIDs)
  Adverse Reactions to Nonsteroidal Antiinflammatory Drugs
Selective Inhibition: Cyclooxygenase (COX-1 and COX-2)
Inflammation
Chronic Inflammatory Response

Understanding rudimentary concepts of the basic science governing the administration of antibiotics, corticosteroids, and nonsteroidal antiinflammatory drugs (NSAIDs) in orthopedic practice is essential for the safe and effective application of rehabilitation interventions. Frequently, infections and inflammatory reactions after surgery, acute trauma, and chronic orthopedic diseases significantly affect recovery and physical therapy administration. It is imperative for all rehabilitation personnel to be aware of local and systemic actions and reactions concerning these compounds and to be able to identify indications for their use in orthopedics.

PHARMACOLOGY: DEFINITIONS

Pharmacokinetics describes four essential processes of how drugs are absorbed, distributed, metabolized, and excreted by the body.[1-5]

The wide variability of the effects of drugs from patient to patient is directly related to genetic differences in these processes. Disease states of major organs of metabolism and excretion also adversely affect pharmacokinetic activity.

Absorption describes various routes of administration of how drugs enter the body. Traditional routes of administration are: mouth; intramuscular (IM) injection; subdermal, subcutaneous, or intradermal injection; inhalation; sublingual; buccal; rectal; topical; or intravenous (IV) injection.[1-7]

The selection of the various absorption routes of administration generally depend on availability, the need for emergency access and delivery, or patient comfort and compliance of drug acceptance. **Bioavailability** describes the percentage or fraction of drugs that actually reaches the body's systemic circulation. An important principle directly related to a drug's bioavailability is the **"first-pass effect."** This principle describes the significant metabolism of drugs as they pass through the liver before absorption in the gastrointestinal (GI) tract. Only a small fraction of the initial GI dose may be distributed in the serum after chemical modification in the liver. It should be recognized that, anatomically, venous return from the bowel and stomach occurs through the liver before reaching the systemic circulation.[1-7] The highest drug bioavailability is achieved through IV injection, which yields 100% bioavailability.

Metabolism is the modification of drugs in the body. Generally the chemical modification of drugs takes place in the liver. However, metabolic activity of drugs also occurs in the kidney, lungs, and bloodstream.[1,5]

Pharmacodynamics is the detailed study of specific drug effects on the molecules, cells, tissues, organs, and systems of the body. Two common terms used to describe antibacterial drug effects are **bactericidal** and **bacteriostatic.**[1,2,5,6] Antibacterial bactericidal activity refers to termination (death) of the offending organism.

Antibacterial bacteriostatic activity refers to the inhibition of organism replication (reproduction). Depending on the dose, some drugs demonstrate both bacteriostatic and bactericidal activity.

CLASSIFICATION OF DRUGS

The United States Food and Drug Administration (FDA) controls the regulation and approval of all therapeutic agents. Over the counter (OTC) or legend (caution: federal law prohibits dispensing without a prescription) are the two general classifications of drug availability under the domain of the FDA.[5]

All legend drugs that have the potential for abuse (physical or psychologic addiction or dependency) are further regulated by the United States Federal Drug Enforcement Agency (DEA). These drugs (narcotics, sedatives, opiates, hallucinogens, and stimulants) bear the term *controlled substances*. The general structure and function of this regulatory system involves the classification, category, or schedule of five subclasses or categories of controlled substances. A category, class, or schedule I drug is defined as having a high potential for abuse with no accepted medical use. A class II drug is also described as having a high potential for abuse that also may lead to severe physical or psychological dependence. All prescriptions for schedule II drugs require inscriptions in ink or type, written with the original signature of the practitioner, with no renewals permitted. A class III drug has some potential for abuse that may lead to low to moderate physical or psychologic dependence. Renewals are permitted with limits of five in 6 months. A schedule IV drug has a low potential for abuse with limited physical or psychologic dependence. Class V drugs with low potential for abuse are subject to local or state regulations, and a physician's prescription may not be required.[1-5]

ANTIBIOTICS

There are five basic mechanisms of bactericidal and bacteriostatic activity of antibiotic drugs: I-inhibition of cell wall synthesis, II-increase in cell membrane permeability, III-inhibition of ribosomes, IV-blocking of DNA metabolism, and V-antimetabolic action.[1-7]

Penicillins

Penicillins are bactericidal agents that act by inhibiting cell wall synthesis, resulting in bacterial cell lysis. Penicillin is a limited spectrum agent that is effective against *Streptococcus pyogenes*, *Neisseria*, and some *Clostridium* species. Second-generation penicillins are ampicillin and amoxicillin, which generally affect the same species as natural penicillin. Third-generation agents are carbenicillin and ticarcillin, which affect the same organisms, as well as *Pseudomonas* species.[1-6]

Synthetic penicillins methicillin, oxacillin, nafcillin, and dicloxacillin are effective against resistant strains of *Staphylococcus aureus*. Clavulanic acid in addition to penicillin broadens the range or spectrum of drug activity.[1-6]

Cephalosporins

Cephalosporins are bactericidal agents that also act by inhibiting cell membrane synthesis. First-generation cephalosporins are essentially antistaphylococcus agents. Common first-generation cephalosporins are cefazolin, cefuroxime, and cefmetazole. Third-generation cephalosporins include cefotaxime, ceftriaxone, and moxalactam. The indications for third-generation cephalosporins include increased gram-negative activity.[1-6]

Aminoglycosides

Aminoglycosides are bactericidal agents that are generally effective against aerobic gram-negative bacteria such as *Escherichia coli*, *Klebsiella* species, and *Pseudomonas* species. Examples are gentamicin, tobramycin, streptomycin, amikacin, and neomycin. Unfortunately, with this class of antibiotics, there is a relatively high level of toxicity associated with their continued use. Gentamicin, tobramycin, and amikacin are systemically delivered drugs, whereas neomycin is a topical agent that generally is used for wound irrigation.[1-6]

Tetracyclines

Tetracyclines are bacteriostatic and include doxycycline, minocycline, and tetracycline, which affect enteric bacteria and various *Chlamydia* species. The narrow range of effect limits the use of tetracycline in the treatment of orthopedic infections.[1-6]

Macrolide and Lincosamide Antibiotics

These agents are also bacteriostatic with activity against *Chlamydia*, *Clostridium*, and *Bacteroides* species and *Staphylococcus aureus*. Examples of antibiotics in this class are erythromycin, clindamycin, azithromycin, clarithromycin, and lincomycin.[1-6]

Fluoroquinolones in Quinolones

These are bacteriostatic agents that are broadly effective against all gram-negative rods (*E. coli*, *Salmonella*, *Klebsiella*, *Proteus*, and *Pseudomonas* species). Examples include ciprofloxacin, norfloxacin, ofloxacin, enoxacin, lomefloxacin, levofloxacin, and trovafloxacin.[1-6]

Miscellaneous Antibiotics

The mechanisms of action of these agents vary; however, they are generally bactericidal. The activity of these drugs includes all gram-negative rods, as well as *S. aureus* and *Clostridium* species. Examples include bacitracin, vancomycin, aztreonam, imipenem, chloramphenicol, metronidazole, and rifampin.[1]

INFECTIONS IN ORTHOPEDICS

Treatment of **infections** is extraordinarily complex considering the number of potential offending organisms, as well as the daunting array of antibiotic agents available to combat these organisms. Generally the most effective antibiotic is the least toxic, directed against a single organism and given for a short period of time.[1-7]

In orthopedics the most common uses of antibiotic agents include preoperative surgical prophylaxis, fracture management with internal fixation, and general bone and joint infections.

Preoperative Prophylaxis

Approximately 25% to 50% of all antibiotic therapy is directed at preventing infections rather than directly treating existing infections.[2-4] Generally the bacteria of greatest concern in elective orthopedic surgical procedures are *S. aureus*, *S. epidermidis*, and *Streptococcus* species.

The rationale for the use of perioperative antibacterial administration in total joint arthroplasty, open fractures with internal fixation, bone graft procedures, and extensive open soft-tissue dissection is well supported. Various studies have validated the use of prophylactic antibiotic therapy in total joint arthroplasty by demonstrating infection rates of less than 1% with preoperative administration of antimicrobial agents compared with 4% with the use of placebo.[2-4]

Antibiotic medication must be present at the time of surgery to effectively prevent infection. It is interesting to note that if antibiotic medications are started several hours before the surgical procedure, their efficacy is actually decreased.[2-4]

Fractures

Infection after open fractures can result in nonunion, amputation, and possibly death from sepsis. The risk of infection after open fracture is related to the severity of the fracture. The most common offending organisms are *S. aureus*, gram-negative bacilli, *Clostridium perfringens* (farm-related accidents), or *Pseudomonas* spp. (fresh water injury exposures). The antibacterial coverage typically is with a second- or third-generation cephalosporin, with or without an aminoglycoside for expanded coverage. In one study, an infection rate of 29% was reported when using a cephalosporin alone compared with a 9% occurrence of infection with the addition of an aminoglycoside.[2-4]

In cases of fracture stabilization with use of open reduction with internal fixation (ORIF), postoperative infection poses confounding priorities for the surgeon; treating the infection often requires surgical removal of the implant, whereas treating the fracture requires retention of the implant to stabilize the fracture.[2-4]

It should be noted that the addition of implant hardware to stabilize a fracture actually can reduce the incidence of infection from 71% to 38%, based on use of an animal model contaminated with *S. aureus*.[2-4] In essence a stable fracture union reduces infection rates, whereas an unstable fracture union does not.

Bacterial Adherence to Orthopedic Implants

Internal fracture fixation devices generally are recognized as increasing infection. Common bacteria are capable of colonizing the surface of metal implant devices for fracture stabilization, as well as those for joint arthroplasty. Patients who do not manifest clinical signs or symptoms of infection may in fact harbor bacteria without causing outward signs of sepsis.[2-4]

The type of implant material determines whether or not microbes will adhere to the surface. Animal studies show infection rates of 75% with stainless steel and 35% with titanium. Density and porosity of the implant surface also contribute to the potential for bacterial adherence. Infection rates generally are higher for porous-coated implants compared with solid material. The geometric design configuration of implants may also contribute to bacterial infection. Animal studies

show higher rates of infection with hollow slotted nails compared with solid materials.[2-4]

If bacteria colonize and adhere to implant surfaces, a protective film referred to as **glycocalyx** "slime" tends to nourish the microbes, reduce phagocytosis, interfere with antibody function, inhibit immune response, and promote further bacterial aggregation (Fig. 14-1).[2-7]

Severe Open Fractures

A technique used to combat infection after severe open fractures is with antibiotic beads. A heat-stable antibiotic or vancomycin is manually impregnated within bone cement-polymethylmethacrylate (PMMA) and molded into small beads that are then placed on heavy nonabsorbable suture or surgical wire and positioned within the wound bed and around the fracture site. This particular mode of delivery provides maximum local antibiotic concentrations. In addition, the antibiotic beads provide adequate coverage to fill "dead space" in open fractures and wounds. The use of this technique has been shown to decrease infection rates from 16% to 4% in patients with severe open tibial fractures.[2-4]

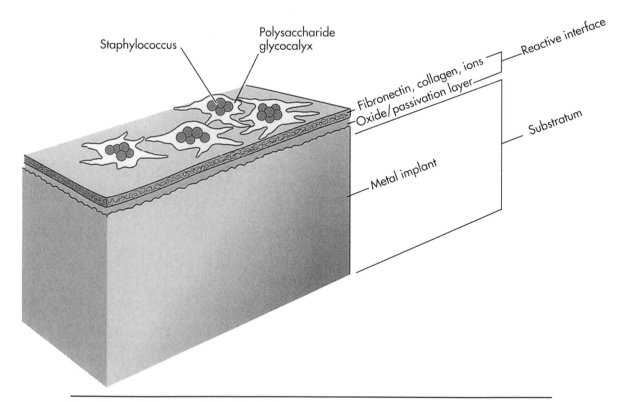

Fig. 14-1 Biofilm containing bacteria on a metal implant. The biofilm or "slime" is made up of the implant passivation layer, host extracellular macromolecules (fibrogen, fibronectin, and collagen), and bacterial extracellular glycocalyx (polysaccharide). Staphylococci are bonded on the implant, which inhibits phagocytosis. Failure of the glycopeptide antibiotics to cure prosthesis-related infection is not caused by poor penetration of drugs into the biofilm but probably by the diminished antimicrobial effect on bacteria in the biofilm environment. (From Browner BD, Levine A, Jupiter J, et al, eds: Skeletal Trauma, 3rd ed, vol 1. Philadelphia, 2003, WB Saunders.)

Infections in Total Joint Arthroplasty

Approximately 500,000 joint replacements are performed annually. Prevention of infection is particularly important to the long-term success of the prosthetic implant. Some surgeons choose to use antibiotic-impregnated bone cement (PMMA) to secure the implant to the bone surface in addition to the standardized preoperative antibiotic therapy. The rationale is to provide local intense concentrations of antibiotics rather than experience morbidity with prolonged systemic administration of antibiotics.[2-7]

CORTICOSTEROIDS

As antiinflammatory agents, **corticosteroids** (a steroid hormone produced by the adrenal glands) are used for moderate to severe painful inflammatory musculoskeletal conditions.[3]

The mechanism of action includes a decrease in lymphocytes, basophils, and monocytes. Corticosteroids also inhibit the migration of leukocytes and suppress production of prostaglandins and leukotrienes through the inhibition of phospholipase.[3]

The specific mechanism of action of corticosteroids differs from NSAIDs by selectively inhibiting the cell membrane enzyme phospholipase, which blocks the immune system's **arachidonic acid** cascade pathways of both **cyclooxygenase** and **lipoxygenase** (Fig. 14-2).

Intraarticular and Paraarticular Corticosteroid Injections

Palliative treatment for moderate to severe musculoskeletal inflammatory painful conditions can be managed effectively with the judicious use of selective injectable corticosteroids. Ideally, steroids are designed to maximize local effects of the drug while minimizing deleterious systemic effects. Generally the following paraarticular conditions can be treated with corticosteroid injections: shoulder bursitis, tendinitis, elbow epicondylitis, greater trochanter bursitis, pes anserine bursitis, plantar fasciitis, and Achilles tendinitis.[3]

Non–weight bearing small joints (acromioclavicular joint, carpometacarpal, and metacarpophalangeal) respond best to intraarticular injection when compared with large weight-bearing joints of the hip and knee. Intraarticular corticosteroid injections of the knee for osteoarthritic pain and inflammation generally are effective at 1 week. However, relief of symptoms is similar to placebo at 4 weeks.[3]

Paraarticular injections are placed into peritendinous tissue and not into the ligament or tendon substance itself.

The most clinically relevant complication of corticosteroid injections are potential ruptures of ligament or tendon after repeated injections. Corticosteroids inhibit collagen synthesis in addition to their known effect as antiinflammatory, antipyretic, and analgesic agents.

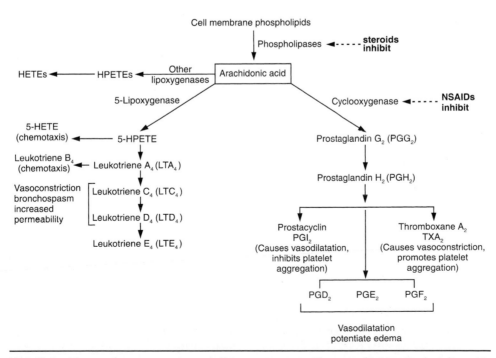

Fig. 14-2 The cyclooxygenase and lipoxygenase pathways. (From Buckwalter JA, Einhorn Ta, Simon SK, eds: Orthopedic Basic Science, Biology, and Biomechanics, 2nd ed. Rosemont, IL, American Academy of Orthopedic Surgeons, 2000:229.)

Responses to corticosteroid injection complications are variable but real when given repeatedly in a short period of time. General recommendations dictate that large weight-bearing joints be rested approximately 24 hours after injection and a minimum of 4 weeks be allowed between injections.[3]

The physician's decision to use various steroids is determined by several factors. Short- to intermediate-acting agents are water soluble (betamethasone, dexamethasone, prednisolone sodium phosphate, and methylprednisolone), whereas others are less soluble (hydrocortisone and triamcinolone) and have longer-lasting action in the body. Typically a combination of short- and long-acting, less soluble corticosteroids is administered.[3]

NONSTEROIDAL ANTIINFLAMMATORY DRUGS

In contrast to corticosteroids, **nonsteroidal antiinflammatory drugs (NSAIDs)** exert their effect by inhibition of the arachidonic acid metabolic enzyme cyclooxygenase (COX), which, in turn, inhibits **prostaglandins** and thromboxane synthesis. Prostaglandins produce pain and also act as mediators of additional pain-producing inflammatory agents.[3] Prostaglandins are strong vasodilators and act to produce increased vascular permeability. The main function of NSAIDs is to inhibit cyclooxygenase and prostaglandin synthesis. However, because of unique mechanisms of inhibition, some NSAIDs also act to inhibit the lipoxygenase enzyme of the arachidonic acid metabolic pathway, which leads to inhibitory action of leukotriene inflammatory agents. Two examples are indomethacin (Indocin) and diclofenac (Voltaren).[3]

Generally, all NSAIDs are superior to placebo for treatment of osteoarthritis. There are no objective differences among available NSAIDs in that choices are largely subjective and based on physician preference, trial and error, and patient tolerance.[3]

Adverse Reactions to Nonsteroidal Antiinflammatory Drugs

GI toxicity is the predominant side effect of NSAID usage.[3] A major contributing factor to GI upset is that these agents typically are prescribed in relatively high dosages and delivered over prolonged periods of time. It is interesting to note that the mechanism of GI upset from NSAIDs is not from erosive action but rather from inhibition of prostaglandin synthesis. Prostaglandins act to inhibit acid secretion in the gastric mucosa and serve to increase GI blood flow. Therefore inhibition of prostaglandins typically may reduce GI vascularity and expose the GI tract to the negative effects of gastric acid.[3]

Unfortunately, an unacceptably high percentage (20% to 30%) of persons 65 years of age and older who develop peptic ulcers from NSAID therapy require hospitalization. Approximately 20% of all patients who use NSAIDs complain of some form of GI toxicity.[3]

SELECTIVE INHIBITION: CYCLOOXYGENASE (COX-1 AND COX-2)

Two forms of COX have been identified: **COX-1** and **COX-2.** As stated, NSAIDs act through various mechanisms to inhibit cyclooxygenase and prostaglandin synthesis. Although NSAIDs effectively reduce proinflammatory mediators (prostaglandins), they also contribute to the demise of gastric mucosa circulation and potential ulceration by exposure to gastric acid.

Specific NSAIDs referred to as COX-2 inhibitors—valdecoxib (Bextra), celecoxib (Celebrex), and rofecoxib (Vioxx)—selectively inhibit prostaglandins, which are produced locally during intense inflammatory episodes, but do not reduce base prostaglandin production that serve a GI protective role.[3]

As such, COX-2 inhibitors are as effective in reducing pain and inflammation as nonselective NSAIDs but have a low incidence of adverse effects because of the role of not inhibiting COX-1 protective prostaglandin secretion.[3]

INFLAMMATION

Acute inflammatory responses after injury or surgery involve vascular permeability, edema with leukocyte exudates, and neutrophil migration to the injury site. Local signs of **inflammation** include redness (rubor), swelling (tumor), heat (calor), pain (dolor), and loss of function (function lata).

Histamine is synthesized and stored in mast cells and basophils. The secretion of histamine after membrane injury causes vasodilation, increased capillary permeability, and smooth muscle contraction.

As cell membranes are broken down, phospholipid degradation releases arachidonic acid, which in turn is converted to prostaglandins, **thromboxanes,** and **leukotrienes** by either the cyclooxygenase or lipoxygenase pathway (Fig. 14-3).[1]

The various factors (cytokines) related to acute inflammation are interleukin-1 (IL-1) and tumor necrosis factor (TNF). In addition to the mediation of cellular activity, IL-1 and TNF are also responsible for systemic manifestations of acute phase inflammatory responses, including fever, loss of appetite, and increased sleep.[1,7]

Prostaglandins and thromboxanes are synthesized from the COX pathway of arachidonic acid metabolism. Prostaglandins are biologically active lipids that exert strong vasodilation activity. Thromboxanes are synthesized from prostaglandins and are responsible for stimulating primary homeostasis. Thromboxanes are potent stimulators of vasoconstriction and smooth muscle contraction.[1,7]

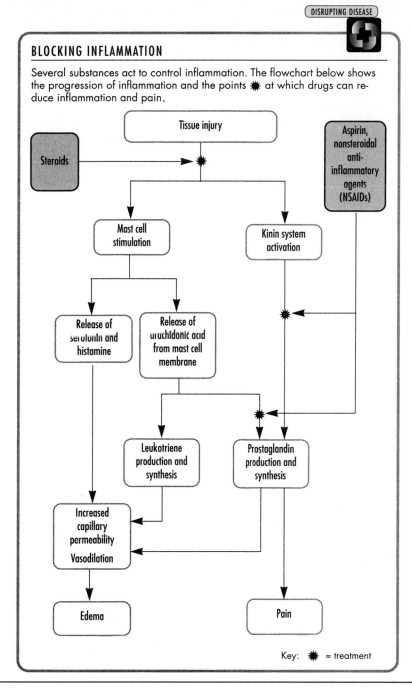

Fig. 14-3 Flowchart that shows pathways of inflammation and points of drug interactions. (From Handbook of Pathophysiology. Springhouse, PA, Springhouse, 64.)

Leukotrienes are synthesized from the lipoxygenase pathway of arachidonic acid metabolism. Generally these cells cause vascular permeability and smooth muscle contraction, resulting in vasoconstriction.

Leukocytes (polymorphonuclear leukocytes, neutrophils, eosinophils and basophils, and monocytes and lymphocytes) are involved with the process of increased vascular permeability and blood flow stasis (margination). Leukocytes also are involved with the process of adhesion with endothelial cells. Chemotaxis describes leukocytes migrating to the injury site by following chemical gradients.[1,7]

CHRONIC INFLAMMATORY RESPONSE

A persistent inflammatory reaction to injury lasting several weeks to months may be defined as chronic inflammation. Classically, the major cells involved with acute inflammation, the hallmark predominant cells, are mononuclear cells (monocytes, macrophages, lymphocytes, and plasma cells).[1] Macrophages and lymphocytes are the cornerstone types of chronic inflammation.

IL-1, interleukin-6 (IL-6), and TNF mediate acute phase reactions, as well as systemic manifestations of chronic inflammation: fever, hypotension, loss of appetite, and increased sleep.[1-4]

Various cellular changes in chronic inflammatory reaction include leukocytosis, neutrophilia (increased neutrophils in circulation), lymphocytosis (increased lymphocytes in circulation), and eosinophils (increased eosinophils).[1-4] Ultimately, acute and chronic inflammatory reactions may incite tissue hypoxia, ischemia, anoxia, necrosis, pain (noxious chemical stimuli), vascular congestion, occlusion, muscular inhibition, atrophy, bone mineral loss, infection, and sepsis.[1]

❖ ADDITIONAL FEATURES

Age: Liver metabolic activity declines with increasing age. The drug dose may have to be reduced in elderly patients.

Bioavailability: The percentage of the drug that reaches the systemic circulation. IV drugs have 100% bioavailability.

Clearance: Measurement of how fast substances are removed from the blood and excreted in the urine.

Distribution: The transfer of drugs from one compartment of the body to another.

Drug Half-life: The time it takes for 50% of the drug dose to be cleared from the body.

Metabolism: Chemical change or modification of drugs in the body. Typically, metabolism takes place in the liver; however, metabolism also takes place in the kidney, lungs, and circulation.

Pharmacokinetics: Four separate areas represent pharmacokinetics: absorption, distribution, metabolism, and excretion.

Steady State: When the rate of drug administration becomes equal to the rate of drug clearance. This maintains the plasma concentration at a constant level.

Tachyphylaxis: Rapid reduction or loss of a drug's effect after administration.

Tolerance: Responsiveness or effect of drugs may be reduced with continued use.

REFERENCES

1. Cell biology. In United States Medical Licensing Examination (USMLE) Step 1. Princeton Review, 3rd ed. New York, Random House, 2000.
2. Garvin KL, et al: Infections in orthopedics. In Buckwalter JA, Einhorn Ta, Simon SK, eds. Orthopedic Basic Science, Biology, and Biomechanics, 2nd ed. Rosemont, IL, American Academy of Orthopedic Surgeons, 2000.
3. Morris CD, Einhorn TA: Principles of orthopedic pharmacology. In Buckwalter JA, Einhorn Ta, Simon SK, eds. Orthopedic Basic Science, Biology, and Biomechanics, 2nd ed. Rosemont, IL, American Academy of Orthopedic Surgeons, 2000.
4. Schmidt AH, Switonkowski MF: Pathophysiology of infections after internal fixation of fractures. *J Am Acad Orthop Surg* 2000; 8:285–291.
5. Pharmacology. In United States Medical Licensing Examination (USMLE) Step 1. Princeton Review, 3rd ed. New York, Random House, 2000.
6. Microbiology. In United States Medical Licensing Examination (USMLE) Step 1. Princeton Review, 3rd ed. New York, Random House, 2000.
7. Immunology. In United States Medical Licensing Examination (USMLE) Step 1. Princeton Review, 3rd ed. New York, Random House, 2000.

REVIEW QUESTIONS

Multiple Choice

1. Pharmacokinetics describes which of the following? (Circle all that apply.)
   A. Absorption
   B. Metabolism
   C. Distribution
   D. All of the above

2. Which of the following describes the highest bioavailability of drug administration and absorption?
   A. Oral (PO)
   B. Intramuscular (IM)
   C. Intravenous (IV)
   D. Inhalation

3. Which of the following describes the activity of antibiotics? (Circle all that apply.)
   A. Inhibition of cell wall synthesis
   B. Increase cell wall permeability
   C. Block DNA metabolism
   D. All of the above

4. The most effective antibiotics have which of the following characteristics?
   A. Potentially most toxic
   B. Prescribed for long periods
   C. Directed against a single organism
   D. None of the above

5. What percent of antibiotic therapy is directed at preventing infections rather than treating existing infections?
   A. 10% to 20%
   B. 25% to 50%
   C. 5% to 15%
   D. 30% to 60%

6. Which of the following describes rates of infection in the preoperative administration of antibiotics compared with placebo?
   A. 3%
   B. 5%
   C. 1%
   D. 4%

7. "Glycocalyx" has which effect on bacterial adherence to metal implants? (Circle all that apply.)
   A. Decreases bacterial aggregation
   B. Promotes immune response
   C. Reduces phagocytosis
   D. None of the above

8. Which of the following best describes the differences between corticosteroids and nonsteroidal antiinflammatory drugs (NSAIDs)?
   A. NSAIDs block both enzyme cascade pathways.
   B. Corticosteroids block only the lipoxygenase pathway.
   C. NSAIDs are used for severe inflammatory conditions.
   D. Corticosteroids inhibit cyclooxygenase (COX) and lipoxygenase.

Short Answer

9. Identify nine routes of drug delivery.

10. Name two common mechanisms of antibacterial effects and define their activity.

11. Identify the three most common offending bacterial organisms in elective orthopedic surgical procedures.

True/False

12. The greatest bioavailability of drug administration is through the PO route.
13. "Bacteriostatic" refers to inhibition of organism reproduction.
14. The most effective antibiotic is the least toxic, directed against single organisms, and given for a short period of time.
15. Various studies validate the use of prophylactic antibiotic administration in elective total joint arthroplasty by demonstrating infection rates of less than 1% compared with 4% with placebo.
16. Preoperative antibiotic therapy must be given several hours or days before surgery to increase its efficacy.
17. Bacteria are unable to colonize a stainless steel or titanium implant.
18. A patient with a metal implant may in fact harbor bacteria without demonstrating outward signs of infection.
19. A method to reduce risks of infection with total joint arthroplasty is with the use of antibiotic-impregnated polymethylmethacrylate (PMMA) bone cement.
20. Corticosteroids inhibit prostaglandins and thromboxanes only.
21. There is a direct relationship between corticosteroid infections and ultimate tissue disruption.

22. The most significant adverse reaction to NSAIDs is gastrointestinal (GI) dysfunction.
23. The erosive action of NSAIDs on the GI tract contributes to ulcers.

Essay Questions

Answer on a separate sheet of paper.
24. Describe the "first-pass effect."
25. Discuss the mechanisms of action of corticosteroids and describe the differences between corticosteroids and NSAIDs.

Critical Thinking Application

You are treating two patients. One patient is a 68-year-old man with a recent 4-week postoperative total hip arthroplasty. The other patient is a 34-year-old woman typist with chronic epicondylitis.

The physician has prescribed a course of antibiotic therapy for the patient with the total hip replacement. His operative note reveals the use of vancomycin-impregnated PMMA for his total hip replacement. In small groups, discuss the rationale for prophylactic antibiotic therapy preceding elective total joint arthroplasty. What is the rationale for the use of antibiotic-impregnated bone cement? Define or describe glycocalyx "slime" and the pathogenesis of bacterial adherence to orthopedic implants. Specifically name various offending bacteria found with elective orthopedic surgery.

The physician had prescribed a course of diclofenac (an NSAID) for the other patient with chronic lateral epicondylitis. Schematically define the arachidonic acid–phospholipase degradative metabolic pathway. Discuss the importance of suppression of COX and inflammatory mediators.

Discuss a significant adverse reaction that is common with the use of COX inhibitors. Describe the potential pathogenesis of GI upset.

PART IV

GAIT AND JOINT MOBILIZATION

In this section, the physical therapist assistant (PTA) is introduced to rudimentary concepts and compulsory scientific principles related to gait mechanics and peripheral joint mobilization techniques.

A basic yet essential component of orthopedic physical therapy management is the instruction and application of proper gait techniques after injury or disease of the musculoskeletal system. To safely and properly instruct patients in the use of assistive devices and effectively apply fundamental gait techniques, the PTA must understand the components of the gait cycle and be able to instruct patients in appropriate gait patterns and identify deviations in gait. Therefore this section clarifies and describes the gait cycle and introduces basic terms, definitions, and concepts. In addition, the PTA is introduced to proper gait-pattern instruction, weight bearing status, and the identification of gait abnormalities.

It is clinically relevant to clearly state that the delegation of selected mobilization techniques is entirely at the discretion of the physical therapist, and the application of peripheral joint mobilization is not universally accepted as a routine domain of clinical practice for the PTA. Therefore the information concerning peripheral joint mobilization is provided as a means of stimulating the PTA's awareness of the rationale for improving motion and for the reduction of pain as identified and prescribed by the physical therapist.

15 Fundamentals of Gait

LEARNING OBJECTIVES

1. Define and describe basic components of the gait cycle.
2. Discuss the two phases of gait.
3. Identify and describe each component of the two phases of gait.
4. Define and describe common gait deviations.
5. Define and instruct appropriate gait patterns.
6. Outline and describe terms used to define weight bearing status during gait.
7. Identify and discuss the appropriate use of assistive devices.

KEY TERMS

Gait	Midstance	Two-point gait pattern
Base of support	Heel off	Non–weight bearing
Center of gravity	Toe off	(NWB)
Step length	Acceleration	Partial weight bearing
Cadence	Midswing	(PWB)
Stride length	Deceleration	Touch down weight
Stance phase	Antalgic gait	bearing (TDWB)
Swing phase	Steppage gait	Toe touch weight bearing
Double support	Trendelenburg gait	(TTWB)
Single support	Abductor "lurch"	Weight bearing as
Pelvic "list"	Calcaneal gait	tolerated (WBAT)
Heel strike	Four-point gait pattern	Full weight bearing
Foot flat	Three-point gait pattern	(FWB)

CHAPTER OUTLINE

Basic Gait Terms, Definitions, and Concepts
   Additional Elements
The Two Phases of Gait
Gait Deviations
Gait Pattern Instruction
Weight Bearing Status
Negotiating Stairs with Assistive Devices
Selection of Assistive Devices

Instructing patients concerning the appropriate use of assistive devices after orthopedic trauma requires an understanding of normal human locomotion and the ability to identify subtle deviations and abnormalities in gait. The physical therapist assistant (PTA) is frequently assigned tasks related to instruction, supervision, and progression of various factors related to gait. Critical analysis of the individual components of the entire gait cycle and the application of gait mechanics as they relate to function are necessary to safely and effectively instruct patients in gait mechanics and readily identify variations and deviations in gait. The PTA must be able to accurately identify changes in a patient's gait pattern and articulate these changes to the physical therapist.

BASIC GAIT TERMS, DEFINITIONS, AND CONCEPTS

Normal human locomotion requires a cyclic, coordinated pattern of motion focused on minimizing energy expenditure.[3] Certain factors are necessary for a normal, synchronous walking pattern. These factors include an adequate base of support, appropriate foot clearance during swing, adequate step length, and conservation of energy.[3] Although these factors are common components of walking, unique differences are seen in everyone's walking pattern or style.

Gait describes various styles of walking.[2] For example, some people have short, quick steps with very little trunk motion, whereas others demonstrate long, slow strides with excessive arm swing and trunk motion.

A person's **base of support** provides both balance and stability to maintain an erect posture.[1] The base of support is the distance between a person's feet while standing and during ambulation. A wide base of support provides greater stability than a narrow base of support.

A person's **center of gravity** is approximately 5 cm anterior to the second sacral vertebra.[1] The center of gravity changes both vertically and horizontally during gait. The center of gravity during gait also contributes to balance and stability. A lower center of gravity (e.g., while squatting) provides greater stability than a higher center of gravity (e.g., while standing on the toes).

In the description of a *gait cycle* (Fig. 15-1) (defined as the mechanical activity that occurs when foot contact is made with the ground and when the same foot contacts the ground again),[2] view each component separately. **Step length** describes the linear distance between the right and left foot during gait. Generally this distance is measured from heel-to-toe contact with the ground of one foot to heel or toe contact with the ground of the opposite foot. **Cadence** refers to the total number of steps per minute. Normal cadence is between 70 and 120 steps or 90 and 130 steps per minute.[1,2]

Stride length is synonymous with the gait cycle. Leg length obviously influences the magnitude of stride length. Individuals with longer legs demonstrate longer stride lengths. Persons with shorter legs have a smaller stride length. Average values for stride length range from 70 to 82 cm.[1]

The **stance phase** of gait represents approximately 60% of the entire gait cycle (Fig. 15-1). Stance phase begins when foot contact is made with the ground and lasts until the same foot leaves the ground.[1,2,5]

The **swing phase** of gait occupies approximately 40% of the gait cycle (Fig. 15-1). During this phase, one limb is entirely non–weight bearing; it applies throughout the gait cycle.

Double support represents the time within the gait cycle in which both feet are in contact with the ground and weight transfer occurs from one foot to the other.[1] **Single support** is defined as that time during the stance phase when only one foot is in contact with the ground.[1,2]

Additional Elements

In addition to the obvious contribution of the lower limbs to gait, other body parts also play a role in gait

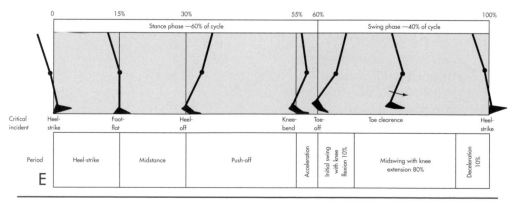

Fig. 15-1 Gait cycle. (From Tachdjian MO: Pediatric Orthopaedics, 2nd ed. Philadelphia, WB Saunders, 1990.)

mechanics. During normal gait, the pelvis rotates approximately 8 degrees within the transverse plane of the body. This 8-degree rotation is broken down as 4 degrees of rotation to the right and 4 degrees of rotation to the left.[1] Pelvic rotation lengthens the femur during the swing phase through initial foot contact and helps to minimize vertical trunk displacement during gait to conserve energy.

The pelvis also rotates within the frontal plane of the body during gait, which is termed **pelvic "list."** This creates a downward motion of the pelvis of approximately 5 degrees on the non–weight bearing limb during stance. The "listing" of the pelvis creates adduction of the weight bearing limb and abduction of the non–weight bearing limb, thereby improving the efficiency of the hip-abductor mechanism (Fig. 15-2).

The trunk, arms, and shoulders also rotate to ensure balance and stability during gait. Knee flexion in stance also contributes to normal mechanics and energy conservation during gait. During stance, the weight bearing knee must flex approximately 15 degrees to decrease impact (Fig. 15-3). Foot and ankle motion produces sequential dorsiflexion and plantar flexion during gait. The dorsiflexors contract eccentrically from initial heel contact with the ground, to keep the foot from "slapping" to the floor. The foot acts as a shock absorber by pronating during the stance phase. During "toe off," the foot serves as a rigid lever (Fig. 15-4).[3]

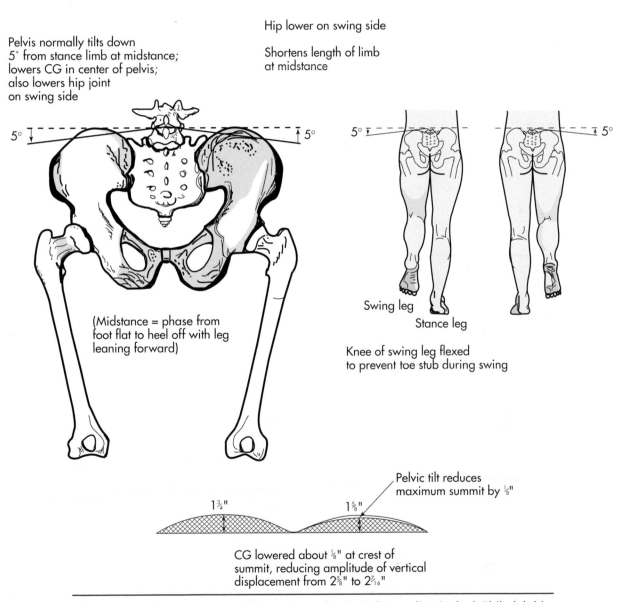

Pelvis normally tilts down 5° from stance limb at midstance; lowers CG in center of pelvis; also lowers hip joint on swing side

Hip lower on swing side

Shortens length of limb at midstance

5°   5°

(Midstance = phase from foot flat to heel off with leg leaning forward)

5°   5°

Swing leg

Stance leg

Knee of swing leg flexed to prevent toe stub during swing

Pelvic tilt reduces maximum summit by ⅛"

1¾"   1⅝"

CG lowered about ⅛" at crest of summit, reducing amplitude of vertical displacement from 2⅜" to 2³⁄₁₆"

Fig. 15-2 Pelvic list. (From Tachdjian MO: Pediatric Orthopaedics, 2nd ed. Philadelphia, WB Saunders, 1990.)

KNEE FLEXION

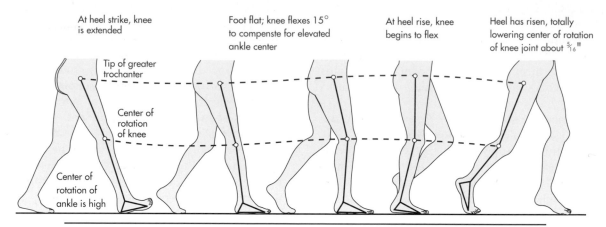

At heel strike, knee is extended

Foot flat; knee flexes 15° to compenste for elevated ankle center

At heel rise, knee begins to flex

Heel has risen, totally lowering center of rotation of knee joint about 5/16"

Tip of greater trochanter

Center of rotation of knee

Center of rotation of ankle is high

Fig. 15-3 Knee flexion during stance. (From Tachdjian MO: Pediatric Orthopaedics, 2nd ed. Philadelphia, WB Saunders, 1990.)

ANKLE ROTATION

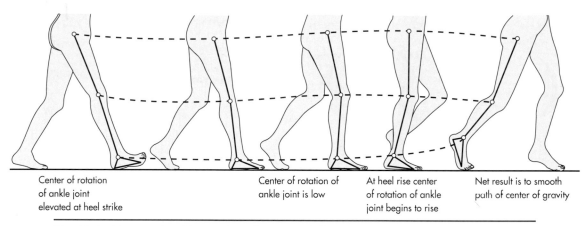

Center of rotation of ankle joint elevated at heel strike

Center of rotation of ankle joint is low

At heel rise center of rotation of ankle joint begins to rise

Net result is to smooth path of center of gravity

Fig. 15-4 Foot and ankle motion. (From Tachdjian MO: Pediatric Orthopaedics, 2nd ed. Philadelphia, WB Saunders, 1990.)

THE TWO PHASES OF GAIT

The swing phase and stance phase of gait are subdivided into eight distinct periods (Table 15-1). The stance phase has five components:

- **Heel strike** or initial contact: The instant foot contact is made with the ground. Ideally the heel initiates contact, but the midfoot or toe will be the point of initial contact in some pathologic gaits.
- **Foot flat** or loading response: The time the entire foot is in contact with the floor. Shock absorption is a primary action during this period.
- **Midstance** or single-leg support: When the body is directly over the weight bearing leg. This action serves to roll the foot over into single-limb support during stance.

- **Heel off** or terminal stance: When the heel of the weight bearing limb initially rises from the floor, weight is unloaded from the weight bearing limb and shifted or transferred to the opposite limb.
- **Toe off** or preswing: When the knee of the weight bearing limb flexes and prepares for the swing phase.

The swing phase has three components:

- **Acceleration,** initial swing, or preswing
- **Midswing:** When the non–weight bearing limb is advanced to where the limb passes directly beneath the body
- **Deceleration** or terminal swing: The limb decelerates and is in a position of extension preparing for heel strike

Most muscle action during the gait cycle is eccentric. When the hip flexors act concentrically to advance the

Table 15-1	*Phases of Gait*			
Phase	**Period**	**Action**	**Percent (%)**	**Cycle**
STANCE			60	
	Heel strike	Foot on ground	—	
	Foot flat	Shock absorption	15	
	Midstance	Roll over foot	15	
	Heel off	Roll beyond foot	25	
	Toe off	Knee flexes	5	
SWING			40	
	Acceleration	Limb begins to advance	5	
	Midswing	Limb advances further	30	
	Deceleration	Limb deceleration/ extension	5	

From Miller MD: Review of Orthopaedics, 2nd ed. Philadelphia, WB Saunders, 1992.

Table 15-2	*Muscle Function During Gait*	
Muscle	**Action**	**Function**
Gluteus medius	Eccentric	Controls pelvic tilt at midstance
Gluteus maximus	Concentric	Powers hip extension
Iliopsoas	Concentric	Powers hip flexion
Hip adductors	Eccentric	Controls lateral sway (late stance)
Hip abductors	Eccentric	Controls pelvic tilt (midstance)
Quadriceps	Eccentric	Stabilizes knee at heel strike
Hamstrings	Eccentric	Controls rate of knee extension (stance)
Tibialis anterior	Concentric	Dorsiflexes ankle at swing
	Eccentric*	Slows plantar flexion rate (heel strike)
Gastrocnemius-soleus	Eccentric	Slows dorsiflexion rate (stance)

*Predominant role.
From Miller MD: Review of Orthopaedics, 2nd ed. Philadelphia, WB Saunders, 1992.

limb during acceleration and midswing, the hamstrings contract eccentrically to control the rate of knee extension. The gluteus maximus and tibialis anterior also contribute concentric contractions during the gait cycle (Table 15-2).

GAIT DEVIATIONS

Gait abnormalities result from injury, muscle weakness, pain, or immobilization. The PTA must be able to accurately identify both obvious and subtle gait deviations and to describe these pathologic characteristics to the physical therapist.

An exceedingly common gait deviation is the **antalgic gait.** It usually occurs in the presence of pain. This gait is characterized by a rapid swing phase of the uninvolved limb, with a reduction of the stance phase of the involved limb. There is an obvious, observable decrease in weight shifting over the stance leg to minimize weight bearing on the painful limb. Cadence is also reduced by the shortened step created by the decreased swing phase.

A **steppage gait** involves muscular weakness of the ankle dorsiflexors (tibialis anterior) and is characterized by extreme hip flexion and knee flexion during swing through to keep from dragging the toes on the floor. This gait is also characterized by the foot "slapping" the ground because the weak dorsiflexors cannot adequately decelerate the foot during contact.

Muscular weakness is responsible for many identifiable gait abnormalities. To appreciate the specific gait deviations, it is best to review each muscle separately.

Weakness of the *gluteus medius* produces a **Trendelenburg** gait pattern, which is characterized by the pelvis dropping toward the unaffected limb during the single-limb support period of the stance phase. The pelvis drops because the gluteus medius cannot produce enough force of contraction (secondary to muscle weakness) from its attachment on the femur to keep the pelvis level during stance. With a weak gluteus medius, a patient also may demonstrate a gluteus medius or **abductor "lurch."** The patient laterally flexes the trunk over the involved limb to keep the center of gravity over the base of support.[1]

Weakness of the *hip flexors* (psoas muscles) produces difficulty in initiating swing-through.[1] To compensate for this specific muscular weakness, the patient externally or laterally rotates the leg and uses the hip adductors for swing-through. This circumduction of the hip exaggerates energy expenditure and produces extreme trunk and pelvis motion.

Gluteus maximus weakness results in rapid hip hyperextension during initial foot contact with the ground.[3] To compensate, the patient quickly extends the trunk during initial foot contact to maintain hip extension of the stance leg.[4]

Weakness of the *quadriceps muscle group* results in knee hyperextension during the stance phase of the gait cycle. Normally, the quadriceps contracts eccentrically to control the knee at heel strike or initial contact.

Table 15-3	Gait Abnormalities Caused by Muscle Weakness			
Muscle	Phase	Direction	Type of Gait	Treatment
Gluteus medius	Stance	Lateral	Abductor lurch	Cane
Gluteus maximus	Stance	Backward	Lurch (hip hyperextension)	
Quadriceps	Stance	Forward	Lurch/back knee gait	AFO
	Swing	Forward	Abnormal hip rotation	
Gastrocnemius-soleus	Stance	Forward	Flat foot (calcaneal) gait	± AFO
	Swing	Forward	Delayed heel rise	
Tibialis anterior	Stance	Forward	Foot drop/slap	AFO
	Swing	Forward	Steppage gait	

From Miller MD: Review of Orthopaedics, 2nd ed. Philadelphia, WB Saunders, 1992.

When the quadriceps is weak, the knee quickly hyperextends at heel strike.

A **calcaneal gait** pattern occurs with weakness of the *gastrocnemius-soleus muscle group*. Because of weakness in the plantar flexion muscles, reduced foot propulsion occurs during the toe-off period of the stance phase. This weakness also creates a delayed rise of the heel at the initiation of swing phase.[3] Table 15-3 outlines the various muscles and resultant gait abnormalities caused by muscular weakness.

GAIT PATTERN INSTRUCTION

Instructing patients in the proper use of assistive devices and identifying appropriate gait patterns are relevant clinical tasks for the physical therapist assistant. Several patterns are outlined here.

A **four-point gait pattern** is described as advancing the crutch opposite the uninvolved limb first, followed by the involved limb, then advancing the crutch toward the uninvolved limb, then finally advancing the uninvolved limb (Fig. 15-5). If the injured limb is the left leg, the four-point gait pattern looks like this:

Right crutch × Left foot × Left crutch × Right foot

The four-point gait pattern attempts to duplicate the normal reciprocal motion that occurs between the upper extremities and the lower limbs during normal gait.

A **three-point gait pattern** is commonly taught using bilateral axillary crutches (Fig. 15-6). The sequence of events begins by advancing both crutches and the involved limb. The noninvolved limb is then advanced forward and the sequence repeated.

A **two-point gait pattern** is described as advancing the left crutch and right lower extremity at the same time, then advancing the right crutch and left lower extremity together (Fig. 15-7). This gait pattern is similar to the four-point gait pattern in which normal reciprocal motion and walking rhythm is encouraged.

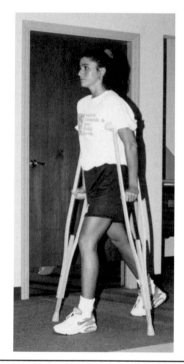

Fig. 15-5 Four-point gait pattern (see text for description).

A tripod gait pattern is used for bilateral nonfunctioning limbs. Crutches are advanced, then the lower body is advanced. With a tripod gait, the body can be lifted and advanced to the crutch or swung through and beyond the crutches.

WEIGHT BEARING STATUS

Depending on the healing constraints of injured tissues (bone, ligaments, tendon, cartilage, and muscle), certain weight bearing restrictions are imposed to protect the injured tissues from excessive stresses and loads, as well as to promote normal physiologic healing. If an injured limb is unable to support any weight, **non–weight bearing (NWB)** status is assigned until sufficient

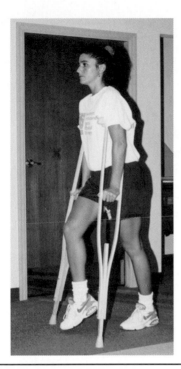

Fig. 15-6 Three-point gait pattern (see text for description).

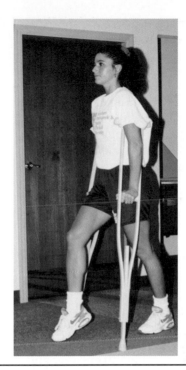

Fig. 15-7 Two-point gait pattern (see text for description).

healing has taken place to allow the limb to safely accept some degree of weight. **Partial weight bearing (PWB)** is frequently graded in a percentage of the patient's weight (20%, 40%, 50%, etc.) or in pounds of pressure applied to the floor from the involved limb. When teaching PWB with orders to apply a certain amount of weight (such as 20 pounds or 50 pounds), a bathroom scale can acquaint the patient with exactly how much weight is necessary to bear on the injured limb. The terms **touch down weight bearing (TDWB)** and **toe touch weight bearing (TTWB)** can be used synonymously to describe minimal contact of the involved limb with the ground. Generally, TDWB is used for balance purposes initially. As healing and pain allow, progressive weight bearing can be instituted. **Weight bearing as tolerated (WBAT)** is assigned to patients in whom pain tolerance is the predominant limiting factor. Then the patient is allowed to bear as much weight on the injured limb as is comfortable. When a patient no longer requires an assistive device to accommodate pain or healing of injured tissues, **full weight bearing (FWB)** status is generally allowed.

Weight bearing status is a progressive process that involves constant assessment and reassessment of pain, joint stability, tissue healing constraints, and function. A patient with severe injuries progresses through each designation of weight bearing as follows:

NWB × TDWB × PWB × WBAT × FWB

Less severe injuries may begin anywhere along the continuum and progress from there.

NEGOTIATING STAIRS WITH ASSISTIVE DEVICES

Ascending and descending stairs, steps, or curbs requires prudent instruction and careful supervision with necessary tactile and verbal cueing. The safety of the patient is the principal concern. Perhaps no other gait training technique elicits as much anxiety as negotiating stairs. Therefore the PTA must accept the responsibility for clearly articulating the fundamentals of climbing and descending the stairs while both validating the patient's fears and providing confidence, encouragement, and a safe environment for instruction.

When instructing patients to ascend stairs using bilateral axillary crutches, the first step is to encourage the use of a handrail, if one is available. As the patient uses the handrail, both crutches are placed in the hand opposite the handrail. If at all possible the patient should be instructed to use the handrail on the side of the injured limb. This may provide an added sense of stability and support. Ascending a step requires the noninvolved leg to step up first. Then the involved limb and crutches are advanced up to the same step.

When descending steps, the same instructions about the use of the handrail next to the injured limb should be repeated. The first step when descending stairs is to advance the crutches or cane to the step. The injured limb is then advanced down to the step, followed by the uninjured limb. It may help patients to remember, "up with the good, down with the bad," when cueing them as to which limb to advance up or down the stairs.

When providing support for the patient during stair climbing, the PTA should stand behind the patient while giving appropriate verbal cues and physical support at the waist. As a safety precaution, an interlocking gait belt should be applied and used during all phases of gait training. When instructing patients during stair descent, it is best to stand in front of the patient. However, enough space must be allowed between the therapist and patient to permit a technically correct and safe descent.

When no handrail is available the patient should follow the same steps, except that both crutches are used as with normal walking with crutches.

SELECTION OF ASSISTIVE DEVICES

The initial selection of assistive gait devices depends largely on the age and activity level of the patient, the severity of the injury, and the weight bearing status. Walkers can be prescribed for an elderly person because they are inherently stable and easy to use. Children may find using a pediatric walker easier and safer than axillary crutches.

Axillary crutches provide less stability than a walker, but compensate with greater mobility. Canes provide the least support of all assistive devices. However, some types of canes provide more support than others. For example, a wide-based quad cane (four points) allows more stability than a narrow-based quad cane or a single-point cane. A hemi-walker provides a wider, more stable base of support than a wide-based quad cane. Hemi-walkers and quad canes are frequently used by patients who have had a cerebrovascular accident (CVA) with resultant hemiparesis.

As with weight bearing status, patients may progress from one form of assistive device to another. As pain, healing, and function allow, a patient may move from using axillary crutches to a cane or from a walker to axillary crutches. Constant reassessment of a patient's balance, coordination, strength, endurance, weight bearing status, and function will guide the PTA in consulting with the physical therapist concerning appropriate gait devices.

❖ ADDITIONAL FEATURES

Antalgic Gait: Reduced stance phase of involved limb with decreased swing phase of noninvolved limb.

Divisions of Stance Phase: Weight acceptance, single limb stance, weight release.

Knee Flexion: At heel strike, is about 10 degrees.

Maximum Hip Flexion: During normal gait, cycle is about 40 degrees.

Phases of Gait Cycle: Stance phase, 60%; swing phase, 40%.

REFERENCES

1. Epler M: Gait. In Richardson JK, Iglarsh ZA, eds. Clinical Orthopaedic Physical Therapy. Philadelphia, WB Saunders, 1994.
2. Lippert L: Normal gait. In Clinical Kinesiology for Physical Therapist Assistants, 2nd ed. Philadelphia, FA Davis, 1994.
3. Miller MD: Review of orthopaedics. Philadelphia, WB Saunders, 1992.
4. Rothstein JM, Roy SH, Wolf SL: Gait. In The Rehabilitation Specialists Handbook. Philadelphia, FA Davis, 1991.
5. Tachdjian MO: Pediatric orthopaedics, 2nd ed. Philadelphia, WB Saunders, 1990.

REVIEW QUESTIONS

Multiple Choice

1. In terms of gait, a wider base of support provides which of the following?
   A. Greater endurance
   B. Less stability
   C. Reduced trunk motion
   D. Greater stability
2. An individual's center of gravity is which of the following?
   A. Unchanged during gait
   B. Approximately 5 cm anterior to the second sacral vertebrae
   C. Unimportant and unrelated to stability
   D. Located in the upper lumbar vertebrae
3. The number of total steps per minute during gait is called which of the following?
   A. Stride length
   B. Cadence
   C. Gait cycle
   D. None of the above
4. Which of the following represents approximately 60% of the entire gait cycle?
   A. Stride length
   B. Stance phase
   C. Swing phase
   D. Double support
5. The swing phase of gait occupies what percentage of the gait cycle?
   A. 10%
   B. 20%
   C. 15%
   D. 40%
   E. 60%
6. The pelvis rotates within the frontal plane of the body during gait. This pelvic rotation is called which of the following?
   A. List
   B. Pitch
   C. Yaw
   D. Pelvic deviation
7. The stance phase of gait has how many components?
   A. Three
   B. Four
   C. Five
   D. Six
8. The swing phase of gait has how many components?
   A. Four
   B. Two
   C. Three
   D. Five
9. During the stance phase of gait, _____ is the instant foot contact is made with the ground.
   A. Foot flat
   B. Heel off
   C. Heel strike
   D. Midstance

10. During the stance phase of gait, _____ is the time when the entire foot is in contact with the ground.
    A. Midstance
    B. Foot flat
    C. Heel off
    D. Toe off

11. What is the name of the period where the body is directly over the weight bearing leg?
    A. Toe off
    B. Heel strike
    C. Midstance
    D. Heel off

12. _____ occurs when weight is unloaded from the weight bearing limb and transferred to the opposite limb.
    A. Toe off
    B. Heel off
    C. Midstance
    D. Heel strike

13. A painful gait pattern is referred to as which of the following?
    A. A steppage gait
    B. An antalgic gait
    C. An abductor lurch
    D. None of the above

14. A rapid swing phase of the uninvolved limb, with a reduction of the stance phase of the involved limb, is characteristic of which type of gait?
    A. Antalgic gait
    B. Steppage gait
    C. Trendelenburg gait
    D. Abductor lurch

15. Weakness of the tibialis anterior and excessive hip flexion and knee flexion during swing-through are characteristic deviations to prevent toe drag. What is this gait pattern called?
    A. Trendelenburg gait
    B. Antalgic gait
    C. Steppage gait
    D. None of the above

16. Weakness of the gluteus medius results in which of the following?
    A. Abductor lurch
    B. Trendelenburg gait
    C. Rapid swing through
    D. Steppage gait
    E. A and B

17. Circumduction of the hip during swing-through is characteristic of weakness to which muscle group?
    A. Quadriceps
    B. Hip flexors (psoas)
    C. Gluteus medius
    D. Hip abductors

18. Weakness of which muscle group demonstrates knee hyperextension during the stance phase of the gait cycle?
    A. Hamstrings
    B. Hip flexors
    C. Hip adductors
    D. Quadriceps

19. Which of the following describes a four-point gait pattern, if the injured limb is the left leg?
    A. Right crutch × left crutch × right foot × left foot
    B. Left crutch × right foot × right crutch × left foot
    C. Right crutch × left foot × left crutch × right foot
    D. Left crutch × right crutch × left foot × right foot

20. Touch down weight bearing is described as which of the following?
    A. Minimal weight bearing (balance only)
    B. Moderate weight bearing
    C. 30% weight bearing
    D. None of the above

21. Weight bearing as tolerated is designed for patients who are limited by which factors?
    A. Muscle strength
    B. Open reduction with internal fixation procedures
    C. Nonsurgical injuries
    D. Pain

22. When ascending stairs with bilateral axillary crutches, which of the following describes the most appropriate sequence?
    A. Involved limb, then crutches
    B. Crutches, then uninvolved limb
    C. Uninvolved limb, then crutches
    D. Crutches, then involved limb

23. When descending stairs using bilateral axillary crutches, which of the following describes the most appropriate sequence?
    A. Crutches first, then the uninjured limb
    B. Involved limb, then crutches
    C. Uninvolved limb, then crutches
    D. Crutches, then involved limb

24. When descending stairs, where should the physical therapist assistant (PTA) should stand and provide support?
    A. To the uninvolved side of the patient
    B. To the involved side of the patient
    C. In front of the patient
    D. Behind the patient

25. When ascending stairs, where should the PTA should stand and provide support?
    A. To the involved side
    B. To the uninvolved side
    C. Behind the patient
    D. In front of the patient

Short Answer

26. What is the term used to describe linear distance between right and left feet during gait?

27. Name the two phases of gait.

28. Name the components of the stance phase of gait.

29. Name the components of the swing phase of gait.

30. Name a primary action of the foot-flat period of the stance phase of gait.

31. A single crutch or cane should be used on which side of the injured limb?

True/False

32. During gait, an individual's center of gravity displaces both vertically and horizontally.

33. Non–weight bearing status allows the patient to place minimal weight on the involved limb.

34. Partial weight bearing status allows the patient to place a prescribed amount of resistance on the involved limb. The amount of weight is determined by the physician and is carried out in physical therapy by grading the resistance by a percentage of the patient's weight (20%, 30%, 50%, etc.).

Essay Questions

Answer on a separate sheet of paper.

35. Define and describe basic components of the gait cycle.
36. Discuss the two phases of gait.
37. Identify and describe each component of the two phases of gait.
38. Define and describe common gait deviations.
39. Define and describe three appropriate gait patterns.
40. Outline and describe terms used to define weight bearing status during gait.
41. Identify and discuss the appropriate use of assistive devices for ascending and descending stairs.

Critical Thinking Application

You are treating a patient with right quadriceps atrophy and a 40% loss of knee extension strength. The physical therapist has asked you to initiate gait instruction using bilateral axillary crutches; a three-point gait pattern and the patient's weight bearing status is WBAT. During which phase of the gait cycle would you anticipate observable clinical manifestations of this patient's problem? What muscle contraction type is required of the quadriceps during heel strike? Which action of the knee does quadriceps strength control? After a few weeks, this patient develops an additional gait deviation, and you notice the pelvis dropping toward the unaffected side during single limb support of the stance phase. Which muscle group(s) is affected, and what is the name of this gait pattern? When instructing this patient to ascend and descend stairs, precisely describe the techniques you would instruct the patient to use if no handrails were available. Where would you position yourself during stair climbing and descent? Why?

16 Concepts of Joint Mobilization

LEARNING OBJECTIVES

1. Discuss the general and applied concepts of peripheral gait mobilization.
2. Define terms and principles of peripheral joint mobilization.
3. Define and describe the convex–concave rule.
4. Define the five grades of mobilization.
5. Identify and describe terms of joint end-range feel.
6. Define and describe capsular and noncapsular patterns.
7. Identify common indications and contraindications for mobilization.
8. Discuss the clinical basics and applications of peripheral joint mobilization.
9. Identify and discuss the role of the physical therapist assistant in assisting the physical therapist with the delivery of peripheral joint mobilization.

KEY TERMS

Mobilization
Glide
Spin
Slide
Roll
Physiologic joint motion
Accessory joint motion
"Joint play"
Joint congruency

Close-packed
Loose-packed
Congruence
Convex–concave rule
Velocity
Oscillation
Amplitude of movement
Traction
Piccolo traction
Bone to bone

Soft-tissue approximation
Hard or springy-tissue stretch
Muscle spasm
Springy block
Empty end-feel
Loose end-feel
Capsular end-feel
Capsular pattern
Noncapsular pattern

CHAPTER OUTLINE

Fundamental Principles of Mobilization
Convex–Concave Rule
Mobilization Grades
Joint End-Feel
Capsular and Noncapsular Patterns
Indications and Contraindications for Mobilization
Clinical Application of Joint Mobilization

Providing comprehensive musculoskeletal rehabilitation requires that the physical therapist assistant (PTA) understand the basic concepts related to joint mobilization. He or she must be able to accurately and skillfully apply the mobilization techniques as delegated by the physical therapist. This chapter focuses primarily on concepts, definitions, and general rationales for peripheral joint mobilization, including mobilization theory and compulsory scientific principles.

FUNDAMENTAL PRINCIPLES OF MOBILIZATION

The term **mobilization** refers to an attempt to restore joint motion or mobility, or decrease pain associated with joint structures using manual, passive accessory-joint movement.[1,7]

The use of passive range of motion (ROM) involves physiologic movements of a joint, which are motions that occur within the active or passive joint ROM. These motions can be visualized and measured by goniometric assessment. Conversely, accessory movements involve motions specific to articulating joint surfaces.[1,7] These joint motions are referred to as **glide, spin, slide**, or **roll**.[1,4] Accessory and **physiologic joint motions** occur together during active ROM. However, **accessory joint motion** cannot be selectively recruited, meaning that a patient cannot selectively perform joint roll, glide, or spin.[1] The application of accessory joint motion is

defined as **"joint play"** or "motion that occurs within the joint as a response to an outside force but not as a result of voluntary movement."[1]

The concept of **joint congruency** and the terms **close-packed** and **loose-packed,** referring to joint position, are pertinent to the discussion of various grades of mobilization. **Congruence** refers to articular position with regard to concave and convex joint surfaces. A joint is congruent when both articulating surfaces are in contact throughout the total surface area of the joint.[1,4] However, the study of arthrokinematics (joint movement) states that joints are rarely in total congruence. As joints move the accessory motions of roll, spin, and glide alter total joint congruence.

MacConaill[4] has described close-packed positions as the most congruent positions of a joint,[1,4] where the joint surfaces are aligned and the capsule and ligaments

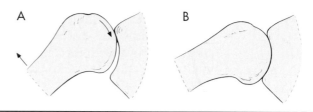

Fig. 16-1 The congruence of articular surfaces: **A,** Loose-packed position. **B,** Close-packed position. (From Gould JA: Orthopaedic and Sports Physical Therapy, 2nd ed. St Louis, Mosby, 1990.)

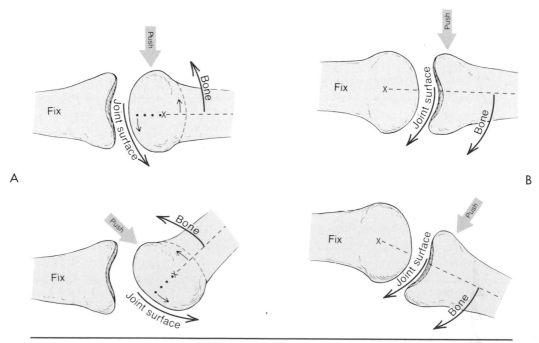

Fig. 16-2 **A,** Convex surface moving on concave surface. **B,** Concave surface moving on convex surface with a combination of roll, spin, and glide occurring in both simultaneously. (From Gould JA: Orthopaedic and Sports Physical Therapy, 2nd ed. St Louis, Mosby, 1990.)

are taut (Fig. 16-1). Generally, a close-packed position is used for testing the integrity and stability of ligaments and capsular structures. However, the close-packed position described by MacConaill[4] is not used for mobilization techniques. When the elbow and knee are fully extended, the ligaments and joint capsule are taut, allowing no freedom of movement. Therefore the knee and elbow in extension serve as two excellent examples of the close-packed position.

Any joint position other than the close-packed position is a loose-packed position. When the knee joint is flexed to 30 degrees, the intracapsular space is increased and supporting ligaments become more relaxed. The loose-packed position is ideal for applying joint mobilization techniques, but painful, stiff, and dysfunctional joints are rarely in "ideal resting positions" for the application of joint mobilization.

CONVEX–CONCAVE RULE

Anatomically, all articular surfaces are either convex or concave,[1,4] although the surfaces of some joints are not overtly of either shape. In these cases, fibrocartilage enhances and modifies the contour of the joint surfaces. On the convex joint surface, more cartilage is found at the center of the surface; on a concave joint surface, more cartilage is found at the periphery.[1]

The **convex–concave rule** specifically states, "When the concave surface is stationary and the convex surface

is moving, the gliding movement in the joint occurs in a direction *opposite* to the bone movement."[1] Conversely, if the convex surface is fixed while the concave surface is mobile, the gliding motion occurs in the *same* direction as the bone movement.[1] This occurs because the convex bone surface always maintains an axis of rotation during joint motion (Fig. 16-2). The concept of accessory joint motions (spin, roll, slide, or glide), as they apply to joint congruency and the convex–concave rule, is clearly illustrated by MacConaill's classification of accessory movements (Fig. 16-3).

MOBILIZATION GRADES

Maitland[6] describes five grades of physiologic and accessory joint motions used in mobilization (Fig. 16-4). The terms **velocity, oscillation,** and **amplitude of movement** describe the degree of force and rate of motion used during any of the grades of mobilization, as follows:

Grade I mobilization: A small oscillation or small amplitude joint motion that occurs only at the beginning of the available range of motion.

Grade II mobilization: A larger amplitude motion occurring from the beginning of the ROM to near midrange.

Grade III mobilization: A large amplitude motion that occurs from midrange of motion to the end of the available range.

Grade IV mobilization: A small oscillation or amplitude of motion that occurs at the very end range of the available joint motion.

Grade V mobilization: "A high velocity thrust of small amplitude at the end of the available range of motion."[1] This grade is not applied to mobilization techniques used by PTAs and is not addressed in this text.

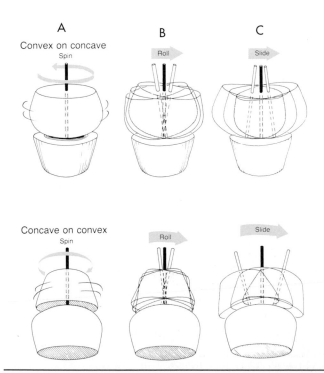

Fig. 16-3 MacConaill's classification of accessory movements: **A,** Spin. **B,** Roll. **C,** Glide. (From Gould JA: Orthopaedic and Sports Physical Therapy, 2nd ed. St Louis, Mosby, 1990.)

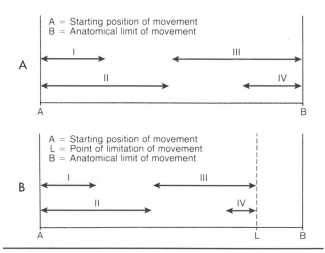

Fig. 16-4 A, Grades of oscillations used in manual therapy. **B,** Grades of oscillations used in manual therapy in relation to a joint with limited motion. (From Gould JA: Orthopaedic and Sports Physical Therapy, 2nd ed. St Louis, Mosby, 1990.)

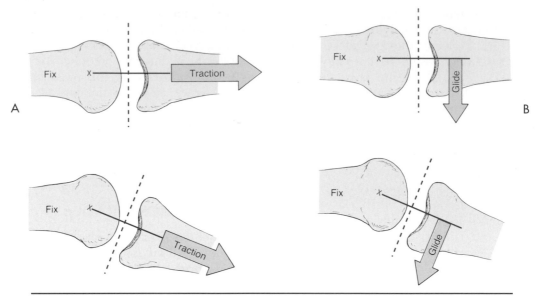

Fig. 16-5 **A,** Traction. **B,** Glide. (From Gould JA: Orthopaedic and Sports Physical Therapy, 2nd ed. St Louis, Mosby, 1990.)

In general terms, a grade I or II small amplitude oscillation is used to treat pain or when joint motion produces pain.[1,7] Therefore mobilization in grades III and IV are used to treat joint restrictions.[1,7]

Traction also is used as a manual therapy technique either by itself or along with various mobilization techniques (Fig. 16-5). Traction can be classified in grades or stages.[3,6] Generally, grade I or stage I traction is used for relief of pain and to minimize compressive joint forces during mobilization. The term **piccolo traction** describes a stage I traction technique. The force used to deliver grade I traction is not enough to actually separate the joint surfaces, but rather only neutralizes joint pressure.[1]

The term *slack* refers to the amount of normal looseness found in nonpathologic joint capsules and describes various degrees of joint tightness with stage II and III traction. Stage II traction is defined as being able to "take up the slack" in the capsule of the joint being stretched; it is commonly used to treat pain. Stage III traction is more substantial and actually involves stretching of the soft tissues. These techniques are performed to stretch out joint tightness.

JOINT END-FEEL

There are various qualities of joint tightness or "play" during the application of passive ROM. Three types of "end-feel" have been defined in normal, nonpathologic joints.[2,5] **Bone to bone** end-feel refers to a sudden, hard, nonyielding sensation felt at the end range of motion. Generally, the end-feel is not painful. Terminal elbow extension provides an example of a sudden bone to bone end-feel.

Another normal end-feel is **soft-tissue approximation.** This type of joint end-feel is characterized by a "yielding compression" typically encountered with knee or elbow flexion.[5] The end-feel that occurs with soft tissue approximation results from muscular tissue compression during joint flexion. The hamstring and calf muscles buttress and compress against each other during knee flexion, delivering a soft-tissue approximation end-feel.

The third normal joint end-feel is described as a **hard** or **springy-tissue stretch.** The characteristic feature of this end-feel is "elastic resistance" or "rising tension."[5] This type of end-feel is the most common normal feel at the end range of joints. Terminal knee extension and wrist flexion provide a "springy" stretch that defines tissue stretch.

The PTA must experience normal joint end-feel and be able to accurately identify distinguishing characteristics between bone to bone end-feel, soft-tissue approximation, and tissue stretch.[2] The PTA performing mobilization encounters abnormal joint end-feel, and its precise identification requires considerable didactic and hands-on experience.[2]

The first type of abnormal end-feel is **muscle spasm.** The major component is pain accompanied by a sudden halt of movement that prevents full ROM.[1,2,5]

In **springy block,** full motion is limited by a soft or "springy" sensation occasionally accompanied by pain. If a meniscus is torn in a knee, frequently the cartilage becomes caught in the joint, preventing terminal knee extension and its characteristic normal tissue stretch and feel.

In an **empty end-feel,** motion is very limited by significant pain without muscle spasm. Clinically, this end-feel is not characterized by any mechanical block or restriction.

Another abnormal end-feel is described as **loose end-feel.**[1] Its primary feature is joint hypermobility, with no resistance typically felt at the end ROM that signifies extraordinary joint looseness.

A **capsular end-feel**[5] is analogous to a normal tissue stretch, but the "elastic resistance" is encountered before the normal ROM. This end-feel is related to a capsular restriction.[5]

CAPSULAR AND NONCAPSULAR PATTERNS

The PTA must be aware that certain limitations of motion can be caused by lesions specific to the capsule or synovial tissues of a joint. All joints controlled by muscle activity possess a characteristic "pattern of proportional limitation."[5] For example, in the shoulder joint, the **capsular pattern** "involves external rotation as the most limited movement, abduction as less limited, internal rotation still less limited, and flexion as the least limited movement."[1,2] Any "characteristic pattern of limitation" is called a capsular pattern.

If a lesion causes a restriction of movement that does not correspond to a characteristic, predetermined capsular pattern, it is called a **noncapsular pattern.**[1,5] Cyriax[2] has identified three possible causes of noncapsular pattern restrictions:

1. *Ligamentous adhesions:* Frequently causes pain and limitation of motion. A noncapsular pattern exists when injury to the capsule or accessory ligaments causes a restriction in one direction, although other motions remain unaffected and pain free.
2. *Internal derangements:* A displaced or loose fragment within the joint. If the medial meniscus becomes wedged in the joint, knee extension is affected although flexion remains normal.
3. *Extraarticular lesions:* Adhesions resulting from injury outside the joint. Muscular adhesions or acutely inflamed structures are examples.

INDICATIONS AND CONTRAINDICATIONS FOR MOBILIZATION

Extreme caution must be employed before applying mobilization techniques in the early stages after trauma, surgery, or immobilization. Although pain is an indication for the use of mobilization, care must be taken to avoid retarding or impairing the sequence of tissue healing during the acute inflammatory phase.

Pain and joint restrictions are rarely separated completely. In many instances of severe joint limitations there may be only mild complaints of pain. Conversely, there may be little or no joint restriction but significant pain. Naturally there are varying degrees of pain and joint limitations occurring as either major or minor components. Therefore pain is a *relative* indication for joint mobilization, depending on which stage of tissue healing is present. If an injury is acute or a patient is recovering immediately after a surgical procedure, mobilization may not be indicated because it is best not to disturb the immature scar. Healing that proceeds in an organized fashion encourages mature collagen formation. When injured tissues have progressed from the acute, intense inflammatory phase to fibroplasia and scar maturation, mobilization is warranted to stress and remodel the scar.[7]

There are a few relative and absolute contraindications to the application of joint mobilization. Extreme caution is needed when considering mobilization in cases of osteoporosis, rheumatoid arthritis, joint hypermobility, and the presence of neurologic symptoms; all are therefore considered relative contraindications.[1,7] In cases of spinal mobilization, pregnancy and spondylolisthesis are relative contraindications. Absolute contraindications include bone diseases of the area treated, malignancy of the area treated, acute inflammatory and infectious arthritis, and central nervous system disorders.[1,7]

CLINICAL APPLICATION OF JOINT MOBILIZATION

Safe and effective joint mobilization requires the patient to be placed in a very comfortable position and the specific joint to be mobilized to be placed in a maximal resting or loose-packed position.[4] Before mobilization is applied, patient compliance and relaxation can be facilitated by the judicious use of moist heat, ultrasound, transcutaneous electrical nerve stimulation (TENS), electrical muscle stimulation, ice, exercise, and the timely use of any physician-prescribed analgesics or muscle relaxant medications. If pain is the predominant feature of the joint to be mobilized, grade I and II mobilization can be employed safely.

Oscillations help modulate or minimize pain when using grade I and II mobilization. Manually applied joint oscillations occur at a rate of two per second, or 120 per minute.[1] Typically, a mobilization grade technique is applied for 20 to 60 seconds only four or five times. This is recommended for the treatment of painful conditions on a daily basis or until pain is reduced.

A program of mobilization is carried out two to three times per week for the treatment of joint restrictions.[1] Piccolo or stage I traction can be used simultaneously with grade I or II mobilization or by itself to reduce pain and "neutralize" joint pressure. When the limitation of joint motion is greater than the complaints of pain, grade III and IV mobilization can be used to help stretch the capsule and soft tissues around the joint.

The pathologic condition of the joint to be mobilized must be thoroughly understood before applying any mobilization technique. For example, it is critical to avoid stressing the anterior capsule of the shoulder after an anterior dislocation, although mobilization to improve shoulder abduction may be warranted.[7]

In every case of joint mobilization, the PTA must constantly observe and document the patient's tolerance, pain response, and swelling to determine whether to halt the procedure, reduce the grade of motion, or consult with the physical therapist about advancing the grade of mobilization.

As stated in the beginning of this discussion, the physical therapist is responsible for delegating selected peripheral joint mobilization techniques to the PTA. Although peripheral joint mobilization beyond active and passive ROM is an area of treatment not usually delegated to the PTA, understanding peripheral joint mobilization techniques and having an awareness of rudimentary concepts and principles of mobilization provide the PTA with a broad understanding of the rationale for the application of certain techniques.

❖ ADDITIONAL FEATURES

Arthrokinematics: Study of motion within the joints. Description of joint typography.

Capsular Pattern: Limitation of movement or a pattern of pain at a joint that occurs in a predictable pattern.

Compression: Occurs when two forces or loads are applied toward each other.

End-Feel Terms: Firm, hard, soft or spongy, loose, capsular, bony bloc, springy bloc, empty end-feel.

Grades of Movement:
Grade I: Small amplitude of motion at the beginning of joint range of motion.
Grade II: Large amplitude of motion that does not affect the limits of available range of motion.
Grade III: Large amplitude of motion that affects the full limits of available range of motion.
Grade IV: Small amplitude of motion at the end range of available joint motion.

Hypermobility Grades:
Grade 3: Considered normal.
Grade 4: Represents slightly increased motion.
Grade 5: Represents significant increased instability.
Grade 6: Represents total instability.

Hypomobility Grades:
Grade 0: Represents ankylosis.
Grade 1: Represents greatly decreased ROM.
Grade 2: Represents minimal decreased ROM.

Joint Motions: Nonaxial, facets. Conaxial, knee. Biaxial, wrist. Triaxial, subtalar joint.

Joint Stability: Two general factors: close-packed position, loose-packed position.

Manipulation: Passive intervention motion of high velocity at end ranges of available joint motion.

Mobilization: Passive intervention motion within and at end range of joint motion with varying degrees of speed and amplitude.

Osteokinematics: Study of movement of bone segments around a joint axis.

Shear: Two parallel forces or loads that slide past each other.

Tension: Occurs when two forces are applied in opposite directions.

REFERENCES

1. Barak T, Rosen ER, Sofer R: Basic concepts of orthopaedic manual therapy. In Gould JA, ed. Orthopaedic and Sports Physical Therapy, 2nd ed. St Louis, Mosby, 1990.
2. Cyriax J: Textbook of Orthopaedic Medicine, Vol 1. Diagnosis of Soft Tissue Lesions, 8th ed. London, Baillière Tindall, 1982.
3. Kaltenborn F: Mobilization of Extremity Joints: Examination and Basic Treatment Techniques. Oslo, Norway, Olaf Norlis Bokhandel, 1980.
4. MacConaill MA, Basmajian JV: Muscles and Movements: A Basis for Human Kinesiology. Baltimore, Williams & Wilkins, 1969.
5. Magee DJ: Orthopaedic Physical Assessment, 2nd ed. Philadelphia, WB Saunders, 1992.
6. Maitland G: Peripheral Manipulation, 2nd ed. Newton, MA, Butterworth-Heinemann, 1978.
7. Wooden MJ: Mobilization of the upper extremity. In Donatelli R, Wooden MJ, eds. Orthopaedic Physical Therapy. New York, Churchill Livingstone, 1989.

REVIEW QUESTIONS

Multiple Choice

1. Which of the following best describes physiologic joint motions of the knee?
   A. Roll
   B. Spin
   C. Flexion-extension
   D. Glide

2. Which of the following best describes accessory movements? (Circle any that apply.)
   A. Flexion
   B. Extension
   C. Spin
   D. Glide
   E. Roll

3. How many grades of physiologic and accessory joint motions has Maitland described?
   A. Three
   B. Five
   C. Six
   D. Eight

4. Which of the following terms is (are) used to describe the degree of force and rate of motion used during the performance of joint mobilization? (Circle any that apply.)
   A. Strength
   B. Power
   C. Velocity and amplitude
   D. Oscillation
   E. Eccentrics

5. A large amplitude motion that occurs from the midrange of motion to the end of the available range is which of the following?
   A. Grade II mobilization
   B. Grade I mobilization
   C. Grade III mobilization
   D. Grade IV mobilization

6. A small oscillation or small amplitude joint motion that occurs only at the beginning of the available range of motion (ROM) is which of the following?

A. Grade III mobilization
B. Grade I mobilization
C. Grade II mobilization
D. Grade IV mobilization

7. A small oscillation or amplitude of motion that occurs at the end range of available motion is which of the following?
   A. Grade IV mobilization
   B. Grade III mobilization
   C. Grade V mobilization
   D. Grade II mobilization

8. A large amplitude of motion that occurs from the midrange of motion to the end of the available range is considered:
   A. Grade I
   B. Grade III
   C. Grade II
   D. Grade V
   E. Grade IV

9. In general terms, which grades of mobilization are used to treat painful joint motions?
   A. Grades II and III
   B. Grades I and III
   C. Grades I and II
   D. Grades II and IV

10. When performing passive ROM to a joint, a sudden nonyielding, hard end-range feel is described as which of the following?
    A. Myositis ossificans
    B. Hard or springy-tissue stretch
    C. Bone to bone end-feel
    D. Soft-tissue approximation

11. Terminal knee extension and wrist flexion describe the most common normal feel at the end range of joints. This is called which of the following?
    A. Bone to bone
    B. Springy-tissue stretch
    C. Soft-tissue approximation
    D. Joint play

12. A characteristic end-range feel during knee flexion or elbow flexion at the end-range of motion is called which of the following?
    A. Soft-tissue approximation
    B. Springy-tissue stretch
    C. Joint play
    D. Rising tension

13. An abnormal end-feel that is characterized by pain and a sudden halt of motion is called which of the following?
    A. Capsular end-feel
    B. Empty end-feel
    C. Springy block
    D. Muscle spasm

14. An abnormal end-feel, which is characterized by a lack of resistance at the end range of motion, signifying extreme joint laxity, is called which of the following?
    A. Empty end-feel
    B. Loose end-feel
    C. Capsular end-feel
    D. Springy block

15. An abnormal end-feel, which is characterized by limited motion, pain without muscle spasm, and without any mechanical block or restriction, is called which of the following?
    A. Capsular end-feel
    B. Elastic resistance
    C. Empty end-feel
    D. Springy block

16. A painful resistance at the end range of motion accompanied by a soft sensation is called which of the following?
    A. Elastic resistance
    B. Springy block
    C. Capsular end-feel
    D. Empty end-feel

17. Elastic resistance is felt before the normal end range of motion. This is called which of the following?
    A. Muscle spasm
    B. Loose end-feel
    C. Capsular end-feel
    D. Springy block

18. All synovial joints under muscular control have unique, characteristic patterns of limitation. This is called which of the following?
    A. Capsular pattern
    B. Noncapsular pattern
    C. Synergistic limitations
    D. None of the above

19. When a lesion causes a restriction of motion that does not correspond to a characteristic, predetermined capsular pattern, this is called which of the following?
    A. Joint laxity
    B. Noncapsular pattern
    C. Joint hypomobility
    D. Nonspecific joint restriction

20. Which of the following are examples of possible causes of noncapsular pattern restrictions? (Circle any that apply.)
    A. Ligament injury
    B. Muscular weakness
    C. Internal joint derangement
    D. Extraarticular lesions
    E. Vascular insufficiency

21. Which of the following is a relative contraindication for the application of joint mobilization?
    A. Local bone disease
    B. Active inflammatory arthritis
    C. Osteoporosis
    D. Malignancy
    E. All of the above

22. Which of the following represent(s) absolute contraindications for the application of joint mobilization? (Circle any that apply.)
    A. Rheumatoid arthritis
    B. Infectious arthritis
    C. Joint hypermobility
    D. Central nervous system signs
    E. Malignancy of the area treated

23. Which of the following can be applied before the application of mobilization techniques to reduce tension and aid in relaxation of the patient?
    A. Hot packs
    B. Ultrasound
    C. Exercise
    D. Transcutaneous electrical nerve stimulation and electrical muscle stimulation
    E. All of the above

Short Answer

24. When the concave surface is stationary and the convex surface is moving, the gliding movement in the joint occurs in a direction _____ to the bone movement.

25. When the convex surface is fixed, whereas the concave surface is mobile, the gliding motion occurs in the _____ direction as the bone movement.

True/False

26. When performing joint ROM, the physical therapist assistant (PTA) should encourage the patient to perform all accessory joint motions.
27. The "closed-packed" joint position is best used for determining joint stability.
28. The "loose-packed" position is best used for joint mobilization techniques.
29. Immediately after surgery, when pain may be significant, it is always appropriate to use grades I and II mobilization to help decrease pain.

Essay Questions

Answer on a separate sheet of paper.

30. Discuss the general and applied concepts of peripheral gait mobilization.
31. Define the terms and principles of peripheral joint mobilization.
32. Define and describe the convex–concave rule.
33. List and define the five grades of mobilization.
34. Identify and describe the terms of joint end-range feel.
35. Define and describe capsular and noncapsular patterns.
36. Identify common indications and contraindications for mobilization.
37. Discuss the clinical basis and applications of peripheral joint mobilization.
38. Identify and discuss the role of the PTA in assisting the physical therapist with the delivery of peripheral joint mobilization.

Critical Thinking Application

You are asked by the physical therapist to prepare a patient for the application of peripheral joint mobilization techniques to the patient's left knee. Using a partner, perform this activity by demonstrating appropriate patient positioning, draping, and limb exposure. List adjunctive techniques that might be appropriate for patient relaxation, pain relief, compliance, and soft-tissue extensibility. Outline and describe closed-packed and loose-packed positions in reference to this case. Before the application of mobilization, the physical therapist instructed you to perform passive joint ROM to this patient's knee. Define and describe the components of physiologic movement and contrast these with accessory joint movements. Give examples of each. Describe the convex–concave rule. During the application of passive ROM, you note a yielding compression during knee flexion. Define and describe this end-feel and give examples of two other distinct nonpathologic end-range feels. Contrast these with three clinically distinct abnormal end-range feels. Discuss capsular and noncapsular patterns.

PART V

BIOMECHANICAL BASIS FOR MOVEMENT

The physical therapist assistant (PTA) is charged with the responsibility of acquiring and demonstrating essential core knowledge of the basic orthopedic sciences. Central to this theme is a fundamental working knowledge of the basis of human movement.

The study of biomechanics supports the application of principles of kinesiology when providing therapeutic interventions. The utility of biomechanics in all clinical settings is demonstrated in the daily provision of gait analysis, manual muscle testing, goniometric assessments, therapeutic exercise modifications, facilitated balance and coordination activities, posture assessment, application and adjustment of prosthetic devices, recognition of abnormal movement patterns, and use of rehabilitation strategies to correct aberrant mechanics.

Biomechanical concepts and specific reference terminology serve to expose the student and practicing clinician to standardized descriptions of body positions, directions of motions, kinematics, kinetics, lever systems, Newton's laws, forces, mechanical loading, energy, and equilibrium.

This section's presentation of introductory mechanics precedes orthopedic pathologies and therapeutic interventions by pulling together essential basics of anatomy, physiology, tissue healing, kinesiology, and principles of therapeutic exercise, thereby providing the student PTA and practicing clinician a sound practical and scientifically based understanding of the essentials of human movement.

17

Biomechanical Basis for Movement

MITCHELL A. COLLINS

LEARNING OBJECTIVES

1. Define and apply biomechanical concepts in the description of rudimentary movement patterns.
2. Discuss the difference between the kinematics and kinetics of movement.
3. Identify and discuss the kinematic principles as related to movement in a rehabilitation setting.
4. Discuss both the linear and angular kinematics and kinetics of movement, and explain how angular motion translates to linear movements.
5. Describe the differences among the different levers, and explain the concept of mechanical advantage as related to levers.
6. Describe Newton's laws of motion.
7. Identify and discuss the different forces that act on objects and how the forces affect movement.
8. Discuss the concepts of mechanical loading, and describe how loading is associated with different types of injuries.
9. Discuss the principles of mechanical energy.
10. Describe the concept of equilibrium and identify the factors that contribute to stability.

KEY TERMS

Biomechanics	Momentum	Ground reaction forces
Kinematic	Time	Friction
Kinetic	Displacement	Law of gravitation
Center of mass	Velocity	Compression
Mass	Acceleration	Tension
Inertia	Moment of force	Shear
Force	Force couple	Mechanical stress
Volume	Lever	Bending
Density	First-class lever	Torsion
Torque	Moment arm	Kinetic energy
Impulse	Mechanical advantage	Potential energy
Work	Second-class lever	Equilibrium
Power	Third-class lever	Balance
Pressure	Newton's laws of motion	

CHAPTER OUTLINE

Reference Terminology
Biomechanical Concepts
Kinematics
Kinetics
  Force
  Levers

Newton's Laws of Motion
  Types of Forces
Mechanical Loading
Energy
Equilibrium

Biomechanics can be defined as the study of the biological and mechanical basis for human motion.[19,20,22] This is accomplished by applying the principles of physics involved in the action of forces—either a push or a pull—on the human body. The mechanics of movement are described under a condition called *static* where there is a state of no motion or constant motion, or *dynamic* where the motion is changing (e.g., acceleration). In addition, motion is analyzed from both **kinematic** and **kinetic** perspectives. Kinematics deals with the description of movement based on alterations in space and time (How did the object move?), whereas kinetics focuses on the actions of forces applied to the body (What caused the object to move in the pattern observed?).

The application of biomechanics is continuously expanding to a variety of settings.[19] Some examples include the biomechanical research conducted to understand the effects of microgravity associated with space flight on the human body.[1,3,12] This research has led to the development of numerous innovations to help prevent the loss of bone mineral and decline in muscular strength that occurs during exposure to a microgravity environment.[2] The field of occupational biomechanics focuses on work-related issues such as prevention of injuries and the enhancement of worker productivity.[7,15,17,23,35] Biomechanics is commonly applied to clinical settings, especially in the area of gait analysis and improvement of mobility.[28,30,33] Research findings have enhanced rehabilitation and intervention strategies that are currently used with elderly or injured people and individuals with medical conditions such as cerebral palsy or limb amputation.[10,13,25,27,34]

The purpose of this chapter is to provide an overview of the basic principles of biomechanics. The major role of a physical therapist assistant (PTA) revolves around human motion. Therefore it is imperative to have a basic understanding of the biologic and mechanical bases for movement.

REFERENCE TERMINOLOGY

To facilitate the process of describing human movement, standardized terminology has been adopted to identify body positions and directions of motion (Box 17-1). Movements are defined based on a reference starting position often referred to as the *anatomic position* (Fig. 17-1), which is a standing position with arms at one's side and palms facing forward. From the anatomic position, three imaginary cardinal planes bisect the body along three dimensions (Fig. 17-2). The *transverse* or *horizontal plane* segments the body into upper and lower parts; the *frontal* or *coronal plane* separates the body into front and back parts; and the *sagittal* or *anteroposterior plane* divides the body into right and left parts. It is important to note that the planes do not necessarily divide the body into equal parts. However, when the segments are equal, the intersection point of the midtransverse, midfrontal, and midsagittal planes is referred to as the **center of mass** (or gravity). Although human movement is not restricted to a single plane, most named movements (e.g., flexion and abduction) are described based on the three cardinal planes.

Movements in the transverse plane occur around the longitudinal axis, which runs superiorly–inferiorly while perpendicularly intersecting the transverse plane. These movements include medial and lateral rotation of the leg, thigh, and shoulder, supination and pronation of the forearm, and horizontal abduction and adduction of the shoulder. Movements in the frontal plane occur around the sagittal axis, which runs anteriorly–posteriorly while perpendicularly intersecting the frontal plane. These movements include abduction and

BOX 17-1

Basic Directional Terms Used to Describe Body Parts or Other Objects in Relation to the Body

Anterior: Toward the front of the body

Posterior: Toward the back of the body

Deep: Toward the inside (core) of the body

Superficial: Toward the surface (skin) of the body

Distal: Away from the body or torso

Proximal: Closer to the body or torso

Inferior: Toward the feet

Superior: Toward the head

Lateral: Away from the midline of the body

Medial: Toward the midline of the body

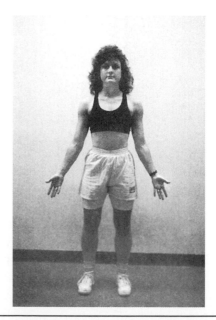

Fig. 17-1 Anatomic reference position for human motion. (From Hall SJ: Basic Biomechanics, 3rd ed. New York, McGraw-Hill, 1999.)

adduction of the shoulder and hip, lateral flexion of the neck and trunk, elevation and depression of the shoulder girdle, and inversion and eversion of the foot. Movements in the sagittal plane occur around the frontal axis, which runs from left to right while perpendicularly intersecting the sagittal plane. These movements include flexion and extension of the knee, hip, trunk, elbow, shoulder, and neck, and dorsiflexion and plantar flexion of the foot. A key role of the PTA is to facilitate patient rehabilitation through the incorporation of various exercises using basic movement patterns. Therefore it is important to be familiar with the appropriate terminology for these movements (Fig. 17-3). (See Appendix F for a description of major body movements and muscle actions, along with an analysis of several basic weight-training exercises.)

BIOMECHANICAL CONCEPTS

A working understanding of various rudimentary concepts is essential to facilitate the discussion of biomechanical principles. The following are definitions of some common terms along with their appropriate unit of

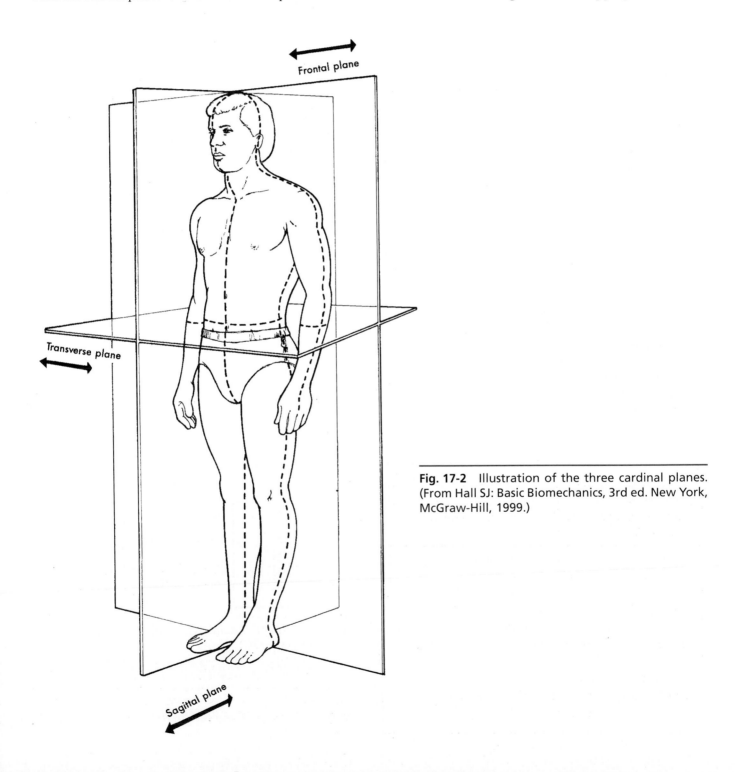

Fig. 17-2 Illustration of the three cardinal planes. (From Hall SJ: Basic Biomechanics, 3rd ed. New York, McGraw-Hill, 1999.)

Wrist—sagittal

Flexion
Exercise: wrist curl
Sport: tennis serve

Extension
Exercise: reverse wrist curl
Sport: racquet backhand

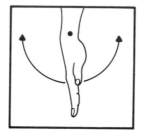

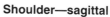

Wrist—frontal

Ulnar deviation
Exercise: specific wrist curl
Sport: baseball batting

Radial deviation
Exercise: specific wrist curl
Sport: golf backswing

Elbow—sagittal

Flexion
Exercise: arm curl
Sport: rowing

Extension
Exercise: triceps pushdown
Sport: boxing jab

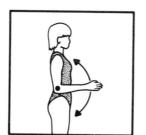

Shoulder—sagittal

Flexion
Exercise: medium-grip military press
Sport: softball pitch

Extension
Exercise: narrow-grip row
Sport: freestyle swimming

Shoulder—frontal

Adduction
Exercise: wide-grip pulldown
Sport: gymnastic rings

Abduction
Exercise: wide-grip military press
Sport: springboard diving

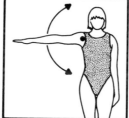

Shoulder—transverse

Internal rotation
Exercise: arm wrestle movement (with dumbbell or cable)
Sport: baseball pitch

External rotation
Exercise: reverse arm wrestle movement
Sport: karate block

Shoulder—transverse
(upper arm 90° to trunk)

Adduction
Exercise: wide-grip bench press
Sport: boxing hook

Abduction
Exercise: row (elbows high)
Sport: tennis backhand

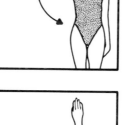

Neck—sagittal

Flexion
Exercise: neck machine
Sport: somersault

Extension
Exercise: neck machine
Sport: wrestling bridge

Neck—transverse

Left rotation
Exercise: neck machine
Sport: wrestling

Right rotation
Exercise: neck machine
Sport: wrestling

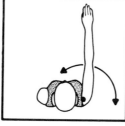

Neck—frontal

Left tilt
Exercise: neck machine
Sport: wrestling

Right tilt
Exercise: neck machine
Sport: wrestling

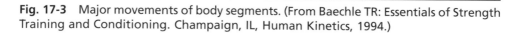

Fig. 17-3 Major movements of body segments. (From Baechle TR: Essentials of Strength Training and Conditioning. Champaign, IL, Human Kinetics, 1994.)

Lower back—sagittal

Flexion
Exercise: weighted sit-up
Sport: somersault

Extension
Exercise: reverse sit-up
Sport: rowing

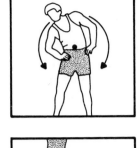

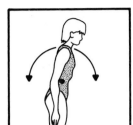

Lower back—frontal

Left tilt
Exercise: side bend
Sport: gymnastics side aerial

Right tilt
Exercise: side bend
Sport: gymnastics side aerial

Lower back—transverse

Left rotation
Exercise: torso machine
Sport: baseball batting

Right rotation
Exercise: torso machine
Sport: baseball batting

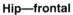
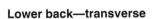
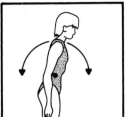

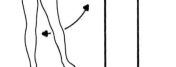
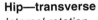
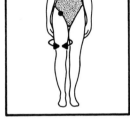

Hip—sagittal

Flexion
Exercise: leg raise
Sport: football punt

Extension
Exercise: squat
Sport: jumping

Hip—frontal

Adduction
Exercise: adduction machine
Sport: lateral movement

Abduction
Exercise: abduction machine
Sport: skating

Hip—transverse

Internal rotation
Exercise: friction rotation
Sport: pivot movement

Extension
Exercise: friction rotation
Sport: pivot movement

Hip—transverse
(upper leg 90° to trunk)
Adduction
Exercise: adduction machine
Sport: karate in-sweep

Abduction
Exercise: abduction machine
Sport: karate out-sweep

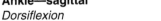
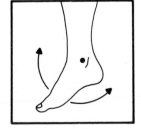

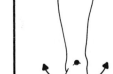
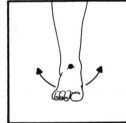

Knee—sagittal

Flexion
Exercise: leg curl
Sport: sprint running

Extension
Exercise: leg extension
Sport: bicycling

Ankle—sagittal

Dorsiflexion
Exercise: dorsiflexion
(weight-resisted)
Sport: running

Plantarflexion
Exercise: calf raise
Sport: jumping

Ankle—frontal

Inversion
Exercise: inversion
Sport: ice skating

Eversion
Exercise: eversion (friction
resisted)
Sport: ice skating

Fig. 17-3, cont'd   Major movements of body segments.

measure. Most of these terms are discussed in more detail as various biomechanical concepts are introduced.

Mass is the quantity of matter that an object possesses. It is expressed in kilograms (kg). It should not be confused with body *weight,* which is a force.

Inertia is the amount of resistance that an object has to change. The inertia of an object is related to its mass, and it is a unitless measure.

Force is a push or pull action on an object. A force has both direction and magnitude. It is commonly expressed in Newtons (N), which is the amount of force necessary to accelerate a 1 kg mass object at a rate of 1 m/s.²

Center of mass (gravity) is the point within which the weight and mass of an object are equally distributed or balanced in all directions. The center of mass is important because when a force is applied to an object, the movement pattern varies based on the relation of the point of force application to the center of mass.

Volume is the amount of space that an object occupies. It is commonly expressed in liters (L).

Density is equal to mass divided by the volume of an object, and is frequently expressed in kilograms per cubic meter (kg/m³).

Torque, or rotary force, is a measure of the rotary effect produced when a force is applied eccentrically (point outside of the center) to an object. Torque is the product of force and the perpendicular distance between the line of action for the force and the axis point of rotation (e.g., moment arm). The unit of measure is Newton-meters (N-m).

Impulse is the product of force and the length of time the force was produced, and it is expressed in Newton • seconds (N • s).

Work is the product of force and the distance the object moves. The unit of measure is a Newton-meter (N-m) or joule (J), which is an equivalent unit (1 N-m = 1 J).

Power is the rate of performing work, and can be expressed algebraically as the product of force and displacement over time. Musculoskeletal activities that involve the application of force over a brief period of time relate to the concept of power. Power is expressed in watts (W): 1 W is equal to 1 J of work per second.

Pressure is a measure of the force distribution over a given area (force/area), and generally is expressed in Newtons per meter² (N/m²).

Momentum is the product of an object's mass and its velocity, which reflects the quantity of motion an object has. A motionless object has no momentum. The unit of measure is kilogram • meters/second (kg • m/s).

KINEMATICS

The **kinematics** of motion deals with describing the changes in space and time that occur during movement.

When sufficient force is applied to an object, motion can result that is *translatory* (linear) and *rotational* (angular). From a kinematic perspective, this motion is described based on four parameters: **time, displacement, velocity,** and **acceleration.**

Time is a key component of movement because of its link to velocity and acceleration. In addition, quantification of a precise measure of time is imperative in describing and understanding quick movements (e.g., sudden reaction movement or throwing an object). **Displacement** is a measure of the change in position of an object. It reflects the change in space of an object from the starting to the ending points, and can be linear (in meters) or angular (in degrees) movement. It is also important to note that displacement is a vector quantity; therefore it must be described based on magnitude and direction. **Velocity,** which also is a vector quantity, is calculated from the ratio of displacement and time. The determination of velocity is a key aspect for any object that is in motion (Fig. 17-4). The rate of change in velocity of an object is termed **acceleration.** Although sometimes the term *deceleration* is used to denote that the velocity of an object is decreasing, acceleration is appropriately used any time the velocity changes, whether increasing (positive acceleration) or decreasing (negative acceleration). If an object is moving at a constant velocity or is motionless, the resulting acceleration is 0: There is no acceleration. Acceleration is a vector quantity that possesses direction along with magnitude.

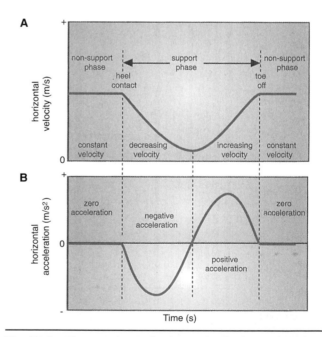

Fig. 17-4 Changes in, **A,** horizontal velocity and, **B,** horizontal acceleration during running. (From Hamill J, Knutzen KM: Biomechanical Basis of Human Movement. Baltimore, Williams & Wilkins, 1995.)

All of the described kinematic concepts apply to both linear and angular motion. The primary difference is the displacement unit of measure: meters versus degrees, respectively. However, it is important to realize that human motion incorporates linear (translation of a wheelchair) and angular (arm movements to rotate wheels) movements to accomplish many common tasks. Therefore there is a mechanical relationship between linear and angular motion:

$$v = r \times \omega$$

where v represents the linear (tangential) velocity of a point along the angular arc, r is the radius of rotation for the point, and ω is the angular velocity of the rotating object expressed in radians/s (1 radian = 57.3°). This relationship is important because it allows quantification of linear movements (e.g., of the foot) as a result of angular motion (e.g., at the knee).

There is also a relationship between linear and angular acceleration, because the angular acceleration of an object has two corresponding perpendicular linear acceleration components (Fig. 17-5). The *tangential acceleration* component during angular motion represents the change in linear velocity along a tangent to the path of motion. The relationship between angular acceleration and tangential acceleration can be expressed as:

$$a_t = r \times \alpha$$

where a_t is the tangential acceleration, r is the radius of rotation, and α is the angular acceleration expressed in radians/s.^{2} A second component during angular movement is the *radial acceleration*, which is perpendicular to

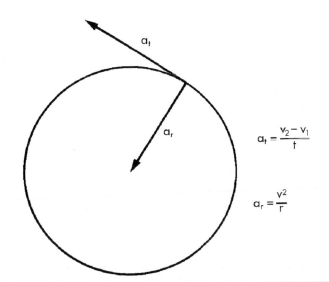

Fig. 17-5 Tangential (a_t) and radial (a_r) acceleration components for angular motion. (From Hall SJ: Basic Biomechanics, 3rd ed. New York, McGraw-Hill, 1999.)

the tangential acceleration and toward the center of rotation. Radial acceleration can be expressed as:

$$a_r = v^2/r$$

where a_r is the radial acceleration, v is the tangential linear velocity, and r is the radius of rotation. From this equation, it is apparent that radial acceleration increases as the radius of rotation decreases.

An understanding of kinematic principles is important for clinicians. Analysis of motion can facilitate the determination of the etiology of injury, extent of damage, along with assessment of the effectiveness of treatment.[11,31] Historically, researchers have studied injuries in sport settings, but the same applications are pertinent to nonathletic settings, such as gait analysis of individuals with knee injury.[8,11,18] Thus it is imperative for PTAs to be knowledgeable about normal movement patterns from a kinematic perspective to facilitate the recognition of abnormal movements of rehabilitating patients.

KINETICS

Although it is important to be able to quantify the nature of motion as discussed related to kinematics, rehabilitation strategies focus on altering movement patterns. Therefore it is critical for a PTA to understand the factors that cause motion. Kinetics is concerned with the forces that act on the body, and how these forces influence movement. Similar to kinematics, motion is addressed from both a linear and angular kinetic perspective.

Force

Because the main aspect of kinetics centers on force, it is important to have an understanding of force and how it is related to movement. As defined, a force is a push or pull action on an object, and is a vector quantity. If the magnitude of the force exceeds the resistance encountered by the object, then positive or negative acceleration (motion) of the object occurs. Forces that are applied directly through the center of an object result in *translatory* or *linear* motion. However, in most instances forces are applied somewhere outside the center of an object, causing the object to move in a *rotational* or *angular* pattern along with translation (e.g., when a ball rolls across the floor, it moves linearly and rotates simultaneously).

One key aspect of a force is the specific *point of application* on an object (Fig. 17-6). Because of variations in the specific *line of application* of the force, the point of application controls the magnitude and nature of motion. Within the human body the point of application can be more than a single point, such as found in multipennated muscles such as the deltoid. Therefore multiple movements may be produced by contraction of a single muscle. Another aspect of force, the *angle of application,* is designated based on the angle between the line of action and bony attachment being moved (Fig. 17-6). This angle is important because for a given force produced at the tendon (point of attachment), the magnitude of the action produced varies based on the specific angle of application, which changes during human movements at a joint.

Most forces in the human body cause rotation. The product of the force and the perpendicular distance from the line of action to the axis point (*moment arm of the force*) is termed torque or **moment of force.** Torque is considered a rotary force, but more specifically a measure of the ability of a force to cause rotation. In Figure 17-7 notice how the torque produced during lifting must be counteracted by a torque produced by the muscles of the back. Therefore the lower back is susceptible to injury when improper lifting techniques result in large amounts of torque in the lower back region. In rehabilitation settings, the concept of torque is used during manual resistance exercise. For example, during knee extension exercise, the PTA might offer resistance to movement by applying a force at the midtibia level. As the patient progresses, the therapist can lower the point of application of the same force to ankle level, which increases the amount of torque the patient must overcome to perform the exercise. Consequently, torque can be increased or decreased easily by altering the length of the moment arm of the force. A **force couple** is formed in situations where there are two torques that are equal in magnitude but opposite in direction. The resultant action of a force couple is rotation without any translation.

Levers

Human movement is accomplished primarily through contraction of skeletal muscle and the resultant action on the bony levers of the skeleton. The PTA should

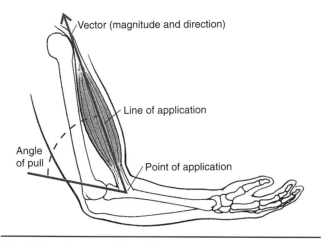

Fig. 17-6 Characteristics of forces within the human body. (From Hamill J, Knutzen KM: Biomechanical Basis of Human Movement. Baltimore, Williams & Wilkins, 1995.)

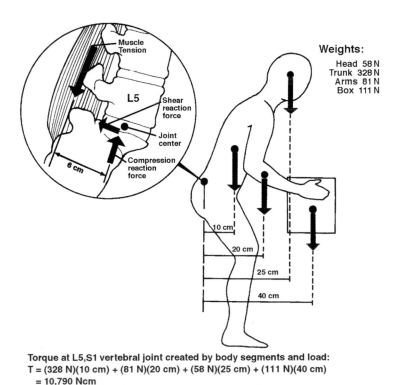

Torque at L5,S1 vertebral joint created by body segments and load:
T = (328 N)(10 cm) + (81 N)(20 cm) + (58 N)(25 cm) + (111 N)(40 cm)
= 10,790 Ncm

Fig. 17-7 Effect of torque produced at L5/S1 during lifting and the counter torque necessary by the muscles in the back. (From Hall SJ: Basic Biomechanics, 3rd ed. New York, McGraw-Hill, 1999.)

understand the mechanical basis for the leverage system. Proper mechanical alignment can facilitate patient motion, and alterations in body position can aid the PTA when assisting a patient.

A **lever** is a simple machine composed of a relatively rigid body (e.g., bone or bodily segment) that is capable of rotation about a fulcrum or axis (e.g., articulation point of two bones). Forces are applied in the human body by contraction of muscle, which pulls on bone that serves as the lever. When forces are applied the lever is capable of moving a resistance about the axis. Levers are designated as one of three classes based on the orientation of the point of force application, the axis, and the resistance (Fig. 17-8).

In a **first-class lever,** the fulcrum is located between the point where the force is applied and the resistance. The perpendicular distance from the line of action of the force to the fulcrum is termed the **moment arm** of the force (M_F). Likewise, the perpendicular distance from the line of action of the resistance is termed the moment arm of the resistance (M_R). This is important because a lever may be evaluated based on the computation of its **mechanical advantage** (MA).

$$MA = \frac{M_F}{M_R}$$

In a first-class lever, when the fulcrum is located halfway between the point of force and point of resistance on the lever, the MA is equal to 1 (e.g., $M_F = M_R$). If the fulcrum is closer to the point of the resistance than the point of force (e.g., $M_F > M_R$), the MA becomes greater than 1; thus a smaller force is necessary to overcome a constant resistance. In the opposite scenario

where the M_F is less than the M_R, the MA is less than 1 and a larger force is necessary to move a given resistance.

In a **second-class lever,** the point of resistance is located between the fulcrum and the point of force. The M_F is always greater than the M_R, yielding a MA greater than 1. Hence this arrangement favors the effort of force, because less force is necessary to cause movement of a given resistance.

In a **third-class lever,** the point of force is located between the fulcrum and the resistance. The M_F always is less than the M_R, yielding an MA less than 1. Therefore this arrangement favors the effort of resistance, because more force is necessary to cause movement of a given resistance. This is the more common type of lever found within the human body (Fig. 17-9). Therefore muscles within the body tend to work under a mechanical disadvantage, resulting in larger internal muscular forces than the mass of the external object (resistance) being moved. It is also important to realize that within some joints of the skeletal system, the actual fulcrum point changes through the range of motion (ROM). Consequently, mechanical advantage and muscle force vary as the length of the moment arm changes.

The resistive force, or more specifically the *resistive torque*, encountered during movements varies based on the length of the resistance arm (moment arm of the resistance). As shown in Figure 17-10, the length of the resistance arm is maximized when the elbow is at a 90-degree angle. As the angle increases or decreases, the length of the resistance arm shortens, thus reducing the magnitude of the resistive torque. Therefore it is important to realize that less force is necessary to lift a given resistance when the resistance is closer to the fulcrum

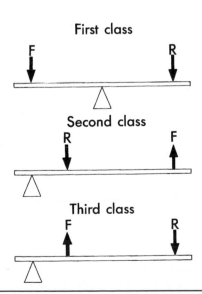

Fig. 17-8 Orientation of the force, resistance, and fulcrum for the three classes of levers. (From Hall SJ: Basic Biomechanics, 3rd ed. New York, McGraw-Hill, 1999.)

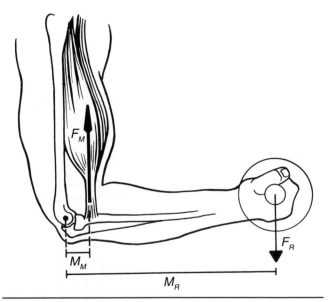

Fig. 17-9 Example of a third-class lever in the human body. (From Baechle TR: Essentials of Strength Training and Conditioning. Champaign, IL, Human Kinetics, 1994.)

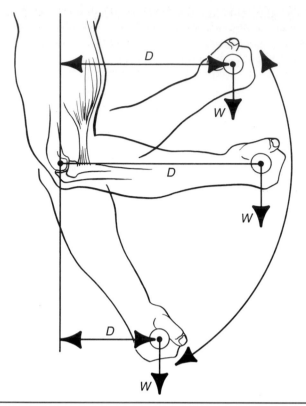

Fig. 17-10 Illustration of how changes in the angle at the elbow alter the length of the resistance arm, thus modifying the resistive torque. (From Baechle TR: Essentials of Strength Training and Conditioning. Champaign, IL, Human Kinetics, 1994.)

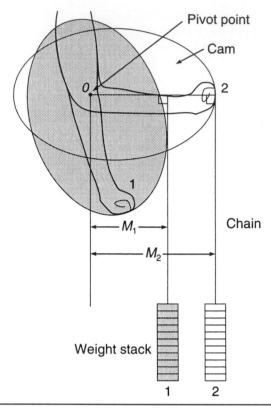

Fig. 17-11 Alterations in the length of the resistance arm during cam-based exercise. (From Baechle TR: Essentials of Strength Training and Conditioning. Champaign, IL, Human Kinetics, 1994.)

(e.g., the resistance arm is reduced). This basic biomechanical principle has numerous applications, including the mechanical function of exercise equipment.[21] Various manufacturers use a pulley system consisting of cam-based pulleys (Fig. 17-11). The unique advantage of a cam compared with a traditional round pulley is the variation in the length of the resistance and force arms during rotation of the pulley. By simply increasing the length of the resistance arm or reducing the length of the force arm, the resistive torque can be increased to provide a variable resistance through the range of motion. This relatively simple alteration in design has enhanced the effectiveness of exercise equipment to provide proper loading on muscles throughout the full ROM.

Newton's Laws of Motion

Much of the basis for kinetics originates from the laws of motion introduced by Sir Isaac Newton (1642–1727) in 1687. Although Newton's theories date back more than 300 years, the basic concepts introduced continue to be used today by biomechanists to provide the explanation for the factors that cause an object to move in a specific manner.

Newton's first law of motion is commonly referred to as the law of inertia, which states:[5]

Every body continues in its state of rest, or of uniform motion in a straight line, unless it is compelled to change that state by forces impressed on it.

Inertia of an object is used to describe the reluctance of an object to change its movement pattern; that is, to stay motionless or to move in a linear path unless a force is applied. The amount of inertia an object possesses is related to the mass of the object. As a result, the larger the mass or inertia of an object, the more difficult it is to alter its motion. We can observe the concept of inertia by examining events that occur during car accidents. When a car strikes an object and is suddenly forced to stop, the passengers continue to move forward because of each person's inertia. This forward motion continues to occur until a force is applied (hopefully seat belts and airbags) to counteract the inertia.

Newton's second law of motion is commonly referred to as the law of acceleration, which states:[5]

The change of motion is proportional to the force impressed and is made in the direction of the straight line in which that force is impressed.

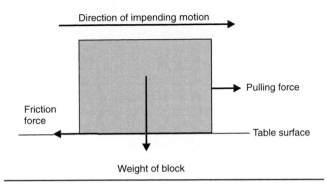

Fig. 17-12 Effect of different forces acting on a sliding object. (From Hamill J, Knutzen KM: Biomechanical Basis of Human Movement. Baltimore, Williams & Wilkins, 1995.)

This law can be expressed algebraically with force (F), mass (m), and acceleration (a):

$$F = m \times a$$

When the equation is rearranged, it yields a useful expression:

$$a = \frac{F}{m}$$

which mathematically illustrates that the acceleration of an object is directly proportional to the force applied and inversely related to mass of the object. Newton's second law is relatively simple, but it has many applications to physical therapy. Because acceleration (motion) is inversely related to mass, it is clear that basic weight bearing movements tend to be more challenging for larger patients. In addition, a greater force application is needed for these patients to accomplish said movement. The difficulty in locomotion is compounded if larger mass of a patient results from too much fat, because fat does not contribute to force production.

Newton's third law of motion is commonly referred to as the law of reaction, which states:[5]

> To every action there is always opposed an equal reaction; or, the mutual action of two bodies upon each other are always equal and directed to contrary parts.

The concept of reaction can be more difficult to visualize than inertia and acceleration, but when a force is applied to an object such as a wall, there is a force opposite in direction and equal in magnitude to the force applied. As the applied force increases, the reaction force likewise increases. From a clinical perspective, reaction forces are of interest during gait analysis. When a patient walks or runs, clinicians may analyze the differences in gait patterns among individuals with varying levels of disability and the subsequent **ground reaction forces** that occur when the foot strikes the floor.[9,29] These forces can achieve three times one's body weight during running, and patterns vary based on

running style.[14] Physicians and therapists use devices such as orthotics to alter ground reaction force patterns to help minimize foot injuries.[36]

Types of Forces

The concept of force has been described from a general perspective. It is important to examine individual forces and discuss how each force affects movement from a kinetic perspective based on Newton's laws of motion. Often forces are classified based on their nature: *contact* and *noncontact*.

When two objects are in direct *contact*, there is a force called **friction** that acts to impede motion of the objects (Fig. 17-12). The frictional force is exerted in the opposite direction of impending motion. Frictional force can be described by the following formula:

$$F_f = \mu \times N$$

where μ is the *coefficient of friction* between the surfaces of the object, and N is the *normal reaction force* perpendicular to the surface. The coefficient of friction, a unitless number, is a measure of the nature of the interface between the surfaces (Box 17-2). The normal reaction force is proportional to the mass of the object. Based on the law of reaction, as a force is applied to the object that is in contact with another, the frictional force increases to oppose the impending movement. When the applied force reaches a point where movement begins, it is called the point of *maximum static friction*. As illustrated in Figure 17-13, once the object begins to move, the frictional force decreases but remains constant even with additional applied force. As one can observe, the effort to sustain sliding motion is less than to initiate the movement because of a change in the frictional force. Also, frictional force can be increased or decreased by adding substances between the two surfaces, such as the installation of tennis balls on the rear support for walkers. Damage caused by chronic exposure to frictional forces can lead to the need for joint replacement.

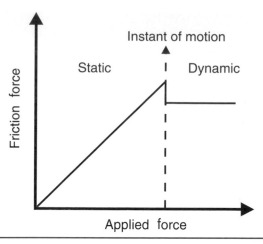

Fig. 17-13 Relationship between the friction force and an applied force acting on an object. (From Hamill J, Knutzen KM: Biomechanical Basis of Human Movement. Baltimore, Williams & Wilkins, 1995.)

Pressure is defined as a measure of the distribution of a force over a given area (force/area). The magnitude of a pressure can be large when the area is small (e.g., high-heeled shoes against a wood floor) or great (e.g., the weight of a car). Although force and pressure are related, the pressure for a given force can be reduced by increasing the contact area. An example of the concept of pressure in a clinical setting is the development of decubitus ulcers that commonly occur among diabetics. Innovations in shoe design help dissipate the forces applied to the foot over a larger area (e.g., reduced pressure) during locomotion, thus minimizing soft-tissue damage and the incidence of ulceration.[6]

The primary *noncontact* force is gravity. The **law of gravitation** states that the force of gravity is inversely proportional to the square of the distance between attracting objects and proportional to the product of their masses. This law can be visualized best when examining the attraction of objects to the earth. The closer an object is to the earth the greater the gravitational force. Also, the more mass an object has, the greater the gravitational force.

MECHANICAL LOADING

Load is defined as an outside force or group of forces that act on an object. For example, when a patient performs an exercise with sandbags on the foot, a load is being applied to the muscles that cause knee extension. Although loads apply to the point of contact (e.g., use of compression bandage), other loads are applied away from the point of contact, as described. Depending on the magnitude of the load (stress), there is a deformation in the object, termed a *mechanical strain*. There are three types of stresses: **compression, tension, and shear** (Fig. 17-14).

Compression occurs when two forces or loads are applied toward each other (Fig. 17-15). A common example is the compression stress on the vertebral column during standing while supporting an object (e.g., dumbbell). Excessive compression stress can lead to contusions, fractures, or herniations.[32]

Tension occurs when two forces or loads are applied in opposite directions. This type of loading is commonly applied to muscles and tendons during stretching activities to improve flexibility (see Chapter 4). When the loading exceeds the ability of the object to resist the stress, injuries such as strains, sprains, and avulsion fractures commonly occur.[26] Figure 17-15 illustrates the compression and tension stresses acting on the vertebrae during movements of the trunk.

Shear occurs when there are two parallel forces or loads in opposite directions, causing adjacent points on the surface to slide past each other. Injuries such as vertebral disk problems, femoral condyle fractures, and epiphyseal fractures of the distal femur in children occur as a result of shear stress acting on the body.[20]

The resulting action of compression, tension, and shear forces is dependent on how these forces are distributed, a concept called **mechanical stress.** Force applied over a smaller surface area results in a greater mechanical stress than force applied over a larger surface area. Given that the lumbar vertebrae typically is more load bearing than the vertebrae in the upper back, one notices that the load bearing surface area in the lumbar vertebrae is greater than that found in the upper vertebrae.[20] Accordingly, the greater surface area for the thoracic vertebrae translates into a lower mechanical stress for a given load.

Another type of loading on an object called **bending** occurs when nonaxial forces are applied, resulting in compressive stress on one side and a tension stress on the other (Fig. 17-14). When an object is forced to twist along the longitudinal axis, a load called **torsion** is produced (Fig. 17-14). Injuries commonly occur because of torsion in activities such as skiing, when a foot is planted and the body begins to twist.[19,20]

Deformation or a change in shape can occur when an object is loaded. The *load–deformation curve* describes the relationship between the loading and corresponding degree of deformation (Fig. 17-16). Within the elastic region, the object deforms in direct relation to the force, and returns to the beginning shape once the force is removed. However, at the *elastic limit point*, the response becomes plastic, resulting in some degree of permanent deformation even when the force is removed. Also within the plastic region, excessive loading can result in a point of failure: For a bone, this is the point where a fracture occurs.

Although excessive acute loading as described in the preceding can result in damage to the object, the effect of chronic or repetitive loading that commonly occurs

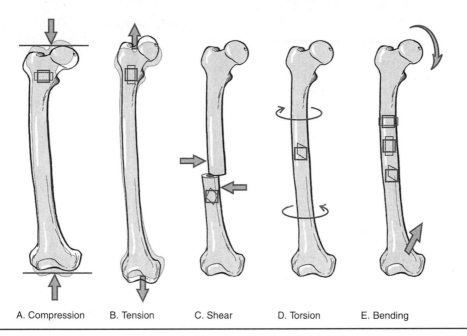

A. Compression   B. Tension   C. Shear   D. Torsion   E. Bending

Fig. 17-14 Illustration of different types of loading. (From Hamill J, Knutzen KM: Biomechanical Basis of Human Movement. Baltimore, Williams & Wilkins, 1995.)

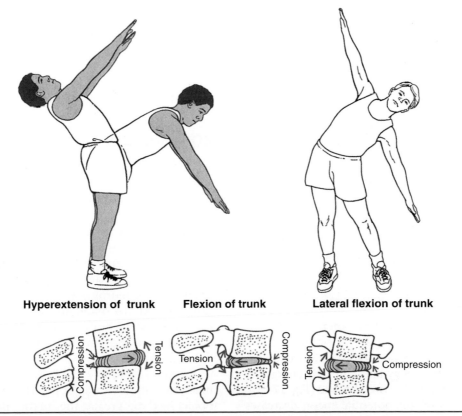

Hyperextension of trunk   **Flexion of trunk**   **Lateral flexion of trunk**

Fig. 17-15 Compression and tension stress acting on the vertebrae during trunk motion. (From Hamill J, Knutzen KM: Biomechanical Basis of Human Movement. Baltimore, Williams & Wilkins, 1995.)

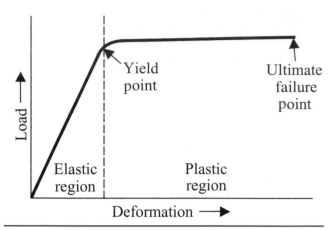

Fig. 17-16 Relationship between load and deformation of an object. (From Hall SJ: Basic Biomechanics, 3rd ed. New York, McGraw-Hill, 1999.)

in occupational settings is equally problematic.[35] Repetitive loading can result in microtrauma to the point of stress. If this persists long enough, a chronic wound, termed a stress-related injury, may occur.[19,20]

ENERGY

From a biomechanical perspective, energy is generally described as the ability to perform mechanical work (e.g., mechanical energy). Mechanical energy can be subdivided into two categories: **kinetic energy** and **potential energy.** Kinetic energy (KE) is the energy consequential to motion. It is expressed algebraically as:

$$KE = \frac{1}{2} \text{ mass} \times \text{velocity}^2$$

An object must be in motion to possess kinetic energy. As can be observed based on the equation, velocity is a key aspect of kinetic energy. The quantity of kinetic energy increases exponentially in relation to the velocity. However, it is important to not overlook the effect of mass, because extremely large objects possess much kinetic energy even under situations where the velocity is extremely low. Potential energy (PE) is the capacity to perform work based on position. It can be defined as the following:

$$PE = \text{mass} \times \text{gravity} \times \text{height from a reference point}$$

Therefore for an object to possess potential energy, it must be positioned above a surface or deformed. The term potential refers to the potential to produce kinetic energy; therefore kinetic energy and potential energy are inversely related for objects that are airborne (Fig. 17-17). As an object nears the ground, potential energy decreases because of the reduction in position, but conversely kinetic energy magnifies because of the increased velocity generated from the gravitational acceleration.

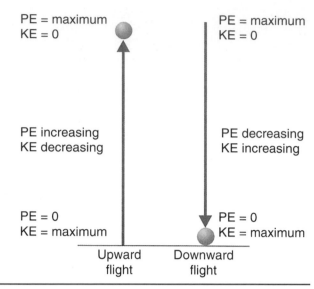

Fig. 17-17 Relationship between potential energy and kinetic energy for objects that are airborne. (From Hamill J, Knutzen KM: Biomechanical Basis of Human Movement. Baltimore, Williams & Wilkins, 1995.)

Kinetic and potential energy concepts also apply to nonprojectile motion. To better understand the nature and severity of an injury, it is useful to evaluate the energy involved in tissue loading.[16] The speed of mechanical loading tends to result in different types of injuries (e.g., bone fractures versus ruptured ligaments). Also, the body provides protection (e.g., intervertebral disks) to absorb energy during tissue loading. However, in some cases the body's natural ability to dissipate energy is compromised, resulting in injuries such as stress fractures from repetitive low energy loading.[35]

EQUILIBRIUM

Balance of all forces and torques in the body (the sum = 0) is referred to as a state of **equilibrium.** Under this condition the body either must be motionless or moving at a constant velocity. An aspect related to equilibrium is the concept of *stability,* which can be operationally defined as the body's resistance to change in the state of equilibrium (Box 17-3). Similarly, **balance** is the ability to control one's state of equilibrium. PTAs in rehabilitation settings routinely assist patients to reeducate the body to maintain a degree of equilibrium by enhancing stability, thus improving balance. This is particularly important for patients who are prone to fall-related injuries.[4]

Based on Newton's first law of motion, we know that mass contributes to stability. The greater the mass an object has, the greater the inertia, thus a greater reluctance to change in motion. A second factor contributing to stability is frictional force. It is easier to maintain stability (e.g., walking on sand versus ice) as frictional

BOX 17-3

Key Principles for Maintaining Stability

1. Increase body mass.
2. Increase friction between contact surfaces.
3. Increase size of the base of support, especially in the direction of an impending external force.
4. Move the center of mass (gravity) closer to the direction of an impending external force.
5. Lower the center of mass.

From Hall SJ: Basic Biomechanics, 4th ed. Boston, McGraw-Hill, 2003.

force increases. Also a larger base of support contributes to greater stability. This can be observed by the variation in assisted walking devices. Those with a larger base of support (e.g., a four-pronged cane versus a single-prong cane) contribute more to a stable walking environment. In addition, the position of the *line of gravity* (line through the center of gravity or mass running perpendicular to the contact surface) affects the degree of stability. Generally, the most stable position is when the line of gravity goes though the center of the base of support. However, when a force is being applied, it is more advantageous for the line of gravity to be nearer to the edge of the base of support closest to where the force occurs. Finally, a more stable environment can be created by lowering the center of mass closer to the base of support.

Balance is a key component for rehabilitation programs, especially in cases of prolonged convalescence.[24] Recovery from an injury necessitates the reeducation of kinesthetic and mechanical control, which is crucial for performing daily tasks such as locomotion and maintaining proper posture. A thorough presentation of balance and its role in orthopedic management can be found in Chapter 7.

❖ ADDITIONAL FEATURES

Abiotrophy: A degeneration or failure of microscopic or macroscopic structure of a body tissue or part.

Articular Cartilage—Biomechanical Function: Acts to increase load distribution and provides a wear-resistant surface that reduces wear.

Biotribology: The division of tribology that focuses on understanding the frictions, lubrication, and wear of diarthrodial joints.

Creep: A constant force increases deformation of a material over time as long as the force is maintained.

Force Couple: A moment created by equal, noncolinear, parallel but opposite directed forces. The moment created is called a couple.

Intrinsic Material Properties: Deformational properties of an object that do not depend on size or shape.

Joint Surface Motions: Rotation, rolling, and gliding.

Lamellar Bone—Biomechanical Function: Lamellar bone increases stiffness and strength of bone with a corresponding increase in brittleness.

Linear Elastic Material: Three fundamental stress–strain characteristics: I-Stress and strain are directly proportional. II-Strain is totally recovered when stress is removed. III-Material is not sensitive to the rate of loading.

Patella—Biomechanical Function: Acts to distribute forces across the distal femur. Lengthens the lever arm of the quadriceps extensor mechanism.

Stress: A force required to maintain the deformation of viscoelastic material. Diminishes with time until equilibrium is reached.

Tibial Stem and Tray—Biomechanical Function: In a total knee arthroplasty, the tibial stem effectively reduces shear forces at the bone–implant interface and distributes loads across the proximal tibia.

Tribology: The science that deals with friction lubrication and wear of interacting joint surfaces in motion.

Velocity: A change of position with respect to time. Velocity is also a vector, possessing both speed and direction.

REFERENCES

1. Antonutto G, Bodem F, Zamparo P, et al: Maximal power and EMG of lower limbs after 21 days spaceflight in one astronaut. *J Gravit Physiol* 1998;5:63–66.
2. Antonutto G, Capelli C, Di Prampero PE: Pedalling in space as a countermeasure to microgravity deconditioning. *Microgravity Q* 1991;1:93–101.
3. Baroni G, Ferrigno G, Anolli A, et al: Quantitative analysis of motion control in long term microgravity. *Acta Astronaut* 1998; 43:131–151.
4. Bloem BR, Steijns JA, Smits-Engelsman BC: An update on falls. *Curr Opin Neurol* 2003;16:15–26.
5. Cajori F: Sir Isaac Newton's Mathematical Principles (translated by Andrew Motte, 1729). Berkeley, CA, University of California Press, 1934.
6. Cavanagh PR, Ulbrecht JS, Caputo GM: New developments in the biomechanics of the diabetic foot. *Diabetes Metab Res Rev* 2000; 16(Suppl. 1):S6–S10.
7. Chadwick EKJ, Nicol AC: Elbow and wrist joint contact forces during occupational pick and place activities. *J Biomech* 2000; 33:591–600.
8. Chen CP, Chen MJ, Pei YC, et al: Sagittal plane loading response during gait in different age groups and in people with knee osteoarthritis. *Am J Phys Med Rehabil* 2003;82:307–312.
9. Coleman KL, Boone DA, Smith DG, et al: Effect of trans-tibial prosthesis pylon flexibility on ground reaction forces during gait. *Prosthet Orthot Int* 2001;25:195–201.
10. Davids JR, Foti T, Dabelstein J, et al: Voluntary (normal) versus obligatory (cerebral palsy) toe-walking in children: a kinematic, kinetic, and electromyographic analysis. *J Pediatr Orthop* 1999; 19:461–469.
11. DeVita P, Hortobagyi T, Barrier J: Gait biomechanics are not normal after anterior cruciate ligament reconstruction and accelerated rehabilitation. *Med Sci Sports Exerc* 1998;30:1481–1488.
12. di Prampero PE, Narici MV: Muscles in microgravity: from fibres to human motion. *J Biomech* 2003;36:403–412.
13. Engsberg JR, Lee AG, Tedford KG, et al: Normative ground reaction force data for able-bodied and trans-tibial amputee children during running. *Prosthet Orthot Int* 1993;17:83–89.
14. Ferber R, McClay D, Williams DS: Gender differences in lower extremity mechanics during running. *Clin Biomech* 2003; 18:350–357.

15. Finsen L, Christensen H: A biomechanical study of occupational loads in the shoulder and elbow in dentistry. *Clin Biomech* 1998; 13:272–279.
16. Fleisig GS, Barrentine SW, Escamilla RF, et al: Biomechanics of overhand throwing with implications for injuries. *Sports Med* 1996; 21:421–437.
17. Garg A: Occupational biomechanics and low-back pain. *Occup Med* 1992;7:609–628.
18. Georgoulis AD, Papadonikolakis A, Papageorgiou CD, et al: Three-dimensional tibiofemoral kinematics of the anterior cruciate ligament-deficient and reconstructed knee during walking. *Am J Sports Med* 2003;31:75–79.
19. Hall SJ: Basic Biomechanics, 4th ed. Boston, McGraw-Hill, 2003.
20. Hamill J, Knutzen KM: Biomechanical Basis of Human Movement, 2nd ed. Philadelphia, Lippincott Williams & Wilkins, 2003.
21. Harman E: The biomechanics of resistance exercise. In Baechle TR, Earle RW, eds. Essentials of Strength Training and Conditioning, 2nd ed. Champaign, IL, Human Kinetics, 2002.
22. Hay JG, Reid JG: Anatomy, Mechanics, and Human Motion, 2nd ed. Englewood Cliffs, NJ, Prentice-Hall, 1988.
23. Hidalgo JA, Genaidy AM, Huston R, et al: Occupational biomechanics of the neck: a review and recommendations. *J Hum Ergol* 1992;21:165–182.
24. Hobeika CP: Equilibrium and balance in the elderly. *Ear Nose Throat J* 1999;78:558–562, 565–566.
25. Jones ME, Steel JR, Bashford GM, et al: Static versus dynamic prosthetic weight bearing in elderly trans-tibial amputees. *Prosthet Orthot Int* 1997;21:100–106.
26. Kirkendall DT, Garrett WE Jr: Clinical perspectives regarding eccentric muscle injury. *Clin Orthop* 2002;403(Suppl.):S81–S89.
27. Laporte DM, Chan D, Sveistrup H: Rising from sitting in elderly people, part 1: implications of biomechanics and physiology. *Br J Occup Ther* 1999;62:36–42.
28. McGinley JL, Goldie PA, Greenwood KM, et al: Accuracy and reliability of observational gait analysis data: judgments of push-off in gait after stroke. *Phys Ther* 2003;83:146–160.
29. Nigg BM: The role of impact forces and foot pronation: a new paradigm. *Clin J Sport Med* 2001;11:2–9.
30. Nolan L, Kerrigan DC: Keep on your toes: gait initiation from toe-standing. *J Biomech* 2003;36:393–401.
31. Perry J: The use of gait analysis for surgical recommendations in traumatic brain injury. *J Head Trauma Rehabil* 1999;14:116–135.
32. Pintar FA, Yoganandan N, Voo L: Effect of age and loading rate on human spine injury threshold. *Spine* 1998;23:1957–1962.
33. Riley PO, Kerrigan DC: Torque action of two-joint muscles in the swing period of stiff-legged gait: a forward dynamic model analysis. *J Biomech* 1998;31:835–840.
34. Singer BJ, Dunne JW, Singer KP, et al: Velocity dependent passive plantar flexor resistive torque in patients with acquired brain injury. *Clin Biomech* 2003;18:157–165.
35. Stock SR: Workplace ergonomic factors and the development of musculoskeletal disorders of the neck and upper limbs: a meta-analysis. *Am J Ind Med* 1991;19:87–107.
36. Tang SF, Chen CP, Hong WH, et al: Improvement of gait by using orthotic insoles in patients with heel injury who received reconstructive flap operations. *Am J Phys Med Rehabil* 2003;82:350–356.

REVIEW QUESTIONS

Multiple Choice

1. Movements such as flexion/extension of the elbow, knee, and hip occur in the _____ plane.
   A. Transverse
   B. Frontal
   C. Sagittal
   D. They can occur in all of the above.

2. A measure of the rotary effect produced when a force is applied eccentrically is called which of the following?
   A. Torque
   B. Impulse
   C. Inertia
   D. Power

3. All of the following kinematic principles are vector quantities *except* which of the following?
   A. Displacement
   B. Time
   C. Acceleration
   D. Velocity

4. Forces applied directly through the center of an object results in which of the following?
   A. Rotation
   B. Translation
   C. A torque
   D. Tangential acceleration

5. Which of the following is the most common lever in the human body?
   A. First-class
   B. Second-class
   C. Third-class
   D. All three are commonly found in the human body.

6. According to _____, objects that are at rest tend to have a reluctance to move until a force is applied.
   A. Newton's first law
   B. Newton's second law
   C. Newton's third law
   D. The law of gravitation

7. Once an object begins to move, the frictional force acting between the object and the contact surface:
   A. Increases slightly
   B. Is reduced by 50%
   C. Decreases slightly
   D. Increases in proportion to the velocity of the object

8. _____ occurs when two forces or loads are applied in opposite directions.
   A. Compression
   B. Shear
   C. Torsion
   D. Tension

9. As the velocity of an object increases, the _____ also increases.
   A. Potential energy
   B. Kinetic energy
   C. Equilibrium
   D. Elastic limit point

10. The ability to control one's state of equilibrium is termed which of the following?
    A. Torsion
    B. Stability
    C. Impulse
    D. Balance

Short Answer

11. What is the point called where the midtransverse, midfrontal, and midsagittal planes intersect?

12. Forces applied outside of the center of an object cause the object to do what?

13. Which lever generally has the greatest mechanical advantage?

14. Which of Newton's laws of motion describes the relationship among force, mass, and acceleration?

15. What types of injuries commonly occur when tension loading exceeds the ability of the object to resist the stress?

True/False

16. Kinematics deals with the description of movements based on alterations in space and time.
17. The majority of human movements are restricted to a single plane of motion (e.g., abduction occurs only in the frontal plane).
18. There is a mechanical relationship between linear and angular motion.
19. A force couple is formed when there are two torques that are equal in magnitude and opposite in direction.
20. When the fulcrum is located somewhere between the point of force and point of resistance, the lever is termed "third class."
21. Newton's third law is the law of inertia.
22. Pressure is a measure of the distribution of a force over a given area.
23. The speed of mechanical loading can influence the nature of different types of injuries (e.g., bone versus ligament).

24. Increased mass can contribute to the stability of an object.
25. Kinetic energy and torque are inversely related when an object is airborne.

Essay Questions
Answer on a separate sheet of paper.
26. Identify and discuss the different forces that act on objects and how the forces affect movements.
27. Discuss the concept of mechanical loading, and describe how loading is associated with different types of injuries.
28. Discuss the principles of mechanical energy.
29. Identify the factors that contribute to stability.
30. Describe Newton's laws of motion.
31. Discuss both the linear and angular kinematics and kinetics of movement, and explain how angular motion translates to linear movements.

Critical Thinking Applications
Select a rudimentary daily activity (e.g., walking, jumping, or standing) and explain how Newton's laws of motion apply to the factors causing the movement patterns observed during the activity.

Select an injury commonly observed in the physical therapy setting. Explain the kinematic and kinetic principles related to the etiology of the injury and the rehabilitation procedures incorporated during the therapy.

PART VI

MANAGEMENT OF ORTHOPEDIC CONDITIONS

This section introduces the physical therapist assistant (PTA) to many of the diseases and injuries that occur in the musculoskeletal system. Each region of the body is surveyed separately, and common and uncommon soft-tissue injuries, fractures, and diseases are outlined. This introduction defines specific orthopedic injuries and identifies criterion-based rehabilitation programs with an emphasis on practical applications.

Clinically, many orthopedic injuries are managed using a traditional protocol approach. This is based on a timetable, which is a written document that outlines and prescribes a progression for therapeutic interventions within the rehabilitation plan. Generally, a protocol lays out a systematic progression based on tissue healing constraints that should fall within certain time frames.

A more progressive way to manage rehabilitation is the criterion-based program, or critical mapping. This method, which is also known as critical treatment pathways, is "a description of the elements of care to be rendered . . . for a particular diagnosis. The pathway often takes the form of a chart or care path/care map that can be followed" by the clinician and patient.* Instead of using a timetable for progression, a set of criteria is developed that the patient must meet before progressing to the next phase of rehabilitation. These are based on tissue healing constraints and the patient's individual tolerance to the program. Therefore a criterion-based progression fosters close scrutiny of all objective and subjective data concerning the individual's performance.

The components necessary for effective management of orthopedic injuries by the PTA are knowledge of musculoskeletal tissue healing principles, familiarity with various rehabilitation programs, skillful application of rehabilitation techniques, and a fundamental understanding of common and uncommon soft-tissue injuries, fractures, and diseases of muscles, bones, and joints. Knowledge of specific indications and contraindications for certain therapeutic interventions also is helpful.

Orthopedic anatomy is not reviewed substantially in this section. Instead, chapters focus on mechanisms of injury, fracture classifications, clinical features of the injury, specific surgical procedures, and rehabilitation programs. Therefore the student clinician is strongly encouraged to review comprehensive musculoskeletal anatomy texts along with the study of each body part and disorder.

---

*APTA Guidelines for Physical Therapists Facing Changing Organizational Structures. APTA BoD, APP 3, 1995.

18

Orthopedic Management of the Ankle, Foot, and Toes*

LEARNING OBJECTIVES

1. Identify common ligament injuries of the foot and ankle.
2. Describe methods of management and rehabilitation of common ligament injuries to the foot and ankle.
3. Identify and describe common tendon injuries to the ankle.
4. Outline and describe common methods of management and rehabilitation of tendon injuries to the ankle.
5. Identify common fractures of the foot and ankle.
6. Discuss common methods of management and rehabilitation of foot and ankle fractures.
7. Identify toe deformities and describe common methods of management and rehabilitation.
8. Describe common mobilization techniques for the ankle, foot, and toe.

KEY TERMS

Inversion ankle sprain	Tendinitis	Plantar fasciitis
Subluxing peroneal tendons	Lauge–Hansen classification	Neuroma
Deltoid ligament	Distal tibia compression fractures (pilon fractures)	Hallux valgus
Mechanical instability	Calcaneal fractures	Hammer toe
Functional instability	Talar fractures	Mallet toe
		Claw toe

CHAPTER OUTLINE

Ligament Injuries of the Ankle
  Lateral Ligament Injuries (Inversion Ankle Sprains)
    Mechanisms of Injury
    Classification of Sprains
  Clinical Examination
    Testing
    Order of Procedures
    Rehabilitation
  Deltoid Ligament Sprains (Medial Ligament)
    Rehabilitation
Chronic Ankle Ligament Instabilities
  Mechanical Instabilities
    Rehabilitation
  Functional Instabilities
    Rehabilitation

Subluxing Peroneal Tendons
  Management
  Rehabilitation
Achilles Tendinitis
  Rehabilitation
Ruptures of the Achilles Tendon
  Management and Rehabilitation
Compartment Syndromes
  Management and Rehabilitation
Ankle Fractures
Distal Tibia Compression Fractures (Pilon Fractures)
Calcaneal Fractures
Fractures of the Talus
Stress Fractures of the Foot and Ankle
Medial Tibial Stress Syndrome

Continued

*Refer to orthopedic anatomy figures on the Evolve website.

259

CHAPTER OUTLINE—cont'd

Plantar Fasciitis (Heel Spur Syndrome)
  Management
Arch Deformities (Pes Planus and Pes Cavus)
Morton's Neuroma (Plantar Interdigital Neuroma)
  Treatment
Hallux Valgus
Lesser Toe Deformities (Hammer Toes, Mallet Toes,
    and Claw Toes)
  Management and Rehabilitation
Common Mobilization Techniques for the Ankle,
    Foot, and Toes
  Ankle Mobilization
  Metatarsal Mobilization
  Proximal Interphalangeal Joint Mobilization

This chapter introduces the physical therapist assistant (PTA) to injuries affecting the ankle, foot, and toes. Included are fractures and specific injuries to structures that influence ankle and foot mechanics.

LIGAMENT INJURIES OF THE ANKLE

Injuries to the lateral ligament complex (the anterior talofibular ligament, fibulocalcaneal ligament, and posterior talofibular ligament) account for approximately 25% of all sports-related injuries,[22] making **inversion ankle sprains** the most common sports injury and one of the common orthopedic injuries seen in the emergency room.[34] Studies report that approximately 95% of all ankle sprains occur to the lateral ligament complex.[35] Therefore only about 5% of all ankle sprains involve the medial structures.

Lateral Ligament Injuries (Inversion Ankle Sprains)

Mechanisms of Injury

Ligament sprains of the lateral aspect of the ankle usually are caused by plantar flexion, inversion, and adduction of the foot and ankle (Fig. 18-1). Large forces are not needed to produce an ankle sprain. Stepping off a curb, stepping into a small hole, or stepping on a rock can produce sudden plantar flexion and inversion motions. During athletic competition, stepping on an opponent's foot is a common occurrence that leads to lateral ligament sprains of the ankle.

Classification of Sprains

Classifying inversion ankle sprains can be difficult and confusing. The standard classification of ligament injuries (e.g., first-, second-, and third-degree sprains) requires elaboration when applied to inversion ankle sprains, specifically addressing grades, degrees, and descriptive severity of the injury (mild, moderate, or severe). A classification model described by Leach[24] is contrasted with the common standard classification of ankle sprains as a means of comparison and to illustrate the potential for confusion about classification of inversion ankle sprains.

First-degree sprain: Single ligament rupture. The anterior talofibular ligament is completely torn. In the standard classification of ligament sprains a complete tear or rupture of a ligament is called a *grade III*, or *third-degree* sprain (Fig. 18-2).

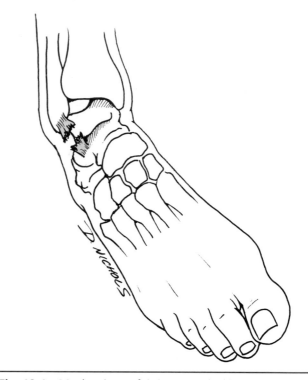

Fig. 18-1 Mechanism of injury to the lateral ligament complex of the ankle. Note the motion of plantar flexion, inversion, and adduction of the foot and ankle.

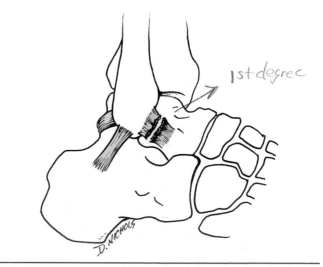

Fig. 18-2 Tear of the anterior talofibular ligament.

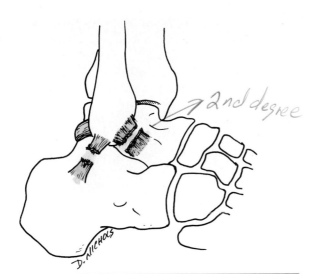

Fig. 18-3 Tears of the anterior talofibular ligament and fibulocalcaneal ligament.

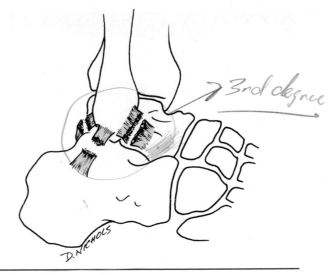

Fig. 18-4 Tears of the anterior talofibular ligament, fibulocalcaneal ligament, and posterior talofibular ligament.

Second-degree sprain: Double ligament rupture. Both the anterior talofibular ligaments and fibulocalcaneal ligaments are completely torn. The standard classification describes a partially torn single ligament as a *grade II* sprain (Fig. 18-3).

Third-degree sprain: All three lateral ankle ligaments (anterior talofibular, posterior talofibular, and fibulocalcaneal) are completely torn. In the standard classification, a single ligament that is completely torn is defined as a *grade III* ligament sprain (Fig. 18-4).

Consequently, it is essential that the system of classification used to describe the severity or complexity of injury be accepted and understood and not confused with another system or model of classification.

Clinical Examination

The PTA must be aware of the organization and administration of examination procedures used to inspect inversion ankle sprains. Throughout rehabilitation, the assistant must communicate changes in the patient's status relative to initial evaluation data and make safe and appropriate modifications to the existing program based on consultation with the supervising therapist.

Testing

Ankle stability tests are used by the physical therapist (PT) to identify and quantify the integrity of the lateral ligament complex. Injury to the anterior talofibular ligament can be assessed clinically by performing the anterior drawer test (Fig. 18-5). The patient must be in a relaxed seated or semirecumbent position with the involved leg flexed 90 degrees at the knee and the involved ankle slightly plantar flexed. Stabilize the distal tibia and support it with one hand, while using the other hand to gently but firmly grasp the calcaneus and

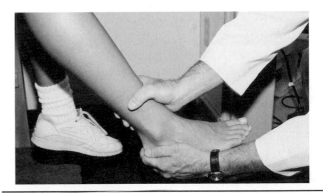

Fig. 18-5 Anterior drawer test of the ankle. With the affected foot slightly plantar flexed, the distal tibia is stabilized with one hand while the other hand grasps the calcaneus and directs an anterior force to manually displace the calcaneus to test the integrity of the anterior talofibular ligament.

attempt to translate or pull the ankle forward. No excessive motion is seen or felt if the ligament is intact. However, the ankle demonstrates excessive forward or anterior motion if the anterior talofibular ligament is torn.

The talar tilt test examines the ankle ligament's resistance to maximal inversion stress (Fig. 18-6). While the patient is in the same position as the anterior drawer test, the ankle is gradually stressed by exertion of constant pressure over the lateral aspect of the foot and ankle while counter pressure is applied over the inner aspect of the lower leg until maximal inversion is reached.[3] The severity of ligament injury should be graded according to the classification system used by the supervising PT.

BOX 18-1

Physical Therapist Initial Evaluation Outline for the Clinical Assessment of Inversion Ankle Sprains

HISTORY

1. How did the injury happen?
2. Where is the pain located?
3. Did you hear or feel a "pop" or "snap"?
4. Have you had a similar injury previously? If yes, explain.

OBSERVATION

1. Note any obvious deformity suggesting a fracture or dislocation.
2. Note the area and degree of swelling.
3. Evaluate complaints of pain.
4. Note any discoloration.
5. Perform a bilateral visual comparison of symmetry.

PALPATION

Always begin palpation by explaining the procedure, then initially performing the procedure on the uninvolved side.

1. Distal tibia-fibula
2. Lateral ligament complex
3. Medial ligaments-deltoid ligament
4. Base of the fifth metatarsal
5. Peroneal tendons
6. Achilles tendon

RANGE OF MOTION

1. Active and passive
2. Dorsiflexion
3. Plantar flexion
4. Inversion
5. Eversion

STRENGTH

1. Manual muscle testing
   a. Dorsiflexion
   b. Plantar flexion
   c. Inversion
   d. Eversion

CLINICAL STABILITY TESTS

1. Anterior drawer test
2. Talar tilt test

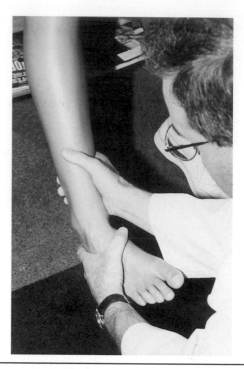

Fig. 18-6 Talar tilt test. The distal tibia is stabilized while the other hand "tilts" the talus to test the integrity of the lateral ligament complex.

Order of Procedures

Box 18-1 outlines the procedure for evaluation of inversion ankle sprains. The mechanism of injury that produces an inversion ankle sprain also may cause other conditions that must be differentiated by the physician[34] and PT, such as fracture of the base of the fifth metatarsal, malleolar fractures, osteochondral fractures, osteochondritis dissecans, midfoot ligament sprains, and **subluxing peroneal tendons.**

Rehabilitation

The specific rehabilitation program used to treat inversion sprains depends on the severity of sprain (first, second, or third degree). Generally first- and second-degree sprains can be effectively managed nonoperatively according to a closely supervised rehabilitation program.

Initial management of acute inversion ankle sprains calls for rest, ice, compression, and elevation (RICE). *Rest* is a relative term used to define avoidance of unwanted stress; it does not necessarily require complete avoidance of *all stress.* The application of ice, compression, and elevation is directed at minimizing and reducing intense inflammatory response, hemorrhage, swelling, pain, and "cellular metabolism" to provide the most conducive environment for tissue healing.[34]

Clinically, the most effective means to reduce swelling are elevation and compression. Elastic compression bandages (Ace wraps) are applied while elevating the injured limb above the heart. A three-phase (phase I, maximum protection; phase II, moderate protection; phase III, minimum protection), criteria-based rehabilitation program is effective for the management of inversion ankle sprains. The maximum-protection phase calls for the RICE program to be used three to five times daily. Application of ice should be encouraged for 15 to 20 minutes, with a 1- to 2-hour rest period between applications. Protecting the torn ligaments from unwanted stress is the cornerstone of this phase. Joint protection and immobilization can be achieved through an array of commercial appliances, tape, casting, and braces; selection is left to the physician or PT. Some physicians choose to use a short-leg walking cast or posterior plaster splint. More commonly, a plastic shell brace with an inflatable air bladder or a leather semirigid ankle support is used. Tape can be used for both compression and ligament support, but it must be applied skillfully and reapplied daily to be effective. The ankle must be positioned correctly during the application and use of all support devices. It should be in a neutral position or slightly dorsiflexed and somewhat everted to closely approximate the torn ligaments. Weight bearing status and ambulation with assistive devices are individualized. A patient's pain tolerance guides the PTA phase. Weight bearing as tolerated should be encouraged.

An active range-of-motion (ROM) program must be used cautiously during the maximum-protection phase. It is imperative to *avoid* plantar flexion and inversion when instructing patients to perform ROM exercises.

Motion exercises are important to help reduce pain and swelling, as well as help increase function of the joint. However, if certain motions (e.g., plantar flexion or inversion) are employed too early in the rehabilitation period, these "unwanted stresses" can disrupt the normal healing process. Electrical galvanic stimulation also can help reduce pain and swelling (see Chapter 3).

Isometric strengthening exercises are initiated as soon as the patient's pain tolerance allows. Isometric dorsiflexion and eversion exercises are performed for two or three sets of 10 repetitions, holding each contraction for 10 seconds. Leg-strengthening exercises (leg extension, hamstring curls, hip abduction and adduction, and hip extension exercises) and general full-body conditioning should be encouraged throughout the course of rehabilitation. Clinically it is vital to view inversion ankle sprains as injuries that affect the whole person, rather than just the injured extremity. Maintaining aerobic fitness and strength during recovery is particularly important in a population involved in sports.

The moderate-protection phase can begin once the patient can bear weight on the injured limb without crutches, perform all ROM and isometric exercises without undue complaints of pain, and control the swelling. This phase encourages the use of the RICE principle, full

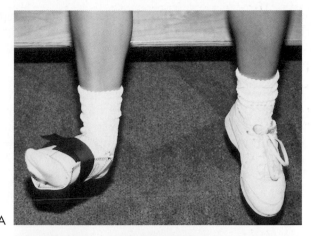

A

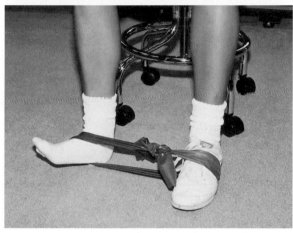

B

Fig. 18-7 A, Concentric and eccentric exercise with ankle weights. As the weight is slowly elevated to a position of dorsiflexion and eversion, the patient is encouraged to emphasize the eccentric or lowering phase of the exercise. **B,** Thera-band elastic band resistance for eversion and dorsiflexion.

weight bearing, and continued ligament support with the use of braces or tape. More progressive exercises are initiated, including concentric and eccentric contractions (Fig. 18-7) (with ankle weights or latex bands), heel cord stretching (Fig. 18-8) (towel stretch, wall stretch, or prostretch), and standing toe and heel raises.

Gradually and cautiously, plantar flexion motions are added as pain allows. Stationary bicycling can be initiated with the seat height lowered slightly to encourage a more neutral ankle position instead of a plantar flexion position.

Proprioception exercises generally are initiated during the moderate-protection phase. Protection of the ligament must be encouraged during these challenging exercises. Balancing on the injured limb on a flat surface is progressed to use of a balance board, and then to a minitrampoline—all excellent exercises that stimulate balance, coordination, and muscular endurance (Fig. 18-9).

The minimum-protection phase can begin once the patient can perform all resistive exercises (ankle weight, Thera-band, and manual resistance) and ambulate without pain or limping, and swelling is reduced.

From 4 to 8 weeks after injury, new collagen formation allows almost-normal stresses to be applied (see Chapter 8).[34] At this point, more functional activities are allowed, including straight-line jogging, large figure-of-eight running, jumping drills, and cutting activities.

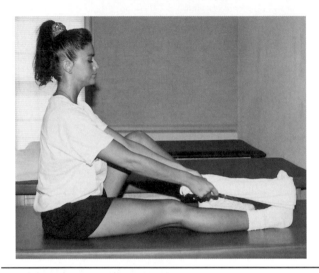

Fig. 18-8 Long-seated towel stretch.

The minimum-protection phase does not imply removal of all supportive devices. Maturation of the injured ligaments can take as long as 6 to 12 months.[34] Therefore it is critical to encourage patient compliance with the use of either tape or a semirigid brace during all running activities.

Box 18-2 outlines a general three-phase rehabilitation program for an inversion ankle sprain. In all instances, if pain, swelling, or irritation persists, the patient is not taken to the next phase until he or she is pain free in the present phase. The ankle must be securely taped or braced when running, jumping, or otherwise performing aggressive, ballistic motions.

The treatment of grade III ankle sprains (using the standard classification) is somewhat controversial.[34] Some authors[3,5,38] report that surgery is needed because "surgical exploration often reveals that the torn ends of the fibulocalcaneal ligament are so widely separated that simple immobilization alone is not sufficient to allow the ligament to heal in a stable position."[3] However, other authors have found that "early controlled mobilization (functional treatment) was the method of choice and provided the quickest recovery in ankle mobility and the earliest return to work and physical activity without compromising the late mechanical stability of the ankle."[34] Therefore depending on the physician's choice of treatment, a grade III sprain can be treated

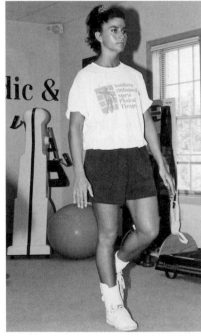
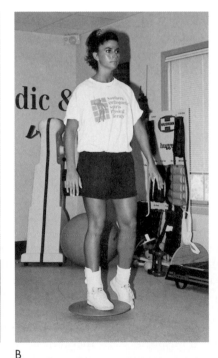
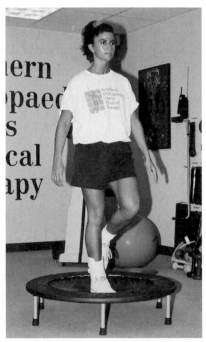

A   B   C

Fig. 18-9 **A,** Single-leg standing proprioception and balancing. Note the continued use of external support during the late stage of recovery. **B,** Single-leg standing proprioception and balancing with use of a wobble board or BAPS (biomechanical ankle platform system) board. **C,** Single-leg standing proprioception and balancing on a minitrampoline. The highly unstable surface provides a challenging balance activity.

BOX 18-2

General Three-Phase Rehabilitation Program for Inversion Ankle Sprains

PHASE I: MAXIMUM-PROTECTION PHASE *light*

1. Rest, ice, compression, and elevation (RICE)
2. Electrical galvanic stimulation (EGS)
3. Weight bearing as tolerated (WBAT)
4. Joint protection (plastic, hinged orthosis, tape, air-cast, semirigid braces)
5. Active range of motion (dorsiflexion and eversion)
6. Isometric exercises
7. General fitness exercises

PHASE II: MODERATE-PROTECTION PHASE

1. RICE
2. Full weight bearing
3. Concentric and eccentric contractors (latex rubber band, ankle weights)
4. Continued joint protection
5. Heel cord stretching
6. Stationary cycling
7. Proprioception exercises
8. General fitness exercises
9. Avoidance of unwanted stresses (inversion and plantar flexion)

PHASE III: MINIMUM-PROTECTION PHASE

1. Joint protection during activities
2. Running
3. Jumping
4. Plyometrics
5. Proprioception exercises
6. General fitness exercises
7. Isotonic exercises
8. Isokinetic exercises

---

either surgically or with immobilization and supervised physical therapy.

Immobilization and joint protection last longer with grade III ankle sprains than with grade I and II sprains. When these injuries are treated surgically, immobilization produces deleterious effects on muscle, bone, cartilage, tendons, and ligaments.

Deltoid Ligament Sprains (Medial Ligament)

Acute isolated sprains of the deep and superficial layers of the **deltoid ligament** are rare,[34] occurring in only 3% to 5% of all ankle sprains.[34,35] It is clinically important to recognize that "complete deltoid ligament ruptures occur in combination with ankle fractures."[34]

Rehabilitation

Partial tears are managed nonoperatively with physical therapy. Because complete ruptures occur with fractures, many authorities[7,10] advocate surgical repair and fixation of the fracture fragments. However, some authors[16] recommend casting, non–weight bearing for 6 weeks, then progressive weight bearing and physical therapy. In either case, rehabilitation focuses primarily on joint protection and the use of a semirigid orthosis.

The use of ice, compression, and elevation assists with pain and swelling. Progressive strengthening follows a three-phase plan of maximum, moderate, and minimum protection. Isometric exercises, latex rubber band strengthening exercises, active ROM (carefully avoiding unwanted stresses), and progressive weight bearing are added as tolerated. Generally, a total body fitness program can be initiated during cast immobilization and non–weight bearing.

CHRONIC ANKLE LIGAMENT INSTABILITIES

The PTA, as an integral part of the rehabilitation team, must be aware of certain short- and long-term complications that may arise from acute or chronic ligament injuries of the ankle. Complications after surgical repair or conservative treatment of ankle sprains are common. Renstrom and Kannus[34] report that 10% to 30% of patients have chronic symptoms of weakness, swelling, pain, and joint instability after inversion sprains. There are two types of instabilities associated with chronic ankle sprains: mechanical and functional.

Mechanical Instabilities

Mechanical instability is defined as laxity of the ankle ligaments. With mechanical instabilities, surgery may be necessary to stabilize the ankle joint. The Watson-Jones,[40] Evans,[15] Chrisman–Snook,[8] and Elmslie[8] procedures are common reconstructive surgical procedures used to help stabilize the lateral ligament complex of the ankle. In general, the peroneus brevis muscle is rerouted through a surgically constructed tunnel in the distal fibula (Fig. 18-10). The rerouting of the peroneus brevis dynamically stabilizes the lateral aspect of the ankle. Another method used to help stabilize chronic ligament laxity is a delayed anatomic repair of the ligaments. The ligaments are surgically cut, shortened, and reattached to the bone with this method (Fig. 18-11).

Rehabilitation

The postoperative course of treatment after surgical correction of chronic ankle instability involves strict, rigid immobilization in a below-the-knee cast for approximately 2 weeks. After the cast is removed the patient's involved limb is placed in a hinged rigid orthosis that allows adjustable limited ROM for 5 or 6 weeks. Passive dorsiflexion and plantar flexion exercises are

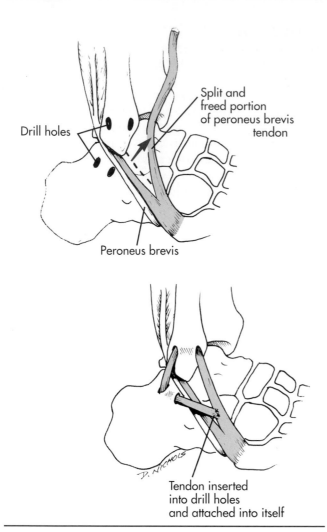

Drill holes

Split and freed portion of peroneus brevis tendon

Peroneus brevis

D. NICHOLS

Tendon inserted into drill holes and attached into itself

Fig. 18-10 Chrisman–Snook procedure used for mechanical ankle instability.

begun after immobilization has ended. Active motion is not permitted initially to allow the rerouted peroneus brevis muscle to scar down and heal properly. When tolerated, active ROM exercises begin with careful avoidance of excessive plantar flexion and inversion motions. A general body fitness program is encouraged throughout the period of immobilization. The use of aerobic exercises (stationary bicycle), leg strengthening exercises (leg extensions and hamstring curls), and proprioception exercises is vital throughout rehabilitation.

Dynamic muscular support is the foundation of various surgical procedures to correct chronic ankle instabilities. Therefore careful and thorough consideration is given to isometric stabilization exercises, Theraband resistive exercises in all directions, manual resistance, isotonic resistance (with ankle weights), and isokinetic strengthening during the minimal-protective phase. In all cases, full ROM exercises with an emphasis on the eccentric contraction phase of each repetition should be encouraged.

In primary delayed repair or anatomic reconstruction, the ligament is surgically shortened and reinserted (imbricated). The healing time for ligaments is slightly longer and more tenuous than that for muscle and tendon reconstructions (tenodesis); therefore the period of immobilization may be prolonged. The progression of rehabilitation is the same as with a tenodesis. Active and passive ROM, control of swelling and pain, isometric and manual resistive exercises (being careful to avoid unwanted excessive plantar flexion and inversion motions), Thera-band and isotonic exercises, and isokinetics are used.

Generally, proprioceptive exercises are used extensively. Single-leg standing exercises, balance board activities, minitrampoline exercises, and heel walking exercises are part of the moderate- and minimum-protection phases of rehabilitation. In all cases, joint protection with tape, braces, or a hinged orthosis is a rudimentary but critical principle throughout rehabilitation.

Functional Instabilities

Functional instability refers to a subjective feeling of giving way without affecting ligament laxity. Unlike mechanical instability, functional instability involves a host of factors, including strength, proprioception, and ligament stability.

Rehabilitation

The primary components of rehabilitation for chronic functional instabilities are closed-chain resistance exercises, proprioception maneuvers, dynamic muscular exercises (concentric and eccentric loads), and bracing for support. Single-leg support proprioception exercises with external resistance (Fig. 18-12) provide dynamic support and balance training. Balance board activities, heel-toe walking, and minitrampoline activities are the cornerstones of proprioception exercises for the ankle throughout all phases of rehabilitation for functional ankle instabilities.

SUBLUXING PERONEAL TENDONS

The PTA must recognize that certain anatomic variations and acute injuries can result in instability of the peroneal tendons and ultimate disability. This injury is classified as acute or chronic. The mechanism of injury involves passive dorsiflexion with the foot slightly everted.[14,27] Acute subluxation of the peroneal tendons can be misdiagnosed as a lateral ankle sprain because of the close anatomic proximity of the tendons to the lateral ligament complex (Fig. 18-13).

Some patients who suffer dislocation of the peroneal tendons have a loose retinaculum (which supports the tendon within the peroneal groove) and also may have a very shallow peroneal groove. Acute injuries result in sprains (grades I, II, and III, using the traditional classi-

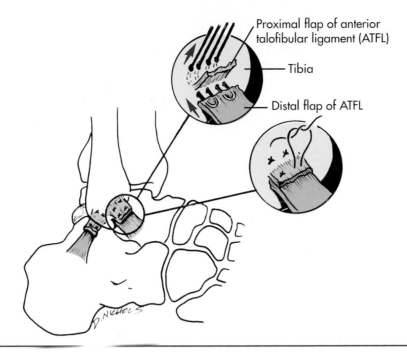

Proximal flap of anterior
talofibular ligament (ATFL)

Tibia

Distal flap of ATFL

Fig. 18-11   Direct delayed primary anatomic repair of torn ligaments.

fication of sprains) to the peroneal retinaculum that cause anterior dislocation of the peroneal tendon over the lateral malleolus with ankle dorsiflexion.[14,27]

Management

Acute injuries usually are treated initially with conservative measures,[39] including rigid-cast immobilization and non–weight bearing gait for approximately 6 weeks.[39] However, in some cases,[21,39] patients ultimately require a surgical repair to correct the disability.[39] Many authorities still recommend cast immobilization and non–weight bearing for 6 weeks for acute injuries,[21] but operative care is the treatment of choice for cases involving recurrent or chronic subluxing peroneal tendons. Keene[21] reports the five basic types of surgical repair procedures for correction of chronic subluxing peroneal tendons:

- Bone block procedures
- Rerouting procedures
- Periosteal flaps
- Groove deepening procedures
- Tendon slings

Rehabilitation

The postoperative care of subluxing peroneal tendons requires excellent communication among the PTA, PT, and surgeon. The exact procedure performed should be explained to the PT, who should articulate the key points of the surgery to the PTA and outline the indications and contraindications for rehabilitation. Usually postoperative care involves the use of immobilization

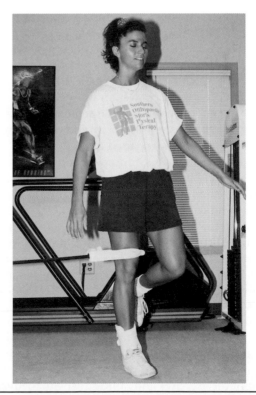

Fig. 18-12   Single-leg standing balance and proprioception exercise with the use of elastic cord to stimulate and encourage strength in a weight bearing closed-chain functional position.

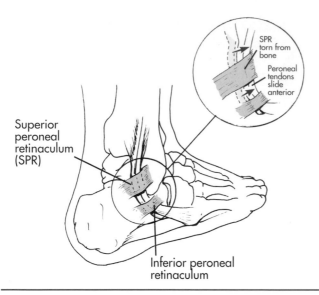

Fig. 18-13 Subluxing peroneal tendons. Note anatomic position of the peroneal tendons in relation to the lateral ligament complex of the ankle.

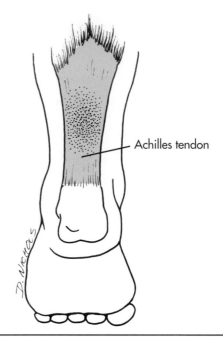

Fig. 18-14 Achilles tendinitis.

for a few weeks and instruction in weight bearing as tolerated. Keene[21] recommends plantar flexion and dorsiflexion exercises 3 weeks after surgery.

All immobilization is terminated 6 weeks after surgery. While immobilized, the patient progresses through a general body conditioning program of aerobic exercise and strengthening. After immobilization, active ROM and isometric strengthening exercises are begun. As pain allows, manual resistive and Thera-band strengthening exercises can be added. Care must be taken with extreme dorsiflexion and eversion maneuvers after surgery. Depending on which procedure was used, soft-tissue and bone healing constraints must be observed carefully to avoid placing excessive stress on the surgically repaired tissues.

Initially, limited ROM dorsiflexion strengthening exercises should be used. As pain, swelling, and strength improve, greater degrees of dorsiflexion motion can be added. Proprioception exercises on a flat surface can be initiated soon after immobilization ends. Progression to balance board activities and minitrampoline exercises depends on the patient's tolerance. Keene[21] recommends that a running program can begin when ROM has been achieved and the involved limb reaches 80% of the strength of the noninvolved limb.

At first, slow straight-line jogging is attempted. Longer distances are tried if there is no pain, swelling, or complaint of instability. As symptoms allow, sprints can be attempted with careful observation of symptoms.

Plyometric exercises and rapid cutting maneuvers can be included for the athletic patient. For example, jumping in place, side-to-side hops, and quick figure-of-eight sprints are progressive functional activities that involve rapid change of direction and ballistic concen-

tric and eccentric open- and closed-chain loading. In most cases, full return to activity can be achieved about 16 weeks after surgery.

ACHILLES TENDINITIS

Achilles **tendinitis** is an overuse injury resulting from repetitive microtrauma and accumulative overloading of the tendon[21] (Fig. 18-14). The primary feature of Achilles tendinitis is localized pain at the midportion, distal third, and insertion on the calcaneus.

Many intrinsic and extrinsic factors can lead to Achilles tendinitis. Intrinsic factors are "decreased vascularity, aging and degeneration of the tendon, anatomic deviations such as heel-leg or heel-forefoot malalignment and poor gastroc-soleus flexibility."[21] Extrinsic factors include variations in training, running-surface changes, and poor or inappropriate footwear.

The general features of Achilles tendinitis include soft-tissue swelling, pain, and crepitus.

Rehabilitation

Most cases of Achilles tendinitis are managed conservatively with various physical agents, oral medications, relative rest, and progressive exercises. Initial management includes the use of ice massage or ice packs for 15 to 20 minutes, three to five times daily. The treating physician may prescribe a nonsteroidal antiinflammatory drug (NSAID) to help reduce swelling and pain. All aggravating motions must be stopped. For example, an athletic patient who runs must stop running temporarily until symptoms subside. A program of aerobic exercise using a stationary bicycle or a swimming program can take the place of the running program. Sometimes a small felt heel-lift can be placed in everyday shoes to help reduce the stress on the tendon. The heel wedge is gradually diminished as symptoms are reduced. It is not advisable to suddenly remove the heel-lift support when symptoms improve because pain and swelling return occasionally.

Ultrasound also can be used to help reduce pain and assist with collagen synthesis.[19] Generally, ultrasound can be used immediately before an exercise program to improve circulation, enhance relaxation of the soft tissues, and reduce pain. Occasionally phonophoresis (ultrasound used with a topical hydrocortisone cream) is used in cases of severe pain.

Flexibility exercises are used to increase dorsiflexion motion and reduce the effects of scarring in prolonged cases of Achilles tendinitis. Researchers have pointed out that a lack of dorsiflexion is a common denominator for patients suffering from Achilles tendinitis.[23]

Initially, active dorsiflexion exercises are used. Towel stretches are added gradually as pain allows. In many cases it may be helpful to apply ice packs or ice massage to the tendon before stretching and strengthening exercises. Standing heel cord stretches can be added to the flexibility program as soon as towel stretches do not cause pain or swelling. In all cases of stretching, it is advisable to avoid any ballistic motions, stretch gently and firmly, and hold each stretch for 10 to 30 seconds.

Standing heel cord stretches can be performed on a small block or with a commercial appliance to produce greater dorsiflexion motion. A soleus stretch is also used for Achilles tendinitis. The patient faces a wall with his or her knees touching the wall while keeping the heels on the floor (Fig. 18-15).

Strengthening exercises often prove very beneficial for patients with Achilles tendinitis. However, most full ROM strengthening and stretching exercises also cause complaints of pain. A safe and effective exercise program focuses initially on limited ROM and submaximal exercises. When the patient can perform all exercises without pain, the next phase of more vigorous exercise can begin.

Initially, Thera-band plantar flexion exercises can be used. Use of the Thera-band for plantar flexion motion should emphasize the eccentric phase of the exercise.[12] Curwin and Stanish[12] advocate eccentric exercises for treatment of many types of tendinitis. For example, when strengthening the gastroc-soleus muscle group using standing heel raises, the patient is instructed to rise up on the balls of the feet using the uninvolved limb. Before the descent phase, the body weight is transferred to the involved limb and then the body is slowly lowered. As symptoms improve, more concentric lifting is allowed gradually, with greater dorsiflexion motion.

In some severe cases of Achilles tendinitis, physicians may prescribe rigid cast immobilization of the ankle for

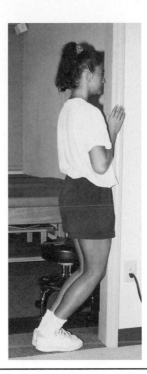

Fig. 18-15 Standing soleus stretch. Flexing the knees enhances the stretch to the gastroc–soleus complex.

10 days.[23] The entire program of rehabilitation after cast immobilization progresses at a slightly slower rate because of the limited ROM and strength loss associated with immobilization. In all cases of Achilles tendinitis, the patient is instructed in a general body fitness program. Aerobic exercise can be achieved with an upper body ergometer (UBE), seated bicycle ergometer with the seat height corrected to prevent plantar flexion, or swimming program. Upper- and lower-body stretching and strengthening exercises are encouraged as long as the tendon suffers no undue stress or pain.

RUPTURES OF THE ACHILLES TENDON

Complete ruptures of the Achilles tendon can occur with excessive sudden plantar flexion (Fig. 18-16). These ruptures usually involve the area "3 to 4 cm proximal to its insertion on the calcaneus, within the area of decreased vascularity" and occur mostly in men 20 to 50 years old.[21] In acute Achilles tendon rupture, palpation reveals a defect or gap in the continuity of the distal third of the tendon. The sensitive Thompson test clinically assesses the integrity of the Achilles tendon. To perform this simple test, the patient lies prone on an examining table with the feet extending off the end. The entire lower leg is exposed, from knee to toes. The belly of the calf of the uninvolved limb is grasped and squeezed so that the foot plantar flexes. If the tendon is ruptured on the involved limb when the calf is squeezed, no plantar flexion motion results (Fig. 18-17).

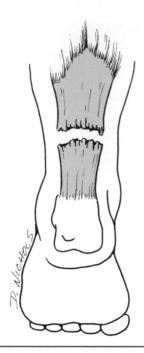

Fig. 18-16 Complete rupture of the Achilles tendon.

Management and Rehabilitation

A ruptured Achilles tendon can be treated surgically or with cast immobilization. Nonoperative treatment of Achilles tendon ruptures requires the patient to be immobilized for as long as 8 weeks.[21] However, with nonoperative treatment, researchers[2,15,20] have documented rerupture rates of 8% to 39%. In addition, there is a greater loss of strength, power, and endurance compared with surgically repaired tendons.[2,17,20,21] Surgically repaired Achilles tendons have a much lower rate of rerupture (0 to 5%), and there is a significant increase in the ultimate recovery of muscular strength, power, and endurance. However, Nistor[33] reports only minor differences between surgical and nonsurgical management. Some surgeons[33] prefer nonoperative management because there are fewer complications related to surgery, reduced complaints, no hospitalization, and no significant differences in function compared with surgically treated patients. Keene[21] reports various techniques used to repair acute Achilles tendon ruptures, including end-to-end primary repair and direct repair and augmentation with tendon or synthetic grafts.[21]

The rehabilitation program used after nonoperative immobilization of an Achilles tendon rupture requires the PTA to appreciate the time-dependent nature of tendon healing and plastic and elastic deformation principles (see Chapter 4). Throughout the course of immobilization, the patient should be instructed in a general body conditioning program that does not stress the involved tissues. The muscles of the noninvolved limb (i.e., quadriceps, hamstrings, gastroc-soleus) should be vigorously strengthened along with the thigh and hamstring muscles of the involved limb. Aerobic exercise also is encouraged. Stationary bike ergometers using only the uninvolved limb (a toe clip is necessary for single-limb cycling) and UBEs are appropriate and safe cardiovascular fitness tools. When the cast is removed and after the initial evaluation by the PT, the PTA proceeds with thermal agents as indicated. Moist heat followed by ultrasound can be used before ROM and flexibility exercises. If pain and swelling are present, a cold whirlpool or ice packs with compression can be applied.

Regaining full dorsiflexion and plantar flexion motion is an exceedingly slow process after cast removal. Gentle active dorsiflexion and plantar-flexion exercises are initiated immediately. Typically, a small heel-lift is used in everyday shoes to minimize stress on the healing tendon. Because the tendon was not surgically repaired, the process of regaining tensile strength and collagen alignment must be approached cautiously (see Chapter 4). Progressive active motion is an essential component for full return to function. However, if the tendon is stressed too soon or vigorously, the tendon may rerupture. The heel-lift is worn for 3 to 4 weeks and gradually reduced in size to prevent sudden excessive stress on the tendon.[21]

Progressive plantar-flexion and dorsiflexion exercises using a latex band are encouraged as pain and motion allow. Proprioception exercises can be employed early, depending on the patient's tolerance. Generally, proprioception exercises begin with the patient in a seated position (Fig. 18-18) and progress as tolerated. If rerupture occurs, it is usually within 4 weeks after immobilization.[21] During this maximum-protection phase, the patient is encouraged to avoid sudden forceful plantar flexion or dorsiflexion motions.

As motion increases gradually, closed-chain resistive exercises can be initiated, based on the patient's ROM, pain tolerance, swelling, and the length of time after cast removal. Seated stationary cycling can be used for aerobic fitness, ROM, and local muscular endurance. The seat must be adjusted to avoid excessive plantar flexion or dorsiflexion, however. Step-ups can be used (with heel-lift) to encourage weight bearing eccentric loading.

Weight bearing plantar flexion can begin gradually once the patient has successfully completed the prescribed program of ROM and strengthening exercises without complications. Standing plantar flexion is initiated without a block to stand on. The patient is instructed to gradually rise up on the toes using primarily the uninvolved limb, then lowers himself or herself using both feet. As strength improves, the patient gradually uses more of the involved limb to rise up on the balls of the feet. Adding a small block of wood on

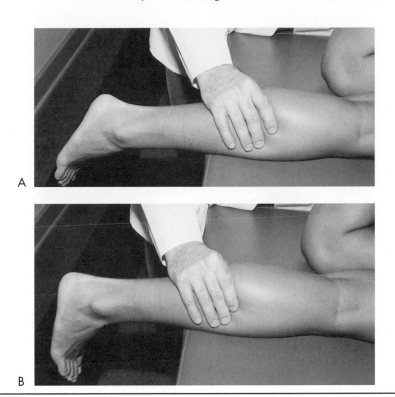

Fig. 18-17 Thompson test to confirm or deny the presence of a ruptured Achilles tendon. **A,** A negative Thompson test is demonstrated by observation of plantar flexion of the foot when squeezing the calf. **B,** A positive Thompson test reveals no plantar flexion of the foot when the calf is squeezed.

which to rise adds greater dorsiflexion stress and motion. Seated calf raises can be performed by modifying a leg extension machine (Fig. 18-19). The seated position may be more comfortable initially.

The PTA reassesses the patient's ROM, strength, pain, and swelling on a daily basis. Modifications are necessary if the patient is having undue pain with any phase of the program. Daily communication with the PT allows continuous restructuring of the rehabilitation plan based on the patient's needs as assessed by the PTA. Isokinetic testing for plantar flexion, dorsiflexion, ROM, strength, power, and local muscular endurance generally is reserved for the minimal-protection phase. However, isokinetic strengthening exercises can be employed early if done at higher speeds and performed submaximally under limited ROM conditions.

Postoperative rehabilitation follows a similar criteria-based rehabilitation program. Keene[21] reports that isokinetic strengthening exercises are begun 2 to 4 weeks after immobilization (which usually lasts 6 weeks). When strength values are at least 70% of the uninvolved limb, a gradual, progressive jogging program can begin.[21] Recovery from a surgically repaired Achilles tendon rupture varies from patient to patient, but generally, good results are seen in 6 months.

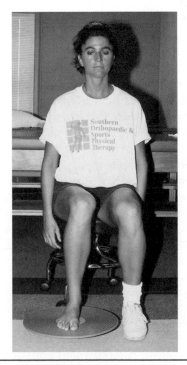

Fig. 18-18 Initial proprioception activities can begin in a seated position using a wobble board.

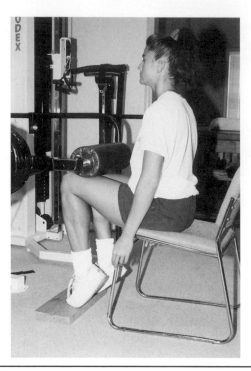

Fig. 18-19 Seated heel or calf raises are performed by modifying and adjusting a knee-extension machine with a range-limiting device.

COMPARTMENT SYNDROMES

Compartment syndromes of the lower leg are defined as either acute or chronic elevated tissue pressure within a closed fascial space, resulting in occlusion of vessels and compromised neuromuscular function.[1,36]

Acute compartment syndromes of the leg are most commonly associated with tibial fractures, direct trauma to the area, muscle rupture, muscle hypertrophy, and circumferential burns.[22,34] **Acute elevated intracompartmental pressure within the lower leg** is considered a medical emergency.

Chronic compartment syndromes also are referred to as exertional compartment syndrome or exercise-induced compartment syndrome. Muscular contractions and exertion have been shown to cause increases in muscle size, leading to increased intracompartmental pressure.[22,34] This results in ischemia and reduced neuromuscular function. To understand this series of events, it is necessary to review pertinent anatomy of the lower leg.

There are four well-defined compartments of the leg, divided by nonyielding fascia.[1,36] The *anterior compartment* of the lower leg contains the tibialis anterior, anterior tibial artery and vein, and foot and toe extensor muscles. The *lateral* **compartment** contains the superficial peroneal nerve and short and long peroneal muscles. The *superficial posterior compartment* contains the soleus muscle and plantaris and gastrocnemius tendons. The *deep posterior compartment* contains the posterior tibial muscle, the peroneal artery and vein, tibial nerve, and posterior tibial artery and vein. If swelling occurs in one or more of these compartments, reduced capillary blood perfusion results in neurovascular and muscular dysfunction.

Clinical symptoms of acute compartment syndrome include pain, palpable swelling or tenseness, and paresthesias.[1,36] The skin may be warm, shiny, and tense. Passive stretching of the muscles of the lower leg may produce severe pain.

Symptoms of chronic or exertional compartment syndromes include a dull aching pain within the muscle during and after long-term exercise. Paresthesias also may develop as the syndrome progresses. The sections most commonly affected with chronic exercise-induced compartment syndromes are the anterior and deep posterior compartments of the lower leg.

Management and Rehabilitation

Acute compartment syndrome is treated with a surgical procedure called a fasciotomy.[1,36] When nerve and muscle ischemia last longer than 12 hours, severe and irreversible damage occurs.[1] If, however, the ischemia can be reduced in less than 4 hours, usually no permanent damage occurs.[1]

A surgical fasciotomy is designed to relieve intracompartmental pressure by opening or releasing the fascial compartment, thus allowing the pressure to be reduced. It is interesting to note that the surgical incision is left open and is managed with sterile dressings.[1] Immediately after surgery, ice packs and leg elevation are necessary to reduce swelling. Walking as tolerated and active and passive gentle ROM of the ankle and knee are begun 2 days after surgery. Treatment with ice and leg elevation is continued after exercise. A general conditioning program can begin with strengthening exercises and aerobic exercises using a single-leg ergometer or UBE. Once the patient shows improved motion and reduced pain and swelling, light resistance exercises can begin for the involved leg. However, very light resistance should be encouraged because heavy and intense exercise, which leads to muscular hypertrophy, is contraindicated after fasciotomy for acute compartment syndromes.

The management of chronic exercise-induced compartment syndromes is similar to that of acute compartment syndromes. However, chronic compartment syndromes do not represent a surgical emergency. Therefore subcutaneous fasciotomy should be used only when pain and symptoms affect function. The postoperative management of fasciotomy after chronic compartment syndromes parallels the rehabilitation program outlined for acute compartment syndromes.

ANKLE FRACTURES

The most widely accepted classification of ankle fractures is described by **Lauge–Hansen.**[29] The organization and classification of ankle fractures frequently involve the direction of force, which results in specific patterns of injury (Fig. 18-20). For example, a Lauge–Hansen pronation-abduction or pronation-lateral rotation injury may result in a malleolar or bimalleolar fracture of the ankle (Fig. 18-21).

Ankle fractures include lateral malleolar fractures, medial malleolar fractures, bimalleolar fractures (combined medial and lateral malleolar fractures), and trimalleolar fractures (bimalleolar fractures plus the

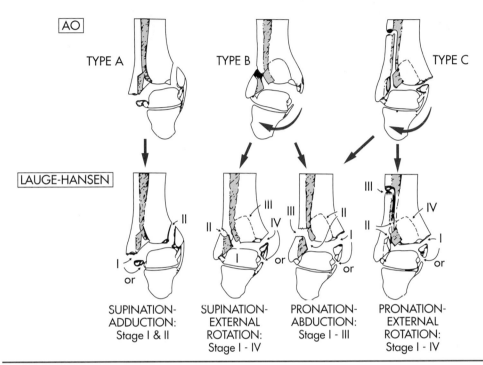

Fig. 18-20 AO and Lauge–Hansen classification of ankle fractures. (From Sangeorzan BJ, Hansen ST: Ankle and foot: trauma. In Poss R, ed. Orthopaedic Knowledge Update III. Park Ridge, IL, American Academy of Orthopaedic Surgeons, 1990.)

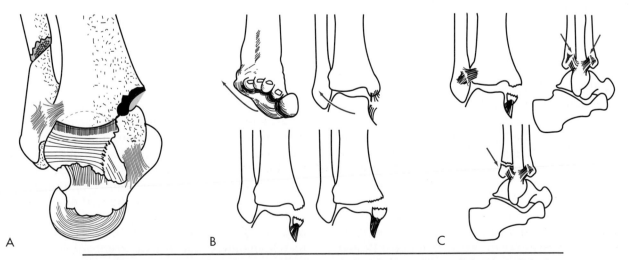

Fig. 18-21 **A,** Pronation-lateral rotation injury; **B,** Pronation-abduction injuries; **C,** Pronation-abduction injury. (From McRae R: Practical Fracture Treatment, 3rd ed. New York, Churchill Livingstone, 1994.)

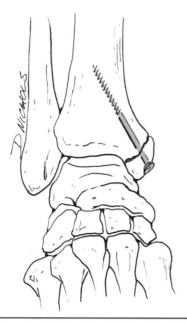

Fig. 18-22 Open reduction with internal fixation screw fixation for medial malleolar fracture.

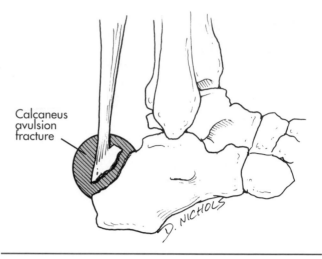

Fig. 18-23 Fractured calcaneus type II with avulsion.

posterior margin of the tibia). Most fractures are managed with an open reduction with internal fixation (ORIF) procedure. Typically, these fractures are fixed with various screws and plates to hold the fragments in place (Fig. 18-22).

In many cases of ankle fractures repaired with an ORIF procedure, the patient is in a semirigid postoperative removable splint for 2 weeks. This splint can be removed to allow for active dorsiflexion and plantar flexion ROM exercises. Because of the mechanism of injury that caused the malleolar fracture and the position of the internal fixation devices, no inversion or eversion exercises are performed.

A walking cast is applied once the patient achieves full plantar flexion and dorsiflexion ROM. Before casting, the surgical wound must be fully closed, sutures removed, infection absent, and no drainage present. A general full-body conditioning program is prescribed throughout immobilization. Both aerobic fitness and strengthening exercises are advocated also.

ROM exercises, isometric strengthening, stationary cycling, and weight bearing exercises are begun once the cast is removed. Progressive exercises employ latex rubber tubing, manual resistive exercises, proprioception exercises, and isokinetic strengthening. The PTA must be acutely aware of the signs and symptoms of possible hardware loosening (increased pain, swelling, crepitus, and motion) so as to swiftly inform the PT and make all necessary modifications in the present program. If, for example, after cast removal following an ORIF procedure for a medial malleolar fracture the PTA

recognized increased swelling and complaints of crepitus when strengthening exercises were increased, stressing inversion of the ankle, the PTA should halt those particular exercises and inform the PT.

DISTAL TIBIA COMPRESSION FRACTURES (PILON FRACTURES)

Distal tibia compression fractures (pilon fractures) occur as a result of vertical or axial loads that "drive" or compress the tibia into the talus. The initial management of these injuries usually involves an ORIF procedure, external fixation, or skeletal traction with a calcaneal pin.[29] Because of the nature of these fractures, weight bearing activities usually are deferred for as long as 12 or more weeks. Weight bearing creates vertical compression and compromises the natural course of healing needed for a stable outcome. Secondary osteoarthritis is a common complication with severe multifragmented compression fractures.[29] Typically throughout immobilization, a general conditioning program is allowed as long as no weight bearing occurs.

After immobilization, active motion and general ankle strengthening exercises are performed to the patient's tolerance. Care is taken to protect the articular surface of the distal tibia and talus. Initially, non–weight bearing strengthening exercises and ROM maneuvers are allowed. Progressive loading (compression) can proceed cautiously using latex surgical tubing for long-sitting plantar flexion strengthening. Partial weight bearing repetitive motion activities, such as a stationary bicycle ergometer, can be used to enhance ankle motion and endurance. Weight bearing activities generally are painful until satisfactory healing has occurred. However, toe-touch weight bearing progressing to partial weight

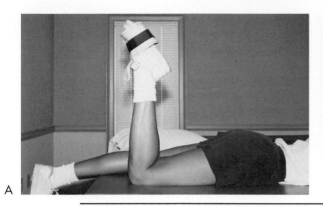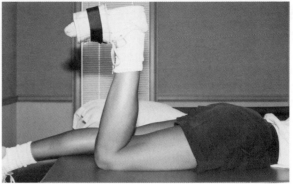

A   B

Fig. 18-24   Prone gastroc-soleus strengthening. **A,** Starting position with the knee of the affected limb flexed to 90 degrees. **B,** The patient actively plantar flexes the foot against gravity and the applied resistance.

bearing is well tolerated, helps restore proprioception, and assists with healing.

CALCANEAL FRACTURES

Calcaneal fractures are intraarticular depression fractures usually caused by falls from a height and resulting in compression of the calcaneus from the talus (Fig. 18-23). McRae[29] describes seven common patterns of calcaneal fractures:
1. Vertical fractures of the calcaneal tuberosity
2. Horizontal fractures
3. Fractures of the sustentaculum tali
4. Anterior calcaneal fractures
5. Fracture of the body of the calcaneus without involvement of the subtalar joint
6. Calcaneal fractures with lateral displacement and involvement of the subtalar joint
7. Central calcaneus crushing fractures

Depending on the type of fracture pattern, the patient can be treated conservatively with casting or an ORIF procedure.[29] Physical therapy management begins when the patient is casted (with or without ORIF) and as pain allows. Active and active assisted plantar flexion with inversion and dorsiflexion with eversion usually are allowed. Supportive measures to control pain and swelling are used as necessary. The cornerstone in recovering from a calcaneal fracture lies in regaining motion and strengthening the plantar flexors. Multiangle isometric plantar flexion can be initiated and progressed to full ROM manual resistance dorsiflexion and plantar flexion. The use of latex rubber tubing for plantar flexion in a long-seated position is an appropriate and challenging calf-strengthening exercise during the moderate-protection phase of rehabilitation. Strengthening of the soleus can be achieved by having

the patient lie prone with the affected leg flexed 90 degrees at the knee and placing ankle weights around the foot of the affected leg (Fig. 18-24).

FRACTURES OF THE TALUS

The talus can be fractured by falling from a height and landing on the foot in a crouched position.[29] This produces an axial compression load between the talus and calcaneus. There are four classifications of **talar fractures:**[29]

Type I: Talar neck fracture without displacement
Type II: Talar fracture with subtalar subluxation (the incidence of avascular necrosis is as high as 50%)[29]
Type III: Talar fracture with further subtalar subluxation (the incidence of avascular necrosis is as high as 85%)[29]
Type IV: The talar head dislocates from the navicular in association with a type III injury

These fractures can be treated with closed reduction and cast immobilization or with an ORIF procedure. To allow for proper healing, these fractures require 3 months of non–weight bearing. The rehabilitation program can proceed during this immobilization period with single-leg stationary cycling, aerobic training, or a UBE. Strengthening exercises include knee extension and hamstring curl maneuvers and non–weight bearing hip abduction, adduction, flexion, and extension. Usually the patient is immobilized in a posterior splint that can be removed for exercise periods. ROM exercises and supportive measures for pain and swelling control can be used during the maximum-protection phase of the rehabilitation program.

Osteoarthritis is a common long-term complication with talar fractures because of the duration of immobilization and non–weight bearing status.

STRESS FRACTURES OF THE FOOT AND ANKLE

A stress fracture is a partial or complete fracture of bone caused by unrelenting stress and force that do not allow for osteoblastic repair of bone and in turn cause accelerated bone resorption. Common sites for stress fractures in the foot and ankle are the metatarsals, lateral malleolus, Os calcis, navicular, and sesamoid.

Clinically, pain is the predominant feature of a stress fracture. The pain usually increases with activity and subsides with rest. The incidence of stress fractures in the foot and ankle is related in part to participation in demanding physical activity. If stress and forces are applied to bone and are not removed to allow the bone to repair, osteoclast activity overtakes the rate of osteoblast activity and stress fractures occur.

The development of stress fractures can be viewed in part as resulting from a linear progression or continuum of excessive external forces that lead to intrinsic reactions of muscle, bone, and periosteum. For example, with increased muscular forces resulting from continued and excessive use (marathon running, recreational jogging, aerobic dance, or occupations that require standing or walking all day) there is an associated increased rate of bone remodeling around the area of increased stress.[37] If the stress is not removed, this increase in bone remodeling is followed by a greater rate of bone resorption. If the stress continues, the bone eventually responds by developing microfractures, periosteal inflammation, and resultant stress fractures.[37] If stressed further, and the bone and soft tissues are not allowed to recover fully and heal properly, the development of linear fractures and ultimately displaced fractures can occur.[37]

There are certain stress fractures that pose a greater risk of delayed union, nonunion, and displacement than others.[28] The base or proximal diaphysis of the fifth metatarsal is described as "no-man's-land" and is "at risk" for delayed union or nonunion after a stress fracture.[28,34] Usually, complete rigid-cast immobilization is indicated for a period of 6 to 8 weeks when conservative, relative rest has failed to arrest symptoms of pain.[28,34,35] Other stress fractures termed *at risk*[22] are tarsal navicular fracture, sesamoid fractures, and all intraarticular fractures.

The management of not-at-risk[28] stress fractures of the foot and ankle can be effectively rehabilitated with activity modification; relative rest; therapeutic agents to relieve pain and swelling; and specific leg, ankle, and foot stretching and strengthening exercises. For example, the therapist may suggest arch strengthening exercises with the use of marbles, gastroc strengthening, dorsiflexion strengthening, ankle eversion-and-inversion exercises, and closed kinetic chain proprioception exercises. Low-impact aerobic exercise is useful in athletic patients who run a great deal. For example, instead of running or jogging, the patient can use a stationary cycle ergonometer, UBE, or stair stepper, or run in a non–weight bearing manner under water.

For stress fractures of the foot and ankle that are at risk[28] (fifth metatarsal, navicular sesamoids, and intraarticular fractures), more caution is necessary during the advancement of closed-chain activities to protect the healing bone from unwanted forces. With at-risk stress fractures, some form of external support can be used to brace the area. Usually some type of bracing, padding, casting, or orthosis is applied to control stress and forces to the healing bone.[28] The application of therapeutic exercises must be approached cautiously. Submaximal isometric exercises are encouraged initially. Active ROM and light concentric and eccentric loads are added as pain allows. Obviously, vertical compressive loads and shearing forces (i.e., jumping, running, cutting) are strictly prohibited to allow proper healing. Modifications in aerobic activity and general physical conditioning can allow the patient to continue to participate in strenuous physical conditioning, provided no stress is applied to the healing tissues. The initiation of closed-chain functional activities must be deferred until radiographic confirmation by the physician documents stable bone healing.

MEDIAL TIBIAL STRESS SYNDROME

Musculoskeletal overuse injuries of the lower leg involving the distal third of the posterior medial border of the tibia have historically been referred to as shin splints. This term has no place in orthopedic management and should be discarded as a nonspecific term used to describe any pain occurring in the lower leg.[1] A more precise and descriptive term is *medial tibial stress syndrome*, which describes pain over the distal and middle thirds of the tibia along the posterior medial border.[3] Differential assessment by the physician and PT includes stress fractures of the tibia and fibula, ischemic disorders, and deep compartment syndromes of the lower leg. Therefore medial tibial stress syndrome includes musculotendinous inflammation and periosteal inflammation of the muscle–tendon–bone interface at the posterior medial border of the tibia.

Specifically, the tissues most often responsible for the pain associated with medial tibial stress syndrome include the posterior tibialis muscle and medial origin of the soleus muscle.[1,30] Investigators have shown through cadaver dissection, electromyographic studies, and bone scans that clinical findings of pain associated with medial tibial stress correlate with the medial origin of the soleus and not the posterior tibialis muscle.[30] However, excessive traction on the posterior tibialis muscle and tendon (which originates at posterior surfaces of the tibia, interosseous membrane, and fibula and inserts into the undersurfaces of the navicular, all three cuneiforms and the second, third, and fourth metatarsals) can occur from excessive foot pronation, thus causing stress and strain on supporting soft tissue of the lower leg.[1]

Because pain is the predominant feature of medial tibial stress syndrome, it is helpful to classify and describe the severity of pain related to the patient's ability to perform activities.[18] Grade I describes pain that is experienced after activities. Grade II defines pain felt both during and after activities that does not affect the actual performance of activities. Grade III pain is felt before, during, and after activities and affects the patient's ability to perform activities. Grade IV pain is so significant that no activities can even be attempted.

In general, grade I pain refers to muscle soreness and minor soft-tissue inflammation. Grade II pain is viewed as a mild or moderate soft-tissue inflammation. Grade III pain involves significant soft-tissue inflammation and bone microfractures. Grade IV pain defines an actual stress fracture.

A patient experiencing minor pain (grade I) typically describes transient muscle soreness and general tenderness after activities. Treatment generally consists of ice packs or ice massage, physician-prescribed NSAIDs, rest, and gradual stretching and strengthening exercises for the entire lower leg.

With grade II pain, the patient is able to localize the exact site of the pain and typically has had symptoms for a few weeks.[18] It is significant to note that along with treatments involving ice, medications, and exercise, the therapist makes a significant attempt to decrease the volume of activity and to modify activities that exacerbate the pain. A reduction of 10% to 25% of the total volume of activity usually is appropriate to allow for sufficient healing.[18]

With a major soft-tissue inflammation (grade III) the patient is able to clearly define an exact or focal area of pain (point tenderness). The patient may demonstrate other evidence of inflammation, including heat, erythema, swelling, and crepitus. Because of the significance of pain and dysfunction associated with grade III pain that is localized to the posterior medial border of the tibia, the physician may order a bone scan in addition to radiographs to determine whether periosteal inflammation and bone breakdown are present. Treatment of major soft-tissue inflammation focuses on pain and swelling reduction. Therapeutic interventions includes ice packs or ice massage, oral analgesics, NSAIDs, complete rest from the aggravating activity, and specific stretching exercises for the gastroc-soleus complex, intrinsic foot musculature, and posterior tibialis. Upon resumption of activities, a 25% to 75% reduction in frequency is warranted until full pain-free motion is achieved. This grade of pain can be considered a prestress fracture syndrome if not managed appropriately. The condition can worsen if stress is not removed.

Grade IV pain usually is constant, and activity is severely affected. In addition to the five cardinal signs of inflammation (redness, swelling, pain, heat, and dysfunction), the patient may demonstrate reduced ROM and muscular atrophy.[18] This level of pain signifies a breakdown of the periosteal–bone interface and a stress fracture. Complete rest, crutches, ice, medications, therapeutic agents, iontophoresis, and phonophoresis may be indicated to control swelling and pain.

In general terms, treatment of medial tibial stress syndrome is highly individualized and specifically related to the comprehensive evaluation performed by the PT. If the PT determines that the patient demonstrates excessive foot pronation, custom molded orthotics may be prescribed to relieve stress on the medial soleus and reduce traction on the tibialis posterior muscle and tendon. Cryokinetics (ice packs or ice massage in conjunction with stretching and strengthening exercises) usually are advocated as a means to control pain and swelling and encourage motion and function. Relative rest is prescribed in most cases of medial tibial stress syndrome. That is, instead of complete rest and immobilization, the patient's activity level is modified to accommodate the patient's complaints of pain and dysfunction. For example, a patient who is an avid jogger may be encouraged to jog in a pool instead. If a UBE is available, the patient can still actively perform aerobic conditioning activities without the associated stress on the lower leg. Overall, modifications in the patient's activity level (relative rest) and the judicious use of physician-prescribed NSAIDs or analgesics, and a highly specific gastroc-soleus stretching program and lower-leg strengthening regimen, prove effective in the management of medial tibial stress syndrome.

PLANTAR FASCIITIS (HEEL SPUR SYNDROME)

Chronic inflammation of the plantar aponeurosis, with or without an associated calcaneal heel spur, is called **plantar fasciitis** (Fig. 18-25). Leach and co-workers[25] describe plantar fasciitis as repetitive microtrauma leading to injury, attempted repair, and chronic inflammation. Brody[6] describes plantar fasciitis as an "inflammatory reaction due to chronic traction on the plantar aponeurosis (fascia) at its insertion into the calcaneus."

Patients frequently complain of pain along the medial border of the calcaneus on the plantar surface. Many patients report that pain is worse in the morning when the foot contacts the floor in getting out of bed. Palpation of the plantar fascia usually reveals tenderness at the medial tuberosity of the os calcis or throughout the entire course of the fascia.[4] Palpation is performed with the toes flexed, which reduces tension on the fascia, or with the toes extended, which increases tension on the fascia.[4]

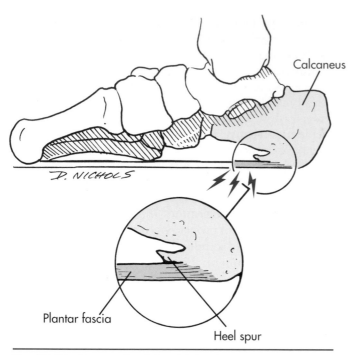

D. NICHOLS

Calcaneus

Plantar fascia

Heel spur

Fig. 18-25 Plantar fasciitis with heel spur.

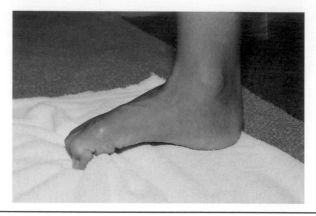

Fig. 18-26 Resistive toe curls are performed by gripping a towel.

Management

Many patients respond well to conservative physical therapy procedures. All causative factors must first be eliminated or modified for healing to proceed. Ice massage or ice packs and physician-prescribed NSAIDs along with a plastic heel cup are initial management procedures used to reduce pain and swelling. Specific stretching exercises are employed to help reduce tension on the plantar fascia. General calf-stretching exercises are initiated and progressed according to the patient's tolerance. Specific soleus-stretching exercises also are used. Occasionally ultrasound, phonophoresis, or iontophoresis is used to reduce pain and swelling. Additional stretching exercises should include toe-extension stretches with a towel. Specific strengthening exercises can be used to strengthen the intrinsic and extrinsic foot muscles as pain and swelling improve.

Toe curls are effective when used in conjunction with stretching, ice, or ultrasound (Fig. 18-26). The picking up of marbles with the toes or the repeated "gripping" with the toes of a towel placed on the floor strengthens the foot muscles.

The physician may inject a local steroid to help decrease pain and swelling in more severe cases. Because many patients complain that the most severe pain is in the morning, some physicians and PTs prescribe night splints, which place the foot in a position that decreases stress on the plantar fascia. In an athletic population, plantar fasciitis occurs from running and competitive sports participation. During recovery from plantar fasciitis, it is imperative to maintain aerobic fitness and general body strength. Aerobic exercises can be performed without weight bearing in a pool or with a UBE to decrease repetitive loading on the plantar fascia. Stationary cycling is an excellent alternative.

With some patients who do not respond to conservative therapy, the physician may decide to correct the problem surgically. Surgical options include plantar fascia release (fasciotomy) and excision of calcaneal exostosis (spur).

ARCH DEFORMITIES (PES PLANUS AND PES CAVUS)

Pes planus (flatfoot) is a congenital or acquired deformity of the foot where the medial longitudinal arch of the foot is reduced, causing the medial border of the foot to contact the ground when a person is standing.[26] The usual cause of acquired pes planus is muscular weakness, laxity of ligaments that support the medial longitudinal arch, paralysis, or a pronated foot.[26] Pes planus deformity can be classified as mild, moderate, or severe.[32]

During the initial evaluation, the PT measures the degree of hindfoot (tibiofibular joints; talocrural joint articulation between the talus, medial malleolus of the tibia, and the lateral malleolus of the fibula; and the subtalar joint) and forefoot (tarsometatarsal joints, intermetatarsal joints, metatarsal-phalangeal joints, and interphalangeal joints) varus, and valgus.[26] A 4- to 6-degree hindfoot valgus and a 4- to 6-degree forefoot varus is classified as a mild pes planus. A moderate pes planus is associated with a 6- to 10-degree hindfoot valgus and a 6- to 10-degree forefoot varus. Severe pes planus results from a 10- to 15-degree hindfoot valgus and an 8- to 10-degree forefoot varus. In addition, the PT assesses the deformity in weight bearing and non–weight bearing positions.[35] With a rigid pes planus deformity, the foot appears to have an abnormally low arch in both weight bearing and non–weight bearing

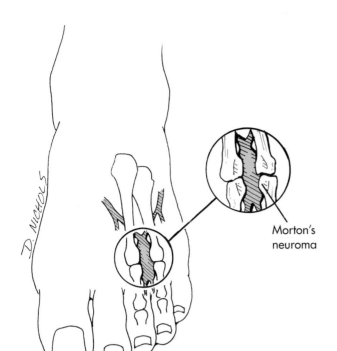

Fig. 18-27 Morton's neuroma.

positions.[35] With a flexible pes planus deformity, the foot appears to have a normal arch in a non–weight bearing position, but an abnormally low or flat arch in weight bearing.

No specific therapeutic interventions are necessary if there is no associated pain or dysfunction. However, because the area is a terminal component of the closed kinetic chain during weight bearing (the arch can affect the knee, hip, and spine in a closed kinetic chain), treatment that is specific to the arch may be indicated if associated pain and dysfunction are experienced in other joints along the kinetic chain. For example, pes planus can affect the normal neutral-to-pronation sequence of the foot during the gait cycle. Because the foot is already pronated (with pes planus), the reduced normalized motion from neutral to pronation is affected during gait. Therefore the knee and other joints along the kinetic chain must compensate for this reduced motion. If pain and resultant dysfunction occur in one or more of these associated joints, then corrective action is necessary to place the foot in a more neutral position to enhance the normal physiologic motion of the entire kinetic chain. Usually the use of a custom-fabricated orthotic is indicated to create a more normal mechanical arch. An orthosis or orthotic device is defined as an "apparatus or appliance that is used to correct or control a structural abnormality of a body part."[9] Materials used in orthotics include cork, leather, rubber, foam, felt, and plastic.[9] The rationale for the use of a custom-molded orthotic to correct a symptomatic pes planus is sup-

ported by the work of D'Ambrosia,[13] who documented that 90% of patients with pes planovalgus reported effective relief of symptoms with the use of orthotics.

Pes cavus, on the other hand, describes an abnormally high arch.[26,35] Pes cavus usually is a result of neurogenic pathologic processes, muscle imbalances, and congenital abnormalities; both medial and lateral longitudinal arches are affected. Clinically, patients may complain of painful calluses beneath the metatarsal heads because of the mechanical friction and pressure that occur with metatarsal heads. Osteoarthritic changes are not uncommon in the tarsal area because of the altered biomechanics of the foot.

Treatment for pes cavus is focused on pain and dysfunction. No treatment is indicated if no symptoms exist, although the PT may document this deformity during a lower-quarter evaluation. Felt pads can be used to control the pain of metatarsal head callosities. Unfortunately, D'Ambrosia[13] found little benefit (25%) from the use of orthotics with patients who have pes cavus.

MORTON'S NEUROMA (PLANTAR INTERDIGITAL NEUROMA)

Patients with a **neuroma** may complain of diffuse, occasionally radiating pain into the toes and proximally to the dorsal or plantar surface of the foot.[11] A neuroma usually occurs at the 3-4 interspace and less frequently at the 2-3 interspace[31] (Fig. 18-27). Morton's neuroma occurs bilaterally only 15% of the time, with the patient complaining of a "burning," "cramping," or "catching" sensation.[11,31] A painful mass can be palpated in approximately one third of the cases.[31]

Treatment

Conservative care calls for the use of a metatarsal pad; change of footwear to a wider, softer shoe; and local corticosteroid injections. Surgical excision of the neuroma may be necessary when all attempts at conservative care fail to relieve pain.

Physical therapy care involves early active motion to limit postoperative stiffness and fibrosis. Postoperative care dictates that the patient be weight bearing as tolerated and progressed to full weight bearing as pain allows. Compression bandages are used with elastic tape to assist with swelling and pain management. Generally, physical therapy care begins 2 to 3 weeks after surgery, once the sutures are removed. Typically, however, patients are encouraged to perform active ankle, foot, and knee ROM exercises during the early healing phase before physical therapy is begun.

Thermal agents used to reduce swelling and pain include whirlpool baths and cryotherapy. In addition, ultrasound can be used under water in conjunction with active motion exercises to improve circulation, reduce tissue congestion, and improve motion. Active ROM

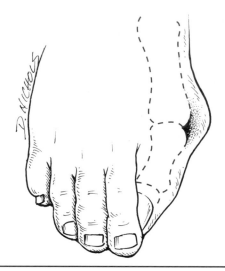

Fig. 18-28 Hallux valgus.

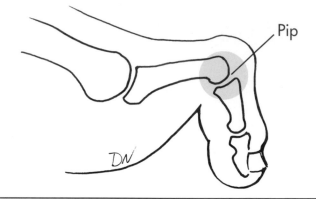

Fig. 18-29 Hammer toe.

exercises include ankle motion in all directions, knee flexion and extension, and specific toe extension exercises with toe curls and splaying of the toes as tolerated. Occasionally, passive mobilization of the metatarsals may be needed to avoid the development of movement limitations. Strengthening exercises can be initiated as soon as the pain allows.

All strengthening exercises for the ankle and knee are included with specific intrinsic foot strengthening exercises. Resistive toe curls can begin as an open kinetic chain exercise and progress to a closed kinetic chain exercise as strength and patient tolerance allow.

General body strengthening exercises and aerobic fitness are encouraged during all phases of recovery from surgical resection of a Morton's neuroma.

HALLUX VALGUS

Hallux valgus is a lateral or valgus deviation of the great toe with both soft tissue and bony deformity (Fig. 18-28). This condition is made worse by improper footwear (narrow toe box), and often the pain can be relieved by removing the shoes. Examination should include assessment of the deformity in a standing position, which often accentuates the deformity,[11,31] and measurement of the hallux valgus angle (normal is <15 degrees) to determine the degree of deformity and angle of deviation.

Management options include both conservative care and operative procedures. Initial care is supportive, with a change in footwear to include a wider toe box (this alone can significantly reduce symptoms), insoles, arch supports (orthotics), and pads to dissipate stress and relieve pain. Modifications in activity may reduce symptoms profoundly. In an athletic population, changing from running activities to swimming or bicycling can

reduce pain caused by the repetitive pounding of running.

Many surgical options are available, depending on the severity of the deformity. General physical therapy management of postoperative bunionectomy is designed to reduce pain and swelling, improve ROM, and increase strength to enable a return to normal daily activities. Generally, the patient wears a wooden-soled shoe, progressing to an open-toed sandal. Gauze padding and toe spacers are used to maintain proper alignment after the surgical procedure. Once the sutures are removed and the wounds closed, whirlpool treatments can begin, with active ROM exercises for both flexion and extension of the great toe. Manual resistive toe extension and toe flexion exercises can begin as pain allows. Gait mechanics must be reviewed carefully and correct walking encouraged after bunionectomy. Usually weight bearing patterns and restrictions of movement affect proper gait mechanics, especially the strength, power, and motion needed for toe-off. Restoration of joint motion and stability, and toe flexion and extension strength, form the foundation of the rehabilitation program.

LESSER TOE DEFORMITIES (HAMMER TOES, MALLET TOES, AND CLAW TOES)

Three distinct types of lesser toe deformities are **hammer toes, mallet toes, and claw toes.** All three deformities are worsened by wearing improper shoes (narrow toe box).

Hammer toe (Fig. 18-29) is characterized by deformity of the metatarsophalangeal (MTP) joint, proximal interphalangeal (PIP) joint, and distal interphalangeal (DIP) joint. The MTP joint is either in neutral position or extension. The PIP joint is held in flexion with the DIP joint in either flexion or extension.

Mallet toe (Fig. 18-30) is characterized by a neutral MTP joint, a neutral PIP joint, and a flexed DIP joint.

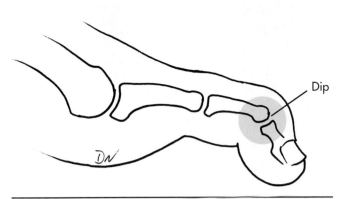

Fig. 18-30 Mallet toe.

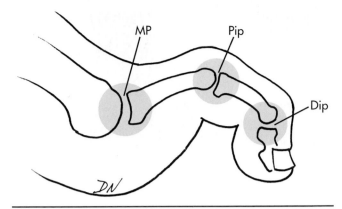

Fig. 18-31 Claw toe.

Claw toes (Fig. 18-31) often are associated with neuromuscular disease and are similar in appearance to hammer toes. Claw toes are distinguished by MTP hyperextension, PIP flexion, and DIP flexion. This deformity usually results from "simultaneous contraction of the extensors and flexors."[31]

The physician or PT determines if the lesser toe deformity is either rigid (fixed) or flexible. Flexible deformities usually are correctable with conservative, passive measures, whereas fixed deformities may require surgery.

Management and Rehabilitation

Nonoperative conservative care of lesser toe deformities focuses on modifying activities that exacerbate pain, changing footwear to a wider, softer toe box (to avoid pressure and the occurrence of soft or hard callus formation over bony prominences), padding areas subjected to blistering and corn formation, and using supportive measures to reduce pain and swelling (such as custom fabricated orthotics or "off-the-shelf" orthotics). Whirlpool baths, ultrasound, stretching exercises for the toes, and foot and ankle strengthening exercises may help reduce pain and swelling.

Surgical repair is reserved for fixed or rigid deformities, although some flexible deformities also require operation. Typically, sutures and pins are removed about 3 weeks after surgery.[11] The patient is weight bearing as tolerated initially, with a progression to full weight bearing as pain allows. The affected extremity is held in a rigid-solid open-toe postsurgical boot to protect the repair from unwanted excessive flexion and extension of the toes.

For approximately 6 weeks after surgery, taping, padding, and protecting the repair are emphasized before progressing to weight bearing toe-off proper gait mechanics. This time is necessary to protect the surgical repair and to allow for the healing of bone and tendons (tenotomies are done for flexible lesser toe deformities). Throughout the rehabilitation program, from the immediate postoperative period until discharge, maintain

strength, flexibility, and aerobic fitness. The affected extremity may be strengthened with open-chain resistive exercises (knee extension and leg curls), and aerobic fitness can be achieved with a stationary bike ergometer with the seat height lowered to maintain a neutral ankle position at the bottom of the pedal stroke. If the patient cannot operate the bike in this fashion, the opposite, uninvolved extremity can be used alone (single-leg pedaling) using toe clips. A UBE also can be an effective aerobic conditioning tool during rehabilitation.

Once the pins and sutures are removed at 3 weeks, physical therapy management can begin. Whirlpool baths, ultrasound, active ROM, and gentle stretching and strengthening exercises (open-chain progressing to closed-chain toe curls with a towel or marbles) can be employed. The toes must be protected from unwanted stress throughout the maximum-protection phase (6 to 8 weeks after surgery) of rehabilitation. Coughlin[11] recommends avoiding all running activities for 9 to 12 weeks after surgery to allow for proper healing.

COMMON MOBILIZATION TECHNIQUES FOR THE ANKLE, FOOT, AND TOES

Limitations of movement resulting from fibrosis after trauma, surgery, or disease of the foot, ankle, or toes frequently require specific mobilization procedures to regain normal joint function. Mobilization techniques typically are used in conjunction with thermal modalities to control pain and swelling and aid in relaxation; these modalities include hot packs, ultrasound, whirlpool baths, and ice packs. Active and passive exercises, specific stretching exercises, strengthening exercises (open progressing to closed chain), and proprioception tasks help the patient regain balance, coordination, and function. The choice of mobilization technique, direction of application, grades, amplitude of force, velocity, oscillations, and distractions is made by the PT based on the specific pathologic condition involved, tissue-healing constraints, and overall appropriateness with

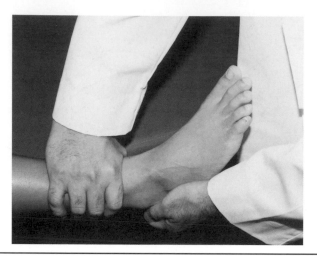

Fig. 18-32   Anterior glide of the calcaneus.

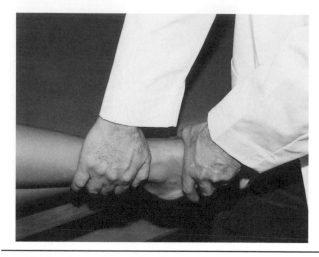

Fig. 18-33   Posterior glide of the talus.

regard to the short- and long-term goals of the rehabilitation program.

The following techniques are general procedures used for a wide variety of specific joint limitations. These techniques can be modified by the PT depending on the specific nature of the limitations involved. This list is not intended to be a comprehensive review of all techniques for each joint of the ankle, foot, and toes. These methods are commonly used, easily practiced, effective procedures for treating a host of joint limitations. It is clinically relevant to restate that the delegation of selected mobilization techniques to be used by the PTA is entirely at the discretion of the PT and peripheral joint mobilization is not universally accepted as a routine domain of practice of the PTA. Information concerning peripheral joint mobilization has been provided as a means to stimulate the PTA's awareness of the rationale for improving motion and for the reduction of pain as identified and prescribed by the PT.

Ankle Mobilization

Anterior and posterior glides are best performed with the patient in a supine or "long-sitting" position with the lower leg firmly and comfortably supported. For anterior glide of the calcaneus, the hand position, stabilization, and direction of force are similar to those for the anterior drawer test for ligament stability testing of the anterior talofibular ligament. One hand should be placed firmly on the distal anterior surface of the tibia and fibula. The application hand should be used to firmly "cup" the calcaneus and provide an anterior-directed force (Fig. 18-32).

The posterior glide technique is performed with the patient in the same position as the anterior glide. The distal tibia and fibula should be stabilized with the palm of one hand. The application hand should be placed on the dorsal surface of the talus to provide a posterior-directed force (Fig. 18-33).

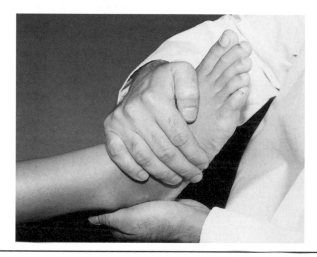

Fig. 18-34   Long-axis distraction of the talus.

Traction is achieved through long-axis distraction of the talus caudally from the tibia and fibula. The patient can be supine or prone with the lower leg firmly and comfortably supported. The dorsal surface of the talus should be firmly grasped with the open palm of one hand, while the other hand is used to firmly grasp and cup the calcaneus. The force should be applied simultaneously with both hands along the long axis of the tibia and fibula (Fig. 18-34), effectively distracting the talus from the mortise.

Metatarsal Mobilization

Distal metatarsal glides are performed while the patient is supine with the lower leg supported. The hand, thumb, and fingers of one hand should be used to stabilize the ray of the second metatarsal while the hand, thumb, and fingers of the application hand firmly grasp the first ray at the metatarsal head. Force should be applied in a plantar and dorsal direction (Fig. 18-35).

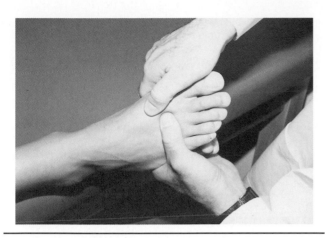

Fig. 18-35 Distal metatarsal anterior-posterior glides.

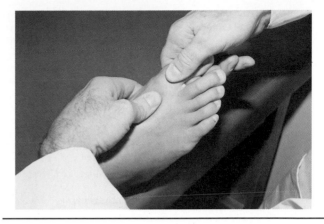

Fig. 18-37 Proximal interphalangeal plantar and dorsal glides.

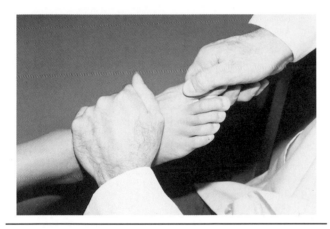

Fig. 18-36 Long-axis proximal interphalangeal distraction.

Proximal Interphalangeal Joint Mobilization

Long-axis distraction of the PIP joint is achieved by stabilizing the affected metatarsal ray with one hand while using the application hand to firmly grasp the affected phalanx. The thumb and fingers apply long-axis traction (distraction) (Fig. 18-36).

Plantar and dorsal PIP glides are performed with the patient supine and the lower leg supported. One hand should be used to firmly grasp the first metatarsal ray at the metatarsal head. The thumb of the stabilizing hand must be placed on the dorsal surface of the metatarsal head. The application hand should be used to grasp the proximal phalanx and apply a plantar and dorsal force while stabilizing the metatarsal head (Fig. 18-37).

❖ ADDITIONAL FEATURES

Calcaneus Fracture: A calcaneus fracture that heals in a varus position locks the subtalar joint in inversion, creating a rigid transverse tarsal joint.

Charcot's Neuropathy: Diabetes is the leading cause of this disorder. Joint destruction, bone resorption, and insensitivity to pain.

Freiberg's Infraction: Avascular necrosis of the metatarsal head.

Lisfranc's Fracture: Ligaments at the base of the second metatarsal connecting the medial cuneiform provide a keystone effect of stability; fracture-dislocation of the tarsometatarsal joint.

Os Trigonum: A nonunited lateral tubercle of the posterior talus. Radiographs demonstrate smooth edges of the os trigonum versus an acute fracture with "rough" edges.

Positive Talar Tilt: Tests integrity of both anterior talo-fibular ligament and calcaneo-fibular ligament. Both must be disrupted for a positive tilt.

Posterior Tibial Artery: Bifurcates into medial and lateral plantar arteries behind the medial malleolus.

Sesamoiditis: Repetitive stress or trauma of sesamoids at the plantar surface of the first (great toe) metatarsal.

Syndesmosis: Ligaments responsible for maintaining stability of the distal tibio-fibular articulation.

Tarsal Tunnel Syndrome: Tibial nerve entrapment with "burning" pain and paresthesias behind the medial malleolus radiating to the planar surface of the foot.

Tibial Nerve: Passes behind the medial malleolus.

Tibialis Posterior Tendon: Rupture results in planovalgus, or "flatfoot."

Talus: No muscle attachment origin or insertion. Has a tenuous blood supply.

REFERENCES

1. Andrish JT: The Leg. In DeLee JD, Drez D, eds. Orthopaedic Sports Medicine, Principles and Practice, vol 2. Philadelphia, WB Saunders, 1994.
2. Beskin JL, Sanders RA, Hunter SC, et al: Surgical repair of Achilles tendon ruptures. *Am J Sports Med* 1987;15:1–8.
3. Black HM, Brand RL: Injuries of the foot and ankle. In Scott NW, Nisonson B, Nicholas J, eds. Principles of Sports Medicine. Baltimore, Williams & Wilkins, 1984.
4. Bordelon RL: Heel pain. In DeLee JD, Drez D, eds. Orthopaedic Sports Medicine: Principles and Practice, vol 2. Philadelphia, WB Saunders, 1994.
5. Brand RL, Collins MDF, Templeton T: Surgical repair of ruptured lateral ankle ligaments. *Am J Sports Med* 1981;9:40–44.
6. Brody DM: Running injuries: prevention and management. *Clin Symp* 39:38, Ciba-Geigy, 1987.
7. Canale ST: Ankle injuries. In Crenshaw AH, ed. Campbell's Operative Orthopaedics, vol 3, 7th ed. St Louis, Mosby, 1987.

8. Chrisman OD, Snook G: Reconstruction of lateral ligament tears of the ankle: an experimental study and clinical evaluation of seven patients treated by a new modification of the Elmslie procedure. *J Bone Joint Surg* 196951A:904–912.

9. Clanton TO: Sport shoes, insoles and orthoses. In DeLee JD, Drez D, eds. Orthopaedic Sports Medicine: Principles and Practice, vol 2. Philadelphia, WB Saunders, 1994.

10. Conrad JJ, Tannin AH: Trauma to the ankle. In Jahss MH, ed. Disorders of the Foot. Philadelphia, WB Saunders, 1982.

11. Coughlin MJ: Conditions of the forefoot. In DeLee JD, Drez D, eds. Orthopaedic Sports Medicine: Principles and Practice, vol 2. Philadelphia, WB Saunders, 1994.

12. Curwin S, Stanish W: Tendinitis: its etiology and treatment. Lexington, MA, Callamore Press, 1984.

13. D'Ambrosia RD: Orthotic devices in running injuries. *Clin Sports Med* 1985;4:611–618.

14. Eckert WR, David EA: Acute rupture of the peroneal retinaculum. *J Bone Joint Surg* 1976;58A:670–673.

15. Evans DL: Recurrent instability of the ankle: a method of surgical treatment. *Proc R Soc Med* 1953;46:343–344.

16. Harper MC: The deltoid ligament: an evaluation of need for surgical repair. *Clin Orthop* 1988;226:156–168.

17. Inglis AE, Sculco TP: Surgical repair of ruptures of the tendon Achilles. *Clin Orthop* 1981;156:160–168.

18. Jackson DW: Shin-splints: an update. *Phys Sports Med* 1978; 6:101–161.

19. Jackson BA, Schwane JA, Starcher BC: Effect of ultrasound therapy on the repair of Achilles tendon injuries in rats. *Med Sci Sports Exer* 1991;23:271–176.

20. Jacobs D, Martens M, Van Audekercke R, et al: Comparison of conservative and operative treatment of Achilles tendon rupture. *Am J Sport Med* 1978;6:107–111.

21. Keene JS: Tendon injuries of the foot and ankle. In DeLee JD, Drez D, eds. Orthopaedic Sports Medicine: Principles and Practice, vol 2. Philadelphia, WB Saunders, 1994.

22. Lassiter TE, Malone TR, Garrett W: Injury to the lateral ligaments of the ankle. *Orthop Clin North Am* 1989;20:629–640.

23. Leach RE, James S, Wasilewski S: Achilles tendinitis. *Am J Sports Med* 1981;9:23–98.

24. Leach R. Acute ankle sprains: vigorous treatment for best results. *J Musculoskel Med* 1983;1:68–76.

25. Leach RE, Seavey MS, Salter DK: Results of surgery in athletes with plantar fasciitis. *Foot Ankle* 1986;7:161–356.

26. Magee DJ: Lower leg, ankle and foot. In Orthopaedic Physical Assessment, 2nd ed. Philadelphia, WB Saunders, 1992.

27. Marti R: Dislocation of the peroneal tendons. *Am J Sports Med* 1977;5:19–22.

28. McBryde A: Stress fractures of the foot and ankle In DeLee JD, Drez D, eds. Orthopaedic Sports Medicine: Principles and Practice, vol 2. Philadelphia, WB Saunders, 1994.

29. McRae R: Practical Fracture Treatment. New York, Churchill Livingstone, 1994.

30. Michael RH, Holder LE: The soleus syndrome: a cause of medial tibial stress (shin splints). *Am J Sports Med* 1985;13:27–94.

31. Miller M: Review of Orthopaedics. Philadelphia, WB Saunders, 1992.

32. Myerson MS: Injuries to the forefoot and toes. In Jahss MH, ed. Disorders of the Foot and Ankle: Medical and Surgical Management, vol 2, 2nd ed. Philadelphia, WB Saunders, 1991.

33. Nistor L: Surgical and nonsurgical treatment of Achilles tendon rupture. *J Bone Joint Surg* 1981;63A:394–399.

34. Renstrom P, AFH, Kannus P: Injuries of the foot and ankle. In DeLee JD, Drez D, eds. Orthopaedic Sports Medicine: Principles and Practice, vol 2. Philadelphia, WB Saunders, 1994.

35. Riddle DL: Foot and ankle. In Richardson JK, Iglarsh ZA, eds. Clinical Orthopaedic Physical Therapy. Philadelphia, WB Saunders, 1994.

36. Riehl R: Rehabilitation of lower leg injuries. In Prentice WE, ed. Rehabilitation Techniques in Sports Medicine, 2nd ed. St Louis, Mosby, 1994.

37. Stanitski CL, McMaster JH, Scranton PE, et al: On the nature of stress fractures. *Am J Sports Med* 1978;6:391–396.

38. Staples OS: Ruptures of the fibular collateral ligaments of the ankle: results study of immediate surgical treatment. *J Bone Joint Surg* 1975;57A:101–107.

39. Stover CN, Bryan D: Traumatic dislocation of peroneal tendons. *Am J Surg* 1962;103:180–186.

40. Watson-Jones R: Recurrent forward dislocation of the ankle joint. *J Bone Joint Surg* 1952;34B:519.

REVIEW QUESTIONS

Multiple Choice

1. What percentage of all ankle sprains occurs to the lateral ligament complex?
   A. 50%
   B. 65%
   C. 95%
   D. 85%

2. What is the primary mechanism of injury to the lateral ligament complex of the ankle?
   A. Eversion, plantar flexion
   B. Plantar flexion, adduction, and eversion
   C. Inversion, plantar flexion, and adduction
   D. Dorsiflexion, abduction, and eversion

3. The anterior drawer test is used to clinically examine which ligaments of the ankle?
   A. Posterior talofibular
   B. Anterior talofibular
   C. Fibulocalcaneal
   D. Deltoid
   E. All of the above

4. Which of the following represents potential pathologies that may be seen in conjunction with an inversion ankle sprain that is produced by inversion plantar flexion and adduction?
   A. Subluxing peroneal tendons
   B. Fracture of the base of the fifth metatarsal
   C. Malleolar fractures
   D. Sprains of the midfoot
   E. All of the above

5. Using the injury classification model described by Leach, which of the following describes a second-degree lateral ligament complex sprain of the ankle?
   A. The anterior talofibular ligament is completely torn.
   B. The anterior talofibular ligament and fibulocalcaneal ligaments are completely torn.
   C. All three ligaments are partially torn.
   D. The anterior talofibular and fibulocalcaneal ligaments are partially torn.

6. Which of the following best describes initial injury management of a grade II inversion ankle sprain?
   A. Short leg cast, crutches non–weight bearing (NWB)
   B. Rest, ice, compression, and elevation (RICE); crutches weight bearing as tolerated (WBAT)
   C. Ligament protection with semirigid external support, RICE, crutches, WBAT
   D. Cold whirlpool, crutches, NWB

7. Which of the following motions should be avoided during the acute and subacute phases of recovery from an inversion ankle sprain?
   A. Dorsiflexion
   B. Plantar flexion and inversion
   C. Eversion and dorsiflexion
   D. Plantar flexion and eversion
   E. All of the above

8. Deltoid ligament sprains of the ankle occur in what percentage of all ankle sprains?
   A. 10%
   B. 15%
   C. 7%
   D. 3% to 5%

9. Which of the following describe the mechanisms of injury for a deltoid ligament sprain of the ankle?
   A. Pronation and abduction
   B. Pronation and external rotation
   C. Supination and external rotation
   D. All of the above

10. What percentage of patients suffer from chronic weakness, swelling, pain, and instability after surgical repair or conservative treatment of inversion ankle sprains?
    A. 10% to 30%
    B. 15%
    C. 25%
    D. 3%

11. Mechanical instability is best defined as which of the following?
    A. Loss of joint proprioception
    B. Ligament laxity
    C. Subjective feeling of ankle giving way
    D. Mechanical block of normal joint motion

12. Functional instability is best described as which of the following?
    A. Ligament laxity
    B. Loss of muscular support
    C. Subjective sensation of joint instability
    D. Loss of gait proprioception

13. After surgery, if the peroneus brevis was used to stabilize the ankle, which of the following is (are) not allowed during the immediate postoperative period of recovery? (Circle any that apply.)
    A. Passive motions
    B. Active motions
    C. Manual resistance
    D. Eccentric contractions
    E. Plyometrics

14. Because functional ankle instabilities are classified as "giving way," a sense of instability without objective ligament laxity, the focus of rehabilitation is centered on which of the following?
    A. Pain relief
    B. Swelling reduction
    C. Proprioception drills and closed-chain resistance exercises
    D. Anaerobic power

15. Which of the following is the treatment of choice in cases of acute subluxing peroneal tendons?
    A. Surgery
    B. Immediate rehabilitation
    C. Immobilization, NWB gait, and progressive rehabilitation
    D. Immobilization followed by full active range of motion (ROM)

16. Chronic subluxing peroneal tendons require which of the following?
    A. Immediate aggressive strengthening
    B. ROM exercises
    C. Casting followed by rehabilitation
    D. Surgery

17. In general, how many weeks of immobilization are necessary after surgery to correct chronic subluxing peroneal tendons?
    A. 2 weeks
    B. 6 weeks
    C. 16 weeks
    D. 9 weeks

18. Which of the following positions should be added cautiously after surgery to correct chronic subluxing peroneal tendons to allow for proper soft tissue and bone healing? (Circle any that apply.)
    A. Plantar flexion
    B. Inversion
    C. Dorsiflexion
    D. Eversion
    E. Terminal knee extension

19. Which of the following represents primary features of Achilles tendinitis?
    A. Muscular weakness
    B. Soft-tissue swelling at the mid-portion of the calf
    C. Specific localized pain at the distal[13] of the tendon and the insertion on the calcaneus
    D. A palpable gap

20. Which of the following is (are) the cause(s) of Achilles tendinitis? (Circle any that apply.)
    A. Sudden trauma (indirect)
    B. Direct trauma to the tendon
    C. Repetitive microtrauma
    D. Acute plantar flexion force
    E. Accumulative overload of the tendon

21. Which of the following represent(s) the most appropriate treatment for Achilles tendinitis? (Circle any that apply.)
    A. Surgery
    B. Cast immobilization
    C. Nonsteroidal antiinflammatory drugs, RICE
    D. Ultrasound, gentle ROM, progressive exercise
    E. NWB for 6 to 12 weeks

22. Which of the following describes the most common cause of a complete rupture of the Achilles tendon?
    A. Excessive, sudden plantar flexion
    B. Inversion
    C. Eversion
    D. Dorsiflexion

23. Where does the Achilles tendon rupture most commonly?
    A. At the musculotendinous junction of the gastrocnemius
    B. Midcalf
    C. 6 to 10 cm proximal to its insertion on the calcaneus
    D. 3 to 4 cm proximal to its insertion on the calcaneus

24. Ruptures of the Achilles tendon occur most commonly in which of the following:
    A. 20- to 50-year-old women
    B. 15- to 20-year-old men
    C. 40- to 60-year-old women
    D. 20- to 50-year-old men

25. Clinically, to examine the affected leg for the presence of a ruptured Achilles tendon, the physical therapist (PT) performs which test?
    A. Anterior drawer test
    B. Talar tilt test
    C. Thompson test
    D. Malleolar compression

26. Which of the following best describes how to perform the Thompson test?
    A. Patient supine, knee flexed, squeeze the affected calf
    B. Patient seated, knee flexed, squeeze the affected calf
    C. Patient prone, knee extended, squeeze the affected calf
    D. Patient prone, knee flexed, squeeze the affected calf

27. Which of the following generally describes the rate of rerupture of the Achilles tendon if it is treated nonoperatively?
    A. 10% to 20%
    B. 8% to 39%
    C. 50%
    D. 5% to 20%

28. The duration of immobilization of a ruptured Achilles tendon treated nonoperatively is usually how long?
    A. 4 to 6 weeks
    B. 8 weeks
    C. 16 weeks
    D. 10 days

29. During the immobilization of a ruptured Achilles tendon, which of the following treatments are employed?
    A. Quad and hamstring strengthening of the involved limb
    B. Total body conditioning
    C. Upper body ergometer (UBE)
    D. Stationary cycle ergometer
    E. All of the above

30. During nonoperative cast immobilization of a ruptured Achilles tendon, the affected ankle is placed in which position?
    A. Dorsiflexion
    B. Inversion
    C. Eversion
    D. Plantar flexion

31. When the cast is removed after nonoperative treatment of a ruptured Achilles tendon, the initial treatment consists of which of the following? (Circle any that apply.)
    A. Vigorous dorsiflexion exercise
    B. Thermal agents, very gradual dorsiflexion range of motion
    C. The use of a felt heel-lift to avoid excessive dorsiflexion
    D. Gentle active plantar flexion range of motion
    E. Ballistic stretching

32. The rehabilitation of postoperative repair of a ruptured Achilles tendon is which of the following?
    A. Much faster than nonoperative treatment
    B. Much slower than nonoperative treatment
    C. Very similar to nonoperative rehabilitation
    D. Much faster and does not follow the same criterion-based rehabilitation program as does operative rehabilitation

33. The organization and classification of ankle fractures described by Lauge–Hansen involve which of the following? (Circle any that apply.)
    A. The direction of force
    B. Specific patterns of injury
    C. The age of the patient
    D. The sex of the patient
    E. All of the above

34. Ankle fractures include which of the following?
    A. Lateral malleolar fractures
    B. Medial malleolar fractures
    C. Bimalleolar fractures
    D. Trimalleolar fractures
    E. All of the above

35. Generally, ankle fractures are treated with which of the following?
    A. Crutch walking, WBAT
    B. ORIF procedures
    C. Compression wraps and NWB
    D. Early active exercise

36. Throughout the duration of cast immobilization after surgery for an ankle fracture, which of the following can be prescribed?
    A. Quad and hamstring strengthening for the involved limb
    B. UBE
    C. Total body conditioning
    D. Single-leg stationary cycling
    E. All of the above

37. Distal tibial compression fractures also are referred to as pilon fractures. These specific fractures occur from which of the following?
    A. Rotational forces
    B. Inversion forces
    C. Axial or vertical loads
    D. Eversion loads
    E. All of the above

38. Because the mechanism of injury involves the articular surfaces of the distal tibia and the talus, weight bearing activities after pilon fractures may be deferred for which of the following?
    A. 8 weeks
    B. 6 weeks
    C. 10 weeks
    D. 12 weeks

39. A common complication after a multifragmented compression fracture of the distal tibia is which of the following?
    A. Severe vascular compromise
    B. Neurologic deficits
    C. Secondary osteoarthritis
    D. Rheumatoid arthritis
    E. All of the above

40. The cornerstone in the recovery from a calcaneal fracture lies in regaining motion and strength of which of the following?
    A. Dorsiflexors
    B. Inversion musculature
    C. Eversion musculature
    D. Plantar flexors

41. There are how many classifications of talar fractures?
    A. Three
    B. Four
    C. Six
    D. Five

42. A type II talar fracture with subtalar subluxation may result in which of the following? (Circle any that apply.)
    A. Osteoarthritis
    B. Neurovascular compromise
    C. Avascular necrosis
    D. Rheumatoid arthritis
    E. Quad atrophy

43. Because talar fractures involve the articular surface, immobilization and NWB may last how long?
    A. 6 weeks
    B. 3 months
    C. 8 weeks
    D. 4 weeks
44. Plantar fasciitis is caused by which of the following?
    A. Acute plantar flexion
    B. Acute dorsiflexion
    C. Chronic traction on the plantar aponeurosis
    D. Chronic inflammation of the flexor tendons
45. The treatment of plantar fasciitis can involve which of the following?
    A. Surgery
    B. Ice
    C. NSAIDs
    D. Stretching and strengthening exercises
    E. All of the above
46. Which of the following are appropriate techniques to be used in the treatment of plantar fasciitis?
    A. Nocturnal splints
    B. Picking up marbles with the toes
    C. Iontophoresis or phonophoresis
    D. Toe extension stretches
    E. All of the above
47. Which of the following is the most common location of Morton's neuroma?
    A. Medial and dorsal aspect of the foot
    B. Third to fourth interspace
    C. Plantar fascia
    D. Second to third interspace
48. Which of the following are various options for the treatment of Morton's neuroma? (Circle any that apply.)
    A. Corticosteroid injections
    B. Metatarsal pad
    C. Cast immobilization
    D. Change of footwear
    E. Surgical excision
49. After surgical correction of hallux valgus, the PT focuses attention on which of the following? (Circle any that apply.)
    A. Proper gait mechanics
    B. Inversion strength of the ankle
    C. Toe flexion and extension
    D. Eversion strength of the ankle
    E. Quad strength
50. Lesser toe deformities generally are made worse by which of the following?
    A. Too much exercise
    B. Kicking a ball
    C. Improper shoe wear (narrow toe box)
    D. High arch

Short Answer

51. Chronic instability may follow an inversion ankle sprain. Name the two types of instabilities associated with chronic ankle sprains.

52. Name the three major ligaments that represent the lateral ligament complex of the ankle.

53. Name the pathology shown in the figure.

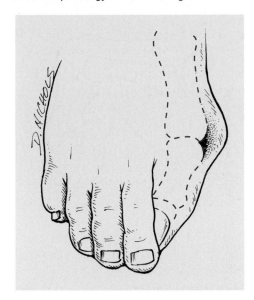

54. Match the following figures with the appropriate name of the deformity: Claw toe _____ Hammer toe _____ Mallet toe _____

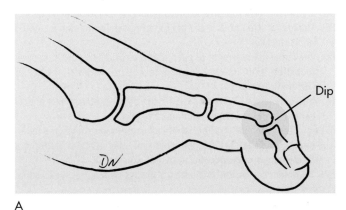

A

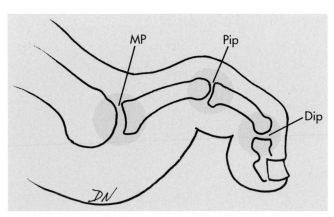

B

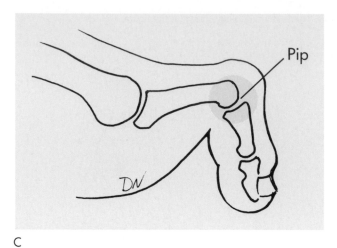

C

True/False

55. During the early recovery (acute phase) period of an inversion ankle sprain, it is imperative to instruct the patient to "write the alphabet" with the injured ankle.
56. Complete deltoid ligament sprains occur in combination with ankle fractures.
57. Mechanical instability may require surgery to stabilize the ankle.
58. Treatment for a ruptured Achilles tendon is always with surgery.
59. The loss of strength is less if the ruptured Achilles tendon is treated nonsurgically.
60. The initial management of pilon fractures usually involves an open reduction with internal fixation procedure, external fixator, or skeletal traction.
61. In severe cases of plantar fasciitis, the physician may inject a local corticosteroid to reduce pain and swelling.
62. In cases of plantar fasciitis where all conservative measures fail to bring significant results, the physician may elect to perform a fasciotomy or excision of a calcaneal exostosis.
63. Treatment of Morton's neuroma is always with surgical excision.

64. The removal of tight shoes may significantly reduce painful symptoms associated with hallux valgus.
65. Lesser toe deformities are characterized as either rigid or flexible.
66. Flexible toe deformities are most commonly corrected with surgery, whereas rigid toe deformities are corrected with conservative measures.

Essay Questions
Answer on a separate sheet of paper.
67. Identify common ligament injuries of the ankle.
68. Describe methods of management and rehabilitation of common ligament injuries to the ankle.
69. Identify and describe common tendon injuries to the ankle.
70. Outline and describe common methods of management and rehabilitation of tendon injuries to the ankle.
71. Identify common fractures of the foot and ankle.
72. Discuss common methods of management and rehabilitation of foot and ankle fractures.
73. Identify common toe deformities and describe methods of management and rehabilitation.
74. Describe common mobilization techniques for the ankle, foot, and toes.

Critical Thinking Application
In small groups, develop two case studies: one related to a patient with a grade II anterior talofibular ligament sprain; the other, a patient with a displaced bimalleolar fracture. In each case develop a criterion-based rehabilitation program (critical pathway or mapping) that follows the maximum-, moderate-, and minimum-protection phase concepts of progression. Be certain to apply your understanding of the mechanisms of soft-tissue and bone healing and the three general phases of the inflammatory response, repair phase, and remodeling of tissues during each protective phase of recovery. Be specific in identifying the appropriate, safe, and effective use of agents to control pain and swelling. List exercises, activities, weight bearing status, muscle contraction types, open versus closed kinetic chain exercises, general physical conditioning, ROM, cardiovascular fitness, balance-coordination-proprioception, and functional activities that are consistent with each phase of healing.

19

Orthopedic Management of the Knee*

LEARNING OBJECTIVES

1. Identify common ligament injuries of the knee.
2. Discuss general methods of management and rehabilitation of common ligament injuries of the knee.
3. Identify and describe common meniscal injuries of the knee.
4. Discuss common methods of management and rehabilitation of meniscal injuries of the knee.
5. Identify and describe common patellofemoral pathologic conditions of the knee.
6. Describe common methods of management and rehabilitation of patellofemoral disease of the knee.
7. Identify and describe common patella, supracondylar femur, and proximal tibia fractures.
8. Describe common methods of management and rehabilitation of fractures about the knee.
9. Identify and describe methods of management and rehabilitation after knee arthroplasty and high tibial osteotomy.
10. Describe common mobilization techniques for the knee.

KEY TERMS

Anterior cruciate ligament (ACL)
Autograft
Allograft
Ligament-augmentation device (LAD)
Meniscus
Posterior cruciate ligament
Medial collateral ligament

Lateral collateral ligament
Arthroscopically assisted technique
Open arthrotomy technique
Meniscal repair
Subtotal meniscectomy
Articular cartilage
Quadriceps angle (Q angle)

Miserable malalignment syndrome
Supracondylar femur fractures
Tibial plateau fractures
Arthroplasty
Constrained
Nonconstrained
Osteotomy

CHAPTER OUTLINE

Ligament Injuries
  Anterior Cruciate Ligament Injuries
    Pertinent History and Physical Examination
    Ligament Stability Tests
    Mechanical Ligament Stability Tests
    Operative Management
    Central One-Third Bone-Patellar Tendon-Bone Autograft

Healing of the Graft after Surgery
Rehabilitation after Anterior Cruciate Ligament Reconstruction
  Maximum-Protection Phase
  Moderate-Protection Phase
  Minimum-Protection Phase

Continued

*Refer to orthopedic anatomy figures on the Evolve website.

CHAPTER OUTLINE—cont'd

Posterior Cruciate Ligament Injuries
   Management and Rehabilitation
   Nonoperative Rehabilitation
   Postoperative Rehabilitation
   Medial Collateral Ligament Injuries
      Ligament Stability Tests
      Rehabilitation
Meniscus Injuries
   Mechanisms of Injury
   Clinical Examination
   Management
   Rehabilitation after Subtotal Meniscectomy
   Rehabilitation after Meniscal Repair
Patellofemoral Pathologic Conditions
   Lateral Patellar Compression and Patellar
         Tracking Disorders
      Nonoperative Rehabilitation of Anterior
         Knee Pain
      Postoperative Rehabilitation of Anterior
         Knee Pain
Fractures
   Fractures of the Patella
   Supracondylar Femur Fractures
   Proximal Tibia Fractures (Tibial Plateau Fractures)
Knee Joint Reconstruction
   Knee Arthroplasty
      Rehabilitation after Total Knee Joint
         Replacement
High Tibial Osteotomy
Common Mobilization Techniques for the Knee
   Mobilization of the Patellofemoral Joint
   Mobilization of the Tibiofemoral Joint

As a vital team member, the physical therapist assistant (PTA) is frequently challenged to safely and effectively manage acute, chronic, and postsurgical orthopedic conditions of the knee. This chapter presents common pathologic conditions of the ligaments, meniscus lesions, patellofemoral diseases, extensor mechanism disorders, and fractures of the knee, as well as rehabilitation procedures related to total knee joint replacement. This chapter gives the PTA an appreciation of various knee ailments, mechanisms of injury, and specific tissue healing constraints, and provides an introduction to the rationale behind criterion-based rehabilitation programs for the knee.

The knee is an extraordinarily complex joint. Therefore the PTA is strongly encouraged to review pertinent knee joint anatomy and functional mechanics before and throughout this study.

LIGAMENT INJURIES

Ligament injuries of the knee refer to various degrees of sprains that may lead to frank ruptures of the ligament, manifested by loss of joint function. Knee ligament sprains and joint instability are complex and sophisticated problems involving various degrees of straight-plane or combined rotatory instability. Knee ligament sprains may be defined as follows:

Mild: Grade I, first-degree ligament sprain: An incomplete stretching of collagen ligament fibers resulting in minimal pain, minimal or no swelling, no loss of joint function, and no clinical or functional instability.

Moderate: Grade II, second-degree ligament sprain: A partial loss of ligament fiber continuity. A few collagen ligament fibers may be completely torn; however, most of the ligament remains intact. This degree of sprain is characterized by moderate (more intense than first-degree) pain, moderate swelling, and some loss of joint function and stability.

Severe: Grade III, third-degree sprain (rupture): The entire collagen ligament fiber bundles are completely torn. There is no continuity within the body of the ligament. This is usually characterized by profound pain, intense swelling, loss of joint function, and instability.

Anterior Cruciate Ligament Injuries

Pertinent History and Physical Examination

The natural history of an **anterior cruciate ligament** (ACL) sprain usually involves combined forces of external rotation, valgus stress, and internal tibial rotation alone or combined with knee hyperextension while the affected foot is planted (Fig. 19-1).[43] In contrast to many other knee injuries, the typical ACL sprain involves a noncontact, deceleration, closed kinetic chain (CKC) mechanism of injury, rather than external forces affecting the ligament. The resultant sprain can rapidly develop a tense hemarthrosis (blood within the joint) requiring arthrocentesis (aspiration of fluid from within a joint). Removal of blood can signal a ligament tear, whereas blood with fat droplets may reveal a fracture or ligament sprain. Removal of synovial fluid without blood may indicate a chronic meniscus lesion or synovitis.[40]

The PTA must recognize that the cruciate ligaments are intracapsular structures, which can produce a joint effusion when injured. This anatomic relationship is contrasted with the medial and lateral collateral ligaments, which are extracapsular structures. When the medial collateral ligament (MCL) is sprained, there is generally less swelling and no intraarticular effusion because the resultant bleeding from the injured tissues can evacuate the area and the fluid is not restrained within the joint capsule.

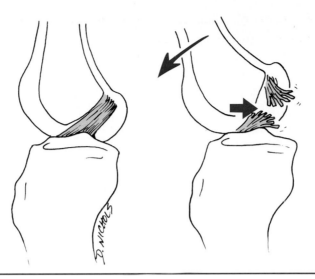

Fig. 19-1 Mechanism of injury to the anterior cruciate ligament (ACL). Typically, the ACL is injured in a noncontact deceleration mechanism of combined forces of external tibial rotation, valgus stress, internal tibial rotation, and knee hyperextension.

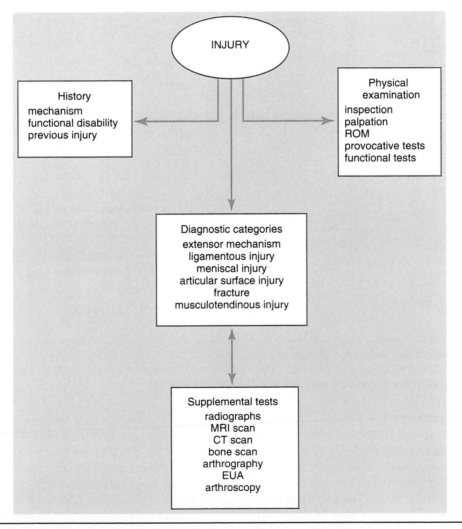

Diagnostic algorithm for the injured knee.
ROM, Range of motion; *MRI,* magnetic resonance imaging; *CT,* computed tomography; *EUA,* examination under anesthesia. (From Browner BD, Jupiter J, Levine A, et al: Skeletal Trauma, 2nd ed, vol 2. Philadelphia, WB Saunders, 2003.)

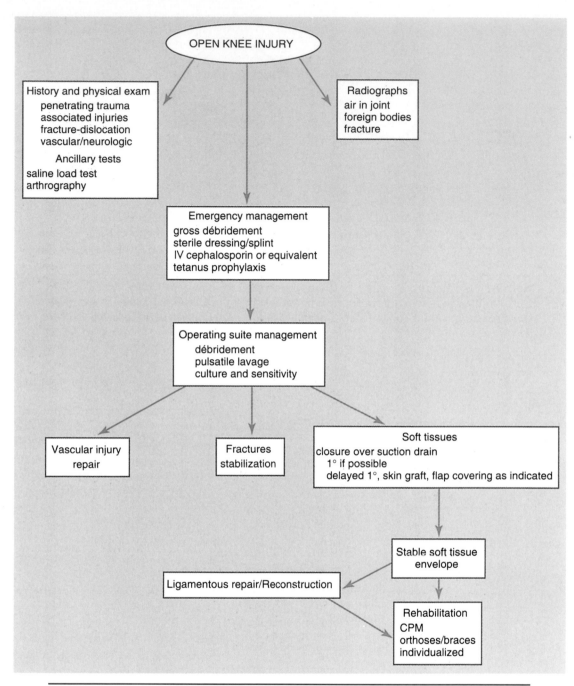

Treatment algorithm for an open knee injury.
CPM, Continuous passive motion. (From Browner BD, Jupiter J, Levine A, et al: Skeletal Trauma, 2nd ed, vol 2. Philadelphia, WB Saunders, 2003.)

Ligament Stability Tests

The PTA must be aware of various clinical ligament stability tests to accurately and effectively communicate changes in a patient's stability to the supervising physical therapist (PT) and physician. Although ligament stability tests are part of the initial evaluation procedures used by the physician and PT, the PTA can better understand the static and dynamic restraints of the knee and develop a more comprehensive view of rehabilitation when exposed to the rudimentary concepts of ligament stability testing.

Degrees of instability are graded similarly to degrees of ligament sprains. Hughston[26] has divided ligament instabilities into three degrees, as follows:

1. *Mild instability:* Graded 1+; characterized by 5 mm or less of joint surface separation
2. *Moderate instability:* Graded 2+; joint surface separation of 4 to 10 mm
3. *Severe instability:* Graded 3+; joint surface separation of 10 mm or more

Perhaps the most common, clinically useful, and easily taught and performed ligament stability test for the ACL

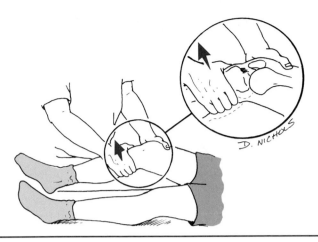

Fig. 19-2 The Lachman examination. This examination tests the stability of the anterior cruciate ligament (ACL) with the knee flexed 25 to 30 degrees. If the tibia can be displaced anteriorly in reference to the stabilized distal femur, then an injured ACL should be considered.

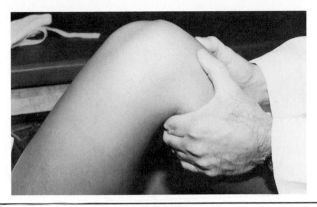

Fig. 19-3 The anterior drawer test. With the injured knee flexed to 90 degrees, the clinician grasps the proximal tibia and provides an anteriorly directed force. If the tibia displaces anteriorly in reference to the stabilized distal femur, then the anterior cruciate ligament may be considered injured.

is the Lachman examination (Fig. 19-2).[26] The patient is supine on an examining table with the affected knee flexed to approximately 25 to 30 degrees. One hand is used to stabilize the distal femur, and the other hand grasps the proximal tibia. An anterior and posterior force is gently directed to the proximal tibia. The integrity (stability) of the ACL should be observed, and the degree of joint motion (5 to 10 mm) present should be noted.

The anterior drawer test (Fig. 19-3) is another clinical examination used to approximate the degree of anterior tibial translation relative to the fixed femur. This examination is used less frequently than the Lachman test and is a less sensitive test to challenge the stability of the ACL. Hughston[26] describes the validity of the anterior drawer test in flexion this way:

> The anterior drawer test in flexion has long been incorrectly perceived to test for a tear of the anterior cruciate ligament, but this ligament is relatively relaxed at 80 to 90 degrees of knee flexion. Instead, the anterior drawer test in flexion assesses the meniscotibial ligaments and the mobility of the menisci on the tibia.

The examination is performed with the patient supine and the affected knee flexed to approximately 90 degrees. The PTA should stabilize the affected limb by sitting on the foot of the affected limb. Both hands should be used to grasp the proximal posterior tibia, with the thumbs of both hands on the anterior joint line of the knee. An anterior and posterior force should be exerted to the proximal tibia, and the amount of joint separation of the tibia relative to the femur should be observed.

Other relevant tests for the stability of the ACL incorporate multidirectional rotation examinations to acknowledge the presence of anteromedial rotatory

instability (AMRI), posteromedial rotatory instability (PMRI), and posterolateral rotatory instability (PLRI). Anterolateral rotatory instability (ALRI) is the more common multiplanar instability encountered.[26,43] The Hughston jerk test and pivot shift test commonly are used examinations to sublux and reduce the tibia relative to the femur.[26]

Mechanical Ligament Stability Tests

Various instrumented ligament stability devices help quantify degrees of instability (Box 19-1). The most common devices used with the greatest reliability are the KT1000 and KT2000 knee ligament arthrometers.[10]

BOX 19-1

Instrumented Knee Ligament Stability Devices

KT1000 and KT2000 knee ligament arthrometers (Medmetric, Inc., San Diego, CA)
Measures: Single-plane anterior and posterior translation

Genucom (Faro Medical Analysis Systems, Faro Medical, Inc., Montreal, Canada)
Measures: All six degrees of tibiofemoral joint

CA-4000 (Orthopaedic Systems, Inc., Hayward, CA)
Measures: Four degrees of freedom of the tibiofemoral joint)

From Greenfield BH. Sequential evaluation of the knee. In Greenfield BH, ed. Rehabilitation of the Knee: A Problem Solving Approach. Philadelphia, FA Davis, 1993.

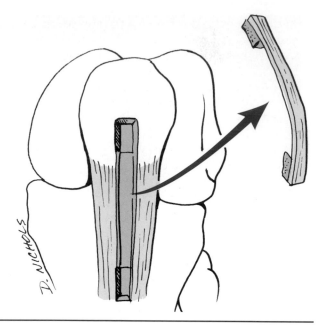

Fig. 19-4 Bone-patellar tendon-bone harvest. A pedicle of bone from the tibial tubercle and patella is removed along with a full-thickness graft of the patellar tendon to be used to anatomically reconstruct the anterior cruciate ligament.

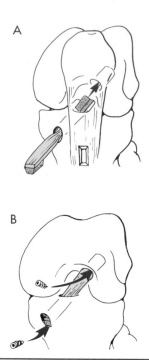

Fig. 19-5 The central one-third arthroscopically-aided bone-patellar tendon-bone autograft procedure. **A,** The placement of the graft within the knee joint, through tunnels drilled in the tibia and femur; **B,** The graft tissue and bone pedicles being secured with anchor screws.

The patient is supine with both knees flexed approximately 20 to 25 degrees over a plastic bolster. The device is attached to the tibia with Velcro straps while the patella is stabilized (seated) with the patella reference pad. A handle is used to direct an anterior and posterior force to the proximal tibia. Audible tones are encountered when various pounds of force are applied to the tibia. The needle on a small dial on the surface of the device deflects in a positive or negative direction, quantifying the degree of tibial translation relative to the stable femur in millimeters of displacement.

Throughout the performance of this examination, complete muscle relaxation of the hamstrings, quadriceps, and gastroc-soleus muscle group must be maintained. Swelling, intraarticular effusion, and muscle spasm falsely stabilize the knee,[29] rendering the examination meaningless.

Operative Management

The PTA must recognize the various surgical procedures used to correct functional instabilities related to injuries of the ACL and be aware of the short- and long-term ramifications of ligament healing to more effectively deliver sound rehabilitation programs and better appreciate the complex nature of surgical repair and rehabilitation. Therefore this section provides a rudimentary description of the most common ACL surgical procedures as they relate to the scope and practice of the PTA.

Central One-Third Bone-Patellar Tendon-Bone Autograft

An **autograft** uses tissue from the body of the patient. Various tissues are used for grafts, including the gracilis tendon, fascia lata, semitendinosus tendon, and quadriceps muscle tendon. The bone-patellar tendon-bone autograft is the strongest one used for ACL reconstructions.[14]

An **allograft** refers to biologic tissue taken from another human body.[14] The major risks of using allograft involve disease transmission (risk of human immunodeficiency virus infection) and problems with effective sterilization procedures.[14]

Artificial ligaments include synthetic devices (Gore-Tex), tissue-scaffold devices, and **ligament-augmentation devices (LAD).** The major disadvantage of using prosthetic ligaments is that this material tends to deteriorate over time and cannot repair itself.[14]

The arthroscopic central one-third bone-patellar tendon-bone autograft procedure involves harvesting the graft from the involved knee (Fig. 19-4) and surgically routing this structure through tunnels placed in the femur and tibia in a way that duplicates normal ACL anatomy, then securing (fixing) the graft to the bone to allow for stable healing (Fig. 19-5). A small stab wound is made in the knee, and a small diameter drainage tube is inserted to help evacuate the joint of residual bleeding, which increases arthrofibrosis if allowed to accumulate. This small drain is usually removed after a few days when the bleeding is controlled. Even with the placement of the drain, postoperative arthrofibrosis is a clinically significant problem that occurs frequently. Sterile bandages are placed over the incisions, and the patient's leg is placed in a brace or knee immobilizer locked in 0 degrees of flexion.

Healing of the Graft after Surgery

Ligament healing processes and revascularization of graft material are vital concerns in the prescribed rehabilitation program designed by the supervising PT. The appropriate progression of the rehabilitation program depends on the PTA's awareness of the various stages of healing after an autograft procedure.

Once the graft is harvested and surgically routed within the knee, it begins a gradual process of avascular necrosis over the first 6 to 8 weeks.[14] The graft gradually loses strength and is quite fragile during the first 2 months after surgery, so excessive loads and forces that would compromise the healing of the graft must be avoided during this phase. The graft slowly revascularizes, and at approximately 3 months the tensile strength of the graft is less than 50% of its original strength.[14,38] Graft strength may take as long as a year to mature and never reaches preoperative levels.

Rehabilitation after Anterior Cruciate Ligament Reconstruction

The rehabilitation program after ACL reconstruction is designed to protect the graft; reduce pain and swelling; increase joint motion while improving strength, endurance (local muscular endurance, as well as aerobic fitness), flexibility, and proprioception; and ultimately return the knee to full function. This task is organized sequentially and is constantly modified, based on the patient's individual response to surgery and rehabilitation. By design, set "cookbook" type protocols for rehabilitation after ACL surgery are rapidly losing favor among rehabilitation specialists. The PT and PTA must work together to assess and adjust programs based on the individual's ability to recover and adapt. As stated by Einhorn and associates,[14] "each patient reacts differently to the surgical intervention. Loss of strength, swelling, and range of motion are unpredictable. Patient personality, attitude, and pain tolerance vary greatly with each case." Therefore the PT and PTA must design and implement a rehabilitation program based on goals and criteria the individual must achieve before advancing to a more challenging phase.

In general terms, ACL reconstruction rehabilitation can be organized into three broad, interconnecting phases:
1. *Maximum-protection phase:* From the first day postoperatively to approximately the sixth week after surgery.[43]
2. *Moderate-protection phase:* From approximately the seventh to the twelfth weeks after surgery.[43]
3. *Minimum-protection phase:* From the thirteenth week after surgery until return to activity.[43]

This section reviews each phase separately and introduces the PTA to the many variables and individual differences among patients. The importance of reassessment of initial evaluation data and the need for open communication and teamwork with the supervising PT cannot be emphasized too strongly.

Maximum-Protection Phase

As the graft slowly loses its strength (6 to 8 weeks after surgery), excessive loads and forces that stress the ACL must be avoided. These forces are controlled primarily by joint protection with range-limiting hinge braces and avoidance of anterior tibial translation and shearing forces, as well as rotatory motions.

Control of swelling is important throughout each phase of rehabilitation. Postoperative swelling can have a profound negative effect on the progress of the patient, even with suction drains inserted at the time of surgery. Swelling inhibits muscle contractions, contributes significantly to pain, limits joint motion, and can stimulate arthrofibrosis. The use of elastic compression wraps along with the application of ice packs and elevation of the limb help to minimize swelling. Commercial cold and compression appliances are available for convenience and ease of application for the patient to use at home.

The patient's ability to achieve early active range of motion (ROM) is an essential component of the maximum-protection phase. While the newly placed graft is struggling to revascularize, it must be protected from anterior translatory and rotatory forces by use of an adjustable range-limiting brace. However, regaining full knee extension and flexion must proceed.

Frequently, patellar motion (caudal, cephalic, medial, and lateral glide) must be an immediate goal for knee flexion and extension to improve. Scarring from the graft harvest site and suprapatellar pouch typically inhibits free patellar motion. Initially the PTA must provide gentle stretching of the patella (Fig. 19-6) and instruct the patient to perform these stretches two to three times daily. Generally, full knee extension is achieved soon after surgery; if not, passive prone or supine knee extension stretches can be used judiciously to gradually increase knee extension (Fig. 19-7). In addition to active and passive knee flexion and extension, some authors[14,39,43] advocate the use of a continuous passive motion (CPM) device for a limited time very early in this phase. The use of a CPM device is based on studies that show that "instituting CPM immediately after surgery helps maintain a normal articular surface and prevent degenerative changes that might occur as a result of ACL reconstruction."[43] Other investigators[14,39]

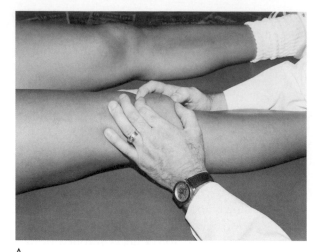

A

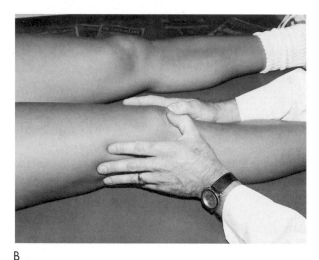

B

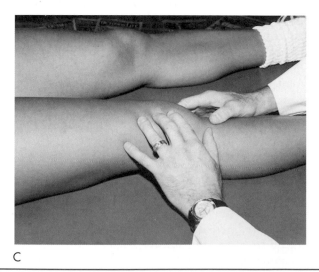

C

Fig. 19-6 Postoperative manual patellar stretching is used to enhance knee motion. If the patella becomes "adhered" to surrounding tissues, then normal knee flexion and extension cannot occur. **A,** A caudal (inferior)-directed force applied to the patella. **B,** A cephalic (superior)-directed force. **C,** The patella being directed medially.

have shown that CPM may help evacuate synovial joint hemarthrosis and aid in the prevention of knee joint contracture. The use of CPM generally is limited to the period immediately after hospitalization and is reserved for daytime use only.[14]

Ambulation and weight bearing status are somewhat controversial in terms of when to allow full weight bearing. In general, weight bearing with crutches is allowed as tolerated as soon as possible after surgery. Daniel and associates[11] advocate weight bearing as tolerated for 5 to 6 weeks with crutches. Einhorn and associates[14] recommend full weight bearing by 2 to 4 weeks. Timm[43] encourages non–weight bearing for the first week postoperatively, progressing to weight bearing as tolerated.

Strengthening exercises during the maximum-protection phase focus on isometric cocontractions of the quadriceps and hamstrings. The PTA must recognize that passive terminal knee extension is allowed, but open-chain active knee extension, with or without resistance, causes an anterior tibial translation force relative to the femur that stresses the new graft. Cocontraction of the quadriceps and hamstring muscles within the hinged brace help stabilize the joint and provide for muscular activity. Open kinetic chain knee-extension exercises may be used during the maximum-protection phase if the resistance is placed proximal to the knee joint and the patient is not allowed to extend the knee in the final 40 degrees of extension "because of the high tensile forces on the ACL."[14] The primary focus of strengthening the postoperative ACL patient during the maximum-protection phase is to encourage quadriceps control (be able to demonstrate active quadriceps-hamstring setting) and hamstring strength. The hamstrings act as dynamic stabilizers to limit anterior tibial shearing forces,[14,38,39,43] and work on hamstring strength begins within the first week postoperatively.[14] Both standing leg curls and supine leg curls can be initiated during this phase if a brace is used. New studies offer the following exercise protocol that does not strain the ACL:[5]

■ Isometric hamstring muscle contraction exercises at 15, 30, 60, and 90 degrees
■ Isometric quadriceps contractions at 60 and 90 degrees
■ Simultaneous contraction of the quadriceps and hamstring muscles at 30, 60, and 90 degrees of knee flexion
■ Active flexion-extension motion of the knee from 35 degrees to full flexion
■ Passive flexion-extension motion of the knee without muscle contraction

Four-way (flexion, extension, abduction, and adduction) hip- and calf-strengthening exercises also are encouraged during this phase. The criteria to be achieved by the patient before advancing to the moderate-protection phase include the following:

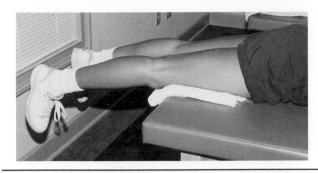

Fig. 19-7 Prone passive knee-extension stretch. Note the application of a folded towel under the thigh to elevate the leg and avoid compression of the patella and patellar tendon against the end of the table.

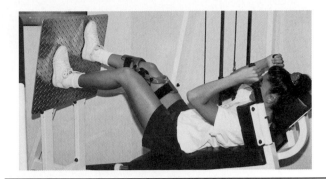

Fig. 19-8 Closed kinetic chain leg press with the knee braced. The uninvolved leg is used to support the weight and provide confidence during the application of the short-arc leg press.

- ROM from 0 degrees extension to 120 degrees of flexion
- Full weight bearing (encourage normal gait mechanics)
- Quadriceps control
- Hamstring control
- Controlled pain and swelling
- A minimum of 6 weeks from the day of surgery

Moderate-Protection Phase

As stated by Malone,[32] "Rehabilitation must degenerate into function!"; therefore the moderate-protection phase begins the process of functional recovery and focuses on CKC tasks and proprioceptive activities.

Progression from one phase to another is a slow, interrelated process with a strong carryover from one phase to the next. For example, at the beginning of the moderate-protection phase, the patient continues with all of the rudimentary exercises initiated in the maximum-protection phase. To advance to the next level at the beginning of the moderate-protection phase requires strong compliance from the patient in performing all stretching and strengthening exercises, as well as demonstrated progress in weight bearing status and proper gait mechanics. Generally, immobilization is discontinued around the fifth or sixth week postoperatively.[11] Control of pain and swelling continues as indicated.

CKC exercises and progressive proprioceptive tasks (to stimulate the afferent neural input system) are initiated and progressed throughout this phase. Studies[1,3] have demonstrated that "the ligaments of the knee have a rich sensory innervation that allows them to act as the first link in the 'kinetic-chain.'" Loss of the mechanoreceptor "stabilizing reflex" may result in reduced afferent neural input system function, which may contribute to "progressive instability and disability."[3] Therefore gradual CKC progressive loads are essential to encourage functional muscle control and confidence in the use of the affected limb during weight bearing (functional) activities. As mentioned (see Chapter 5), CKC exercises are a system of interdependent articulated links in which motion at one joint produces motion at all other joints in the system in a predictable manner. CKC activities are used early in the rehabilitation process because these exercises are more functionally relevant, stimulate neuromuscular coordination, enhance joint approximation, and influence the joint mechanoreceptor system.

Initial instruction in CKC exercises begins with the patient braced to protect the healing graft. Standing and shifting of body weight from the nonaffected limb to the affected limb is a safe and appropriate introduction to CKC exercises. Once the patient can demonstrate confidence, muscle control, and stability, the brace is removed (with prior consultation and concurrence from the supervising physical therapist) and the patient is allowed to shift weight without braced support. The leg press is used as a CKC exercise in a short-arc motion early in the moderate-protection phase while the patient is braced (Fig. 19-8). Progressive ROM exercises are allowed as the patient tolerates them. Standing wall slides also are introduced during the moderate-protection phase if the affected limb is braced and the tibia is kept as vertical as possible to avoid an anterior tibial translation force (Fig. 19-9). The short-arc step-up is an excellent exercise used to stimulate quadriceps control and strength. Often a biofeedback system is used in conjunction with step-ups to encourage appropriate quadriceps control (Fig. 19-10).

Stationary cycling also is encouraged throughout the moderate-protection phase of ACL rehabilitation. The height of the seat may require adjusting to accommodate the limited knee flexion ROM. The stationary cycle is used primarily to encourage ROM, but during the middle and later stages of this phase the cycle can be used as an aerobic conditioning tool if the patient has achieved the required ROM, strength, and stability to perform endurance activities. Stair-steppers also can be introduced during this phase if the ROM and intensity of the resistance on the apparatus are modified and controlled initially to allow for protected joint motion (Fig. 19-11).

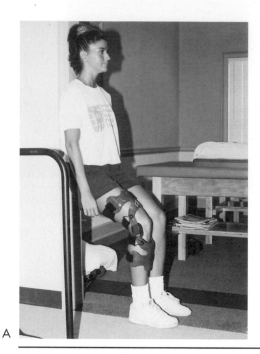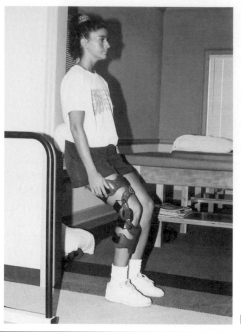

A   B

Fig. 19-9 Closed-chain short-arc wall slides. As the knee is braced to avoid unwanted anterior tibial translation, the patient is introduced to quadriceps strengthening (concentrically, eccentrically, and isometrically) in a vertical weight bearing position. **A,** A partial wall slide with the patient holding an isometric position. **B,** Note the use of a small ball placed behind the patient to encourage greater balance and control.

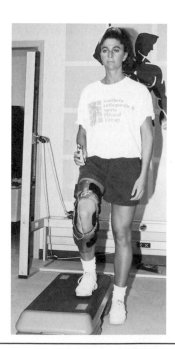

Fig. 19-10 The use of portable biofeedback or electrical muscle stimulation can be used to enhance greater quadriceps control during short-arc step-ups.

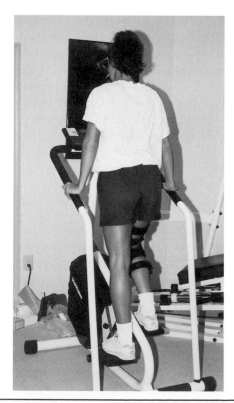

Fig. 19-11 Stair-steppers can be used as a closed-chain functional (stair climbing) exercise, provided the knee is braced and the intensity controlled to avoid excessive unwanted forces.

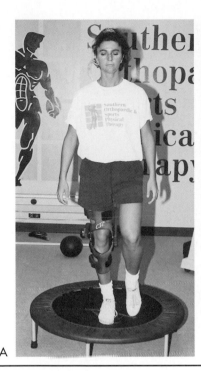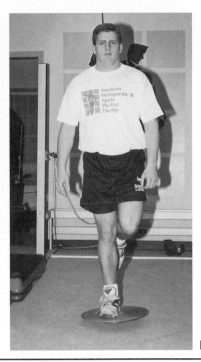

A   B

Fig. 19-12   Closed kinetic chain balance and proprioception exercises. **A,** Use of the minitrampoline is a challenging and effective balancing exercise. **B,** Single-leg standing on a wobble board.

To stimulate greater strength and local muscular endurance of the quadriceps, the patient can be instructed to perform the stair-stepper in a reverse manner. Throughout this phase the patient is encouraged to maintain patellar-stretching, hamstring-stretching, and quadriceps-stretching exercises, normal gait mechanics, a general fitness program of strength and endurance activities that do not stress the affected limb, ice application after exercises, and joint-protection principles.

Criteria that must be met by the patient before progressing to the next phase include the following:

- Full ROM (flexion, extension, and patellar mobility)
- Normalized full weight bearing gait and removal of brace as indicated
- Improved quadriceps strength
- Improved hamstring strength
- Continued control of pain and swelling
- A minimum of 12 to 13 weeks from the day of surgery

Minimum-Protection Phase

The minimum-protection phase signals the return to more normalized activities and the introduction of more challenging functional activities.

Isolated knee ligament stability tests, including manual clinical examinations (e.g., Lachman test, anterior drawer test, and pivot shift test) and instrumented stability examinations (KT1000 knee ligament arthrometer) are performed at the discretion of the PT and physician, usually during the moderate-protection and minimum-

protection phases of rehabilitation. Ongoing documentation of the stability of the affected limb is essential to justify progression to more challenging exercises and quantify the clinical results of the surgery. The use of isokinetic testing of the involved limb is also left to the judgment of the PT and physician. Generally, isokinetic examinations are reserved for the moderate-protection and minimum-protection phases. Certain precautions must be taken to minimize these forces and protect the graft because of the long-term nature of graft healing and the tibial translation forces produced with isokinetic testing and training. Timm[43] states that isokinetic exercise "requires the use of an antishear device or a proximally positioned input pad to protect the reconstructed ACL against excessive anterior tibial translation forces."

More progressive proprioceptive exercises can be initiated because clinical testing demonstrates improved strength, neuromuscular control, and stability of the ligament. The use of a balance board and minitrampoline further challenges the mechanoreceptor system (Fig. 19-12). Standing knee extension with resistance provided by elastic tubing is an excellent CKC exercise that encourages quadriceps control in more functional positions (Fig. 19-13). Slide board activities usually are reserved for a more athletic population but can be modified for the general population to be less intense and less sports specific. Straight-line jogging progressing to faster running is initiated for patients inclined toward participation in sporting activities.

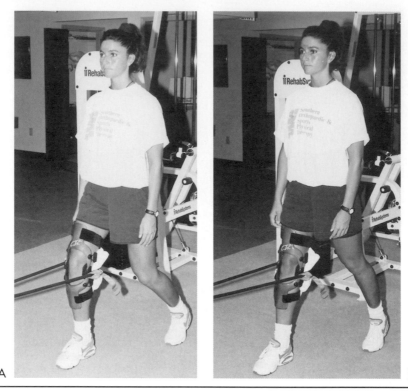

Fig. 19-13 Functional closed-chain resistive knee extension in the standing position. **A,** Starting position with affected knee flexed. **B,** End position with affected knee extended.

Progressive strengthening of the entire lower extremity includes isokinetic velocity spectrum training, isotonic eccentric quadriceps strengthening, leg presses, and squatting exercises. The PTA must be constantly aware that rehabilitation after ACL reconstruction involves the entire body and not just the affected limb. Care must be taken to involve all muscle groups, as well as the sensory input systems and aerobic system throughout each phase of rehabilitation. Returning the patient to functional activities is the primary focus of the rehabilitation team.

Frequently, other structures are injured along with the ACL. The rehabilitation plan outlined does not account for possible injury to the **meniscus, posterior cruciate, medial or lateral collateral** ligaments, or joint capsule; associated fractures; or impaired neurovascular structures. The complex nature and vast array of combined injuries dictates modifications at each level of rehabilitation and prolongs the healing process.

The PTA also must be aware that isolated single or partial ACL injuries and various circumstances may dictate a nonsurgical course of treatment. The physician must decide if the patient is best suited for surgery or should be treated nonoperatively. If the patient is treated nonoperatively, the rehabilitation program progresses at a faster pace, although the injured ligament must still be protected and allowed to heal. There-fore absence of surgery does not mean the patient is allowed unprotected motion and nonrestricted activities. Daniel and Fritschy[11] suggest approximately 12 weeks for a return to running for patients treated nonoperatively for a single-ligament ACL injury.

Posterior Cruciate Ligament Injuries

Isolated posterior cruciate ligament (PCL) injuries occur less often than ACL injuries.[3,9,12] Four specific injury mechanisms can produce a PCL injury, with the most common being a "posteriorly directed force on the anterior aspect of the flexed knee."[12] Hughston[26] describes a second mechanism in which a patient falls on a flexed knee, making contact with the tibial tuberosity and forcing the tibia posteriorly (Fig. 19-14). A third mechanism of injury can occur from hyperflexion of the knee without a resultant force on the tibia.[12] A fourth mechanism usually results in both an ACL and PCL injury and involves knee hyperextension with the foot planted.

Clinical examination of the PCL can be confusing. While assisting the PT with the initial evaluation data, the PTA may observe two distinct tests used to define the presence and degree of a PCL injury. In the first examination, if the PCL is torn—the anterior and posterior drawer test—the tibia "sags" or subluxes posteriorly relative to the femur (Fig. 19-15). The examiner may produce a "false-positive" anterior drawer sign, wherein

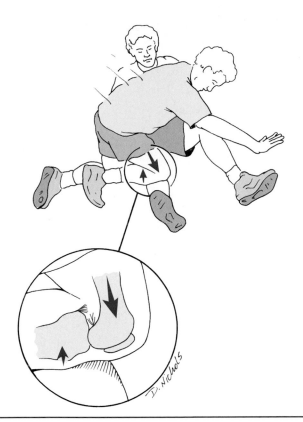

Fig. 19-14 Mechanism of posterior cruciate ligament injury. With the knee flexed, the proximal tibia is driven in a posterior direction.

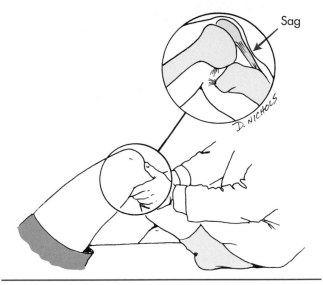

Fig. 19-15 Starting position of the anterior drawer test. If the posterior cruciate ligament injury is torn, the proximal tibia will be in a posterior tibial sag initial reference position.

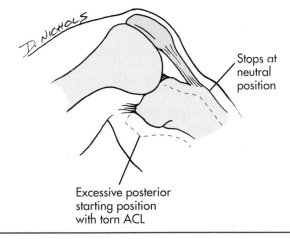

Fig. 19-16 A false-positive anterior drawer test can be seen when the tibia translates forward during the drawer test because the torn posterior cruciate ligament injury places the tibia posterior to the femur; therefore when the clinician directs an anterior force, the tibia appears to actually displace anterior to the femur.

the posterior tibial sag actually is being reoriented to the neutral position rather than a true anterior translation occurring (Fig. 19-16).

A more sensitive test is the Godfrey posterior tibial sag test. The patient is supine with the hip and knee of the affected limb held at 90 degrees. Hold the heel of the affected limb and allow the tibia to translate, sublux, or sag posteriorly by gravity (Fig. 19-17).

Management and Rehabilitation

Many straight-plane and combined rotatory instabilities exist with ligament injuries. Various circumstances, including acute trauma, chronic instability, isolated ligament injury, and complex combinations of injury to multiple structures, profoundly alter the course of rehabilitation. As stated by Hughston,[27] "It must be understood that there is no way the knee can be subjected to a force sufficient to tear the PCL without simultaneously tearing other ligamentous structures about the knee." Hughston[27] elaborates by saying the resultant accessory ligament instabilities are "no greater than mild." Therefore this discussion focuses on the care and rehabilitation of defined straight-plane isolated single-ligament PCL injury and does not delve into the complex nature of the many PCL injuries identified.

There is much disagreement about how best to manage a PCL injury. Some patients appear to respond well to surgical repair, whereas others do very well without surgery.[12,15,27] One common denominator that exists in both groups is the high incidence of articular cartilage degeneration that results from various degrees of instability.[9,12,15,27]

Nonoperative Rehabilitation

The single most significant factor in the rehabilitation of PCL injuries treated nonsurgically is quadriceps

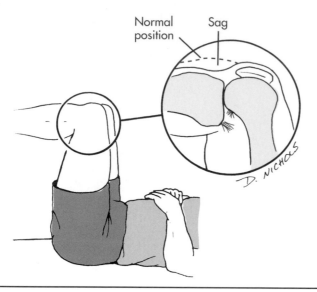

Fig. 19-17 Godfrey tibial sag test. This is a clinically sensitive test to view the reference of the proximal tibia in relation to the distal femur with the leg flexed to 90 degrees.

strengthening.[15,37] Studies demonstrate[37] that satisfactory results can be achieved when the quadriceps strength of the affected limb exceeds the quadriceps strength of the uninvolved limb. Less than satisfactory results are seen when the strength of the quadriceps is less than 100% of the quadriceps strength of the uninvolved limb.[37]

In the acute phase a knee immobilizer or hinged knee brace is used for patient comfort. Rest, ice, compression, and limb elevation (RICE) are used to minimize swelling and control pain. The treating physician may prescribe nonsteroidal antiinflammatory drugs (NSAIDs) in some cases. Full weight bearing is allowed as soon as the patient is able. Isometric quadriceps sets and straight-leg raises can commence immediately. The immobilizer is removed to allow active and passive ROM exercises of the knee on a daily basis.

As swelling, pain, and quadriceps control improve, the brace is removed and the patient is instructed in CKC quadriceps-strengthening exercises. No open-chain resistive hamstring exercises are allowed during the early or maximum protection phase because of the posterior tibial translatory forces provided by the hamstrings, which stress the healing PCL.

Short-arc leg-press exercises, step-ups, and wall squats are initiated early to stimulate quadriceps strength and balance, cocontraction of the quadriceps and hamstrings, and the joint mechanoreceptor system. Gradually, short-arc eccentric hamstring curls are added when ROM has improved and the patient can demonstrate good quadriceps strength and control during all open- and closed-chain exercises. Quadriceps strength is tested isokinetically to determine when to initiate more advanced functional exercises. An excellent CKC exercise is the stair-stepper used in reverse fashion. Quadriceps

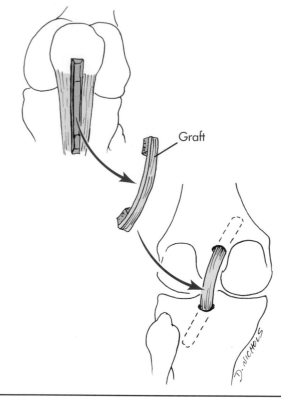

Fig. 19-18 Central one-third arthroscopically aided bone-patellar tendon-bone autograft for posterior cruciate ligament reconstruction. As with the anterior cruciate ligament, the patellar tendon, along with pedicles of bone from the patella and tibial tubercle, is harvested and then surgically routed through tunnels drilled through the femur and tibia.

strength and cocontraction of the hamstrings are enhanced. The stair-stepper used in the forward position allows the patient to push off on the balls of the feet, minimizing the work of the quadriceps. A reverse motion eliminates the plantar flexors and encourages greater quadriceps work. Standing knee extensions using rubber tubing placed behind the knee help encourage strong quadriceps control in a weight bearing position.

After acute isolated PCL injuries treated nonoperatively, DeLee and associates[12] suggest patients can return to full activity within 8 weeks.

Postoperative Rehabilitation

Common graft choices used to surgically reconstruct the PCL include the medial gastrocnemius tendon,[27] central one-third bone-patellar tendon-bone autografts, and Achilles tendon allografts.[12,15] Depending on the surgeon and the procedure used, either an arthroscopically assisted or open arthrotomy technique can be performed (Fig. 19-18).

A postoperative knee immobilizer or hinged range-limiting brace is applied and maintained until the patient demonstrates quadriceps control, full extension, and full weight bearing. Some authors[15] recommend a conservative approach to weight bearing after PCL reconstruction, advocating limited full weight bearing for 4 to 6 weeks or longer in some cases. Other authorities[12] encourage full weight bearing initially. Although early range of motion is encouraged for the patellofemoral joint and knee extension, minimizing full knee flexion to 50 to 60 degrees is necessary to protect the healing graft. Generally, full knee-flexion ROM can be achieved in 2 months after surgery.[12]

The maximum-protection phase of rehabilitation focuses on early isometric and progressive resistive exercises for the quadriceps. Goals throughout the early phases of rehabilitation include patellar-mobility exercises, early knee extension, controlled-limited knee flexion, weight bearing as tolerated, and control of pain and swelling with RICE and thermal agents as prescribed.

Progressive exercises employ CKC activities to stimulate quadriceps control and cocontractions of the quadriceps and hamstring muscle groups. Engle and associates[15] do not advocate isolated resisted hamstring exercises until 12 weeks after surgery. Others[12] suggest that isometric hamstring exercises can be performed early if cocontractions of the quadriceps are performed. Hamstring exercises are progressed to limited-range (10 to 60 degrees) prone, eccentric resistance exercises (while braced during the early postoperative phase).[12]

The moderate-protection phase of rehabilitation defined by Timm[43] begins at the thirteenth week after surgery and progresses to the twenty-fourth week. This phase focuses on weight bearing CKC exercises. Generally, stair-climbers, step-ups, leg presses, and partial squats are advanced throughout this phase. Progression within this phase is dictated by the patient's individual tolerance to exercises, as well as clinically documented objective findings from the KT1000 knee ligament arthrometer, manual clinical stress tests (drawer sign, tibial sag), and isokinetic testing.

The PTA must constantly be aware of the healing constraints of repaired or reconstructed tissues throughout each phase of rehabilitation. The early or maximum-protection phase coincides with the fibroplasia stage of healing.[15] Timm[43] suggests this phase lasts approximately 6 weeks and is characterized by the following goals:

- Protect the articular cartilage of the healing knee.
- Reduce the possibility of scar tissue adhesion formation.
- Ensure adequate circulation to the surgery site and the remodeling tissues.
- Reestablish normal tibiofemoral and patellofemoral arthrokinematics.
- Attain voluntary control over joint forces through muscle reconditioning.

The moderate-protection phase generally corresponds with the early maturation and late-fibroplasia stages of healing.[15] Similar goals during the early phase of the moderate-protection rehabilitation program include the following:

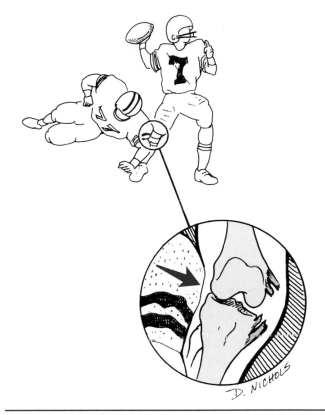

Fig. 19-19 Medial collateral ligament (MCL) sprain from an external force contacting the lateral aspect of the knee, causing the medial knee structures (MCL) to be torn.

- Control forces while protecting the graft.
- Stimulate collagen fiber maturation and remodeling.
- Promote revascularization of the graft.
- Obtain normal functional ROM and strength.[43]

The minimum-protection phase is directed at returning the patient to the premorbid functional state. The late stage of healing is collagen maturation, which signals the initiation of more vigorous, functional activities that are the hallmark of the minimum-protection phase. Because controversy exists among physicians and PTs concerning when to initiate motion, weight bearing, and various functional activities after PCL reconstructive surgery, the PTA must recognize that the cornerstone of any prescribed rehabilitation program comprises tissue healing principles and the patient's ability to attain certain criteria before beginning more advanced activities.

Medial Collateral Ligament Injuries

Injuries to the MCL are the most common ligament injuries seen in the knee.[17,30,47] The MCL can be injured by a direct external force or a noncontact abduction or rotational stress. In contact sports, the MCL is often injured by a valgus-directed force to the lateral aspect of the knee, causing injury to the medial structures (Fig. 19-19). Non–contact-related MCL sprains occur frequently as the lower leg is fixed, the tibia is rotated

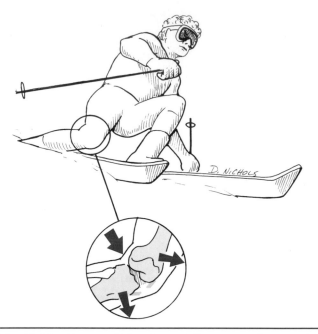

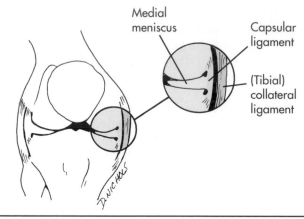

Medial
meniscus

Capsular
ligament

(Tibial)
collateral
ligament

Fig. 19-21 The medial meniscus can also become injured in conjunction with the medial collateral ligament (MCL) because of its intimate anatomic relationship with the MCL.

Fig. 19-20 The medial collateral ligament also can be sprained from noncontact forces.

externally, and a valgus force is directed through the knee (Fig. 19-20).

Injury to other ligaments (ACL or PCL) and associated structures (medial meniscus and lateral meniscus) are often seen in more severe MCL injuries. Studies[16] show an increasing correspondence of associated ligament injuries (most frequently the ACL) with the more severe grades of MCL injuries. Fetto and Marshall[16] demonstrated a 20% occurrence of associated ligament injuries with grade I MCL sprains, 52% in grade II sprains, and 78% with grade III sprains.

There is an intimate anatomic relationship between the MCL and medial meniscus of the knee. O'Donoghue[36] is credited with describing the "unhappy triad" as combined injury to the MCL, ACL, and medial meniscus. Because the MCL and medial meniscus are strongly attached to one another (Fig. 19-21), it is clear that the meniscus may become injured along with more severe MCL injuries. However, the more common triad is the MCL, ACL, and lateral meniscus.[34]

Ligament Stability Tests

The severity of ligament injury can be classified as follows:[34]

Grade I: 0 to 5 mm of joint opening with no instability

Grade II: 5 to 10 mm of joint opening with some degree of instability

Grade III: 10 to 15 mm of joint opening with moderate instability

Grade IV: Greater than 15 mm of joint opening with gross ligament instability

Others report a slightly different classification model:[30]

Grade I: 1 to 4 mm

Grade II: 5 to 9 mm

Grade III: 10 to 15 mm

Specific end-feel classifications during MCL stress testing help clarify the significance of joint injury (see Chapter 16). For example, Linton and Indelicato[30] describe grades I and II as having a definite end-feel to the stress tests, whereas grade III tears have a soft or "loose" end point. The end point, or "feel," is what the PT is looking for during the examination.

The most sensitive test to describe the severity of an MCL sprain is the valgus stress test. This test is performed with the patient supine on an examining table while the examiner stands to the side of the affected limb at the level of the distal tibia. The affected knee is tested in 30 degrees of knee-flexion. The medial aspect of the distal tibia is firmly grasped with one hand, while the other hand is used to apply a valgus-directed force to the lateral proximal joint line, in effect causing the medial joint line to gap or "open." This test also should be performed with the knee in full extension. If the knee gaps open in terminal extension, there is a significant injury to the MCL, ACL, PCL, and posterior capsule. However, even with a complete rupture of the MCL if the PCL and posterior capsule of the knee are not injured, the knee may not demonstrate significant instability when tested in full extension.[30] This clearly shows the ultimate stabilizing effect of the PCL and capsule in terminal extension.

Rehabilitation

Although some authorities[36] advocate surgical repair of selected MCL tears, most physicians now treat isolated grade I, II, and even III MCL tears nonsurgically.[17,30,34,47] However, protection of the ligament during healing is paramount if full function and stability are to be achieved. Wilk[47] outlines four critical conditions that must be observed for MCL healing, as follows:

- Maintenance of the torn fibers in close continuity
- Intact and stable ACL and other supporting ligaments of the knee
- Immediate controlled motion and stresses to the healing ligament
- Protection of the MCL against deleterious stresses (valgus and external rotation stresses)

The concept of early protected motion is the foundation for rehabilitation of MCL sprains. Generally, a three-phase (maximum, moderate, and minimum protection) criteria-based program is used. A knee immobilizer or range-limiting hinged brace is used initially to control unwanted valgus and rotational stress. Ice, elastic compression wraps, and elevation are used to control pain and swelling. Isometric quadriceps sets, straight-leg raises, and ankle pumps are initiated as soon as the patient can tolerate execution of the exercises. Weight bearing with crutches as tolerated generally is prescribed. The immobilizer is removed daily for active and passive knee flexion and extension exercises. Seated assisted knee flexion and supine wall slides are used to assist with painful knee flexion. Clearly all valgus forces and rotational stresses must be avoided to protect the healing ligament. The crutches are discarded as pain lessens and quadriceps strength increases. Wilk[47] suggests nonassisted ambulation by the eighth day after injury. When strengthening the nonoperated MCL, care must be taken to protect the medial structures from all valgus and rotational forces. Hip adduction strengthening can be achieved by placing resistance above the joint line if the knee is protected with a functional brace. Bracing for knee support generally is organized into three distinct categories,[13] as follows:

1. Prophylactic
2. Rehabilitative
3. Functional

In some cases a prophylactic hinged brace can be used during the moderate- and minimum-protection phases of MCL injury rehabilitation because these braces allow for full flexion and extension and may limit valgus stresses to the knee.

CKC exercises are gradually added as pain allows. Stair-steppers, leg presses, step-ups, and wall squats can be instituted as ROM and pain tolerance dictate. Patient compliance with home exercises and joint protection are significant factors that must be reinforced by the PTA during each phase of rehabilitation.

Active knee flexion range should progress steadily without increased complaints of pain and swelling. If the patient does not regain knee flexion or has increased complaints of pain and swelling, the possibility of a torn meniscus must be examined. Daily communication with the PT quickly identifies the necessary modifi-

cations in the rehabilitation program. In addition, through daily communication, the PTA can establish a cycle of scheduling physical therapy reevaluations based on clinical observation.

As with all injuries, the whole patient, not just the injured body part, must be treated. A full-body fitness program that does not produce unwanted valgus or rotation forces is encouraged beginning with the maximum-protection phase. In an athletic population of patients, adding lateral slide board activities and running drills during the minimum-protection phase is appropriate to allow a functional return to sporting activities.

A general set of criteria can be applied for a safe and effective progression from one phase of recovery to the next. Holden and associates[24] believe that the requirements for advancing through the early stages of recovery (2 to 3 weeks) should include the following:

- No significant effusion
- Decreasing tenderness
- Full ROM

Clinically significant warning signs during recovery through the second week are as follows:[24]

- Persistent effusion
- Continued pain
- Reduced ROM

Criteria for advancing through the third week, according to Holden and associates[24] include these points:

- No effusion
- No femoral condyle or tibial tenderness
- Full ROM
- No change in valgus stability test

Other signs to be aware of during the early (maximum- to moderate-protection phases) recovery period as outlined by Holden and associates[24] include the following:

- Subjective complaint of knee giving out with increased stress
- Locking

MENISCUS INJURIES

The functions of the meniscus include:[8,22,23,25]

- Stability
- Shock absorption
- Load transmission
- Nutrition
- Lubrication
- Control of motion

The menisci are fibrocartilaginous tissues containing primarily (90%) type I collagen.[2] The medial and lateral menisci of the knee serve as "extensions of the tibia"[2] and provide for reception of the femoral condyles onto the surface of the tibia (Fig. 19-22).

Injury to the meniscus can result in many patterns of tears (Fig. 19-23). Five main types have been identified,[18] as follows:

- Horizontal tears
- Longitudinal tears
- Degenerative tears
- Flap tears
- Radial tears

Longitudinal tears account for 50% to 90% of meniscus tear patterns in younger patients, whereas horizontal tears are more common among older patients.[18]

Mechanisms of Injury

The meniscus can be injured by sudden trauma or gradual degeneration.[2,8,18,23] Traumatic meniscus injuries are most common in a younger, active population, whereas degenerative tears occur more frequently to individuals over 40 years old.[2] Noncontact, weight bearing injuries to the meniscus usually involve combined forces of knee flexion, rotation, compression, and shear (Fig. 19-24).[2,8,18] Degenerative tears can be subtle

and do not usually involve a history of sudden overt trauma. Generally with degenerative tears, some type of insignificant activity (squatting or getting out of a car) precedes the symptoms of pain, swelling, and locking of the knee.

Clinical Examination

A history of some type of twisting injury followed by symptoms of pain, swelling, locking, or "catching" may indicate meniscal injury. While assisting the PT during the initial clinical examination, the PTA observes various manually applied stress tests to identify if a meniscal lesion is present.

Apley's compression and distraction test[40a] is used to determine if the injury is ligamentous or meniscal. To perform this test, the patient is prone with the affected knee flexed to 90 degrees. The distal femur is stabilized with a strap or hand. The free hand is used to grasp the

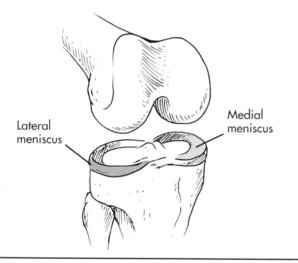

Fig. 19-22 Anatomic relationship of the medial and lateral meniscus to the tibia and femur.

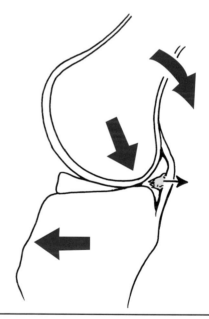

Fig. 19-24 Mechanism of injury to the meniscus. Combined forces of flexion, rotation, and compression can tear the meniscus.

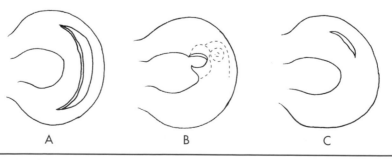

Fig. 19-23 Various patterns of tears can occur to the meniscus. **A,** Bucket-handle tear. **B,** Parrot-beak tear. **C,** Longitudinal tear.

distal tibia and provide a distraction and internal-external rotation force to the tibia. Pain signifies the possibility of a ligament tear. The compression component of this examination is performed in the same manner, except that the free hand applies a compression and rotational force to the distal tibia. Pain with compression and combined internal and external rotation on the flexed knee signifies the presence of a meniscal lesion.

The McMurray test[18,40a] also is used to reproduce symptoms of a torn meniscus. The patient is supine with the hip and knee of the affected limb fully flexed. To test for the presence of a medial meniscus lesion, a valgus force to the knee is applied with one hand while an external rotation force is applied and the knee is extended by holding the distal tibia with the other hand. To test for a lateral meniscus tear, a varus force with internal tibial rotation is provided. With either internal or external rotation of the knee, if a tear is present, the patient may experience pain and an audible or palpable snap or "pop."

The "bounce home" test[40a] is designed to determine if a torn meniscus is preventing knee extension. The patient is supine with the affected knee flexed and supported by the examiner's hand. The knee is passively extended to full extension. If the meniscus is torn, the knee may not fully extend because the torn tissue blocks extension and creates a rubbery, springy end-feel.[32]

Management

The rationale for treatment options is directly related to the location of the tear in the meniscus and the ability of the meniscus to repair itself. The vascular anatomy of the medial and lateral meniscus is reserved for the peripheral 10% to 30% of its width (Fig. 19-25).[2] The remaining portions are relatively avascular and aneural. Researchers and surgeons[2,22,23,40a] recognize a zone classification of injury related to the vascular supply of the meniscus. The injured meniscus may or may not heal or repair itself, depending on the location of the tear. A zone I tear is recognized as "red-on-red" because the location of the tear is vascular on both sides (Fig. 19-26). Injuries in this area may heal better than those in other areas because of the blood supply. A zone II tear is located in the "red-on-white" area of the meniscus (Fig. 19-27). A tear in this area has a vascular supply on only one side. These tears also may heal because of the communication with a blood supply.

A zone III tear is located in the nonvascular central body of the meniscus called the "white-on-white" area (Fig. 19-28). An injury in this area does not heal because there is no blood supply to support the healing process.

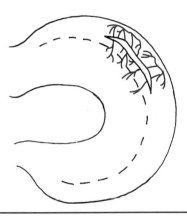

Fig. 19-26 Tear of the meniscus in the "red-on-red" zone of the meniscus. This zone I tear refers to the tear being vascular on both sides. This is a reparable tear.

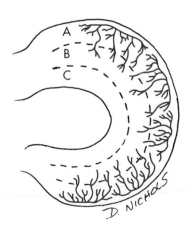

A-Red-on-red zone
B-Red-on-white zone
C-White-on-white zone

Fig. 19-25 The vascular anatomy of the meniscus. The vascular supply to the meniscus is reserved for the peripheral 10% to 30% of the meniscus.

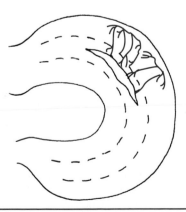

Fig. 19-27 Tear of the meniscus in the "red-on-white" zone. This zone II tear refers to the tear being vascular on only one side. This is a reparable tear.

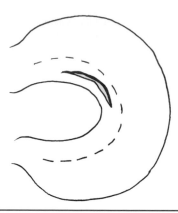

Fig. 19-28 Tear of the meniscus in the "white-on-white" zone. This zone III tear refers to the tear being avascular on both sides. This tear is considered not reparable.

The rationale for management is clearly supported by the severity and location of the tear in the meniscus. Surgical options include total meniscectomy (removal of the entire meniscus), subtotal or partial meniscectomy (removal of only the torn portion of the cartilage), and **meniscal repair** (suturing the torn meniscus together). If the tear is located in the "red-on-red" area, some surgeons elect a nonsurgical course of treatment. Fu and Baratz[18] identify a few variables to consider—the age of the patient, the stability of the knee, the location of the tear, and the integrity of the meniscus—when deciding on the course of treatment.

Degenerative arthritic changes, joint space narrowing, and osteophyte formation[2,18,40a] are common problems associated with total meniscectomy. These destructive changes also occur in a significant number of patients after **subtotal meniscectomy.**[18] The goal of surgical care for meniscal tears is to maintain as much viable tissue as possible by avoiding total meniscectomy and investigating the possibility of surgical repair.

Rehabilitation after Subtotal Meniscectomy

Preservation of the load-bearing functions of the meniscus is the foundation for a partial meniscectomy. Rehabilitation after subtotal meniscectomy focuses initially on management of pain and swelling using RICE, transcutaneous electrical nerve stimulation (TENS), thermal agents, and NSAIDs as prescribed by the physician. ROM is progressed by using a number of techniques:
- Supine wall slides
- Stationary cycle for ROM
- Seated assisted knee flexion
- Standing wall squats
- Prone knee-extension hangs

Early weight bearing as tolerated is progressed to full weight bearing as pain allows. Progressive strengthening

exercises during the early phases of recovery focus on isometric quadriceps control, hamstring isometrics, straight-leg raises, hip abduction-adduction, and hip extension.

The PTA must carefully oversee the advancement of CKC exercises; observe, document, and communicate any objective or subjective changes in pain or swelling; and report to the PT regularly concerning each positive or negative change.

Many patients can tolerate a progressive program of early weight bearing, ROM activities, and strengthening exercises and may develop a chronic effusion that necessitates a significant modification in the rehabilitation plan.

In general, these patients are allowed to advance quickly through the maximum-protection phase. An older, less active population of patients may require a slower progression, depending on whether there is **articular cartilage** degeneration. Some surgeons advocate the use of a knee immobilizer during the first week after surgery to assist with early weight bearing and provide support for the quadriceps.

The patient may begin with more functional CKC exercises during the moderate-protection phase (the fourth to the eighth week).[43] Step-ups, wall squats, leg presses, and stair-steppers promote cocontraction of the quadriceps and hamstrings and stimulate the joint mechanoreceptor system to allow improved support. Proprioceptive exercises, including single-leg standing, balance board activities, and the minitrampoline, can begin during this phase, as can isokinetic velocity spectrum training (sets of exercises at progressively faster speeds).

The minimum-protection phase begins at the ninth postoperative week and advances to the twentieth week.[43] The goal of this phase is to normalize gait, attain full ROM, and enhance functional activities.

The fact that many meniscal injuries occur in conjunction with injuries to other structures (ACL, MCL, or joint capsule) is significant and must be fully appreciated by the PTA. The rehabilitation program for combined subtotal meniscectomy and the presence of other joint pathologic conditions must be modified to account for the healing of other structures.

The long-term consequences of subtotal meniscectomy must be clearly understood when addressing functional activities (activities of daily living, [ADLs]) and a return to athletics. Early degenerative changes are seen with both total and partial meniscectomy,[2,18] and include narrowing of the tibiofemoral joint space, formation of bone spurs (osteophytes), and degeneration of the femoral articular surface on the side of the surgery. Counseling and education of the patient focus on modifying ADLs related to stair-climbing and repetitive vertical compressive loading.

Rehabilitation after Meniscal Repair

The PTA must understand the fundamental differences between complete and partial removal of the meniscus and meniscal repair. Because many meniscal injuries occur in conjunction with associated ligament injuries (ACL, PCL, and MCL), as well as in isolated cases, the ultimate course of treatment for combined meniscal repairs and associated ligament injuries depends largely on the surgical procedure used to correct the ligament instability. In one study,[42] meniscal repairs done in conjunction with reconstruction of the ACL actually healed better (90%) than meniscal repairs done on stable knees (57%). Here discussion includes concepts involving isolated meniscal repair. Associated ACL reconstruction and meniscal repairs generally follow a more progressive program focusing on the principles of ACL rehabilitation, as well as enhancing recovery from the meniscal repair. Combined surgical repairs for the ACL and meniscus require highly individualized rehabilitation programs in which the surgeon and PT carefully consider many short- and long-range issues for the patient, including age, level of activity, and joint stability.

The foundation and contrasting difference between meniscectomy and meniscal repair rehabilitation is allowing the surgically repaired (sutured) meniscus to heal by avoiding (limiting) loads and stresses (ROM) that compromise the repair site.

Initially, after the repair of isolated meniscal injury without ACL reconstruction, the patient is non–weight bearing, gradually progressing to full weight bearing in 4 to 6 weeks.[18,25,40a,42] This delay in weight bearing status for meniscal repairs is necessary to avoid vertical compressive loads that may disrupt the suture site.[25] The patient also may be immobilized in a range-limiting brace for approximately 4 weeks.[18] Limiting knee flexion to approximately 90 to 100 degrees for 4 to 6 weeks is necessary to avoid excessive motion at the suture site. Pain and swelling management is essential throughout the maximum-protection phase.[43] The use of ice, elastic compression bandages, elevation, and electrical stimulation may reduce symptoms related to the surgery.

Regaining quadriceps control and controlled ROM can be initiated immediately after surgery. Quadriceps sets, straight-leg raises, hamstring sets, short-arc knee extensions, hip abduction-adduction and extension, and calf pumps are initiated and progressed from the first day after surgery throughout the maximum-protection phase. ROM activities (prone knee flexion and supine wall slides) are progressed gradually and limited to approximately 100 degrees for the first 4 to 6 weeks. The initiation of isotonic exercises (knee extension and leg curls) can begin during the later stages of the maximum-protection phase (3 to 4 weeks) and throughout the moderate-protection phase (4 to 8 weeks).[43]

Stationary cycling to increase ROM begins during the later stages of the maximum-protection phase (3 weeks) and progresses as tolerated through the moderate-protection phase. These patients cannot begin CKC exercises (e.g., leg presses, squats, step-ups, and stairclimbers) until at least 8 weeks after repair. As motion improves, swelling and pain are controlled and full weight bearing without crutches is achieved at 6 weeks. Then a very gradual program of short-arc leg presses, treadmill walking, and step-ups can begin. Access to an underwater treadmill is advantageous because the buoyancy of the water allows for limited weight bearing and normalized gait mechanics before full weight bearing. To reduce injury to the repaired meniscus, weighted and full squats must be strictly avoided for up to 3 to 6 months after repair.[18] Although the general concepts of regaining lost motion and improving strength and function are the same after subtotal meniscectomy and meniscal repairs, obvious delays in initiating weight bearing, full ROM, and CKC exercises are necessary to enhance healing of the repaired meniscus.

As mentioned, meniscal repairs also are seen in conjunction with ACL reconstruction. The program of recovery for these patients may be different to address both ligament and cartilage healing. Tenuta and Arciero[42] compared protocols involving ACL rehabilitation with meniscal repairs and rehabilitation programs with cruciate-stable knees. Their study shows a "significant decrease in the completely healed meniscal repairs in patients who followed an aggressive rehabilitation program after ACL reconstruction that made little effort to protect the meniscal repair." To minimize postoperative problems associated with ACL reconstructions, the rehabilitation program calls for accelerated weight bearing and motion. With this in mind, it is clear to see why some meniscal repairs may fail to heal completely if the principles of non–weight bearing and controlled motion are not followed.

PATELLOFEMORAL PATHOLOGIC CONDITIONS

Injuries and diseases of the patellofemoral joint and the extensor mechanism (quadriceps, quadriceps tendon, patella, patellar tendon, and patellofemoral articulation) are complex. The PTA must understand the anatomic relationships and rudimentary mechanics of the patellofemoral articulation and extensor mechanism to fully appreciate the rationale for rehabilitation of the many problems that can occur in this area. This requires careful review of the anatomy and kinesiology of the knee and extensor mechanism to gain a broad understanding of the relationships between mechanical deviations and resultant patellofemoral abnormalities.

This section outlines the more commonly encountered problems affecting the patellofemoral joint, focusing mainly on fundamental rehabilitation concepts involving lateral patellar compression and patellar tracking disorders, retropatellar articular cartilage arthrosis, patellar subluxation, and rehabilitation programs related to proximal and distal surgical realignment procedures.

Lateral Patellar Compression and Patellar Tracking Disorders

Often the underlying cause of anterior knee pain[25] is mechanical deviations of patellar tracking during knee flexion and extension. The resolution of pain and dysfunction related to patellar tracking problems is centered on therapeutic exercises that strengthen the quadriceps, stretching exercises to gain flexibility in the hamstrings and lateral knee structures, supportive bracing and taping, NSAIDs, thermal modalities, and various surgical interventions.

Before discussing specific rehabilitation procedures, one must see the relationship between the posture of the patella relative to the femur; the effect of hamstring tightness on patellofemoral compression; and the anatomic alignment of the lower extremity as these relate to patellar tracking dysfunction, patellar subluxation, and anterior knee pain.

In general, the patella is referenced to the femur in three positions (Fig. 19-29). A patellar posture that is more superior than normal is referred to as patella alta[28,34,46] and is associated with greater patellar instability.[34]

In addition to patellar posture, the **quadriceps angle (Q angle)** is a significant clinical assessment that relates directly to patellar tracking deviations and variations in the line or angle of pull of the quadriceps on the patella.[46] The Q angle refers to a line drawn from the anterior superior iliac spine through the center or axis of the patella and distally to the insertion of the patellar tendon on the tibial tubercle (Fig. 19-30). The Q angle can be increased by proximal tibial external rotation or distal tibia varus.[28,46] Figure 19-31 shows the various angles of muscular pull on the patella and how an increased Q angle can profoundly affect the tracking mechanisms of the patella during flexion and extension. Anatomic alignment of the lower extremity also can be a mechanism for patellar tracking dysfunction.

The **miserable malalignment syndrome** (Fig. 19-32)[26,28,34,46] is assessed with the patient in the standing position and provides objective data for the physician and PT about the entire lower-extremity kinetic-chain, patellar tracking dysfunction, and pain. This syndrome is characterized by femoral anteversion (internal femoral rotation), "squinting" patellae (patellae facing toward each other), proximal external tibial torsion (which results in what is called the "bayonet sign"), and foot pronation.[4,46] If the affected lower extremity demonstrates the miserable malalignment syndrome when the patient is in a standing position, then it is easy for the PTA to understand how the extensor mechanism can be changed and result in lateral tracking of the patella.

In addition to mechanical malalignment, muscle forces also can contribute to symptoms of anterior knee pain or retropatellar compression. Excessive hamstring tightness can increase patellofemoral compression because patellar excursion through knee extension is resisted by the hamstrings, requiring more quadriceps force (Fig. 19-33).[28]

In light of this information concerning patellar posture, Q angle, lower extremity malalignment, and muscle forces acting on the patella, the PTA must recognize that the result of these abnormalities is pain and dysfunction related to femoral and retropatellar articular cartilage (hyaline cartilage) degeneration from excessive wear, buttressing, and compression of the patella that tracks abnormally.

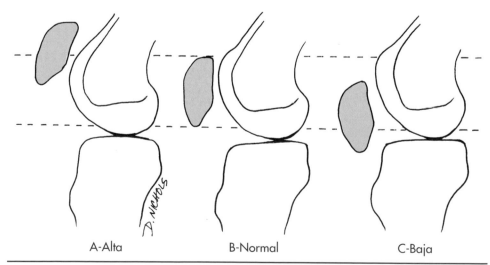

A-Alta   B-Normal   C-Baja

Fig. 19-29 Patella reference positions. **A,** Patella alta. **B,** Normal patella reference position. **C,** Patella baja.

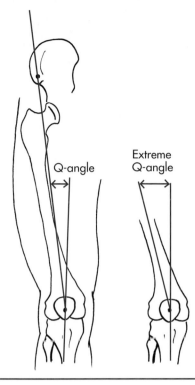

Fig. 19-30 The quadriceps angle is measured from the anterior superior iliac spine, through the axis of the patella, and distally to the insertion of the patellar tendon on the tibial tubercle.

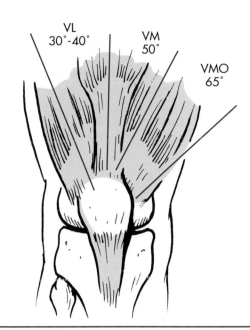

Fig. 19-31 Angles of muscular pull on the patella. Patellar reference positions and the quadriceps angle can affect mechanical tracking of the patella because of muscular angles of pull.

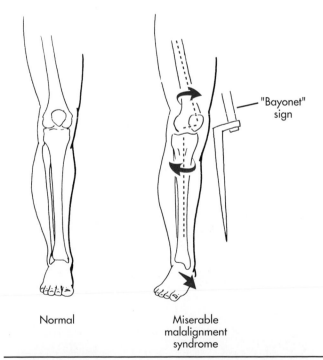

Fig. 19-32 Miserable malalignment syndrome. Anatomic alignment is assessed in the standing position. The miserable malalignment syndrome is characterized by combined femoral anteversion, "squinting patellae," external tibial torsion, and foot pronation.

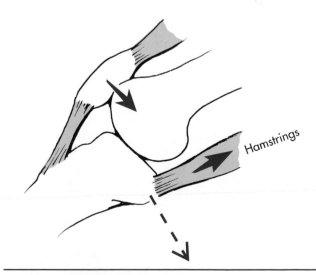

Fig. 19-33 Excessive hamstring tightness can contribute to increased patellofemoral compression.

Nonoperative Rehabilitation of Anterior Knee Pain

The initial course of treatment focuses primarily on controlling pain and swelling and initiating quadriceps strengthening exercises. Any activities that cause the patient discomfort are modified to accommodate pain and dysfunction. For example, stair climbing (descending more often than ascending) can reproduce symptoms of pain. The PTA can counsel the patient to use the non-affected limb in a straight-leg gait pattern when climbing or descending stairs. Ice packs, NSAIDs, and limb elevation may be needed in the acute phase. However, the use of elastic compression bandages should be avoided to prevent continued patellofemoral compression.

Among the classic symptoms of retropatellar pain are signs of inflammation, crepitus (audible, palpable gritty sandpaper, and cracking under the patella), pain, and a laterally tracking patella. The ultimate challenge for the rehabilitation team is the focused selection of appropriate and effective quadriceps-strengthening exercises that act to counter the effects of tight lateral structures, a lateral tracking patella related to the Q angle and malalignment, and quadriceps weakness.

Strengthening of the quadriceps muscle group is initiated by introducing isometric sets that do not produce pain. In some instances, submaximal isometric quadriceps sets are necessary at the beginning of the program to accommodate for pain. The vastus medialis oblique (VMO) is the focus of attention when addressing quadriceps strengthening. Bennett[4] suggests that "these muscles are emphasized because of their ability to stabilize the patella superiorly and, more importantly, medially. The superior medial pull of the vastus medialis muscle complex directly counteracts lateral tracking syndromes." Therefore progressive quadriceps sets serve as the foundation of the initial rehabilitation program.

In conjunction with quadriceps strengthening, the tight lateral structures that act to pull the patella laterally must be addressed. Stretching the hamstrings, stretching the iliotibial band (ITB) (Fig. 19-34), and performing manual patellar-stretching exercises (Fig. 19-35) are essential to counteract anterior knee pain that results from a lateral-tracking patella. Short-arc terminal knee extensions gradually are introduced in the early stages of rehabilitation to regain active quadriceps control. Care must be taken to begin this exercise with a very limited ROM (approximately 10 to 20 degrees of flexion) to avoid pain from lateral patellar compression and accommodate the weakened quadriceps muscles, which cannot control the patella adequately.

In keeping with strengthening of the extensor mechanism, attention also should be turned to the hip adductors, which may influence a medially directed pull on the patella.[4] During quadriceps sets, short-arc terminal knee extensions, and straight-leg raises, the affected limb should be slightly rotated (approximately 10 to 15 degrees) externally to take advantage of the medial pull of the adductors and minimize the potential for the patient to slightly internally rotate the affected leg to help substitute for the weakened quadriceps. Isometric hip adduction (Fig. 19-36) exercises gradually are advanced to isotonic hip adduction exercises (Fig. 19-37). Isometric static holds can begin in the early stages of rehabilitation, as the strength of the quadriceps improves and pain allows.

Functional CKC quadriceps-strengthening exercises are introduced to the program as pain and strength allow. In some instances, patients may tolerate limited

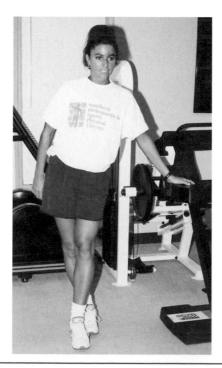

Fig. 19-34 Standing iliotibial band stretching. Stretching the lateral structures of the hip and knee can aid in minimizing lateral tracking of the patella and lateral compressive forces.

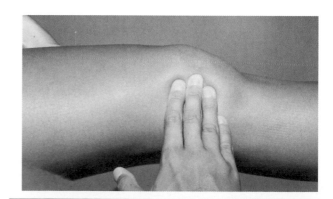

Fig. 19-35 Manual lateral patella stretching. The patient is instructed in "auto-stretching" of the patella. If the lateral retinaculum of the knee is tight and is causing the patella to track laterally, the patient can gently stretch the patella medially to stretch tight lateral structures.

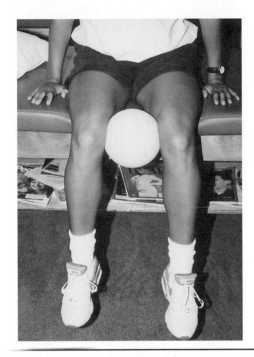

Fig. 19-36 Seated isometric hip adduction.

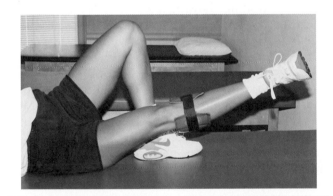

Fig. 19-37 Hip adduction strengthening exercises can be progressed from isometrics to side-lying concentric and eccentric loading.

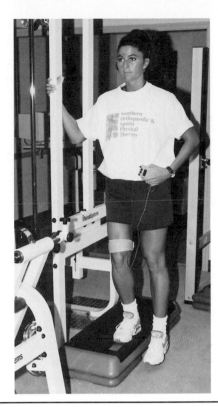

Fig. 19-38 Shallow step-ups with portable biofeedback or electrical muscle stimulation over the vastus medialis obliques is an excellent closed-chain functional drill to enhance control of the quadriceps.

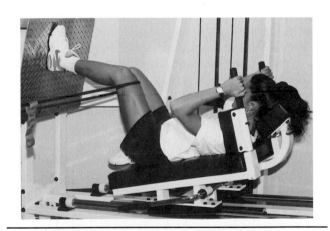

Fig. 19-39 Closed-chain leg-press exercise with elastic tubing to simultaneously enhance hip adduction control with concentric and eccentric loading of the quadriceps.

ROM leg presses, wall squats, and step-ups, as well as open-chain quadriceps isolation exercises. Shallow step-ups using biofeedback (Fig. 19-38) over the VMO are excellent CKC functional quadriceps-strengthening exercises. Limited ROM leg presses using elastic tubing to strengthen the hip adductors can further facilitate quadriceps strengthening (Fig. 19-39).

Supportive devices can help dynamically stabilize the patella. Commercially available patellar stabilizing sleeves provide a lateral buttress support to the patella to minimize lateral tracking. Dynamic patellar stabilization also is aided by adhesive taping techniques.

Postoperative Rehabilitation of Anterior Knee Pain

The basic goal of operative management for anterior knee pain related to lateral patellar tracking disorders (patellar subluxation) is to reestablish appropriate extensor mechanism function and reduce patellofemoral contact forces.[20]

Surgical management of patellofemoral disorders can be classified as proximal realignment procedures, distal realignment procedures, various patellofemoral articular cartilage shaving procedures, and perforation or abrasion chondroplasty.[46]

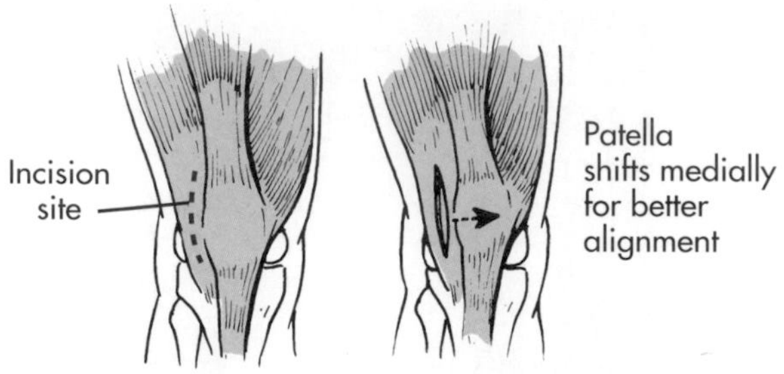

Fig. 19-40 Lateral retinacular release surgical procedure is designed to "free up" or release tight lateral structures and to allow the patella better anatomic alignment.

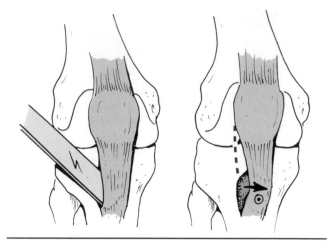

Fig. 19-41 Elmslie-Trillat surgical procedure for radical distal extensor mechanism realignment.

Proximal realignment procedures involve lateral retinacular release with VMO advancement (Fig. 19-40).[45] Rehabilitation after proximal realignment procedures is essentially the same as for nonoperative treatment of anterior knee pain. However, pain and swelling after surgery, as well as specific tissue healing and time constraints, must be addressed carefully. Therefore the initial course of management after proximal realignment procedures is focused on the use of ice, a lateral patellar compression and buttress pad, limb elevation, temporary immobilization and weight bearing as tolerated, and NSAIDs as prescribed by the physician. Control of pain and swelling is essential to reduce the quadriceps inhibition they produce.

Temporary immobilization is specifically related to management of the lateral retinacular release procedure. Because the rationale behind this procedure is to reduce the pull of the vastus lateralis muscle and related lateral structures by surgically cutting (releasing) portions of their attachment on the superolateral aspect of the patella, long-term immobilization of the patellofemoral joint and tibiofemoral articulation helps "scar in" and reattach the release of these tissues and counteract the desired surgical goal of reduced lateral pull. Therefore in this specific procedure, early lateral patellar stretching exercises and early knee flexion ROM exercises are needed to ensure that the lateral structures are maintained in an "opened" or released position. In some cases the VMO is surgically cut and advanced to a more mechanically advantageous angle to help produce a more midline pull of the patella. Early flexion exercises may stretch the advancement of the VMO; therefore extreme caution is needed when encouraging motion after lateral retinacular release with advancement of the VMO. When the VMO has been advanced, early active quadriceps-strengthening exercises must be delayed to allow for appropriate scarring and healing at the suture site.

Supine wall slides, stationary cycling, prone leg flexion, and manual patellar stretching exercises are introduced as pain and swelling allow. Quadriceps strengthening is the foundation for a successful outcome

after this surgical procedure. Open-chain remedial exercises (quadriceps sets, short-arc terminal knee extensions, straight-leg raises, and hip adduction exercises) give way to CKC functional exercises as soon as pain and tissue healing allow.

Step-ups with biofeedback over the VMO, wall squats, leg presses, stair-steppers, and normalized gait mechanics are encouraged during the early stages of postoperative rehabilitation. As with nonoperative management, hip abduction exercises are avoided initially to minimize the lateral pulling influence of this muscle group on the patella.

Distal realignment procedures are also termed *radical* surgeries by Bennett.[4] The goal behind these surgeries is to reduce severe patellofemoral compression loads and significant patellar subluxation by surgically removing the extensor mechanism's insertion (patellar tendon attachment on the tibial tubercle) and elevating and reattaching the tibial tubercle to a more mechanically advantageous site to improve the pull of the quadriceps.[4] The PTA encounters the Hauser, Maquet, and Elmslie-Trillat (Fig. 19-41) surgical procedures. Each is a variation designed to realign the distal extensor mechanism.

Significant modifications in rehabilitation are necessary with distal realignment procedures based on bone and soft-tissue healing and promotion of quadriceps strength. Generally, immobilization in plaster or a hinged range-limiting brace is used for 4 to 6 weeks.[4,46] Crutches are encouraged for about 6 weeks,[46] with initial non–weight bearing progressing to touch-down weight bearing and then to full weight bearing over the full 6 weeks of immobilization.[4,46] Bennett advocates advancing ROM measurements to approximately 100 degrees of knee flexion for the first 2 weeks and progressing to 120 degrees of knee flexion by 6 weeks.[4]

Individual circumstances, surgical procedures, and the wishes of the physician dictate variations in this initial management plan. Isometric quadriceps sets, straight-leg raises, and short-arc quadriceps exercises are encouraged once pain, swelling, and tissue healing allow. With extensor mechanism repair, as well as radical distal realignment procedures, a few weeks' delay is necessary before initiating quadriceps sets and straight-leg raises so as not to endanger the surgical repair site.

Many remedial quadriceps-strengthening exercises can be performed in the brace during the early phases of recovery. ROM, CKC strengthening, and proprioception exercises are progressed according to the proximal realignment plan discussed.

Occasionally arthroscopic procedures are used to directly address the condition of the articular cartilage on the undersurface of the patella and the femoral condyles in cases of anterior knee pain. The term *chondromalacia* describes retropatellar articular cartilage degeneration or softening. The diagnosis of chondromalacia only can be made at the time of surgery because visualization of the articular surfaces is necessary.[34,46]

Various surgical procedures are used to smooth rough articular surfaces and stimulate an inflammatory response to enhance healing. Perforation or abrasion of subchondral bone (chondroplasty and abrasion arthroplasty)[4,7] stimulates a communication between the damaged articular surface and vascular supply of subchondral bone. Pain and swelling after these procedures are significant concerns and require ice, compression dressings (being careful to avoid excessive patellofemoral compression), limb elevation, and antiinflammatory medications prescribed by the physician. Limited weight bearing (non–weight bearing progressing to touch-down weight bearing) is encouraged for 4 to 6 weeks to accommodate the pain and healing of the articular cartilage surface.[4] Regaining quadriceps strength by using isometrics, straight-leg raises, short-arc terminal knee extensions, hamstring stretching, manual patellar stretching, and stretching of the iliotibial band begins during the early recovery stages of rehabilitation. The PTA must pay close attention to complaints of pain and objective signs of swelling and articular cartilage degeneration (crepitus) during all stages of recovery, particularly with knee extension exercises. The angle of short-arc knee extension perhaps should be reduced to eliminate pain. Modifying the angle of the leg press also may limit pain and articular wear. Occasionally a change from open-chain exercises to limited ROM CKC exercises is appropriate (in consultation with the PT) to minimize patellofemoral compression loads and encourage continued quadriceps strengthening.

FRACTURES

This section briefly introduces management and rehabilitation programs associated with fractures of the patella, distal femur **(supracondylar femur fractures)**, and proximal tibia **(tibial plateau).**

Fractures of the Patella

Fractures of the patella can occur with direct or indirect trauma.[46] The most common injury involves the patella making contact with a hard surface. Less frequently the patella can be fractured by a violent contraction of the quadriceps.[33,46] Avascular necrosis (AVN) can result in either case if a transverse fracture occurs, because the vascular supply to the patella is reserved for the central portion and distal pole, leaving the proximal segment of the transverse fracture prone to it.[33] Nondisplaced patellar fractures often are treated conservatively with immobilization of the affected limb in full extension.[31,33,46]

Some controversy exists concerning the recovery of motion and duration of immobilization.[33,46] Some authors advise plaster immobilization for 6 weeks. Other authorities state, "There is no place in modern practice for the traditional 6 weeks immobilization of a nondisplaced patellar fracture." [46]

Rehabilitation management of nondisplaced patellar fractures treated with immobilization is primarily supportive throughout immobilization and limited weight bearing. The nonaffected limb can maintain strength and flexibility using quadriceps strengthening exercises (e.g., knee extensions, leg presses, and leg curls), and aerobic fitness can be enhanced with the use of single-leg stationary cycling or an upper body ergometer (UBE). Ankle pumps are encouraged for the affected immobilized limb throughout immobilization. Quadriceps sets, short-arc knee extensions, and straight-leg raises are introduced gradually once sufficient bone healing has occurred. If quadriceps-strengthening exercises and knee flexion exercises are begun too soon, the force of muscle contraction and knee flexion stretching may separate and stress the fracture site, slowing the healing process and leading to fracture displacement.

The treatment of displaced patellar fractures is based on ranges of acceptable fracture fragment separation exceeding 3 to 4 mm.[31] Stabilization of displaced patellar fractures is best accomplished with an open reduction and internal fixation (ORIF) procedure. Figure 19-42 portrays various patellar fracture patterns.

The most common fixation devices are tension band wiring and cerclage wiring (Fig. 19-43). The tension band wire is a dynamic compression device that approximates and compresses the patellar fragments. The additional use of cerclage wiring adds to the stability of the repair and allows early joint motion without redisplacing the fracture fragments.[46]

When tension band wiring is used with cerclage wiring, the immediate postoperative positioning of the patient calls for the prevention of full passive knee extension to maintain tension and compression of the patellar fracture fragments. Generally, the knee is immobilized in 20 degrees of knee flexion to support dynamic compression of the tension band wiring procedure. One week after surgery, active knee extension, submaximal

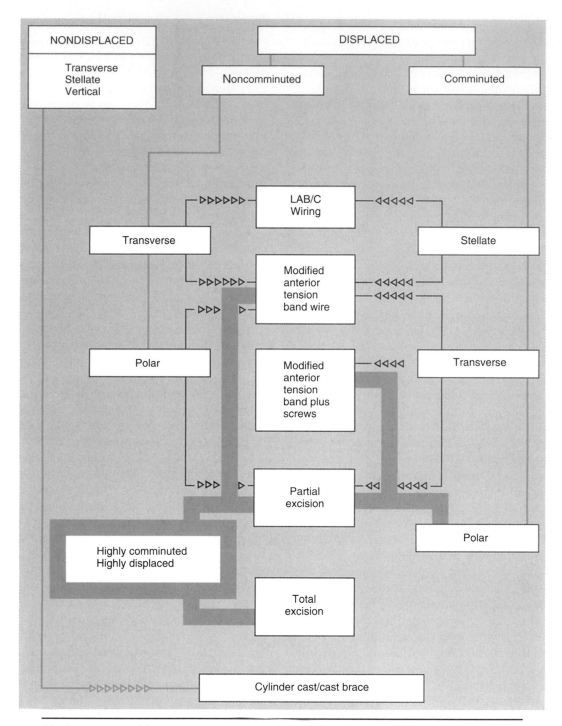

Displacement and fracture pattern guide choice of treatment with which to obtain the two primary goals of quadriceps mechanism continuity and a stable anatomic reduction of the patellar articular surface. Nondisplaced fractures are managed nonoperatively. Displaced articular fractures are repaired, if possible, using tension band wiring techniques with or without screws or interosseous wiring. Polar avulsion fractures may be excised, but a secure reattachment of the quadriceps or patellar tendon is required. If comminution prevents satisfactory repair, total patellectomy may be the only option to restore the quadriceps. (From Browner BD, Jupiter J, Levine A, et al: Skeletal Trauma, 2nd ed, vol 2. Philadelphia, WB Saunders, 2003.)

LAB/C, Longitudinal anterior band plus cerclage.

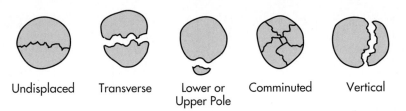

Fig. 19-42 Types of patellar fractures. (From Wiessman B, Sledge CB: Orthopaedic Radiology. Philadelphia, WB Saunders, 1986.)

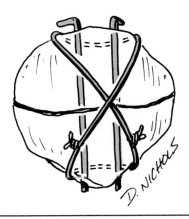

Fig. 19-43 Transverse fracture of the patella. Stabilization is achieved with tension band wiring and cerclage wiring.

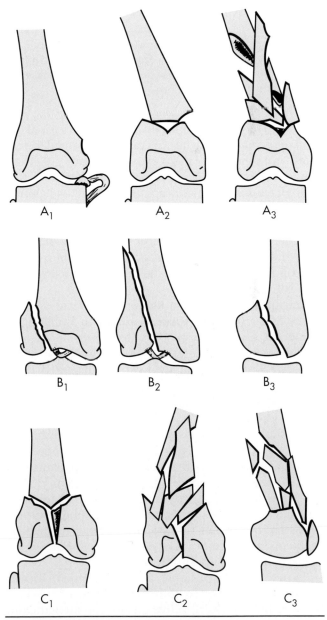

Fig. 19-44 AO/ASIF classification of supracondylar fractures. (From Johnson KD: Orthopaedic Knowledge Update III. Rosemont, IL, American Academy of Orthopaedic Surgeons, 1990.)

quadriceps sets, and straight-leg raises can be initiated. Flexion of the knee out of the immobilizer usually is limited to approximately 100 degrees for at least 6 weeks to allow for proper bone healing. Weight bearing as tolerated with assistive devices is encouraged during the first few weeks after surgery, then progressed to full weight bearing by the third week. The long progression of quadriceps-strengthening exercises and the advancement of full knee flexion correlate with normal bone healing and individual tolerance. Care must be taken not to force aggressive knee extension strengthening exercises with heavy isotonic loads too early in the program. Isokinetic quadriceps and hamstring strengthening at submaximal effort with fast to moderate speeds of contraction can be used when immobilization is discontinued and the patient demonstrates good quadriceps control, improved knee flexion motion, nonpainful performance of the rudimentary quadriceps strength program (quadriceps sets, straight-leg raises, short-arc quadriceps exercises), and appropriate bone healing.

Supracondylar Femur Fractures

Distal femur fractures generally are classified as extraarticular, unicondylar, or bicondylar[33,34] (Fig. 19-44). These fractures usually are managed with an ORIF procedure, immobilization, and non–weight bearing to allow for healing. Various internal fixation devices are used, depending on the position and severity of the fracture.

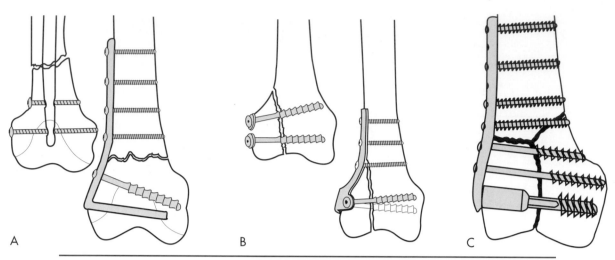

Fig. 19-45 Various methods of open reduction with internal fixation for, **A,** transverse supracondylar fractures, **B,** unicondylar fractures, and, **C,** T- and Y-condylar fractures. (From McRae R: Practical Fracture Treatment, 3rd ed. New York, Churchill Livingstone, 1994.)

Figure 19-45 demonstrates fixation devices used for transverse supracondylar fractures, unicondylar fractures, and type C (T- and Y-pattern) fractures. Because of the location, pattern, and severity of supracondylar femur fractures, the quadriceps, hamstrings, and gastrocnemius muscle groups contribute to posterior angulation and fracture displacement.[31,33] Therefore the method of fixation focuses on fracture site stabilization and fragment apposition while minimizing the pull on the fracture site by the quadriceps, hamstrings, and calf muscles.

Fractures of the distal femur can create vascular injury to the popliteal fossa secondary to swelling and significant forces.[31] Displaced supracondylar fractures can be treated nonoperatively at the discretion of the surgeon. Physicians usually treat nondisplaced distal femur fractures nonoperatively with closed reduction of the fragments and tibial traction for approximately 8 to 12 weeks.[31]

Physical therapy management of supracondylar fractures is guided extensively by the healing process of bone and associated soft tissue. Generally, patients have limited weight bearing for 10 to 12 weeks. Non–weight bearing is followed strictly until subsequent radiologic assessment determines secure bone healing. Arthrofibrosis and quadriceps adhesion to the bone are frequent problems, with significant bleeding and associated tissue damage in distal femur fractures.

Therefore early postoperative management focuses on patellar mobility (within the confines of the knee brace or immobilizer), active quadriceps-strengthening exercises (quadriceps sets and straight-leg raises), and active knee flexion to minimize knee contractures. It is imperative to encourage strengthening and flexibility exercises for the uninvolved limb and instruct the patient in a general fitness program that does not compromise the healing of the injured limb. As bone healing progresses, appropriate normalized gait mechanics are encouraged and CKC-strengthening exercises are added cautiously. Throughout the course of healing, all fundamental quadriceps, hamstring, hip, and calf exercises are maintained, including quadriceps sets, straight-leg raises (all four positions), short-arc terminal knee extensions, leg curls, ankle pumps, gluteal sets, and knee flexion ROM exercises.

When to begin CKC-strengthening and proprioception exercises is determined by the healing of the stabilized fracture site, pain, swelling, improved ROM, improved quadriceps strength, and physician and PT judgment.

As with many fractures about the knee, associated soft-tissue injuries (ligaments, tendon, cartilage, and muscle) are common. Thus the use of various exercises and rate of healing are strongly influenced by bone and soft-tissue healing.

Proximal Tibia Fractures (Tibial Plateau Fractures)

The general treatment of nondisplaced tibial plateau fractures (Fig. 19-46) is described by Loth[31] as follows:

> These patients should be treated with early motion and protected weight bearing to prevent displacement. Traction, a knee immobilizer with intermittent motion, or a fracture brace with protected weight bearing may be appropriate for various fracture patterns. . . .

Associated knee ligament damage may be present;[31] therefore rehabilitation must address bone healing and repair of associated soft-tissue structures. Quadriceps-strengthening exercises (quadriceps sets, and straight-leg raises in all four positions) in an immobilizer can commence as soon as the patient can tolerate them.

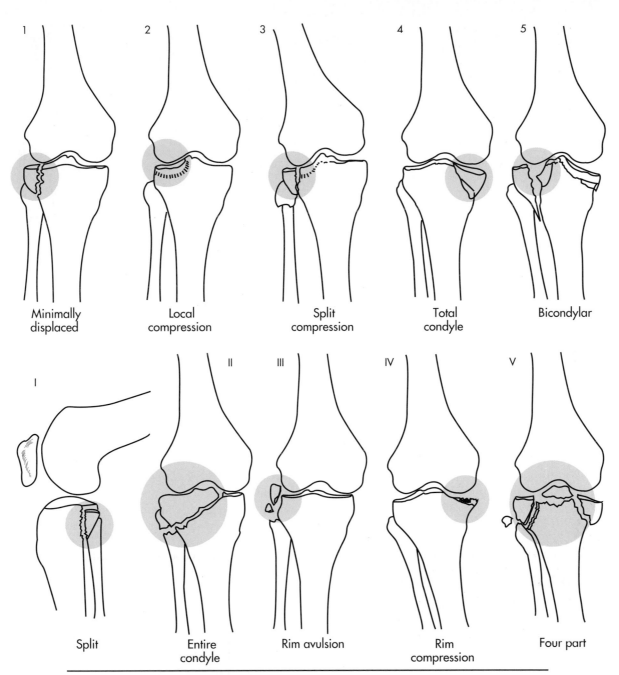

Fig. 19-46 Classification of proximal tibial plateau fractures. (From Loth T: Orthopedic Boards Review. St Louis, Mosby, 1993.)

Knee flexion motion is progressed as bone healing, swelling, and pain allow. Weight bearing activities, proprioception, and CKC-strengthening exercises are deferred until secure bone healing and stabilization occur.

Displaced proximal tibial fractures are treated with an ORIF procedure. Figure 19-47 illustrates various internal fixation devices used with different fracture patterns. Postoperative management and rehabilitation of tibial plateau fractures follow the course of bone and soft-tissue healing.

First, the patient is placed in a leg immobilizer or fracture brace in full extension. Active quadriceps sets are performed and the patient is generally non–weight bearing or partial weight bearing, depending on the severity of the fracture. After initial surgical wound healing has occurred, knee flexion exercises can begin based on the patient's tolerance.

Straight-leg raises can be taught during the first week postoperatively. Active ankle ROM and pumping are encouraged immediately, and hamstring-stretching exercises are safely taught with the limb immobilized. A general conditioning program is advocated early, with specific strengthening exercises for the uninvolved limb and single-leg stationary cycling for aerobic fitness.

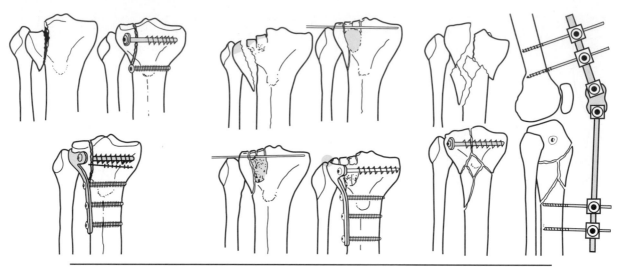

Fig. 19-47 Various methods of internal fixation of tibial plateau fractures. (From McRae R: Practical Fracture Treatment, 3rd ed. New York, Churchill-Livingstone, 1994.)

As bone healing progresses (10 to 12 weeks), verified by radiographic examination by the physician, increased weight bearing, and normalized gait mechanics are encouraged.

Advanced strengthening exercises using isotonic knee extension and leg curl exercises, CKC functional exercises (stair-steppers, short-arc step-ups, wall squats, and leg presses), and proprioception exercises (balance boards and minitrampoline) are added cautiously as the patient demonstrates improved quadriceps strength, increased knee flexion motion, and reduced pain and swelling, and as the necessary healing of bone and soft tissue occurs.

KNEE JOINT RECONSTRUCTION

This section introduces terminology consistent with total knee replacement (TKR) surgery, prosthetic design, and rehabilitation after surgery. In addition to discussing physical therapy management as it pertains to the PTA, tibial osteotomy procedures and recovery are addressed.

Knee Arthroplasty

The indications for TKR are primarily to eliminate or reduce pain and improve functional activities in severely disabled patients.[19,21,34] Osteoarthritis (degenerative joint disease [DJD]) and rheumatoid arthritis contribute significantly to unicompartmental (medial or lateral), bicompartmental (both medial and lateral joint compartments), and tricompartmental (medial, lateral, and patellofemoral compartments) pain and dysfunction.[19,21,34,44]

Authorities define basic contraindications for TKR as active or recent septic arthritis, a "nonfunctioning extensor mechanism or severe neurologic dysfunction that prevents extension or control of the knee," and a neuropathic joint.[31,34] The age of many patients with rheumatoid arthritis who undergo TKR is under 60 years.[21] Patients with osteoarthritis who seek the same procedure are usually over 60 years of age.[21]

TKR generally involves removing the degenerated articular surfaces of the tibia, the femur, and occasionally the articular surface of the patella, and replacing these structures with metal, plastic, or a combination prosthesis. The goals are to relieve pain, uniformly transmit forces across the joint, create a horizontal joint in the stance phase of gait, restore anatomic and mechanical axes, provide adequate stability, and improve function.[21,31,34,44]

The PTA must be aware of common prosthetic designs, as well as methods for securing these devices to bone, because this information affects the rehabilitation program. Two types of implants are used:

Constrained or *conforming implants* sacrifice the cruciate ligaments (ACL, PCL, or both) but rely on the "complete conformity between the components" for stability.[21,34,44]

Nonconstrained (*cruciate-sparing*) or *resurfacing implants* retain the soft-tissue stabilizing restraints (ACL and PCL).[21,34,44]

Miller[34] suggests that the nonconstrained implant is "rarely used due to exacting surgical technique and soft tissue balancing. . . ." Surgical techniques that sacrifice the cruciates (particularly the PCL) may cause problems with stair climbing.[34] The surgeon may elect to perform a nonconstrained procedure on the articular surface of the patella, depending on the severity of joint degeneration involving the patellofemoral joint. With patellofemoral compression forces one to one and a half times body weight while walking on level ground and three to four times body weight while ascending or descending stairs,[31] it is easy to appreciate the rationale for replacing a painful, degenerated retropatellar surface during TKR. One study[6] recommends that:

the patella be resurfaced when an unconstrained prosthesis of this type is used in patients who have inflammatory arthritis or osteoarthritis. Failure to resurface the patella in patients who have these diagnoses may result in an increased rate of revision, including early revision, for the treatment of chronic patellar pain.

In addition, improved stair climbing can be expected after patellar resurfacing because of the reduced patellofemoral pain.[34] Patellar resurfacing components are plastic materials because metal-backed implants lead to wear fracture and create metallic debris particles in the joint.[34]

Securing the various components (tibial, femoral, and patellar) to bone has a direct effect on the progression of weight bearing status after surgery.[21] The prosthesis can be secured with bone cement, usually polymethylmethacrylate (PMMA),[19,34] or a porous-coated cementless prosthesis can be inserted, in which the surrounding bone actually grows into and adheres to the prosthesis, creating a "direct biologic fixation."[21]

Cemented components may loosen over time in more active patient populations,[21] whereas the noncemented prosthesis has no cement debris and a highly organized fibrous ingrowth adhering to the implant.[44] However, some authorities[31] suggest that uncemented knee prostheses are associated with a higher reoperation rate than cemented components. In addition, Loth[31] reports that total implant loosening is more frequent in noncemented prostheses.

Rehabilitation after Total Knee Joint Replacement

Weight bearing may be restricted longer in the noncemented group to allow for firm bone growth to the component.[21] Cemented components demonstrate a more secure fit earlier than the noncemented group, thus allowing earlier progression in weight bearing.

Immediate postoperative care uses a compression dressing with a knee immobilizer in full extension with the involved limb elevated 30 to 40 degrees to minimize swelling. The maximum-protection phase of recovery focuses on reducing unwanted stresses that may loosen the prosthesis, while stimulating muscle strength, increasing ROM, and reducing pain and swelling. Remedial exercises that are initiated immediately after surgery include quadriceps isometrics, ankle pumps, gluteal sets, active assisted straight-leg raises, and short-arc terminal knee extensions out of the immobilizer. As the surgical wound heals (2 to 3 days postoperatively), it is imperative to regain active control over knee flexion. Some authors report that CPM may be beneficial in regaining knee flexion immediately after TKR surgery.[19,21] However, there appears to be no significant difference in the rate of wound healing and the incidence of thromboembolism in patients not receiving CPM during the immediate postoperative period.[31] The

knee immobilizer can be removed to perform supine heel slides and supine hip and knee flexion exercises (Fig. 19-48). The appropriate time to begin weight bearing depends on the fixation used, but generally the patient is instructed in a partial weight bearing gait with a walker or crutches.[19] Supine wall slides and active-assisted wall slides (Fig. 19-49) can be added as pain allows. Usually, the knee immobilizer is discarded by 4 weeks, but an ambulatory assistive device is retained for support until strength and a normalized gait are achieved.

The moderate-protection phase described by Timm[43] extends over 7 to 12 weeks postoperatively and is characterized by enhanced gait mechanics for patients with a cemented prosthesis. Timm[43] recommends 50% weight bearing by the eighth week, 75% weight bearing by the tenth week, and full weight bearing without an assistive device by the twelfth week for patients with noncemented components.

Patellar mobility must be allowed during the early phases of recovery. As the midline surgical incision heals, the patella should be mobilized in a caudal-cephalic motion to reduce patellofemoral adhesions.

Generally, by 13 weeks after surgery the patient can progress to isotonic knee-extension exercises, isokinetic knee flexion and extension,[43] stationary cycling for improved knee ROM, stair-climbers, treadmill walking, and various CKC functional activities (balance board and minitrampoline) as long as pain, swelling, quadriceps strength, joint stability, and tissue healing improve.

It is common for the elderly population receiving TKR to demonstrate reduced cardiovascular fitness and strength; therefore a general conditioning program should be started as soon as the patient can tolerate it. Early single-leg stationary cycling or UBE can be safely and effectively used to maintain or improve cardiovascular fitness. Because a TKR was performed to reduce pain and dysfunction related to osteoarthritis or rheumatoid arthritis, care must be taken to protect other affected joints during the initiation of a general conditioning program. In some cases, a swimming program

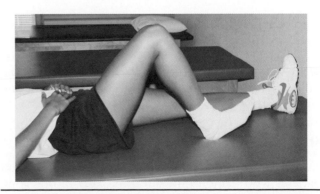

Fig. 19-48 Active supine knee flexion range-of-motion exercises are performed daily with the immobilizer removed.

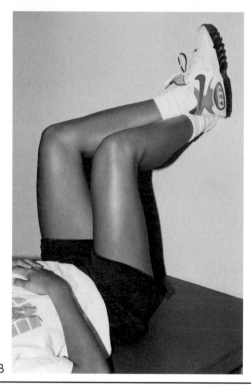

Fig. 19-49 **A,** Supine wall slides. **B,** Supine active-assisted wall slides for gaining knee flexion.

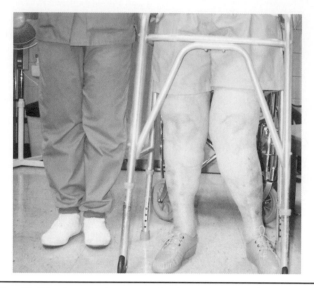

Fig. 19-50 Severe degenerative joint disease of the lateral compartment of the knee. Note the severe valgus deformity of the knee.

may be more appropriate than either open- or closed-chain resistive exercises.

Throughout the course of recovery, the judicious use of ice, compression, whirlpool, and electrical stimulation may help control pain and swelling before and after the prescribed exercise program.

HIGH TIBIAL OSTEOTOMY

A tibial **osteotomy** procedure can be performed on patients who demonstrate advanced DJD of one compartment of the knee.[34] Most commonly, this is the medial joint compartment and is characterized by a varus (bow-legged) deformity that creates abnormal

loads on the medial aspect of the tibiofemoral joint.[35] Less frequently, the lateral compartment is involved and creates a valgus deformity (knock-knees) (Fig. 19-50). Although this procedure is commonly performed on elderly patients (average age 60), one study[35] reports a mean age of 32 years, with a range of 16 to 47 years. This procedure is generally considered a temporary solution, lasting 7 to 10 years, before a TKR is considered.[34]

High tibial osteotomy (HTO) attempts to realign the tibiofemoral joint by surgically creating a wedge in the proximal tibia or distal femur, depending on varus or valgus deformity, and redistributing the forces and compressive loads more evenly across the joint (Fig. 19-51). In valgus deformity associated with lateral tibiofemoral compartment destruction (see Fig. 19-50), a distal femur (supracondylar) closing-wedge osteotomy is performed and is stabilized with a plate.[34,41] Depending on the wishes and training of the surgeon, some patients use CPM immediately postoperatively to facilitate early flexion motion.[41]

Usually the knee is placed in an immobilizer in full extension with a suction drain inserted to help evacuate the excessive accumulation of blood. Initially, strengthening exercises (quadriceps sets, straight-leg raises in the splint, and gluteal sets) are performed and advanced from the first day postoperatively. Manual patellar stretching is encouraged once initial surgical wound healing has occurred, especially with distal femoral wedge osteotomy (preoperative valgus deformity caused lateral joint compartment disease) because the procedure involves extensive invasion of the quadriceps.[41] If CPM is not used, the patient is allowed out of the immobilizer a few times a day to perform active knee flexion exercises. As patellar mobility (caudal-cephalic motion) improves, progressive knee flexion ROM

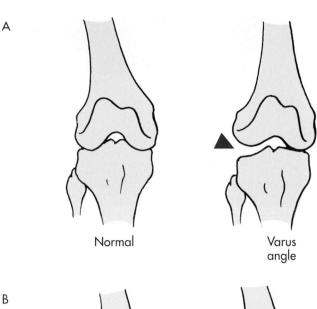

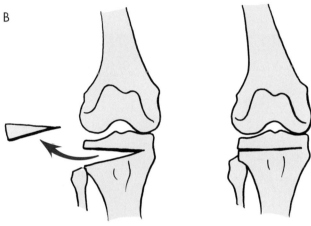

Fig. 19-51 High tibial osteotomy surgical procedure to redistribute compressive loads more evenly across the joint. **A,** Normal and abnormal varus angle. **B,** Wedge removed to change the angle of joint.

exercises are added with the patient in a sitting position to allow gravity to influence the flexion range of the affected limb. Care must be taken to manually assist the affected limb from sudden flexion and encourage quadriceps relaxation. Weight bearing status after HTO is guided primarily by the mechanism and time constraints of bone healing, as well as the type of fixation used to secure the bone.[41] Sisk[41] reports that blade or plate fixation "improves the rigidity of fixation of both tibial and femoral osteotomies, making supplemental casts unnecessary." Usually touch-down weight bearing is allowed after surgery with the aid of crutches or a walker. Progressive ambulation follows bone-healing constraints; therefore protective weight bearing is encouraged for up to 12 weeks.[41] Progressive resistive exercises for the quadriceps and hamstrings are initiated gradually within the first 3 to 4 weeks after surgery. Usually ankle weights, Thera-Band resistance, seated isotonic quadriceps and hamstring exercises, and cables and pulleys can be added cautiously during

the moderate-protection phase of recovery (7 to 12 weeks), as described by Timm.[43] Knee flexion ROM improvement is encouraged by using supine wall slides, seated knee flexion, prone knee flexion, and stationary cycling.

The initiation of functional CKC resistance exercises is deferred until the physician receives radiographic confirmation of secure bone union. Assistive devices for ambulation are discontinued once a minimum of 8 to 12 weeks has passed, fixation of the bone has occurred, and the patient demonstrates good quadriceps strength, improved knee flexion ROM, and confidence in a normalized gait pattern.

COMMON MOBILIZATION TECHNIQUES FOR THE KNEE

The PT may prescribe appropriate directions of force and amplitude, as well as specific mobilization techniques, depending on which specific knee condition is present, the amount of pain, and which motions are limited (see Chapter 16). The patient must be placed in the most comfortable position that allows for maximum relaxation of the affected limb. Patient relaxation and compliance can be enhanced through thermal agents and positioning before applying mobilization techniques.

The techniques presented here are generally safe, effective, and easily performed by the PTA. It is important to recognize that there are many techniques used to modulate pain and improve motion of the knee. The following examples demonstrate the most common techniques used for the patellofemoral and tibiofemoral joints.

Mobilization of the Patellofemoral Joint

With the patient supine on an examination table, the patella should be mobililzed in a caudal direction by firmly grasping the proximal or superior pole of the patella with an open palm or fingertips (Fig. 19-52). Care should be taken to avoid patellofemoral compression while the patella is gently pushed or glided in an

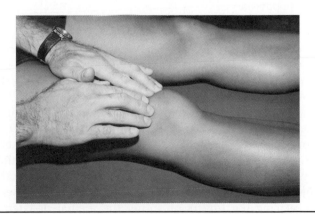

Fig. 19-52 Manual caudal glide of the patella.

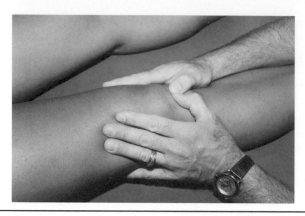

Fig. 19-53 Manual cephalic glide of the patella.

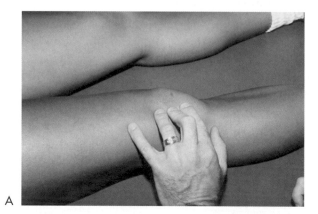

A

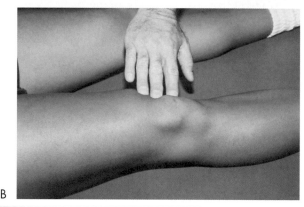

B

Fig. 19-54 **A,** Medial glide of the patella. **B,** Lateral glide of the patella.

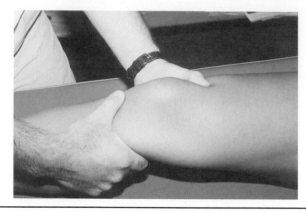

Fig. 19-55 Manual anterior-posterior glide of the tibio-femoral joint with the affected knee flexed approximately 30 degrees. This position parallels the Lachman examination position.

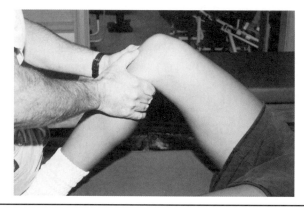

Fig. 19-56 Manual anterior-posterior glide of the tibio-femoral joint with the knee flexed 90 degrees. This position parallels the anterior-posterior drawer examination.

inferior direction (caudally). When the PTA is teaching the patient this technique, he or she should be instructed to use the thumbs of both hands to stretch the patella "toward the foot."

To achieve a superior glide motion (cephalic), one hand should be placed at the inferior pole or distal border of the patella as described. Care should be taken to avoid patellofemoral compressive load while the patella is gently stretched superiorly (Fig. 19-53). Both medial and lateral glides of the patella can be achieved by placing the fingers on either the medial or lateral aspect of the patella and gently pushing either medially

or laterally (Fig. 19-54). A compressive force to the patellofemoral joint should be avoided.

Mobilization of the Tibiofemoral Joint

Anterior and posterior glide motions described by Wooden[48] are similar to the Lachman examination and the anterior and posterior drawer tests previously described. To perform an anterior and posterior glide motion directed to the tibiofemoral joint, the patient's affected limb is held in approximately 30 degrees of flexion. The distal femur is stabilized with one hand, while the other hand to firmly grasps the proximal tibia. Gentle anteriorly and posteriorly directed force is applied (Fig. 19-55).

An anteriorly and posteriorly directed mobilization force can be performed with the affected limb held at approximately 90 degrees of flexion. The PTA stabilizes the foot of the affected limb by sitting on the dorsum of the foot. Both hands are used to grasp the proximal tibia, with the thumbs of the hands directly on the anteromedial and anterolateral joint lines of the

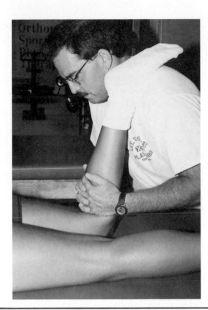

Fig. 19-57 Prone "scooping" of the tibiofemoral joint.

tibiofemoral joint. Gentle anteriorly and posteriorly directed force is applied to the tibia (Fig. 19-56).

In another common mobilization technique, the patient is prone on an examination table with the affected limb flexed 60 degrees to 90 degrees. The PTA places the foot of the affected limb on his or her shoulder and firmly grasps the proximal posterior tibia with open palms over the proximal calf muscles. With a very gentle anterior "scooping" motion of the hands, the PTA rocks the tibia forward and away from the femur (Fig. 19-57).

❖ ADDITIONAL FEATURES

ACL Graft Selection: Autographs are most frequently used. Bone-patellar tendon-bone, semitendinosus, quad tendon, distal ITB, and gracilis.

ACL Mechanoreceptor Function: ACL is a rich sensory organ. ACL sensation is a source of proprioception and kinesthetic ability. Reflex afferent information is provided by mechanoreceptors, which assist in maintaining joint stability when ligaments are loaded.

ACL Postoperative Considerations: Some stress is desirable for healing and remodeling of graft. Graft failure location is usually at the fixation site during the first 2 to 4 weeks.

Causes of Varus Angulation: Primary varus, double varus, and triple varus.

Complications after Supracondylar Fractures: Fat embolism, delayed union, nonunion, malunion, limb shortening, knee stiffness, and infection.

Consequences of Meniscectomy: Early degenerative changes. Narrowing of the tibiofemoral space, bone spurs, osteophytes, and degenerative changes of femoral articular surface, which are collectively referred to as Fairbanks's signs.

Degenerative Tears of the Meniscus: No history of specific trauma, such as squatting or getting out of a car. Degree of stress is considered minor attrition frequently associated with articular cartilage degeneration.

Double Varus: Tibiofemoral osseous alignment, lateral compartment separation, lateral ligamentous laxity, and lateral condylar "lift-off" with gait.

Examination of the ACL: History and mechanism of injury. Clinical examination includes stability tests, radiographs, magnetic resonance imaging, arthrocentesis, arthrography, crossover test, and functionality examination.

Femoral Anatomy: Excessive torsion deformity at the hip causes significant trochlear orientation alterations at the knee. Internal femoral torsion or femoral neck anteversion produces malfunction of extension mechanics that act to displace the patella laterally.

High Tibial Osteotomy: Unicompartmental degenerative arthritis. Designed to transfer loads to uninvolved tibiofemoral joint. Most commonly used for varus deformity.

Knee Stiffness after Supracondylar Fractures: Common complication. Quad tethering; quad tendon and proximal extensor mechanism becomes adherent to the femoral shaft and patella. Bony mechanical block. Prolonged immobilization.

MCL Examination: Valgus test at 0 and 30 degrees of flexion. End-feel is critical. Grades I and II have a firm, definite end-feel; grades III and IV have a softer, loose end-feel.

MCL Injuries: The most common knee ligament injury. Valgus-external rotation and noncontact mechanism of injury. Deep MCL fibers are attached to medial meniscus.

MCL Treatment: Generally successful after rigid nonsurgical critical pathway. Knee must be stable in extension. There must be firm end-feel with less than 3 mm of opening with valgus stress. Local, not diffuse tenderness. No massive effusions.

Meniscus Repair: Isolated repairs may be non–weight bearing, progressing to full weight bearing by 6 to 8 weeks. Avoid vertical compression and shearing forces that may disrupt the suture site. May have range-limiting orthosis for 4 weeks, limiting flexion to 90 degrees or 100 degrees for 4 weeks.

Meniscus Trauma: Generally occurs in younger, more active individuals. Trauma is associated with torque and acceleration forces. Commonly associated with ACL injury.

Patella Fractures: Displaced or nondisplaced; transverse or displaced fractures are prone to avascular necrosis of proximal segment due to disruption of blood supply.

Patella Postures: Patella baja, patella alta, "grasshopper" eyes, and squinting patella.

Patellofemoral Pathology and Femoral Anatomy: An important factor in patellofemoral mechanics is that the anterior projection of the femoral head and neck is called anteversion; the posterior projection is called retroversion. The version angle is created by the long axis of the femoral neck and a line drawn between the femoral condyles.

Patellofemoral Subluxation: Pain descending stairs in about 76% of patients; pain with knee flexion, 75%; quadriceps weakness, 73%; joint effusion, 60%.

Primary Varus: Physiologic genu varum, tibiofemoral geometry, primary osseous alignment of the tibiofemoral joint.

Signs of Patellofemoral Subluxation: Dysplastic VMO occurs in 91% of patients; patella alta, 68%; tight lateral retinaculum, 66%; apprehension sign, 66%; increased Q angle, 21%.

Soft-Tissue Influences: VMO inserts at an angle between 55 and 65 degrees into the proximal one third to one half of the medial patella.

Surgical Options for Meniscus Injury: Generally, total or subtotal meniscectomy and repair.

Tibial Anatomy: Tibial tuberosity anatomic variations; tibial rotational configuration contributes significant mechanical influences. Variations influence Q angle. Q angle = anterior superior iliac spine to center of patella to tibial tuberosity.

Total Knee Arthroplasty: Indications include disabling knee pain, decreased function, and involvement of at least two compartments. All nonoperative care has failed. Complications include patella fracture, patella dislocation, component loosening, peroneal nerve palsy, supracondylar fracture, and decreased ROM.

Traumatic Tears of the Meniscus: Vertical or longitudinal tears are the most common. Medial tears outnumber lateral tears 2.5 to 1. Peripheral tears generally are unstable and require surgery.

Treatment of Patella Fractures: Nondisplaced fractures are treated conservatively, with the knee in extension with knee orthosis or immobilizer. Displaced fractures are treated with ORIF and soft-tissue repair. Limited flexion for 6 weeks.

Triple Varus: Tibiofemoral osseous and geometric alignment. Lateral compartment separation with lateral ligament laxity, increased external tibial rotation, and knee hyperextension.

REFERENCES

1. Abbott LC, et al: Injuries to the ligaments of the knee joint. *J Bone Joint Surg* 1944;26:503–521.
2. Arnoczky S, et al: Meniscus. In Woo SL-Y, Buckwalter JA, eds. Injury and Repair of the Musculoskeletal Soft Tissues. Park Ridge, IL, American Academy of Orthopaedic Surgeons, 1988.
3. Barrack RL, Skinner H, Buckley SL: Proprioception in the anterior cruciate deficient knee. *Am J Sports Med* 1989;17:1–6.
4. Bennett JG: Rehabilitation of patellofemoral joint dysfunction. In Greenfield BH, ed. Rehabilitation of the Knee: A Problem Solving Approach. Philadelphia, FA Davis, 1994.
5. Beynnon BD, et al: Anterior cruciate ligament strain behavior during rehabilitation exercises in vivo. *Am J Sports Med* 1995;23:124–134.
6. Boyd AD Jr, Ewald FC, Thomas WH, et al: Long-term complications after total knee arthroplasty with or without resurfacing of the patella. *Update,* Nov/Dec, 1994.
7. Buckwalter J, et al: Articular cartilage: injury and repair. In Woo SL-Y, Buckwalter JA, eds. Injury and Repair of the Musculoskeletal Soft Tissues. American Academy of Orthopaedic Surgeons Symposium, American Academy of Orthopaedic Surgeons, Rosemont, Ill, 1987.
8. Carlson TJ: The rationale behind meniscus repair, postgraduate advances in sports medicine. Forum Medicus, Inc., Course Outline, Rosemont, Ill, 1987.
9. Clancy WG, Shelbourne DK, Zoellner GB: Treatment of knee joint instability secondary to rupture of the posterior cruciate ligament. *J Bone Joint Surg* 1983;65A:310–322.
10. Daniel DM, Stone ML, Sachs R, et al: Instrumented measurement of anterior knee laxity in patients with acute anterior cruciate ligament disruption. *Am J Sports Med* 1985;13:401.
11. Daniel DM, Fritschy D: Anterior cruciate ligament injuries. In DeLee JC, Drez D, eds. Orthopaedic Sports Medicine: Principles and Practice, vol 2. Philadelphia, WB Saunders, 1994.
12. DeLee JC, et al: The posterior cruciate ligament. In DeLee JC, Drez D, eds. Orthopaedic Sports Medicine: Principals and Practice, vol 2. Philadelphia, WB Saunders, 1994.
13. Drez D, ed. Knee braces. American Academy of Orthopaedic Surgeons, Seminar Report, Rosemont, Ill, 1985.
14. Einhorn AR, Sawyer M, Tovin B: Rehabilitation of intra-articular reconstructions. In Greenfield BH, ed. Rehabilitation of the Knee: A Problem Solving Approach. Philadelphia, FA Davis, 1993.
15. Engle RP, Meade TD, Canner GC: Rehabilitation of posterior cruciate ligament injuries. In Greenfield BH, ed. Rehabilitation of the Knee: A Problem Solving Approach. Philadelphia, FA Davis, 1993.
16. Fetto JF, Marshall JL: Medial collateral ligament injuries of the knee: a rationale for treatment. *Clin Orthop* 1978;132:206–217.
17. Frank C, Woo SL, Amiel D, et al: Medial collateral ligament healing: a multi-disciplinary assessment in rabbits. *Am J Sports Med* 1983;11:379–389.
18. Fu FH, Baratz M: Meniscal injuries. In DeLee JC, Drez D, eds. Orthopaedic Sports Medicine: Principles and Practice, vol 2. Philadelphia, WB Saunders, 1994.
19. Goldstein TS: Geriatric orthopaedics, rehabilitative management of common problems. In Lewis CB, ed. Aspen Series in Physical Therapy. Gaithersburg, MD, Aspen Publishers, 1991.
20. Grana WA, Kriegshauser LA: Scientific basis of extensor mechanism disorders. In Larson RL, Singer KM, eds. *Clin Sports Med* 1985;4:247–257.
21. Greene B: Rehabilitation after total knee replacement. In Greenfield BH, ed. Rehabilitation of the Knee: A Problem Solving Approach. Philadelphia, FA Davis, 1993.
22. Hammesfahr R: Surgery of the knee. In Donatelli R, Wooden MJ, eds. Orthopaedic Physical Therapy. New York, Churchill-Livingstone, 1989.
23. Henning CE, Lynch MA: Current concepts of meniscal function and pathology. *Clin Sports Med* 1985;4:259–265.
24. Holden DL, Eggert AW, Butler JE: The nonoperative treatment of grade I and II medial collateral ligament injuries to the knee. *Am J Sports Med* 1983;11:344–540.
25. Hughston JC: Patellar subluxation in patellofemoral problem. *Clin Sports Med* 1989;8:162–253.
26. Hughston J: Knee Ligaments: Injury and Repair. St Louis, Mosby, 1993.
27. Hughston J: Posterior cruciate ligament instabilities. In Hughston J, ed. Knee Ligaments: Injury and Repair. St Louis, Mosby, 1993.
28. Jacobson KE, Flandry FC: Diagnosis of anterior knee pain. *Clin Sports Med* 1989;8:195–279.
29. Jensen JE, et al: Systematic evaluation of acute knee injuries. In Larson RL, Singer KM, eds. Clinical Sports Medicine. Philadelphia, WB Saunders, 1985.
30. Linton, RC, Indelicato PA: Medial ligament injuries. In DeLee JC, Drez D, eds. Orthopaedic Sports Medicine, vol 2. Philadelphia, WB Saunders, 1994.
31. Loth TS: Orthopaedic Boards Review. St Louis, Mosby, 1993.
32. Malone T: Rehabilitation of the surgical knee: the therapist's view of surgery. In Davies G, ed. Rehabilitation of the Surgical Knee. Ronkonkoma, NY, Cybex, 1984.
33. McRae R: Practical Fracture Treatment, 3rd ed. Ronkonkoma, NY, Churchill-Livingstone, 1994.
34. Miller M: Review of Orthopaedics. Philadelphia, WB Saunders, 1992.
35. Noyes FR, Barber SD, Simon R: High tibial osteotomy and ligament reconstruction in varus angulated, anterior cruciate ligament-deficient knees. *Am J Sports Med* 1993;21:1.
36. O'Donoghue DH: Surgical treatment of injuries to the ligament of the knee. *JAMA* 1959;169:142–151.
37. Parolie JM, Bergfeld JA: Long-term results of nonoperative treatment of isolated posterior cruciate ligament injuries in the athlete. *Am J Sports Med* 1986;14:35–38.
38. Paulos LE, Noyes FR, Grood E, et al: Knee rehabilitation after anterior cruciate ligament reconstruction and repair. *Am J Sports Med* 1981;9:140.
39. Paulos LE, Payne FC, Rosenburg TD: Rehabilitation after anterior cruciate ligament surgery. In Jackson DW, Drez D, eds. The Anterior Cruciate Deficient Knee: New Concepts in Ligament Repair. St Louis, Mosby, 1987.
40. Schenck RC, Heckman JD: Injuries of the knee. Presented at clinical symposia, Ciba-Geigy, 1993.
40a. Seto JL, Brewster CE: Rehabilitation of meniscal injuries. In Greenfield BH, ed. Rehabilitation of the Knee: A Problem Solving Approach. Philadelphia, FA Davis, 1993.
41. Sisk TD: Knee realignment and replacement in the recreational athlete. In DeLee JC, Drez D, eds. Orthopaedic Sports Medicine: Principles and Practice, vol 2. Philadelphia, WB Saunders, 1994.

42. Tenuta JJ, Arciero RA: Arthroscopic evaluation of meniscal repairs: factors that effect healing. *Am J Sports Med* 1994;22:697–802.

43. Timm K: Knee. In Richardson JK, Iglarsh ZA, eds. Clinical Orthopaedic Physical Therapy. Philadelphia, WB Saunders, 1994.

44. Tippett SR: Total knee arthroplasty: An overview, physical therapy implications and rehabilitation concerns. Course Notes, 1994.

45. Turba JE: Formal extensor mechanism reconstruction. *Clin Sports Med* 1989;8:297–317.

46. Walsh WM: Patellofemoral joint. In DeLee JC, Drez D, eds. Orthopaedic Sports Medicine: Principles and Practice, vol 2. Philadelphia, WB Saunders, 1994.

47. Wilk KE: Rehabilitation of medial capsular injuries. In Greenfield BH, ed. Rehabilitation of the Knee: A Problem Solving Approach. Philadelphia, FA Davis, 1993.

48. Wooden MJ: Mobilization of the lower extremity. In Donatelli R, Wooden MJ, eds. Orthopaedic Physical Therapy. New York, Churchill-Livingstone, 1989.

REVIEW QUESTIONS

Multiple Choice

1. "A partial loss of ligament continuity, where a few ligament fibers may be completely torn and there is moderate pain, swelling, and some loss of joint function" is a description of what kind(s) of sprain? (Circle any that apply.)
   A. Grade I sprain
   B. Grade II sprain
   C. Grade III sprain
   D. Second-degree sprain

2. External rotation, valgus stress, internal tibial rotation, or combined knee hyperextension defines mechanism of injury to which ligament?
   A. Posterior cruciate ligament (PCL)
   B. Medial collateral ligament (MCL)
   C. Anterior cruciate ligament (ACL)
   D. Lateral collateral ligament (LCL)

3. Blood within the joint is referred to as which of the following?
   A. Swelling
   B. Effusion
   C. Hemarthrosis
   D. Blood clot

4. Arthrocentesis is which of the following?
   A. Joint arthrotomy
   B. A test for stability
   C. A test for vascular compromise
   D. Aspiration of fluid from a joint

5. Blood and fat seen on examination from arthrocentesis may represent which of the following?
   A. A meniscal tear and ligament tear
   B. An MCL sprain
   C. A ligament sprain and possible fracture
   D. Articular cartilage injury

6. The cruciate ligaments are which of the following?
   A. Extracapsular
   B. Rarely injured
   C. Always torn in isolation
   D. Intracapsular

7. If the MCL is sprained, there is usually which of the following?
   A. A great deal of swelling
   B. A tense hemarthrosis
   C. Minimal swelling
   D. Minimal pain and significant swelling

8. A clinically relevant ligament stability test used to examine the integrity of the ACL when the knee is flexed 25 to 30 degrees is called which of the following?
   A. Anterior drawer test
   B. Valgus stress test
   C. Pivot shift test
   D. Lachman test

9. An instrumented ligament stability testing device commonly used in the clinic to quantify anterior-posterior laxity is which of the following?
   A. PTS-Turbo 1000
   B. KT1000
   C. Quantum 2000
   D. A-P Tester

10. Tissue that is used from the body of the patient having surgery is called which of the following?
    A. Allograft
    B. Xenograft
    C. Autograft
    D. Gore-Tex

11. The central one-third bone-patellar tendon-bone autograft surgical procedure describes a reconstruction of which ligament? (Circle any that apply.)
    A. MCL
    B. ACL
    C. PCL
    D. LCL

12. Which of the following tissues is (are) used for reconstruction of the ACL? (Circle any that apply.)
    A. Gracilis tendon
    B. Quadriceps tendon
    C. Semitendinosus tendon
    D. Fascia lata
    E. Achilles tendon

13. An allograft refers to which of the following?
    A. Synthetic tissue
    B. Biologic tissue from another human body (cadaver)
    C. Augmentation device
    D. Prosthetic ligament

14. The major risks of surgery using an allograft are which of the following? (Circle any that apply.)
    A. Disease transmission
    B. Ineffective sterilization
    C. Reduced vascular ingrowth
    D. Rejection
    E. Neurologic compromise

15. Which of the following tissues represents the strongest tissue available for autograft reconstruction of the ACL?
    A. Gracilis tendon
    B. Fascia lata
    C. Bone-patellar tendon-bone
    D. Quadriceps tendon

16. An important point to remember is that the tissue used to surgically reconstruct the ACL goes through which of the following processes?
    A. Gradual vascular ingrowth during the first 6 to 8 weeks after surgery
    B. Rapid collagen alignment, maturation, healing, and strength
    C. Avascular necrosis in the first 6 to 8 weeks after surgery
    D. Rapid strengthening, then gradual loss of vascularity

17. While the newly placed graft is struggling to revascularize, it is essential to avoid which of the following? (Circle any that apply.)
    A. Knee flexion
    B. Terminal extension
    C. Rotational forces
    D. Anterior tibial translation forces
    E. Ballistic closed kinetic chain exercises

18. Typically, scarring from the graft harvest site and suprapatellar pouch after an ACL reconstruction inhibits which of the following? (Circle any that apply.)
    A. Patellar mobility
    B. Knee flexion
    C. Weight bearing
    D. Neurovascular status
    E. Quad strength

19. During the maximum protection phase of recovery after ACL reconstruction, which of the following are allowed? (Circle any that apply.)
    A. Passive terminal extension
    B. Active short-arc knee extensions
    C. Isometric cocontraction of the quads and hams
    D. Lightweight short-arc knee extensions
    E. Plyometrics

20. Which of the following exercises/exercise equipment are appropriate for closed kinetic chain (CKC) exercises for a postoperative ACL reconstruction patient 14 weeks after surgery? (Circle any that apply.)
    A. Depth jumps
    B. Stair-steppers
    C. Leg press
    D. Treadmill
    E. Horizontal bounding

21. Which of the following is a general criterion for the patient's readiness to progress from the moderate protection phase to the minimum-protection phase after ACL reconstruction? (Circle any that apply.)
    A. Full knee range of motion (ROM)
    B. Squat with two times body weight
    C. Single-leg plyometric hops
    D. Jog one-quarter mile

22. If the PCL is ruptured, the clinician performs an anterior and posterior drawer test, and the tibia is confirmed to translate or displace anteriorly. This examination might be considered which of the following?
    A. Positive for ACL tear
    B. False-negative
    C. False-positive for ACL tear
    D. Negative PCL tear

23. A common denominator that exists between groups of patients treated surgically and those receiving conservative care for PCL tears is which of the following?
    A. Significant long-term dysfunction
    B. Vascular compromise
    C. Articular cartilage degeneration
    D. Meniscal tears

24. The most significant factor in rehabilitation of PCL injuries treated nonsurgically is which of the following?
    A. Gait dysfunction
    B. Quadriceps strengthening
    C. Hamstring strengthening
    D. Balance and coordination

25. Which of the following is not advocated during the maximum protection phase of recovery after an acute PCL tear treated surgically or nonoperatively?
    A. Quadriceps strengthening
    B. Terminal passive extension
    C. Open kinetic chain resistance hamstring exercise
    D. Closed-chain quadriceps exercise

26. A primary goal of recovery after PCL injuries is to strengthen which of the following?
    A. Hamstrings
    B. Quadriceps to exceed the strength of the noninjured limb
    C. Quadriceps equal to the noninjured limb
    D. Quadriceps and hamstrings equal to the noninjured limb

27. Common tissues used to reconstruct the PCL are which of the following? (Circle any that apply.)
    A. Achilles tendon
    B. Medial gastrocnemius tendon
    C. Semitendinosus tendon
    D. Patellar tendon
    E. Rotator cuff tendons

28. The most common ligament injury seen in the knee is which of the following?
    A. ACL
    B. MCL
    C. PCL
    D. LCL

29. What percentage of associated ligament injuries occurs in conjunction with a grade II MCL sprain?
    A. 20%
    B. 52%
    C. 75%
    D. 78%

30. The most common "unhappy triad" is which of the following?
    A. PCL, ACL, LCL
    B. ACL, MCL, lateral meniscus
    C. ACL, MCL, medial meniscus
    D. ACL, PCL, lateral meniscus

31. The MCL has direct anatomic attachment to which of the following?
    A. Semitendinosus tendon
    B. Medial meniscus
    C. Medial gastrocnemius tendon
    D. Adductor magnus tendon

32. Which of the following is the most sensitive clinical examination to test the stability of the MCL?
    A. Lachman test
    B. Anterior drawer
    C. Varus stress test
    D. Valgus stress test

33. The foundation of rehabilitation after MCL tears is which of the following?
    A. Use non–weight bearing (NWB) and cast immobilization.
    B. Perform isometric exercises only during the maximum-protection phase of recovery.
    C. Use early protected motion.
    D. Do not use bracing and encourage early plyometric exercise.

34. Which of the following should be done when prescribing hip adduction exercises after MCL injury?
    A. Use 5 pounds or less of resistance.
    B. Place the resistance distal to the joint line.
    C. Place resistance proximal to the joint line.
    D. Use 1 to 3 pounds of resistance.

35. Which of the following highlight(s) the differences between rehabilitation and healing of the extracapsular MCL and intracapsular ACL and PCL? (Circle any that apply.)
    A. MCL has a high propensity to heal.
    B. MCL has greater potential to heal because of its blood supply.
    C. MCL is much stronger than the ACL.
    D. Rehabilitation progresses much slower with MCL injuries.
    E. Resistive knee flexion and extension exercises are prescribed earlier with MCL sprains as compared with ACL and PCL sprains.

36. Which of the following may indicate a meniscal tear? (Circle any that apply.)
    A. History of twisting knee injury
    B. Hemarthrosis
    C. Valgus instability
    D. Swelling; locking of the knee
    E. Pain and "catching"

37. A test used to reproduce symptoms of torn meniscus is called which of the following?
    A. Smith test
    B. McMurray test
    C. Pivot shift test
    D. Lachman test

38. A test used to determine if the meniscus is preventing knee extension is called which of the following?
    A. Bounce home test
    B. Tibial sag test
    C. KT1000 test
    D. Anterior drawer test

39. Which of the following surgical procedures leads to limited early weight bearing, early limited full knee flexion, and generally slower advances with closed-chain exercises in rehabilitation?
    A. Total meniscectomy
    B. Meniscal repair
    C. Subtotal meniscectomy
    D. Lateral release

40. Which of the following represent(s) long-term sequelae after total and subtotal meniscectomy? (Circle any that apply.)
    A. Muscle atrophy
    B. Joint space narrowing
    C. Gait dysfunction
    D. Degenerative arthritic changes
    E. Neurologic dysfunction

41. After subtotal meniscectomy, weight bearing status during the first week is usually which of the following?
    A. NWB
    B. 20% partial weight bearing (PWB)
    C. Weight bearing as tolerated (WBAT)
    D. 10% PWB

42. Which of the following describes the weight bearing status after meniscal repair immediately postoperative?
    A. PWB
    B. NWB progressing slowly to full weight bearing (FWB) at 4 to 6 weeks postoperative
    C. NWB progressing to FWB at 2 weeks postoperative
    D. FWB

43. Closed kinetic chain resistance exercises (e.g., leg press, squats, step-ups, stair-steppers, etc.) generally are not allowed for _____ after meniscal repair.
    A. 3 to 4 weeks postoperative
    B. 4 to 6 weeks postoperative

    C. 8 weeks or longer postoperative
    D. 2 to 5 weeks postoperative

44. Which of the following patellar positions is associated with a higher incidence of patellar instability?
    A. Patella baja
    B. Normal alignment
    C. Patella alta
    D. Patella infera

45. A line drawn from the anterior superior iliac spine (ASIS) through the center or axis of the patella and distally to the insertion of the patellar tendon on the tibial tubercle is called which of the following?
    A. Varus deformity
    B. Genu valgus
    C. Quadriceps angle (Q angle)
    D. Genu recurvatum

46. Which of the following describe(s) the miserable malalignment syndrome? (Circle any that apply.)
    A. External femoral rotation
    B. Squinting patellae
    C. External tibial torsion
    D. Bayonet sign
    E. Hypertrophy of the vastus medialis oblique (VMO)

47. Which of the following are common recognizable signs and symptoms of anterior knee pain? (Circle any that apply.)
    A. Crepitus
    B. Laterally tracking patella
    C. Pain
    D. Vastus lateralis weakness
    E. VMO weakness

48. The cornerstone in the rehabilitation of a painful laterally tracking patella is which of the following?
    A. Hamstring stretching
    B. Stretch lateral retinaculum
    C. Strengthen quadriceps
    D. Pain and swelling management
    E. All of the above

49. In addition to strengthening the quadriceps (with anterior knee pain), which of the following muscle groups contribute to improving the appropriate line of pull on the patella?
    A. Hip extensors
    B. Hip adductors
    C. Hip abductors
    D. Hip flexors
    E. All of the above

50. Which of the following is a proximal realignment surgical procedure for correction of anterior knee pain and a lateral tracking patella?
    A. Elmslie-Trillat procedure
    B. Hawser procedure
    C. Lateral retinacular release
    D. Maquet procedure

51. Which of the following are surgical procedures used to reduce severe patellofemoral compression loads and significant lateral patellar subluxation by surgically realigning the distal extensor mechanism?
    A. Distal-realignment procedures
    B. Elmslie-Trillat procedure
    C. "Radical" surgeries
    D. Hauser procedure
    E. All of the above

52. Which of the following procedures is used to directly address retropatellar and femoral condyle articular cartilage degeneration? (Circle any that apply.)
    A. Perforation chondroplasty
    B. Abrasion arthroplasty
    C. Articular shaving
    D. Reefing
    E. Proximal realignment

53. If a transverse fracture of the patella occurs, a complication of the proximal fracture segment may be which of the following?
    A. Malunion
    B. Nonunion
    C. Avascular necrosis
    D. Osteomalacia
    E. All of the above

54. Stabilization of displaced patellar fractures is best accomplished with which of the following?
    A. Rigid cast immobilization for 6 to 8 weeks
    B. Range limiting hinge-type knee brace for 6 to 8 weeks
    C. An open reduction with internal fixation (ORIF) procedure
    D. NWB for 4 to 6 weeks without immobilization

55. With tension-band wiring after a displaced patella fracture, the knee should be immobilized in which position?
    A. Terminal extension
    B. Knee flexion of 90 degrees
    C. Range-limiting hinge brace set at 0 to 75 degrees
    D. 20 degrees of knee flexion

56. Distal femur fractures are classified as which of the following?
    A. Extraarticular
    B. Bicondylar
    C. Unicondylar
    D. Transverse supracondylar
    E. All of the above

57. Because of the proximity of the knee joint with a distal femur fracture, which of the following represents potential complications? (Circle any that apply.)
    A. Vascular injury
    B. Arthrofibrosis
    C. Adhesions
    D. Gait dysfunction
    E. Recurrent patellar subluxation

58. The purpose of a total knee replacement (TKR) is which of the following? (Circle any that apply.)
    A. Correct deformity
    B. Improve function
    C. Eliminate or reduce pain
    D. Increase gait speed
    E. Reduce swelling

59. What is the most common age of persons with rheumatoid arthritis who undergo TKR?
    A. Less than 60 years old
    B. Less than 30 years old
    C. 75 years or older
    D. 60 to 75 years old

60. Which of the following is the goal of recovery after TKR?
    A. Relief of pain
    B. Restoration of mechanical axis of the knee
    C. Restoration of anatomic axis of the knee
    D. Provision of adequate stability
    E. All of the above

61. A cruciate sparing implant is also referred to as which of the following? (Circle any that apply.)
    A. Conforming
    B. Constrained
    C. Nonconstrained
    D. Resurfacing implant
    E. Compression implant

62. Patellofemoral compression forces are estimated to be _____ times body weight while a person is walking on level surfaces.
    A. 1 to 1.5
    B. 2.5 to 3.0
    C. 5
    D. 4 to 5

63. What is the estimated patellofemoral compression force while a person is ascending or descending stairs?
    A. Five times body weight
    B. Three to four times body weight
    C. Six times body weight
    D. Two to three times body weight

64. Which of the following describes the weight bearing status of a patient after a TKR that is fixed with noncemented prosthetic components?
    A. Limited weight bearing early with slow progression to FWB by 12 weeks
    B. WBAT for 4 weeks, then FWB
    C. NWB for 6 weeks, then progressing to FWB by 8 weeks
    D. FWB by 6 weeks

65. What is the name of the surgical procedure performed for patients who have severe unicompartmental osteoarthritis of the knee?
    A. Hauser procedure
    B. High tibial osteotomy
    C. Watson-Jones procedure
    D. Chondral shaving

66. A high tibial osteotomy attempts to do which of the following?
    A. Lengthen the femur
    B. Lengthen the tibia
    C. Shorten the tibia
    D. Evenly distribute forces and compressive loads across the tibiofemoral joint

Short Answer

67. Which injury does this figure represent?

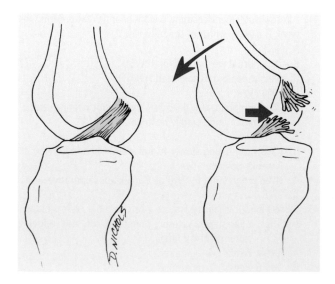

68. Identify the ligament and name the examination being performed in the following figure.

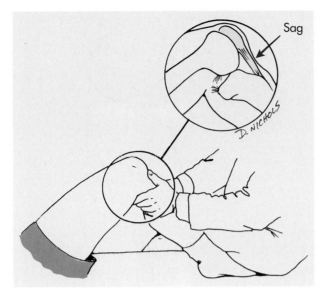

69. Name the mechanism of injury and identify the torn structure in the following figure.

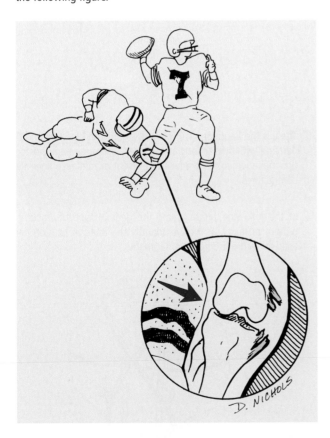

70. Match the names of meniscal lesions with the appropriate diagrams in the following figure. Select from these names: flap tear, longitudinal tear, parrot beak tear, bucket handle, and radial tears.

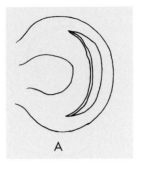

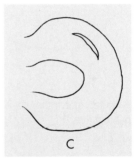

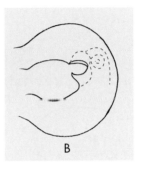

71. Match the following terms with the appropriate diagram: red-on-red zone, red-on-white zone, and white-on-white zone.

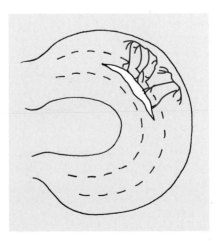

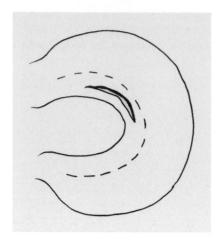

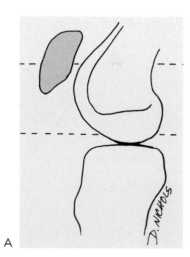

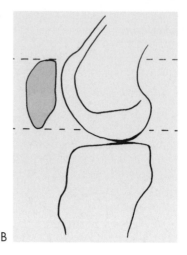

B

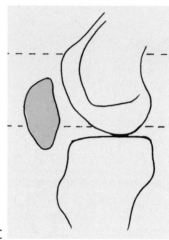

C

72. In the following figures, match the patellar reference description with the appropriate figure.

_____ Patella baja

_____ Patella alta

_____ Normal

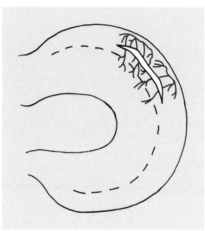

A

73. There is the frequent occurrence of significant bleeding and tissue damage with supracondylar fractures. List three early postoperative management techniques to prevent or minimize knee flexion contractures.

74. In the following figure, name the general type of fracture and pattern of injury, as well as identify the internal fixation devices used to secure the fracture fragments.

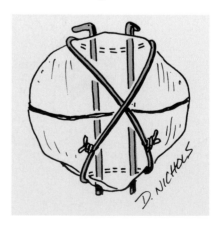

75. Name the two general types of implants used in a TKR.

True/False

76. The MCL is an extracapsular structure.
77. The concept of CKC exercise is not advocated during the moderate-protection phase (seventh to twelfth week after surgery) after ACL reconstruction.
78. When instructing a patient to perform a short-arc leg press after a central one-third bone-patellar tendon-bone autograft, ACL reconstruction at 13 weeks postoperative, it is not essential that the patient wear a brace.
79. Isolated PCL tears occur more frequently than ACL tears.
80. A grade I MCL sprain always occurs as an isolated injury.
81. Grade III MCL tears always must be treated surgically.
82. Apley's compression and distraction test is used to determine if the meniscus or ligament is injured.
83. Preservation of the load-bearing functions of the meniscus is the foundation for a subtotal meniscectomy.
84. Closed kinetic chain exercises are used during the fourth to the eighth postoperative week after subtotal meniscectomy.
85. Full knee ROM is allowed after meniscal repairs as soon as the patient can tolerate it.
86. Excessive hamstring tightness may contribute to increased patellofemoral compression.
87. In the case of a lateral retinacular release without VMO advancement, it is generally appropriate to encourage early postoperative knee flexion range of motion to keep the deep surgically cut tissues "open."
88. Early quadriceps strengthening and knee flexion must be encouraged in cases where a lateral retinacular release was performed in addition to a VMO advancement.
89. The treatment of nondisplaced patellar fractures is with rigid immobilization in terminal extension.
90. After immobilization of a nondisplaced patellar fracture, early quadriceps strengthening and full knee flexion ROM are encouraged.
91. Nondisplaced tibial plateau fractures always are treated with an ORIF procedure.
92. The method of implant fixation of patellar, femoral, or tibial components of a TKR has no direct impact on immediate postoperative rehabilitation.
93. Prosthetic implant fixation of the components of a TKR can be achieved in two ways: bone cement (polymethylmethacrylate) or a porous-coated, cementless prosthesis.
94. The most common compartment affected with severe osteoarthritis of the knee is the lateral knee joint compartment, which results in a valgus deformity.

Essay Questions

Answer on a separate sheet of paper.

95. Identify common ligament injuries of the knee.
96. Discuss common methods of management and rehabilitation of common ligament injuries of the knee.
97. Identify and describe common meniscal injuries of the knee.
98. Discuss common methods of management and rehabilitation of meniscal injuries of the knee.
99. Identify and describe common patellofemoral pathologies of the knee.
100. Describe common methods of management and rehabilitation of patellofemoral disease pathologies of the knee.
101. Identify and describe common fractures of the patella, supracondylar femur fractures, and proximal tibia fractures.
102. Describe common methods of management and rehabilitation of fractures about the knee.
103. Identify and describe methods of management and rehabilitation after knee arthroplasty and high tibial osteotomy.
104. Describe common mobilization techniques for the knee.

Critical Thinking Application

You are treating a patient with a diagnosis of postoperative ACL reconstruction using the central one-third bone-patellar tendon-bone autograft. In addition, the patient also had a repair of the medial meniscus. It is 1 week after surgery. Develop a continuum of progressive rehabilitation (critical-pathway, -criterion-based rehabilitation program) that follows the maximum-, moderate-, and minimum-protection phase concept of recovery. Based on your knowledge of soft-tissue injury and repair, be certain your program of rehabilitation is consistent with the overlapping phases of injury repair. For each phase of healing, identify and recommend appropriate agents for pain and swelling management. For each phase, list exercises, ROM, muscle contraction types, weight bearing status, open and closed kinetic-chain exercises, cardiovascular fitness, general physical conditioning, balance-coordination-proprioception drills, and return to functional activities. What effect does the meniscal repair have on the development of this particular rehabilitation program? How would this program be different if the meniscus were not injured? What modifications in this program would be necessary if the ACL were not injured and just the meniscus was repaired?

20

Orthopedic Management of the Hip and Pelvis*

LEARNING OBJECTIVES

1. Identify common hip fractures.
2. Outline and discuss common methods of management and rehabilitation of ordinary hip fractures.
3. Identify and describe common methods of management and rehabilitation after hip arthroplasty.
4. Identify and describe common soft-tissue injuries of the hip.
5. Outline and describe common methods of management and rehabilitation of soft-tissue injuries of the hip.
6. Identify common fractures of the pelvis and hip.
7. Discuss methods of management and rehabilitation for fractures of the pelvis and acetabulum.
8. Describe common mobilization techniques for the hip.

KEY TERMS

Avascular necrosis (AVN)
Open reduction and internal fixation (ORIF)
Degenerative joint disease (DJD)

Proximal femoral intertrochanteric osteotomy
Hemiarthroplasty
Total hip replacement (THR)

Total hip precautions
Legg-Calvé-Perthes (LCP) disease
Trochanteric bursitis
Strains
Contusions

CHAPTER OUTLINE

Hip Fractures
   Rehabilitation after Hip Fractures
Proximal Femoral Osteotomy
   Rehabilitation after Proximal Femoral Intertrochanteric Osteotomy
Hemiarthroplasty of the Hip
Fixation of Prosthetic Hip Components
Total Hip Replacement
   Rehabilitation after Total Hip Replacement

Legg-Calvé-Perthes Disease
Soft-Tissue Injuries of the Hip (Bursitis, Strains, and Contusions)
Fractures of the Pelvis and Acetabulum
Common Mobilization Techniques for the Hip
   Long-Axis Distraction
   Lateral Distraction of the Hip
   Anterior and Posterior Mobilization
   Inferior Glide of the Hip

*Refer to orthopedic anatomy figures on the Evolve website.

The practicing physical therapist assistant (PTA) is exposed to many orthopedic problems involving the hip and pelvis. This chapter focuses attention on the more common classifications, management, and rehabilitation of hip fractures, joint reconstructive surgery (total hip arthroplasty), rehabilitation after hip replacement, and management of various pelvic fractures and soft-tissue injuries of the hip.

HIP FRACTURES

The clinical significance of hip fractures is reflected in the annual rate of fractures and the financial burden to the economy that hip fractures produce.[4,8] Goldstein states that more than 300,000 fractures occur annually with an associated cost of $10 billion.[4] Other authorities[2,8] report that 267,000 fractures occur annually, with a price tag of $33.8 billion.[2] Although fractures in general occur to all age groups, hip fractures are most common among elderly women.[2,8,9] Hip fractures in women can be attributed in part to the higher incidence of osteoporosis in this group;[9] with regard to age, hip fractures represent the most common acute orthopedic injury in the geriatric population.[8]

The classification of hip fractures is clinically significant for the PTA because the severity and location of the fracture profoundly affect surgical management and physical therapy interventions. The vascular supply to the femoral head and neck may be significantly compromised with certain fracture patterns and levels of severity (Fig. 20-1).[9] LeVeau[9] states, "The extent of the supply of blood to the head of the femur determines remodeling and healing after femoral neck fracture or hip dislocation."

Generally, hip fractures can be classified by location and described by severity (simple or comminuted).[3] Fractures of the hip can be located in the following areas:

■ Extracapsular or trochanteric[3,4,13] (Fig. 20-2)
■ Femoral neck or subcapital areas[5] (intracapsular) (Fig. 20-3)
■ Proximal femoral shaft or subtrochanteric areas[5]

Secondary to the location and severity of hip fracture, the most significant complication is related to osteonecrosis and the loss of blood supply to the femoral head leading to **avascular necrosis (AVN).** Gross and associates[5] affirm, "any fracture of the neck (femoral) can disrupt this tenuous blood supply. As a result, there is an exceedingly high incidence of avascular necrosis of the

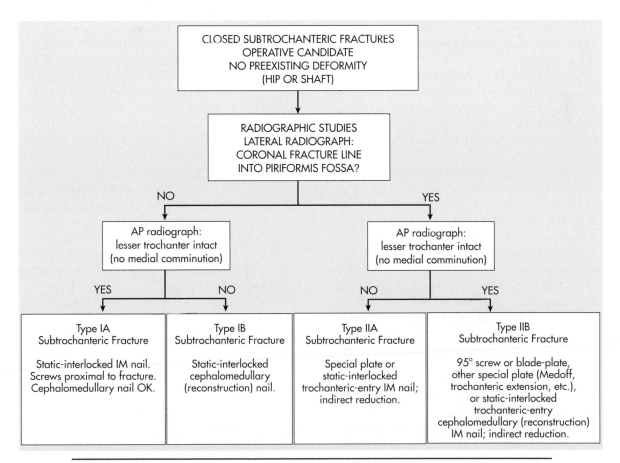

Algorithm for operative treatment of closed subtrochanteric fractures with use of the Russell-Taylor classification. (From Browner BD, Jupiter J, Levine A, et al: Skeletal Trauma, 2nd ed, vol 2. Philadelphia, WB Saunders, 2003.)

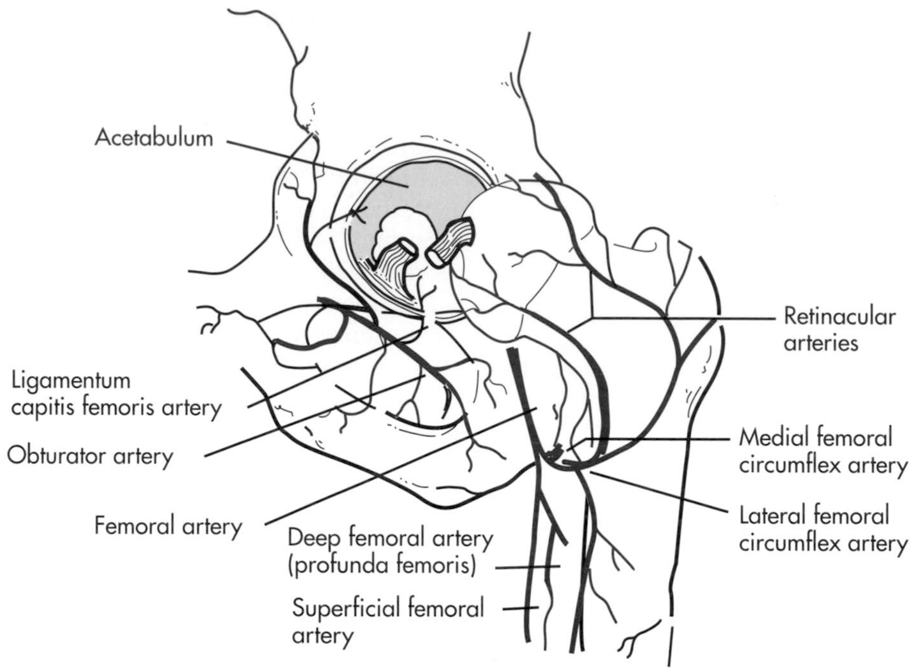

Fig. 20-1 Vascular supply to the femoral head and neck. (From Richardson JK, Iglarsch JK, eds: Clinical Orthopedic Physical Therapy. Philadelphia, WB Saunders, 1994.)

femoral head after hip fractures." LeVeau[9] states, "avascular necrosis may occur after hip fracture in about 65% to 85% of the patients."

Three main clinical complications are noted with subtrochanteric fractures: malunion, delayed union, and nonunion.[10] Two factors are associated with malunion and nonunion of subtrochanteric hip fractures:

■ The subtrochanteric area of the proximal femur is cortical bone, which has a decreased blood supply.
■ The subtrochanteric area is prone to large biomechanical stresses that can lead to loosening of various fixation devices.[10] This complication must be considered by the PTA when treating patients with this type of fracture.

Many options are available in treating hip fractures: The choice depends on the patient's age, location of the fracture, quality of bone, severity of the fracture (simple, displaced, or comminuted), activity level of the patient, associated soft-tissue injuries, and specific goals for the patient's return to activity. Generally, hip fractures are managed surgically with an **open reduction and internal fixation (ORIF)** procedure that secures the fracture fragments with various rods, nails, pins, screws, and plates.[3,4,8] Some hip fractures can be managed conservatively with bed rest, traction, and protected weight bearing.[10] For example, in a fractured greater trochanter where the displaced fracture fragment is less than 1 cm (as evaluated by the physician radiographically), the treatment could be bed rest for several days, range-of-motion (ROM) exercises, and limited weight bearing for 4 weeks.[10]

With an isolated lesser trochanteric fracture (most common in adolescents), the physician bases treatment on the amount of fragment displacement. If the fracture is displaced more than 2 cm, the physician could perform an ORIF procedure; if the fragments are in closer apposition, the physician may elect rest, protected weight bearing, and limited exercise for 3 to 4 weeks.[10] Figure 20-5 depicts common fixation devices used to secure fracture fragments using an ORIF procedure.

While treating patients with hip fractures, the PTA must be aware that venous thrombosis is a potentially critical complication after hip surgery. Without prophylactic medications to minimize thrombosis, statistics show that 40% to 90% of patients develop this condition after hip surgery.[10] Venous thrombosis is the most common complication after hip fracture in the elderly population of patients.[10]

Hip fractures and dislocations can occur in combination, as well as isolated events. Usually hip dislocations are either anterior or posterior (Fig. 20-6). Isolated hip dislocations generally are treated conservatively with bed rest, traction, and protected limited weight bearing for up to 12 weeks.[10] For example, with an anterior hip dislocation, bed rest with traction is prescribed, with specific precautions to strictly avoid extreme hip abduction and external rotation to prevent redislocation. Usually protected weight bearing is allowed when the patient can achieve painless hip ROM around 3 to 4 weeks after the incident.[10] Conversely an isolated posterior hip dislocation is treated with bed rest and traction in abduction with precautions to prevent hip

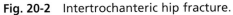

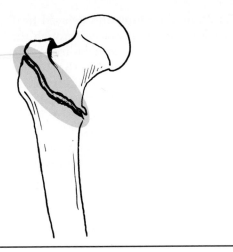

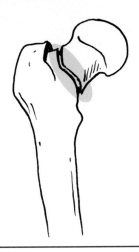

Fig. 20-2 Intertrochanteric hip fracture.

Fig. 20-3 Femoral neck fracture.

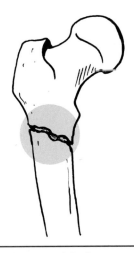

Fig. 20-4 Subtrochanteric hip fracture.

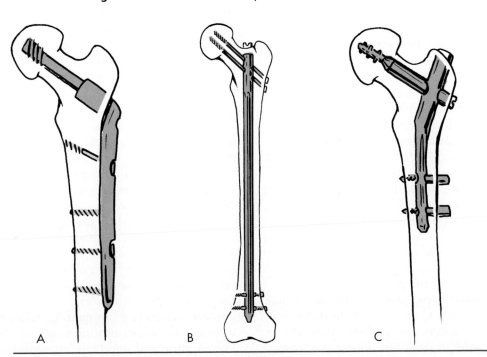

A   B   C

Fig. 20-5 Various methods of internal fixation for hip fractures. **A,** Screws and sideplate. **B,** Rod. **C,** Nails.

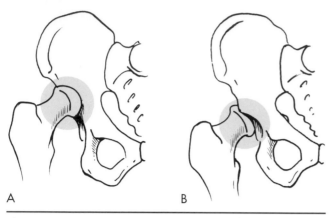

Fig. 20-6 Dislocation of the hip. **A,** Anterior dislocation. **B,** Posterior dislocation.

abduction, flexion, and internal rotation to protect the joint from dislocation.[10]

Rehabilitation after Hip Fractures

Any rehabilitation program used to treat hip fractures is highly individualized. The nature of the fracture type, classification, location, and method of internal fixation (if any) are considered, and the treatment program is adjusted to the patient's ability to cope with specific identified criteria. These criteria are established by the physical therapist (PT) and carried out by the PTA.

The progression from maximum to minimum protection closely follows the rate of bone healing. However, other factors are considered in safely and effectively providing an environment for the return to functional activities. In the maximum-protection phase of recovery (phase 1 to 21 days postoperatively, as described by Goldstein),[3] the fracture site is protected; pain and swelling are reduced; and isometric exercises, gentle protected ROM, and limited weight bearing begin.[3,9]

The general goals of recovery are to increase muscular strength specific to the surgery, improve overall conditioning, increase ROM of the affected hip, enhance aerobic fitness, increase local muscular endurance, reduce pain and swelling, reestablish normalized gait mechanics, and protect the healing structures from internal and external forces that can impede healing.[3,9]

During the maximum-protection phase the exercises used include active ankle pumps for both lower extremities, isometric quadriceps sets, gluteal sets, heel slides, hip abduction and adduction, and supine internal and external hip rotation. These exercises must be done at submaximal levels at first, and then progressively made more difficult according to the patient's tolerance.

Goldstein[3] identified a few major complications that occur, particularly during the maximum-protection phase of recovery. Generally, no combined diagonal or rotary forces are used in exercises during this phase.

Hardware loosening and delayed healing may occur if increased torque is placed through the healing fracture site by excessive unwanted forces.[3] No active straight-leg raises or supine hip bridges should be performed during the first 6 to 8 weeks after surgery. Goldstein states, "The power generated by the massive hip muscles is so great during those exercises that there is a danger of displacing the fractured segments."[3]

In addition to rudimentary isometric quadriceps sets, gluteal sets, ankle pumps, and gentle hip-motion exercises, authorities advocate adding the exercises described in Fig. 20-7 progressively during the first 3 weeks after surgery.[3]

Early protected weight bearing is encouraged soon after surgery. Generally, touch down weight bearing (TDWB) or partial weight bearing (PWB) is allowed by the second day postoperatively. Weight bearing status increases as dictated by the rate of bone healing (more than 8 to 12 weeks), which should be verified radiographically by the physician. Avoiding torque through the affected limb during standing minimizes loosening of the fixation device.

More demanding exercises are added as the bone and associated soft tissues heal. Closed-chain functional exercises are added as full weight bearing (FWB) is achieved. Partial wall squats and step-ups are usually initiated to regain concentric and eccentric muscle control of the quadriceps and hip extensors. A restorator or bike ergometer can be used during the early recovery phase if the patient can tolerate sitting, and depending on restrictions about hip flexion, ROM, and precautions.

The moderate-protection phase, defined as 3 to 6 weeks after surgery,[3] provides for more challenging exercises directed at regaining hip and knee motion, improving quadriceps and hamstring strength, and increasing strength to the hip extensors, abductors, and adductors. Standing four-position hip strengthening can be achieved using a cable system (Fig. 20-8). The initiation of limited ROM leg presses can commence during this phase as well.

The late healing phase (after 6 to 8 weeks) is characterized by normalized gait mechanics and reduced use of assistive devices for ambulation. A treadmill can be used, with step cadence and stride length adjusted, to enhance gait and provide a stimulus for greater hip and quadriceps strength.

More advanced hip strengthening exercises can be added cautiously for more active patients. The stair-stepper stimulates hip extension strength and local muscular endurance, but extreme caution must be used when initiating various open- and closed-chain exercises after surgery for hip fractures. A fine line must be applied to avoid excessive forces (e.g., straight-leg raises or hip bridges), torque, and weight bearing while stimulating hip and knee motion and improving strength and function.

Sitting
  1. Knee extension (kicking)
     Slowly extend knee fully, hold for 1 second, and return slowly to flexed position under control.

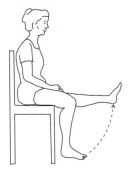

  2. Hip flexion (marching)
     Lift alternate knees to chest, as if slowly marching in place while sitting.

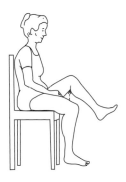

  3. Forward bending of trunk
     Slowly reach hands down along the insides of the legs. Stop at the first pulling sensation. Return slowly to erect posture.

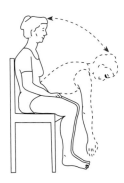

  4. Armchair push-ups
     Place hands on armrests (or push-up blocks) and extend both elbows, lifting torso from chair seat. Feet should be placed on floor for balance, support, and assist.

Supine Lying
  5. Hip rotations
     With hips slightly abducted and knees extended, slowly roll legs in and out.

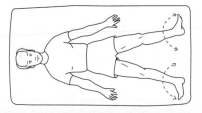

Fig. 20-7 Progressive hip exercises are employed during the first 3 to 4 weeks after surgery. (From Goldstein T: Geriatric Orthopaedics. Gaithersburg, MD, Aspen Publishers, 1991.)   *Continued*

6. Heel slides
   Slide heel along mat toward the buttocks
   and slowly return to original position.

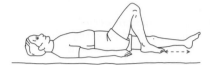

7. Knee to chest
   Flex hip, bringing knee toward the chest,
   and slowly return limb to extended position.

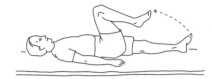

8. Hip abduction/adduction
   Slowly spread legs apart and pull them
   together, keeping the knees extended and
   the toes pointed upward.

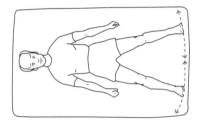

9. Terminal knee extension

Prone Lying
10. Hip flexor stretch
    Lie prone for up to 20 minutes daily. Place pillow or bolster under ankles for comfort.

11. Knee flexion
    Flex knee and bring heel toward buttocks.
    Return to extended position.

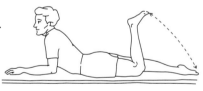

12. Hip extension
    With knee flexed to 90°, lift knee slightly
    off mat without rotating pelvis and slowly
    lower knee to mat.

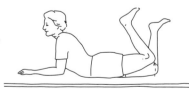

Fig. 20-7, cont'd Progressive hip exercises are employed during the first 3 to 4 weeks after surgery.

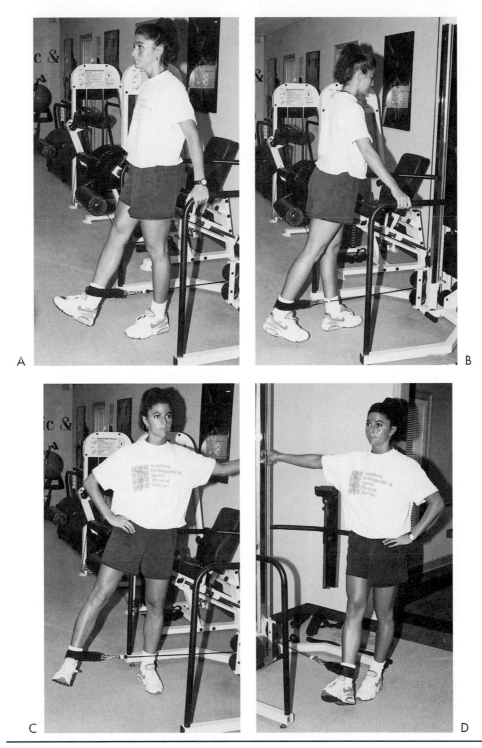

Fig. 20-8 Standing four-way hip strengthening exercises using a cable column system. **A,** Hip flexion straight-leg raise. **B,** Hip extension. **C,** Hip abduction. **D,** Hip adduction.

PROXIMAL FEMORAL OSTEOTOMY

Intertrochanteric osteotomy may be performed when **degenerative joint disease (DJD)** is extensive and results in hip pain associated with subchondral bone erosion, articular cartilage fibrillation and fissuring, and

hip joint incongruity.[7] The goal of this surgical procedure is to reduce pain and improve function related to advanced osteoarthritis by surgically changing the femoral neck-shaft angle so that healthy cartilage is exposed, thus "improving joint surface congruity."[7] Figure 20-9 illustrates this procedure and shows the

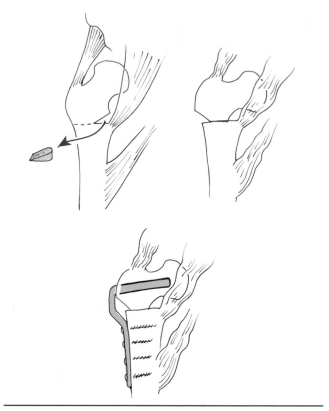

Fig. 20-9 Proximal femoral osteotomy.

changed neck-shaft angle relationship, reduced ligamentous and muscular tension, and improved joint articulation occurring after surgery.[7]

Rehabilitation after Proximal Femoral Intertrochanteric Osteotomy

Because a **proximal femoral intertrochanteric osteotomy** is performed to reduce symptoms related to advanced osteoarthritis (DJD) of the hip, the rehabilitation program must focus on joint protection principles (unloading forces through the hip) and postsurgical bone healing precautions. During the maximum-protection phase of recovery, avoiding unwanted forces, managing pain (with thermal agents or pain medication), using protected weight bearing (to unload the hip from repetitive articular cartilage destruction), restoring hip motion, and improving strength are stressed. Quadriceps-setting exercises, gluteal sets, ankle pumps, and gentle active hip ROM exercises are allowed from the first day after surgery.

Weight bearing status is highly individualized but generally is progressed according to the rate and quality of bone healing. Typically, a walker or crutches reduces compressive loads through the hip during TDWB, PWB, and non–weight bearing (NWB) gait techniques. In most cases, protected weight bearing is strictly enforced for 8 to 12 weeks after this procedure.[7]

The contralateral hip, bilateral knee joints, and spine are targets of joint protection related to osteoarthritis. The PTA must fully recognize that the whole person—not just the affected joint—should be addressed during all phases of recovery. In keeping with joint protection, once the surgical incision has healed and the patient is allowed PWB status, an underwater treadmill is useful to enhance normalized gait mechanics in a protected weight bearing environment. The buoyancy of the water allows reduced compressive loads through the hip.

Once radiographic evidence suggests secure bone healing, more challenging and intense strengthening exercises gradually are added. Isotonic knee extensions, leg curls, and standing hip abduction, adduction, flexion, and extension motions are strengthened through use of a cable system or wall pulleys. Extreme caution must be used with closed-chain strengthening exercises. Minimizing joint compressive loads, which may contribute to articular cartilage degeneration, is the cornerstone in the long-term care of severe osteoarthritis. Therefore functional weight bearing exercises must be added judiciously and without increased pain.

A limited ROM leg-press exercise can be used as the first closed-chain activity. As healing progresses, mini step-ups, short-arc wall squats, and treadmill walking are added. A general conditioning program that encourages weight control, specifically using aerobic exercise (unloaded, upper body ergometer, or recumbent or semirecumbent stationary cycle ergometer), strengthening (while minimizing joint compressive loads and shearing joint motions), and flexibility should be implemented as soon as the patient can tolerate these activities.

HEMIARTHROPLASTY OF THE HIP

For femoral head osteonecrosis or severe femoral head fractures, **hemiarthroplasty** is used to eliminate pain and improve function. This procedure replaces the damaged femoral head with a bipolar prosthesis. Because hemiarthroplasty requires a normal acetabular surface,[7,14] it is rarely used for arthritis.[14] This is considered a "conservative" procedure[7] when compared with a total hip replacement. Hemiarthroplasty can be converted at a later date to total hip replacement if symptoms persist and the joint degenerates.[14] The term *bipolar* refers to two separate snap-fit components of one femoral prosthetic unit. A bipolar prosthesis is usually a large-diameter femoral head component that snap-fits snugly onto a smaller diameter femoral head, which is part of the total prosthetic unit.[3,7] A unipolar femoral prosthesis is a self-contained femoral head and shaft without additional components. The bipolar prosthesis usually produces less wear caused by friction and reduced impact loading of the acetabulum.[12]

FIXATION OF PROSTHETIC HIP COMPONENTS

As discussed in Chapter 10, the method of fixation of various prosthetic components directly affects the short- and long-term course of rehabilitation after hip arthroplasty. Both femoral and acetabular components usually can be secured to the bone with a cement, polymethylmethacrylate (PMMA), which is not actually an adhesive, but rather provides a strong interference fit between the prosthesis and the bone,[12] or with a noncemented biologic tissue ingrowth prosthesis. Miller[14] recommends that cemented femoral stems be used only for patients over age 65, and that noncemented prosthesis be used for younger patients.[14] Weight bearing precautions are related to the specific type of fixation procedure used to secure the prosthesis. Weight bearing generally is deferred for longer periods of time with a noncemented biologic tissue fit prosthesis so that the bone can grow into the porous coated femoral stem. Weight bearing with cemented devices can progress at a slightly faster rate. However, in either case, rotational forces (torque) must be strictly avoided to minimize the loosening of components.

TOTAL HIP REPLACEMENT

Total hip arthroplasty **(total hip replacement, [THR])** involves replacing both the femoral head and the acetabulum, as contrasted with a hemiarthroplasty, which replaces only the femoral head. Indications for the use of THR include the following:

- Rheumatoid arthritis
- Osteoarthritis (both femoral head and acetabulum)
- Osteonecrosis
- Fractures
- Juvenile rheumatoid arthritis (the most common indication for THR in adolescents)[12]
- Pain
- Reduced ambulation
- Significant alterations in activities of daily living (ADLs)[14]

Before discussing rehabilitation procedures, this chapter reviews pertinent complications and component designs related to THR because these issues influence specific physical therapy interventions and precautions.

Surgeons must select a proper femoral head size for each patient. In theory, a large-diameter femoral head may provide for greater ROM and inherent stability.[12,14] This makes sense because greater forces are necessary to dislocate a large-diameter head from the acetabulum. In practice, large-diameter femoral head components do not reduce the incidence of dislocation after surgery. Therefore the most commonly used head size is moderate (26 to 28 mm) rather than overly large (32 mm).[12,14]

One of the most common complications related to THR, using a noncemented femoral stem component, is persistent thigh pain with an antalgic gait (painful limp-gait) pattern. This thigh pain may last for 1 or 2 years after surgery and is reported in approximately 20% of all patients with this fixation type.[12,14]

The most significant complication after THR, with the highest mortality, is thromboembolic disease.[12]

Because the method of fixation is directly related to the initiation and progression of weight bearing after surgery with uncemented components, some authorities recommend TDWB on the second day postoperatively, gradually progressing to FWB by 8 weeks postoperatively.[3] With a cemented (PMMA) prosthesis, Goldstein[3] suggests TDWB 2 days after surgery, progressing to FWB by the third week postoperatively. These timetables for weight bearing are directed by the biologic rate of bone healing and the wishes of the physician and are applied under the direction of the PT. A cemented component generally allows earlier motion and weight bearing than an uncemented prosthesis.

Loosening of the components has been estimated at 10% to 40% by 10 years postoperatively.[14] Loosening is more common among younger, more active patients, obese patients, patients with rheumatoid arthritis, and patients with previous hip surgery.[14] The PTA must be acutely aware of these factors when treating THR patients and recognize the increased potential for component loosening.

Postoperative dislocation of the hip after THR is another clinically significant complication occurring at rates between 1% and 4%.[14] These dislocations are multifactorial, requiring an awareness of the basic concepts of hardware design, fixation procedures, and surgical approaches and patient compliance with specific total hip precautions to avoid dislocation. The most immediate concern during the recovery from THR is teaching and reinforcing precautions to the patient, nursing staff, family, and other caregivers.

The PTA also should be familiar with the surgical approach used to gain exposure to the hip. Universal **total hip precautions** are intended to avoid the exact position the surgeon used to expose and dislocate the hip to carry out the procedure. Usually these precautions are as follows:

- Avoid hip adduction. This is usually accomplished by using an abduction wedge or pillow.
- Avoid hip internal rotation. The affected limb can be supported medially with pillows or a wedge to maintain the limb in neutral or slight external rotation.
- Avoid hip flexion greater than 90 degrees.
- Avoid the combination (simultaneous performance) of hip flexion, internal rotation, and adduction for up to 4 months after surgery.[3]

The preceding precautions apply when a posterolateral or lateral approach is used. If an anterior surgical approach is used, combined hip extension and external rotation should be avoided.[3] Again, this variation is needed because the surgeon had to extend and externally rotate the limb to dislocate the hip and gain exposure for replacement.

Rehabilitation after Total Hip Replacement

Recovery from the significant trauma of THR requires extensive bone and soft-tissue healing. Following THR precautions, recovery may take up to 4 months in some cases.

The rehabilitation program can be divided into maximum-, moderate-, and minimum-protection phases of recovery. The time frames associated with each phase depend on the individual patient's ability to achieve certain criteria of improved motion (being careful not to compromise THR precautions), increased strength, weight bearing status (taking into account whether the replacement has been secured with cement or a porous coated biologic ingrowth component), reduced pain, compliance with THR precautions, bed mobility, transfers, and improved confidence.

In the maximum-protection phase of recovery, the patient is instructed in bilateral ankle pumps, isometric quadriceps sets, gluteal isometrics, and active knee flexion (being careful to avoid excessive hip flexion) exercises. The contralateral limb can be exercised with active straight-leg raises, quadriceps sets, hamstring sets, ankle pumps, and full knee and hip mobility exercises. To ensure primary healing, all universal hip precautions must be enforced. (Avoid hip flexion, adduction, and internal rotation with a posterolateral or lateral surgical approach, and avoid hip extension and external rotation with an anterior approach.) In addition, the patient should be strongly cautioned to avoid the following positions and actions, as outlined by LeVeau:[9]

■ Do not sit in low chairs.
■ Do not cross your legs.
■ Do not sleep on your side.
■ Do not bend forward at your hip (causes excessive hip flexion).
■ Do not squat.

Transfer training and bed mobility must be addressed immediately after surgery. The affected limb should be maintained in a stable, secure position during all transfers from bed to commode or wheelchair. A raised toilet seat is a basic requirement during the early phase of recovery. In addition, a raised and rigid (although padded) seat cushion is necessary to eliminate the sling effect of the wheelchair seat, which places the hip in an internally rotated position.[3]

The use of crutches or a walker is advocated for TDWB or PWB, depending on how the prosthesis is secured. A

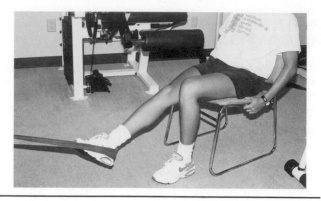

Fig. 20-10 Seated hamstring strengthening using elastic band.

cemented prosthesis requires TDWB on the second day after surgery, with the patient gradually progressing to FWB by 3 weeks. An uncemented THR can begin with PWB; then the patient can progress to FWB up to 8 weeks after surgery.

The moderate-protection phase can begin when the patient has demonstrated improved quadriceps control, active knee flexion, reduced pain, compliance with all precautions and exercises, independent bed mobility and transfers, and improved gait (with necessary weight bearing precautions). Moderate protection does not imply reduced THR precautions in any way. During this phase, more challenging exercises are added to more closely approximate functional activities. Light resistance exercises for quadriceps strengthening in a semirecumbent position and elastic tubing (Thera-Band) also can be used to strengthen the hamstrings and hip extensors in a semirecumbent or seat-elevated position (Fig. 20-10). Standing exercises stress active hip motion (straight-plane motions, no combined rotational forces, THR precautions strictly enforced) and strengthening.

To enhance aerobic fitness, a recumbent bucket-seat bicycle ergometer or an upper body ergometer (UBE) can be used. The addition of increases in weight bearing is determined by component fixation, tissue healing constraints, and the wishes of the physician. Closed-chain functional activities begin between 3 and 8 weeks postoperatively[4] for cemented prostheses, with increased weight bearing orders by the physician. These activities can include sit-to-stand exercises with an elevated seat, partial supported knee bends (for concentric and eccentric quadriceps control), weight-shifting exercises, treadmill walking, mini step-ups, and standing resisted hip and knee extension (Fig. 20-11). For an uncemented prosthesis, closed-chain functional activities are deferred for 2 or 3 weeks longer than for cemented prostheses. However, standing straight-plane resistance exercises (hip extension, adduction, abduction, and flexion) are allowed between 3 and 8 weeks postoperatively.

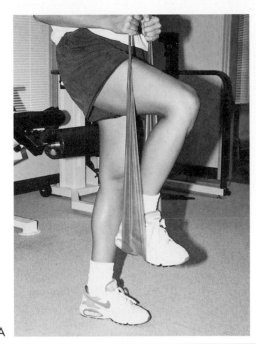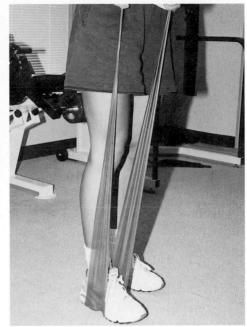

A   B

Fig. 20-11 Standing hip and knee extension press-down using elastic band. **A,** Starting position. **B,** Finish.

The minimum-protection phase of recovery is initiated 12 to 16 weeks after surgery. Depending on individual cases, the physician may elect to discontinue THR precautions during this phase. A great deal of soft-tissue and bone healing must take place and muscular strength must improve dynamic stability before THR precautions are relaxed.

The minimum-protection phase is classically characterized by a return to normalized gait patterns without assistive devices, and by instruction in balance, coordination, proprioception, and advanced closed-chain functional activities that duplicate the patient's specific ADLs. Most patients recover most of their hip motion during the first year after surgery.[12] Therefore at this phase of recovery (approximately 4 months after surgery) the patient may still demonstrate decreased motion, but must be reassured that more time is needed before assessing the ultimate degree of hip motion attainable.

While addressing proprioception, coordination, and balance after either knee or hip replacement (single-leg standing, eyes open and eyes closed, single-leg standing on a minitrampoline or balance board), the PTA must recognize that certain afferent neural input mechanoreceptors (type I, Ruffini; type II, pacinian; types III and IV, free nerve endings) will be lost because of the removal of the articulating joint surfaces. However, the joint capsule surrounding the joint replacement remains essentially intact and well supplied with mechanoreceptor feedback organs, which can be retrained and enhanced via appropriately applied weight shifting activities, balance board exercises, and closed-chain functional strengthening exercises.

LEGG-CALVÉ-PERTHES DISEASE

In 1910, three researchers identified a hip condition that usually affects children between the ages of 4 and 8 years.[5] (According to LeVeau, the range is 2 to 12 years of age with the most common age being 6 years.)[9] This condition, which is referred to as **Legg-Calvé-Perthes (LCP) disease** or *coxa plana*, is characterized as a noninflammatory, self-limiting (can heal spontaneously with or without specific treatment) syndrome in which the femoral head becomes flattened at the weight bearing surface[5] as a result of disruption of the blood supply (AVN) to the femoral head in the growing child.[5,9] The long-term complications of the flattened femoral head lead to an incongruous joint surface and advanced DJD (Fig. 20-12).[5,9,11]

Throughout the management of this disease, the primary focus is on maintaining the femoral head within the confines of the acetabulum, regaining motion, and reducing pain and dysfunction.[5,9,11] In the acute or maximum-protection phase, reducing pain and dysfunction is generally accomplished using physician-prescribed nonsteroidal antiinflammatory drugs (NSAIDs), bed rest, and traction to take the load off the hip and restore motion in abduction.

Keeping the femoral head seated within the acetabulum can be accomplished using an abduction orthosis (Fig. 20-13).[5,9] To aid healing and reduce unwanted

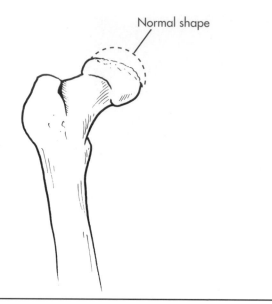

Normal shape

Fig. 20-12 Legg-Calvé-Perthes disease.

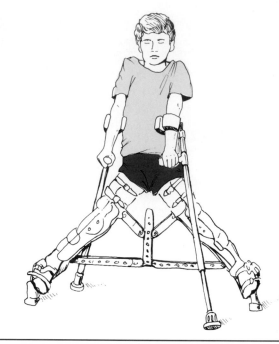

Fig. 20-13 An abduction orthosis can be used during the treatment of Legg-Calvé-Perthes disease to help maintain the femoral head seated within the acetabulum.

stress on the affected hip, the abduction orthosis can be worn as long as 2 years.[9] During this time, the brace can be removed for short periods each day to exercise the limb and attend to personal hygiene.[9] With the brace removed, the patient must maintain hip abduction during ROM exercises for the knee (flexion and extension), internal rotation of the hip, quadriceps strengthening, hip abduction, and hip extension strengthening exercises (gluteus medius and gluteus maximus).[9]

SOFT-TISSUE INJURIES OF THE HIP (BURSITIS, STRAINS, AND CONTUSIONS)

Trochanteric bursitis is a common soft-tissue injury affecting the hip in an active population of patients. The greater trochanter of the femur is most commonly affected. The trochanteric bursa may become irritated and inflamed because of excessive compression and repeated friction as the iliotibial band snaps over the bursa while lying superior to the greater trochanter (Fig. 20-14).

Treatment for greater trochanteric bursitis is centered on relieving pain and inflammation while addressing the underlying cause of the condition. Rest, ice, and anti-inflammatory medications are commonly used first to arrest the symptoms of pain and swelling. Any specific motions or activities (e.g., running) that may exacerbate the pain must be modified or eliminated. Typically a program of stretching is essential to reduce the compression and friction from the iliotibial band (ITB) over the greater trochanter. After ice is applied directly over the affected hip, either standing or side-lying ITB stretches should be used slowly as long as the patient does not complain of pain. In addition, hamstring, quadriceps, and hip adductor stretching can be used as a total program

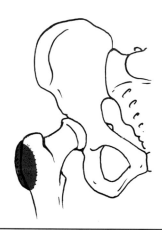

Fig. 20-14 Greater trochanteric bursitis.

to improve hip flexibility in all planes and to maintain proper balance among these muscle groups.

A comprehensive program of care focuses on all aspects of the disorder. Strength must be addressed, taking care not to stress the affected hip and reproduce the symptoms of pain, swelling, and tightness of the lateral hip structures. Specific strengthening exercises include quadriceps strengthening, hamstring curls, hip adduction, hip extension exercises (partial squats, leg press), and hip abduction exercises. Aerobic fitness can be maintained using a stationary cycle, UBE, treadmill, or stair-climber. In any case, the ROM must be modified

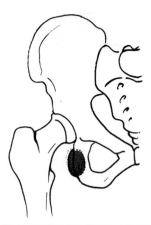

Fig. 20-15 Ischial bursitis.

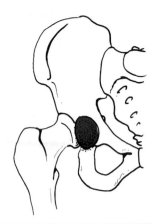

Fig. 20-16 Iliopectineal bursitis.

to limit hip and knee motion and avoid repeated snapping of the ITB over the trochanter. Ultrasound and hydrotherapy also may be useful during the acute phase of recovery.

Two other areas of bursitis commonly affecting the hip are ischial bursitis and iliopectineal bursitis. *Ischial bursitis* (Fig. 20-15) is characterized by pain over the ischial tuberosity underlying the gluteus maximus. It can be caused by direct contusion of the ischial tuberosity or extended periods of sitting.[5,15] Occasionally this condition can mimic a hamstring strain at the origin of the muscle at the ischial tuberosity.[5,15] Management is similar to other forms of bursitis: rest from the aggravating activity, ice packs, NSAIDs, and a judiciously applied program of stretching exercises that do not aggravate the symptoms. Generally, hamstring stretches are encouraged along with quadriceps-strengthening exercises. Occasionally, conservative care fails and the physician may elect to inject the area with corticosteroids.[5]

Iliopectineal bursitis is characterized by either local tenderness over the iliopsoas muscle and tendon or diffuse radiating pain into the anterior thigh (Fig. 20-16).[15] Because the iliopectineal bursa lies deep to the tendon of the iliopsoas muscle, tightness of the iliopsoas alone and in conjunction with excessive hip extension can cause compression and frictional wear of the iliopectineal bursa. Specific care centers on reducing pain and irritation using a program of rest, ice, antiinflammatory medications, and physical therapy interventions such as thermal agents, stretching, and strengthening exercises.

Unfortunately, in some cases of iliopectineal bursitis, stretching the tight iliopsoas muscle group increases pain over the bursa. Stretching of the psoas muscle perhaps should be deferred in cases where pain is exacerbated by such activity. The use of ice, hydrotherapy, ultrasound, and physician-prescribed NSAIDs can minimize the pain and allow for the initiation of quadriceps-strengthening exercises, hamstring stretches, ITB stretches, hip adductor stretches, and the beginning of an aerobic

fitness program, as long as the symptoms do not increase. Specific stretching of the iliopsoas is indicated once initial healing has occurred and the acute inflammatory process is arrested.

Most acute injuries affecting the hip are musculotendinous **strains** of the hamstrings, iliopsoas, adductors, and rectus femoris.[5,15] Injuries to the hamstrings at the origin (ischial tuberosity) can be caused by sudden, forceful contraction of the hamstrings or by decelerating the lower leg against the concentric contraction of the quadriceps during running as the hamstrings contract eccentrically (Fig. 20-17).

Initial injury management involves the application of cold packs for 20 minutes, three to five times daily. Wrapping the affected limb with a compression bandage also can help relieve stress on the limb. Motions that produce pain and interfere with the healing process should be avoided. Two motions should not be attempted during the acute or maximum-protection phase of recovery: full knee extension combined with forward trunk flexion and full leg flexion.[1,2]

The use of crutches may be indicated during this phase to limit stress on the hamstrings. The PTA can significantly aid the patient in coping with a difficult problem during the early recovery phase. Sleeping may be extraordinarily painful. The PTA should counsel the patient to sleep supine with pillows under both knees to support the injured limb and to reduce passive nocturnal stretching by placing the hamstrings in a relaxed position. As pain and swelling are reduced, active knee extension and leg flexion are encouraged (if the patient remains pain free) to help influence the direction of immature collagen fibers (see Chapter 4). The PTA must recall the intrinsic nature of muscle and tendon healing time constraints and avoid the temptation to encourage an aggressive stretching program for the hamstrings during the early maximum-protection phase of recovery. Sufficient time must be allowed for the torn tissue to scar and reorganize itself before subjecting the fragile

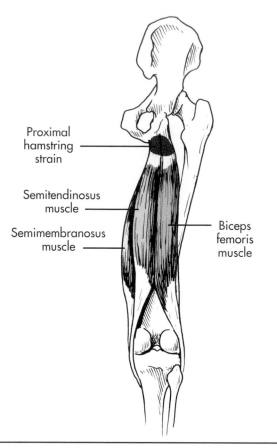

Fig. 20-17 Anatomy of posterior thigh musculature. Note proximal hamstring strain just inferior to the origin at the ischial tuberosity.

Proximal hamstring strain

Semitendinosus muscle

Semimembranosus muscle

Biceps femoris muscle

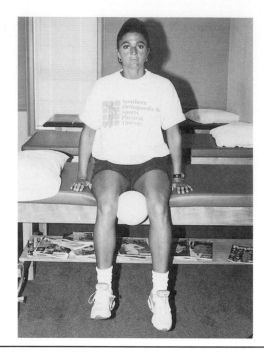

Fig. 20-18 Seated hip adduction isometrics.

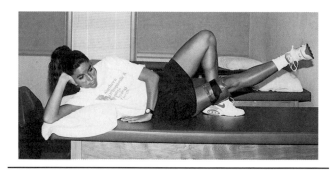

Fig. 20-19 Side-lying hip adduction concentric and eccentric contractions. Note the proximally placed resistance.

immature collagen to excessive tensile loads that may impede healing. However, flexibility certainly must be addressed and is the focus of long-term recovery during the moderate- and minimum-protection phases of recovery, as defined by the significance of the injury; the patient's ability to achieve improved motion, strength, and pain-free gait; the physician's wishes; and the PT's direction.

Strength training proceeds according to the patient's individual situation and is strongly influenced by muscle and tendon healing constraints. Initially, isometric quadriceps sets and submaximal multiangle hamstring sets can be done as pain allows. Progressive strengthening can be achieved with prone manual resistive leg curls, ankle weights, or sitting Thera-Band leg curls. (This particular exercise strongly encourages slow eccentric hamstring muscle contractions.) An excellent, dynamic, and fun exercise to perform is "scooting" with a rolling adjustable-height stool. This exercise encourages knee flexion against resistance at various controllable speeds. Supine hip bridges can be added as function increases.

An adductor muscle strain (usually the adductor longus) is termed a *groin pull*. A classic program of protection, ice, compression bandaging, crutches, and protected weight bearing during the acute or maximum-

protection phase should be followed. As with other muscle and tendon strains, early aggressive stretching should be avoided. Once pain subsides, active hip flexion, gentle hip abduction and adduction motion, and knee ROM exercises should begin. Specific hip abduction stretching can be initiated, instructing the patient to perform the seated "butterfly" stretch, with a strong caution to proceed slowly without pain. Some authorities suggest waiting 3 to 6 weeks before instructing the patient in progressive resistance exercises.[5] However, resistance exercises can begin earlier, depending on the severity of the strain. To specifically strengthen the hip adductors, submaximal isometrics (Fig. 20-18) can give way to proximally placed resistance in various positions (Fig. 20-19).

Progression to more dynamic strengthening exercises depends on the specific goals established by the patient and PT. For example, in a young athletic population of

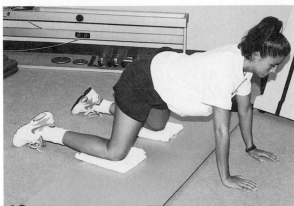

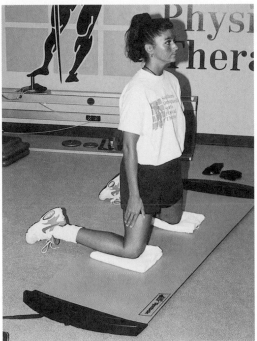

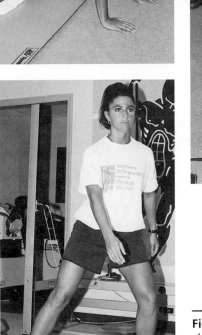

Fig. 20-20 Progressive slide board activities for dynamic closed-chain hip abduction and adduction. The series of exercises are begun. **A,** On hands and knees for support; the patient then slowly abducts and adducts both hips. **B,** Kneeling position is slightly more challenging. **C,** Standing position.

patients eager to return to sports activities, a slide board can be an effective tool to introduce dynamic hip adduction and abduction motions (Fig. 20-20).

An iliopsoas muscle strain also is referred to as a "hip flexor pull." This injury can occur from sudden, forceful extreme hip extension or by forced hip flexion against resistance.[15] A standard program of protection, rest, ice, and compression bandages with crutches and limited weight bearing is encouraged in the acute phase. Sleeping comfort can be enhanced by sleeping supine with pillows under the knees to reduce hip extension. Gentle, active hip flexion and extension exercises are begun once the initial healing phase has ended and the patient no longer complains of pain. A prolonged period of time may be needed to avoid hip extension (e.g., push-off during gait running or hip extension past neutral) and encourage healing. Gentle active stretching of the hip flexors can begin with the patient supine and the nonaffected knee and hip flexed. In addition, a hurdler's

stretch can be initiated once the patient demonstrates improved hip extension motion without pain. The PTA should strongly encourage the patient to perform these stretches in a slow, static fashion without pain. Very close supervision is needed to guard against any ballistic, forceful, or violent motions that could impede healing and reinjure the affected limb.

The most common **contusion** affecting the hip and pelvis involves the subcutaneous tissues of the iliac crest and is commonly termed a *hip pointer*.[6] Typically this injury can occur in one of two ways:

1. The iliac crest is contused by direct contact from an external force or falling on the exposed iliac crest.
2. There is a sudden forceful contraction or overstretching of the muscles attached to the iliac crest.[6] This seemingly minor injury can be severe, causing extreme pain and dysfunction.

First, the patient is treated with protection, rest, ice, gentle compression wraps, crutches, and partial weight

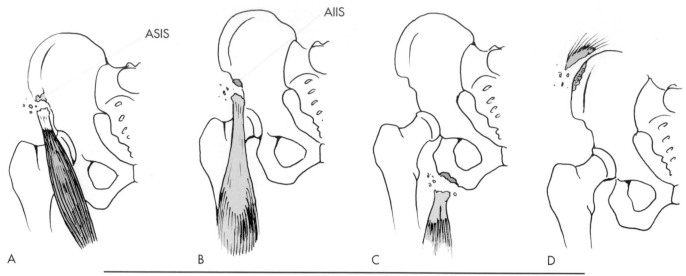

ASIS

AIIS

A   B   C   D

Fig. 20-21 **A,** Avulsion fracture anterior superior iliac spine. **B,** Avulsion fracture anterior inferior iliac spine. **C,** Avulsion fracture ischial tuberosity. **D,** Avulsion fracture iliac crest.

bearing. Initial soft-tissue healing must proceed without delay, so extreme caution is warranted to guard against unwanted forces or stress to the affected area. Stretching and strengthening of the affected hip commence once soft-tissue healing has progressed and pain is controlled. Usually in the moderate-protection phase, ultrasound, hydrotherapy, electrical stimulation, phonophoresis, or iontophoresis can be used at the discretion of the physician and PT to help control pain and swelling.

FRACTURES OF THE PELVIS AND ACETABULUM

General principles dealing with pelvic fractures and their classification with acetabular fractures dramatically show the PTA the extensive and potentially life-threatening nature of these injuries.[5,13,14] This discussion outlines the profound complications that may occur with pelvic fractures, giving the PTA a better understanding of the long-term rehabilitation needed in many cases of severe fractures.

The most basic classification of pelvic fractures refers to the injury as either stable or unstable.[5,13,14] *Stable* fractures include avulsion-type fractures of the anterior superior iliac spine, anterior inferior iliac spine, ischial tuberosity, and iliac crest (Fig. 20-21).[5,13] Avulsion fractures of the pelvis can be treated conservatively with rest, protected weight bearing, crutches, and avoidance of premature stretching and resistive exercises, which may delay bony union (usually within 6 weeks).[5]

McRae advocates an ORIF procedure with avulsion fractures of the ischial tuberosity and fragment separation greater than 2 cm by saying, "Non-union is an appreciable risk, and if this occurs there may be prob-

lems with chronic pain and disability."[13] Usually avulsion fractures of the ischial tuberosity can be treated with rest, keeping the hip extended and externally rotated to avoid continued stress on the healing bone, and enforcing protected weight bearing for approximately 6 weeks.[5] Once secure bone healing has been established, the PT may direct the assistant to carry out a gentle, progressive flexibility program to regain hip flexion. Strengthening exercises are added when the physician confirms radiographic evidence of secure union of the avulsion.

Other stable pelvic fractures include fractures of the superior pubic ramus, superior and inferior pubic rami on one side, and ilium (Fig. 20-22).[13] In general, stable fractures of the pelvis are treated nonsurgically with protection, bed rest (2 to 3 weeks),[13] and progressive motion and exercise once stable bone union has been confirmed.

Unstable pelvic fractures usually can be defined as either rotationally unstable but vertically stable, or rotationally and vertically unstable.[13] These severe injuries can be treated with an external fixator, ORIF procedure, or extended convalescence involving bed rest.[5,13,14] The PTA must be aware of complications after unstable pelvic fractures that can influence the time to begin rehabilitation procedures and can require protracted periods of recovery before physical therapy interventions. Box 20-1 outlines complications associated with these potentially life-threatening injuries.

The rehabilitation program employed after pelvic fractures is individualized and specific to the type and severity of fracture and the methods used to stabilize the fracture (ORIF, external fixator, and long-term convalescence). Because of the fragile hemodynamic

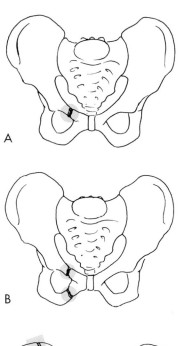

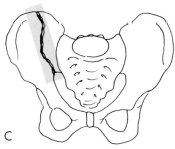

Fig. 20-22 **A,** Fracture of superior pubic ramus. **B,** Fracture of superior and inferior pubic ramus on one side. **C,** Fracture of the ilium.

BOX 20-1

Complications after Pelvic Fractures

1. Hemorrhage (significant blood loss, shock)
2. Gastrointestinal injury
3. Diaphragm rupture
4. Bony malunion (limb length shortening)
5. Nonunion
6. Neurologic damage
7. Degenerative joint disease
8. Infection (sepsis)

From Miller M: Adult reconstruction and sports medicine. In: Review of Orthopaedics. Philadelphia, WB Saunders, 1992; McRae R: Practical Fracture Treatment, 3rd ed. New York, Churchill-Livingstone, 1994.

nature of significant pelvic fractures, weight bearing of any kind is deferred for 8 weeks or longer.[13]

Initially the patient may be introduced to the vertical position using a tilt table. Pulse, respiration, and blood pressure are carefully monitored by the PTA as directed by the PT. Postural hypotension can be adequately addressed by gradually increasing the duration of elevation by small increments under the PT's direction. Maintenance of joint mobility is addressed early after surgery and during long periods of immobilization.

Active bilateral upper-extremity ROM begins as soon as the patient's condition is stable. Lower-extremity motion is limited to bilateral ankle pumps, gentle knee motion, and limited hip motion, depending on the nature of the fracture, fixation techniques used, stabilization of visceral damage (if any), and direction of the physician and PT. By far, the most significant clinical features associated with pelvic fractures are the potentially life-threatening complications, which can be acute or arise during early recovery or just after the acute phase of the injury. The PTA must closely supervise all vital signs before, during, and after all rehabilitation procedures. Once the physician has determined that the fracture site is stable and healed and the patient is medically stable, the PT may direct the PTA to follow a gradual program of general strength and fitness (a high priority with all patients requiring protracted periods of immobilization), quadriceps strengthening, hip motion, gait training, bed mobility, and transfer training.

The PTA must be aware that fractures of the pelvis also can involve the acetabulum. The acetabulum has an articular cartilage surface that allows for articulation between the femoral head and acetabulum. Care of this area is extremely important because the hip joint is a major weight bearing structure.

The classification system used to identify specific patterns of acetabular fractures is defined by Loth[10] as the Letornel classification model (Fig. 20-23). Generally, these fractures are treated according to the severity of the fracture, usually with an ORIF procedure or, conservatively, with bed rest and traction to reduce compression of the joint.[13] Conservative management of acetabular fractures is reserved for severely fragmented acetabular floor fractures in which surgery cannot realign the fragments to anatomically reconstruct the articular surface.[13] An ORIF procedure is used to stabilize the fracture in all other cases.[10]

Protected weight bearing is encouraged for 8 to 10 weeks; in cases of nonsurgical management, weight bearing is permitted at 9 weeks. A lower-extremity strength program is initiated immediately after surgery and involves ankle motion, quadriceps sets, hamstring sets, gentle submaximal gluteal sets, and active knee and hip motion. As with all fractures, as bone healing progresses and the patient achieves individualized criteria (e.g., strength, motion, reduced pain, minimal swelling, increased weight bearing, and normalized gait), the rehabilitation program can be advanced, gradually incorporating more challenging functional exercises.

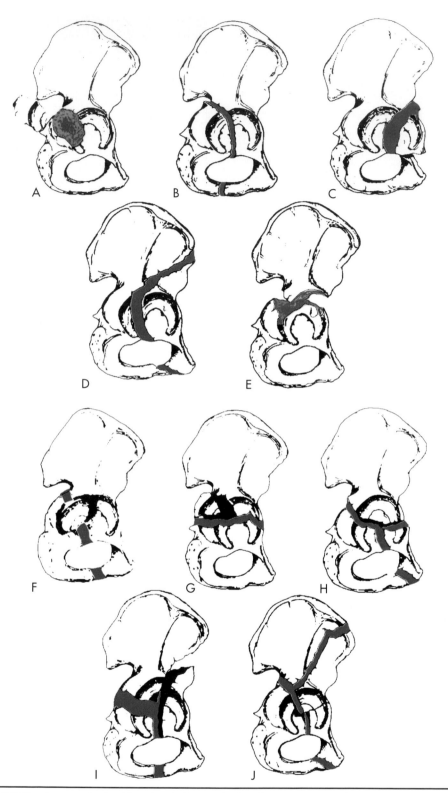

Fig. 20-23 Letornel classification of acetabular fractures. *Simple:* **A,** Posterior wall; **B,** posterior column; **C,** anterior wall; **D,** anterior column; **E,** transverse. *Combined:* **F,** Posterior column and posterior wall; **G,** transverse and posterior wall; **H,** T fracture; **I,** anterior column and posterior hemitransverse; **J,** both columns. (From Loth TS: Lower extremity. In Orthopaedic Boards Review. St Louis, Mosby, 1993.)

The PTA must remember the nature of specific acetabular fractures, since these fractures involve articular cartilage and bone. Therefore the initiation of closed-chain functional activities, which naturally require vertical loads, may be deferred for longer periods to allow for appropriate articular cartilage healing. If premature loads are directed through the weight bearing surface of the affected articular cartilage of the acetabulum, delayed union may result.

COMMON MOBILIZATION TECHNIQUES FOR THE HIP

Reduced motion secondary to pain and fibrosis after fractures, soft-tissue injuries, and various hip arthroplasty techniques may warrant mobilization in conjunction with thermal agents, strengthening, stretching, and functional activities. The techniques presented here are identified by the PT as appropriate techniques to use based on pathology, the presence of pain, or defined limitations of movement. As with all mobilization techniques, the PT selects which techniques to use and the direction of force, amplitude, grades, velocity, and distractions (see Chapter 16).

Most important, patient comfort and compliance with relaxation before and throughout the treatment are of paramount concern. Before each treatment session, the patient should be placed in the most comfortable position with attention paid to supporting the affected limb. The application of thermal agents (e.g., hot packs or ultrasound) to the affected limb and surrounding structures may be helpful to compose and relax the patient before treatment. If the patient has physician-prescribed pain medications or muscle relaxants, it may be helpful to consult with the PT to suggest that the patient take these medications in a timely fashion before treatment to further enhance relaxation.

Long Axis Distraction

With the patient supine, the affected limb should be placed in various degrees of abduction, depending on the specific limitation of movement and the defined goals of the PT. Hands should be placed securely around the dorsum of the affected limb and the calcaneus. The knee of the affected limb should be flexed or held straight. The direction of applied force is in a caudal direction, following the long axis of the femur (Fig. 20-24). The result is distraction of the head of the femur away from the acetabulum.

Lateral Distraction of the Hip

With the patient supine, the hip and knee of the affected limb should be flexed approximately 90 degrees.[1] The PTA should stand on the lateral aspect of the affected limb. The affected limb should be carefully supported against the PTA's chest. Both hands should be placed around the proximal femur while a laterally directed force is applied (Fig. 20-25).

Anterior and Posterior Mobilization

The patient should be placed in a side-lying position on the unaffected side. The hips and knees should be flexed with a pillow between the legs, supporting the thigh, knee, and lower leg. The PTA should stand in front of or behind the patient. Both hands should firmly grasp the greater trochanter. In this position, an anteriorly and posteriorly directed force is applied,[1] effectively translating the head of the femur away from the acetabulum (Fig. 20-26). The force is applied directly anteriorly and posteriorly. If performed casually, the femur is internally and externally rotated instead of appropriately translated forward and backward.

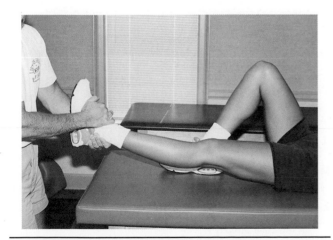

Fig. 20-24 Long-axis distraction of the hip.

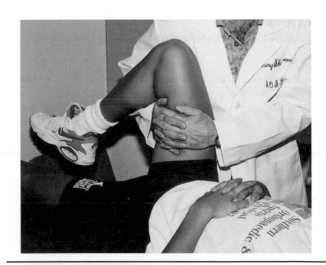

Fig. 20-25 Lateral hip distraction.

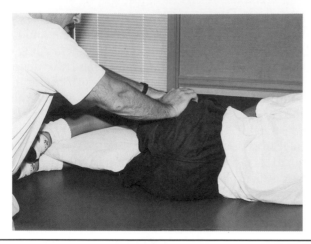

Fig. 20-26 Side-lying anterior-posterior mobilization of the hip.

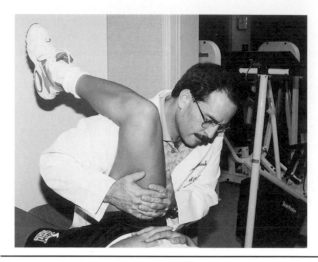

Fig. 20-27 Inferior glide of the hip.

Inferior Glide of the Hip

With the patient supine, the affected hip should be flexed approximately 90 degrees. The PTA should place the knee of the affected limb over his or her shoulder. With both hands (in an open-palm position), the proximal femur should be grasped and a "pulling" or "scooping" directed force applied. The head of the femur should be glided from the acetabulum inferiorly (Fig. 20-27).

❖ ADDITIONAL FEATURES

Bipolar Hip Prosthesis: Advantages—reduced friction forces to acetabular cartilage, polyethylene liner may decrease vertical compressive loading forces.

Femoral Head Blood Supply: Medial femoral circumflex artery, lateral femoral circumflex artery, ligamentum teres artery.

Hip Arthritis: The earliest motion that is lost with arthritic conditions of the hip is internal rotation.

Hip Dislocation—Complications: Avascular necrosis, post-traumatic arthritis, recurrent dislocations, sciatic nerve injury, heterotopic bone formation.

Hip Dislocation—Neurologic Injury: Loss of sensation of lateral calf and dorsum of foot, motor strength dorsiflexion of foot and toes. Risk of sciatic nerve and peroneal branch injury.

Osteonecrosis: Subchondral bone necrosis secondary to vascular insufficiency.

Postoperative Total Hip Arthroplasty ROM: Majority of patients regain most of their motion within 1 year postoperatively.

Slipped Capital Femoral Epiphysis (SCFE): Major complications include chondrolysis and avascular necrosis.

Subtrochanteric Hip Fractures: Clinical problems include malunion, delayed union, and nonunion. Reasons include the fact that the subtrochanteric area is cortical bone with a decreased blood supply, and large physiologic forces in this area may lead to hardware failure.

REFERENCES

1. Corrigan B, Maitland GD: The hip. In Practical Orthopaedic Medicine. Newton, MA, Butterworth-Heinemann, 1992.
2. Cummings S, Nevitt III M: A hypothesis: the cause of hip fractures. J Gerontal Med Sci 44:407, 1989.
3. Goldstein TS: Treatment of common problems of the hip joint. In Goldstein TS, Lewis CB, eds. Geriatric Orthopaedics: Rehabilitative Management of Common Problems. Gaithersburg, MD, Aspen Publishers, 1991.
4. Goldstein TS: The adult and geriatric hip. Continuing Education Course Notes. Boston, Quest Seminars, 1994.
5. Gross ML, Nasser S, Finnerman GAM: Hip and pelvis. In DeLee JC, Drez D, eds. Orthopaedic Sports Medicine: Principles and Practice, vol 2. Philadelphia, WB Saunders, 1994.
6. Henry JH: The hip. In Scott WN, Nisonson B, Nicholas JA, eds. Principles of Sports Medicine. Baltimore, MD, Williams & Wilkins, 1984.
7. Kozinn SC, Wilson PD: Adult hip disease and total hip replacement. Clinical Symposia. Ciba-Geigy, 1987.
8. Lewis CB, Bottomley JM: Orthopaedic treatment considerations. In Geriatric Physical Therapy: A Clinical Approach. New York, Appleton & Lange, 1994.
9. LeVeau B: Hip. In Richardson JK, Iglarsh ZA, eds. Clinical Orthopaedic Physical Therapy. Philadelphia, WB Saunders, 1994.
10. Loth TS: Lower extremity. In Orthopaedic Boards Review. St Louis, Mosby, 1993.
11. MacEwen GD, Bunnell WP, Ramsey PL: The hip. In Lovell WW, Winter RB, eds. Pediatric Orthopaedics. Philadelphia, JB Lippincott, 1986.
12. McDonald D, et al: Total joint reconstruction. In Orthopedic Boards Review. St Louis, Mosby, 1993.
13. McRae R: Practical Fracture Treatment, 3rd ed. New York, Churchill-Livingstone, 1994.
14. Miller M: Adult reconstruction and sports medicine. In Review of Orthopaedics. Philadelphia, WB Saunders, 1992.
15. Saudek CE: The hip. In Gould JA, ed. Orthopaedic and Sports Physical Therapy, 2nd ed. St Louis, Mosby, 1990.

REVIEW QUESTIONS

Multiple Choice

1. Which of the following represent(s) the most significant complication after hip fracture? (Circle any that apply.)
   A. Avascular necrosis
   B. Muscular atrophy
   C. Venous thrombosis
   D. Endurance
   E. Gait dysfunction

2. Avascular necrosis may occur after hip fracture in approximately what percentage of patients?
   A. 10% to 20%
   B. 50% to 60%
   C. 65% to 85%
   D. 5% to 15%
3. Which of the following describe(s) clinical complications noted with subtrochanteric fractures of the hip? (Circle any that apply.)
   A. Muscular atrophy
   B. Malunion
   C. Delayed union
   D. Nonunion
   E. Decreased hip abduction
4. Without prophylactic medications, what percentage of patients may develop thrombosis after hip surgery?
   A. 20%
   B. 10% to 15%
   C. 40% to 90%
   D. 5% to 10%
5. Which of the following exercises must be avoided during the first 6 to 8 weeks after a hip fracture secured with an open reduction with internal fixation (ORIF) procedure?
   A. Quad sets
   B. Heel slides
   C. Supine straight-leg raises
   D. Gluteal sets
6. Which of the following exercises must be avoided during the early recovery phase of healing after a hip fracture (6 to 8 weeks)?
   A. Knee flexion with hip flexion
   B. Rotary or diagonal hip patterns of movement
   C. Knee flexion
   D. Hip extension
   E. All of the above
7. Which of the following procedures is used in cases of femoral head osteonecrosis or severe femoral head fractures?
   A. Femoral osteotomy
   B. Hemiarthroplasty
   C. Tibial osteotomy
   D. Plate and screw fixation
8. Which of the following is (are) generally the goal(s) after hemiarthroplasty of the hip?
   A. Increase muscle size
   B. Improve neuromuscular endurance
   C. Reduce pain and improve function
   D. Increase hip range of motion
9. Which of the following are indications for total hip replacement (THR)?
   A. Rheumatoid arthritis
   B. Osteoarthritis
   C. Severe fractures
   D. Osteonecrosis
   E. All of the above
10. Which of the following represents one of the more common complications of total hip arthroplasty using a noncemented femoral stem component?
    A. Quadriceps weakness
    B. Quadriceps atrophy
    C. Persistent thigh pain and related antalgic gait
    D. Reduced hip range of motion
11. After THR, which of the following is the most significant complication with the highest mortality rate?

   A. Malunion
   B. Thromboembolic disease
   C. Avascular necrosis
   D. Nonunion
12. Postoperative dislocation of the hip after THR, according to Miller, is a clinically significant complication that occurs in approximately what percentage of patients?
    A. 10%
    B. 50%
    C. 15%
    D. 1% to 4%
13. Which of the following generally describe(s) universal hip precautions after THR? (Circle any that apply.)
    A. Avoid hip adduction
    B. Avoid external rotation
    C. Avoid hip flexion greater than 90 degrees
    D. Avoid hip internal rotation
    E. Avoid knee flexion greater than 80 degrees
14. Which of the following are appropriate exercises during the immediate postoperative recovery after a THR? (Circle any that apply.)
    A. Partial squats
    B. Short-arc step-ups
    C. Quad sets
    D. Gluteal isometrics
    E. Hamstring sets
15. With a cemented hip prosthesis, how soon can closed kinetic chain functional activities be initiated?
    A. As soon as pain allows
    B. When hip range of motion (ROM) improves
    C. Between 3 and 8 weeks postoperative and with increased weight bearing orders by the physician
    D. Between 8 and 10 weeks postoperative
16. A noninflammatory, self-limiting syndrome in which the femoral head becomes flattened at the weight bearing surface as a result of disruption of the blood supply to the femoral head in the growing child is called which of the following? (Circle any that apply.)
    A. Coxa plana
    B. Avascular necrosis
    C. Legg-Calvé-Perthes disease
    D. Osteoporosis
    E. Capsulitis
17. In cases of acute hamstring strain, which position provides the greatest support at night?
    A. Supine, knee extended
    B. Prone, knee extended
    C. Supine, knee flexed with pillow for support
    D. Side-lying
    E. All of the above
18. What is a "hip pointer"?
    A. A contusion to the ischial tuberosity
    B. A contusion of the rectus femoris
    C. A contusion of the iliac crest
    D. An indirect strain of the rectus femoris
19. In general, stable pelvic fractures are treated with which of the following? (Circle any that apply.)
    A. An ORIF procedure
    B. Protected weight bearing
    C. Bed rest
    D. Progressive motion
    E. Closed-chain eccentric exercise

20. Unstable pelvic fractures are considered as which of the following? (Circle any that apply.)
    A. Easily treated
    B. Not complicated
    C. Severe and potentially life-threatening
    D. Not medically challenging
    E. Common pediatric fractures

21. Because of the fragile vascular and potentially unstable hemodynamic nature of significant pelvic fractures, weight bearing of any kind is deferred for how long?
    A. 2 to 4 weeks
    B. 3 to 5 weeks
    C. 8 weeks or longer
    D. 4 to 6 weeks

22. Why are fractures of the acetabulum significant? (Circle any that apply.)
    A. They are always unstable.
    B. The acetabulum is an articular weight bearing surface.
    C. Acetabular fractures can result in osteoarthritis of the hip.
    D. These injuries always lead to a THR.
    E. Usually they are treated with an ORIF procedure.

Short Answer

23. Name the type of injury in the following figure.

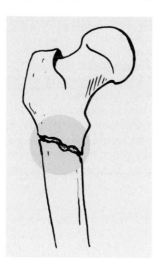

24. Name the type of injury in the following figure.

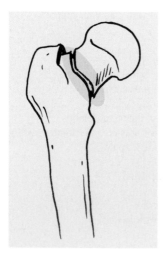

25. Name the type of injury in the following figure.

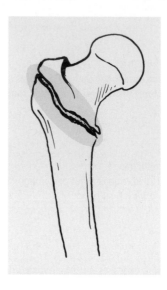

26. Name the soft-tissue injury in the following figure.

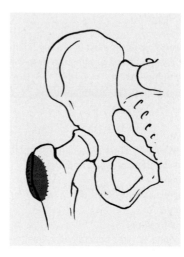

27. Name the soft-tissue injury in the following figure.

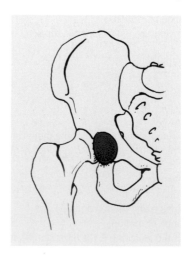

28. Name the soft-tissue injury in the following figure.

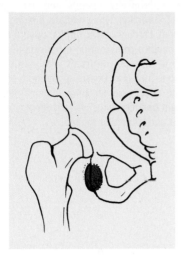

29. Label each muscle in the following figure.

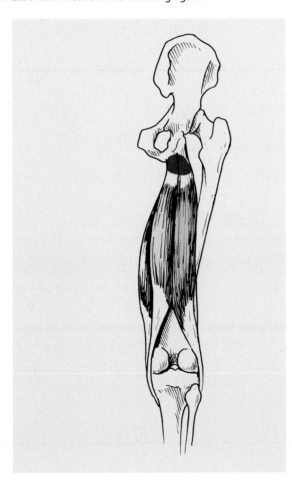

30. Identify the fracture type and location of injury in the following figure.

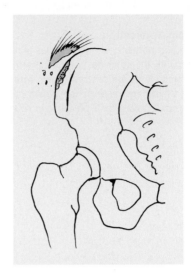

True/False
31. Hip fractures represent the most common acute orthopedic injury in the geriatric population.
32. The subtrochanteric area of the hip is prone to large biomechanical stresses, which can lead to loosening of various internal fixation devices.
33. The treatment of a fractured greater trochanter of the hip is always done with an ORIF procedure.
34. The general progression of weight bearing status after hip fractures usually parallels the rate of bone healing.
35. The method of fixation of various prosthetic hip components has a direct impact on the short- and long-term course of rehabilitation after hip arthroplasty.
36. Noncemented biologic tissue ingrowth prostheses require longer periods of limited weight bearing than cemented prosthetic hip components.
37. It is clinically significant that the simultaneous performance of hip flexion, internal rotation, and adduction be avoided for up to 4 months after THR surgery.
38. It is appropriate to actively encourage full knee extension after a hamstring strain during the first 3 weeks after injury.
39. Unstable pelvic fractures generally are defined as either rotationally unstable but vertically stable, or rotationally and vertically unstable.
40. Closed kinetic chain exercises are advocated during the early healing phases of recovery after acetabular fractures.

Essay Questions
Answer on a separate sheet of paper.
41. Identify common hip fractures.
42. Outline and discuss common methods of management and rehabilitation of common hip fractures.
43. Identify and describe common methods of management and rehabilitation after hip arthroplasty.
44. Identify and describe common soft-tissue injuries of the hip.
45. Outline and describe common methods of management and rehabilitation of soft-tissue injuries of the hip.
46. Identify common fractures of the pelvis and hip.

47. Discuss methods of management and rehabilitation for fractures of the pelvis and acetabulum.
48. Describe common mobilization techniques for the hip.

Critical Thinking Application

You are treating two patients: one patient has a subtrochanteric hip fracture with an ORIF, the other has a total hip arthroplasty in which the prosthetic components are secured (fixed) with cement. In small groups, contrast the differences in rehabilitation progression, weight bearing status, complications, and precautions related to these two cases. Specifically, define and contrast hip precautions related to hip fractures and hip arthroplasty. Identify and list appropriate ROM exercises, muscle contraction types, weight bearing status, general physical conditioning, cardiovascular fitness, open and closed kinetic chain activities, balance-coordination-proprioception drills, and a progressive return to function consistent with your understanding of soft-tissue and bone healing. Does the method of prosthetic hip component fixation affect your recommendations related to motion, strength, and weight bearing status? Clearly identify all complications related to fractures and surgery of the hip.

21

Orthopedic Management of the Lumbar, Thoracic, and Cervical Spine*

LEARNING OBJECTIVES

1. Outline and describe basic mechanics of the lumbar spine.
2. Discuss and apply the principles of fundamental mechanics of lifting.
3. Identify common sprains and strains of the lumbar spine.
4. Discuss common methods of management and rehabilitation of lumbar spine sprains and strains.
5. Identify and describe injuries to the lumbar intervertebral disk.
6. Discuss methods of management and rehabilitation for injuries to the lumbar intervertebral disk.
7. Define and describe methods of quantifying back strength.
8. Define and describe components of the back school model.
9. Define ergonomic and functional capacity evaluations.
10. Define spinal stenosis and describe methods of management and rehabilitation.
11. Define and contrast the terms *spondylolysis* and *spondylolisthesis*.
12. Describe methods of management and rehabilitation for spondylolysis and spondylolisthesis.
13. Identify common lumbar and thoracic spine fractures.
14. Define kyphosis, lordosis, and scoliosis.
15. Identify and describe methods of management and rehabilitation for kyphosis and scoliosis.
16. Identify and describe common cervical spine injuries, and discuss methods of management and rehabilitation.

KEY TERMS

Disk	Sequestrated disk	Functional capacity
Annulus	Radicular signs	evaluations (FCEs)
Nucleus pulposus	Peripheralization	Kyphosis
Prone extension	Centralization	Scoliosis
Spine stabilization	Spinal stenosis	Cervical spondylosis
Herniated nucleus	Spondylolysis	Thoracic outlet (inlet)
pulposus (HNP)	Spondylolisthesis	syndrome
Disk protrusion	"Back schools"	
Extruded disk	Ergonomics	

*Refer to orthopedic anatomy figures on the Evolve website.

CHAPTER OUTLINE
Lumbar Spine
    Basic Mechanics
    Fundamental Mechanics of Lifting
    Quantifying Back Strength
    Muscle Strains
    Ligament Sprains
    Injuries to the Lumbar Intervertebral Disk
    Invasive Management of Lumbar Disk Herniation
    Spinal Stenosis
    Spondylolysis and Spondylolisthesis
    Lumbar Spine Fractures
    Prevention and Education for Back Dysfunction:
        The Back School Model
    Ergonomics and Functional Capacity Evaluations
The Thoracic Spine
    Thoracic Spine Muscle Injuries
    Thoracic Disk Injuries
    Kyphosis
    Scoliosis
The Cervical Spine
    Acute Sprains and Strains
    Cervical Disk Injuries
    Cervical Spondylosis
    Thoracic Outlet Syndrome
Mobilization of the Lumbar, Thoracic, and
        Cervical Spine

In this chapter the physical therapist assistant (PTA) is introduced to injuries that affect the spine. Common soft-tissue injuries (e.g., muscle, ligament, or disk) and fractures of the lumbar, thoracic, and cervical spine are listed, with specific therapeutic interventions, back testing procedures, functional (or physical) capacity evaluations, and injury-prevention techniques (patient education through back school training).

THE LUMBAR SPINE

Perhaps no other medical condition draws as much attention from researchers and clinicians as the identification, treatment, and rehabilitation of lumbar spine injuries. The estimated aggregate financial burden to the United States economy ranges from 7.2 billion[1] to more than 40 billion[12] and almost as high as 100 billion dollars[32] annually for the care of low–back-related problems. Lumbar spine injuries also account for literally millions of lost work days per year in the United States and England.[14,32] The rate of disability from injuries to the low back was estimated over a 10-year period to be a staggering 14 times greater than the rate of population growth for that same period.[1,7] Overall, lumbar spine injuries are the second leading cause of all physician visits in the United States.[1]

Some studies suggest that nonspecific low back dysfunction may affect 80% of the adult population in the United States at some point in their lives.[33] Although acute management and criteria-based rehabilitation programs for low back dysfunction can prove effective, some authorities point out that more than half of the patients with back pain recover in 1 week and 90% improve within 1 to 3 months from the onset of injury.[27]

Currently, there is no universally accepted philosophic agreement about the most efficient, effective, and economical method for treating low back dysfunction. Historically, absolute bed rest, medications, thermal agents (e.g., hot packs or ultrasound), and a series of rudimentary lumbar flexion exercises (e.g., pelvic tilts, single knee-to-chest, double knee-to-chest, and partial direct and oblique sit-ups) were the components of a typical protocol for lumbar sprains, strains, and disk-related pathologic conditions (Fig. 21-1). However, with sophisticated long-term studies and the development of advanced evaluation technology (e.g., computed tomography [CT], magnetic resonance imaging [MRI]), improved understanding of the mechanics of the lumbar spine has led to significant advances in the care of soft-tissue and bony injuries to this area.

Basic Mechanics

Understanding the principles of intradiscal pressure and fluid mechanics related to motion of the disk helps to clarify the rationale for using specific therapeutic measures for individual low back conditions.

The lumbar spine is composed of five anterior convex segments and posterior concave segments that produce the recognizable lordotic curve. Between each vertebral body lies a **disk** (Fig. 21-2). The outer wall of the disk is called the **annulus** and comprises 12 to 18 concentrically arranged rings of fibroelastic cartilage.[14,30] Contained within the annulus is the **nucleus pulposus.** Nuclear material is a mucopolysaccharide gel[14] that transmits forces, equalizes stress, and promotes movement.[29] As well as containing the nucleus, the annulus provides stability, enhanced movement between vertebral bodies, and shock absorption.[29] The disk provides stability between the vertebral bodies, permits movement within each vertebral segment, and transmits motion.[30] The disk is an avascular and aneural[25] (although the outer fibers of the annulus are innervated)[14] structure that obtains nutrition by diffusion from the vascular supply of the vertebral bodies.[7,14,25,30]

Allman[1] describes lumbar motion and postural alterations as producing significant pressure within the disk (intradiscal pressure). The compressive forces that influence intradiscal pressure are as follows:[1]

- *Standing:* Disk pressure is equal to 100% of body weight
- *Supine:* Disk pressure is less than 25% of body weight
- *Side-lying:* Disk pressure is less than 75% of body weight
- *Standing and bending forward:* Disk pressure is approximately 150% of body weight

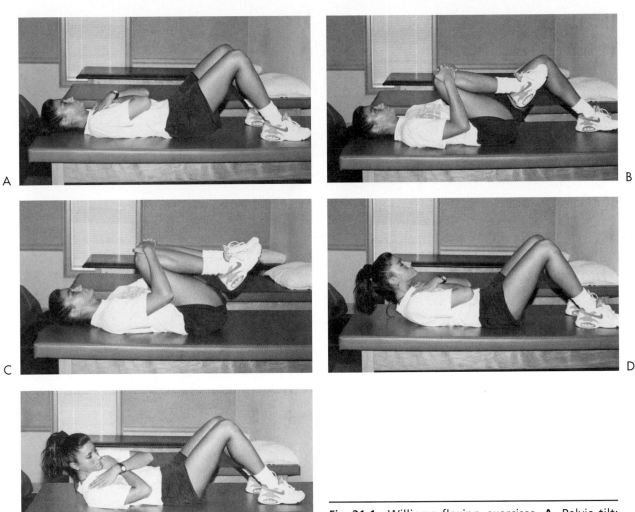

Fig. 21-1 Williams flexion exercises. **A,** Pelvic tilt; **B,** single knee to chest; **C,** double knee to chest; **D,** partial direct sit-ups; **E,** partial oblique sit-ups.

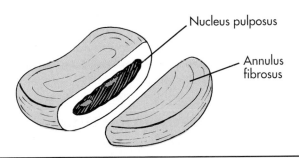

Fig. 21-2 Intervertebral disk.

- *Supine with both knees flexed:* Disk pressure is less than 35% of body weight
- *Seated in a flexed position:* Disk pressure is approximately 85% of body weight
- *Bending forward in a flexed posture and lifting:* Disk pressure is close to 275% of body weight

Intradiscal pressure also can be expressed in terms of pressure or load measured within the intervertebral lumbar disk. Cailliet[4] reports that isometric abdominal sets produce approximately 110 kg of pressure within the disk, whereas walking produces 85 kg, sitting 100 kg, bilateral straight-leg raises in supine position 120 kg, and lifting with a flexed torso and knees held straight an astounding 340 kg of intradiscal pressure. This information may help clarify the rationale for protective postures, lifting protocols, and appropriate body mechanics, as well as prescribed exercises for specific lumbar spine conditions.

The fluid mechanics of the disk (nucleus pulposus) itself also are influenced strongly by the motion of the lumbar vertebral segments. McKenzie[25] describes flexion and extension motion of the spine as having clinically significant effects on the nucleus's direction of movement. When positional changes occur in the lumbar spine, from flexion to extension, the nucleus moves anteriorly (Fig. 21-3).[25] Conversely, when the spine moves from extension to full flexion, the nucleus tends to displace or move posteriorly (Fig. 21-4). Thus it is necessary to fully understand the individual nature of each

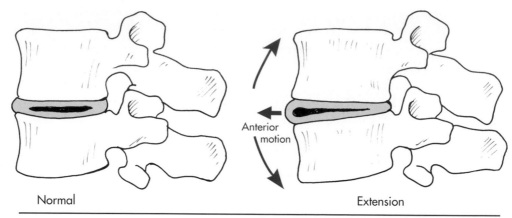

Fig. 21-3 Movement of the spine from a position of flexion into extension causes the nucleus to move in an anterior direction.

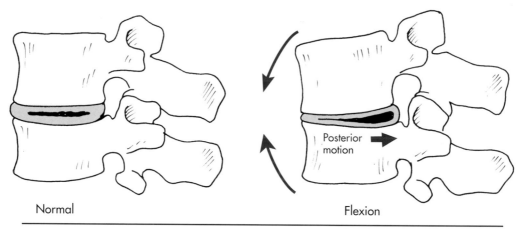

Fig. 21-4 Movement of the spine from a position of extension into flexion causes the nucleus to move in a posterior direction.

injury and avoid or enhance certain motions and postures as directed by the physical therapist (PT).

Positive sciatic and femoral nerve-root tension signs seen during the initial evaluation performed by the PT should be confirmed or denied.[37] Pain that radiates into one or both lower extremities early in the initial evaluation could signify nerve root compression from an adjacent herniated intervertebral disk. A sensitive test for nerve root compression requires the patient to be supine while one leg is raised passively with the knee completely extended (straight-leg test). The opposite leg is tested in the same manner. The test is considered positive only if radicular pain is increased,[11] which indicates stretching of the sciatic nerve. Anterior radiating thigh pain can be evaluated by the PT as follows: The patient assumes the prone position with one knee flexed to 90 degrees. Then the hip is passively extended and any increase in radiating anterior thigh pain is documented.[11] This test (the femoral nerve tension sign) is not considered positive if back pain occurs.

Gould[14] suggests that muscle spasm in the thoracolumbar spine muscles actually may be a compartment syndrome in which swelling accumulates (after injury) within the defined series of compartments formed by the fascia and muscles of the spine. This occurs as the spine is straightened and the lordotic curve reduced.

Fundamental Mechanics of Lifting

Forces and stresses related to lifting, sitting, standing, walking, sleeping, and twisting are common to all activities of daily living (ADLs). O'Sullivan, Ellis, and Makofsky[28] have identified a novel concept to instruct patients in proper lifting mechanics, listing the "five Ls" of lifting: load, lever, lordosis, legs, and lungs.

The *load* to be lifted is central to all concepts of lifting mechanics. The amount of weight to be hoisted should be appropriate for the task and for the individual attempting to lift it. The *lever* refers to keeping the object as close to the body as is functionally possible throughout the lift. If the object is held away from the body, the

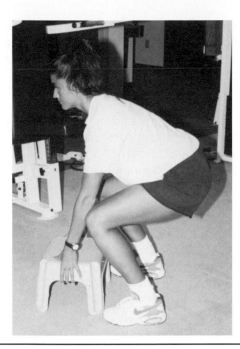

Fig. 21-5 In a flat back lifting position, the abdominals are shortened, lumbar paravertebral muscles show little or no electromyelographic activity, the posterior ligaments are stretched, the nucleus is forced posteriorly, and the center of gravity is posterior to the base of support.

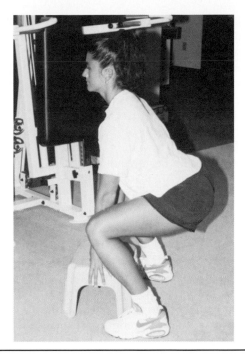

Fig. 21-6 Maintenance of lumbar lordosis during the lift. In this position the abdominals are in normal anatomic length, lumbar paravertebral muscles are contracted, posterior ligaments are relaxed, the posterior annular wall is protected, the nucleus is in a normal position, and the patient's center of gravity is over the base of support.

increased force (both intradiscal pressure and muscle strain) may strain the lumbar spine. *Lordosis* refers to maintaining a normal anatomic lordotic curve while lifting any object. Teaching the patient (and the PTA) to lift with the *legs* is basic to all lifting procedures. The muscles of the legs should be conditioned to fully participate during the lifting of any object from the floor. If the legs are not used fully, the muscles of the back may be necessary to absorb increased stress. The *lungs* refer to the use of proper breathing techniques during lifting. The Valsalva maneuver (closed glottis during attempted expiration) should be avoided and instruction given on exhaling during the actual lift.

Kaiser, Rose, and Apts[20] have identified a lumbar stabilization model comparing two lumbar spine postures during lifting. In the first posture (tested electromyographically) the starting position is characterized by a posterior pelvic tilt. The abdominal muscles are in a shortened position, the lumbar paravertebral muscles show no electromyographic activity, the posterior ligaments and posterior annular wall are stretched, the nucleus is forced posteriorly, the knees are in a position of decreased leverage, and the patient's center of gravity is posterior to the base of support.[20] In the second posture, the patient's lumbar lordosis is maintained during the lift. The abdominal muscles are in their normal anatomic length, the paravertebral muscles contracted, the posterior ligaments relaxed, the poste-

rior annular wall protected, the nucleus in a "normal" position, the knees in an optimal leverage position, and the patient's center of gravity over the base of support. Figures 21-5 and 21-6 graphically describe these two contrasting lifting postures.

Quantifying Back Strength

Beginning with the initial evaluation process and continuing throughout rehabilitation and discharge from formal physical therapy, quantifying back function is paramount for developing an individualized recovery program. Usually the PT directs the PTA to help in patient setup, testing procedures, and data accumulation (the PT is responsible for all data evaluation and interpretation) using various commercially available testing devices.

At present there is controversy concerning the most efficient, effective, meaningful, and economical method of isolating and quantifying lumbar strength. Tan[35] outlines and describes common lumbar testing devices, as follows:

- Isometric (cable tensiometers, strain gauge, Med-X lumbar extension)
- Isokinetic (Cybex, Lido, Kin-Com, Biodex)
- Isoinertial (Isotechnologies Isostation B-200)

Although isometric exercise in general provides appropriate stress, as well as morphologic and functional changes in skeletal muscle, the advantages of isometric strengthening have been identified as follows:[6]

- Increases muscle strength
- Is position dependent, with strength gains (isometrically) that are joint-angle specific
- Reduces muscle atrophy
- Produces muscle hypertrophy

The negative aspects of isometric training are as follows:[6]

- Fatigues muscles rapidly
- Can profoundly increase blood pressure, heart rate, and cardiac output
- Hypertensive response can lead to a marked increase in left ventricular wall stress.

Based on this information, isometric lumbar extension strength testing must be highly selective and applied to patients who can tolerate these activities. The advantages are simplicity of application and "ease of interpretation."[35] Some authorities point out that there are clinically significant strength gains realized by isolating, training, and testing lumbar extension.[12] Fulton reports that "lumbar muscles will respond only to specific, isolated exercise . . . with specific exercise, increases in strength of the lumbar muscles of more than 100% are below average, increases of several hundred percent are common, and increases of several thousand percent are not rare."[12]

Isometric testing may appear very attractive if the single, primary cause of dysfunction is muscle weakness. The fundamental disadvantage is the "poor correlation with real life dynamic activities."[35] The physician and PT determine if isometric strength testing is a safe and appropriate means of quantifying back strength for a particular patient.

Isokinetic training and testing have been validated by a select group of orthopedic surgeons as efficient to develop strength in a normal individual, allowing for exercise throughout a velocity spectrum, producing strength gains at high speeds that carry over to slower speeds, and able to document and reproduce performance testing.[1-4,6] However, Tan[35] suggests that there are inherent limitations with isokinetic lumbar strength testing, primarily that isokinetics "does not simulate real life because we do not move at constant velocity."

The only currently available isoinertial (defined by Tan as a muscle exertion on a constant inertial mass)[35] testing device is the Isostation B-200 (Isotechnologies, Hillsborough, NC). This device is a three-axis dynamometer that measures motion, velocity, and torque simultaneously in three planes.[33] Tan suggests that isoinertial back testing may more closely duplicate functional real-life activities in which the load lifted remains constant.[35]

Regardless of which type of device is available (isometric, isokinetic, or isoinertial), the physician and PT must identify specific patient candidates who are appropriate for testing. Not all patients should be tested isometrically, nor do all spinal dysfunction pathologies require isolated lumbar extension strength testing. The criteria for using the various lumbar spine testing procedures have been identified as follows:[35]

1. Clinical use (objective findings, measure groups, and reinforcement)
2. Medicolegal use (identification of maximum effort, consisting of effort, documentation, and assessment of physical impairment)
3. Occupational use (ergonomic and rehabilitation guidelines, job screening, and work site evaluations)
4. Research use (standardization)

The PTA must become familiar with a wide variety of testing implements, as well as indications (objective documentation of strength, range of motion [ROM], local muscle endurance, and fatigue resistance) and contraindications (acute injury, unstable fractures, spondylolisthesis, and sequestrated nucleus pulposus) for static (isometric) or dynamic (isokinetic or isoinertial) lumbar extension strength testing.

Muscle Strains

Injury to the muscles of the lumbar spine can be caused by sudden, violent contraction (e.g., attempting to lift a heavy object), rapid stretching, combined lumbar extension and rotation (torque), eccentric loading, and repetitive overuse resulting in microscopic damage to the muscle. Although some authorities[12] point out that most low back–related dysfunction results from soft-tissue injury, many other structures are involved with back pain (ligaments, disk, nerve tissue, and bone) and many other causes of nonspecific lumbar spine dysfunction are possible. The function of the lumbar spine muscles contributes to dynamic stability.[29] Panjabi and co-workers have identified the need for specific low back strengthening to reduce injury and "to stabilize the spine within its normal physiologic motions."[29]

Muscle strains of the lumbar spine are common and treatment goals are as follows:[37] Reduce or eliminate inflammation (pain and swelling), restore muscle strength, restore flexibility, enhance aerobic fitness (weight management), restore function, and protect the affected area from further injury through education and supervised practice of proper lifting mechanics.

In general, the initial care of muscle strains focuses on the control of pain and swelling. In addition to any physician-prescribed medications (nonsteroidal antiinflammatory drugs [NSAIDs], analgesics, and muscle relaxants), the PT can employ a wide range of agents to reduce pain and swelling. Therapeutic heat, cold (cryotherapy), electrical stimulation, pharmacophoresis (iontophoresis and phonophoresis), and massage are common agents used to control symptoms of inflammation after soft-tissue injury.[31] The affected area also must be protected from unwanted stresses. Through a detailed and comprehensive evaluation, the PT identi-

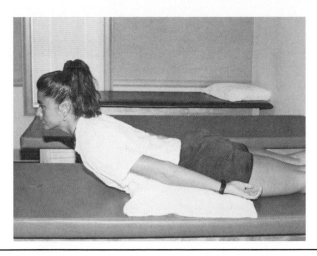

Fig. 21-7 Prone lumbar and thoracic extension with arms at the sides.

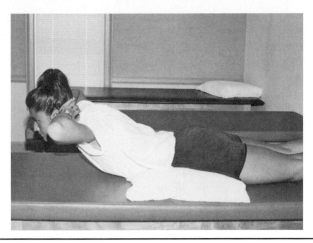

Fig. 21-8 Lumbar and thoracic extension with hands behind the head. In this position the lever arm is extended, requiring greater strength of the lumbar paravertebral muscles and scapular adductors to lift the trunk.

fies the most comfortable resting position for the patient and attempts to place the affected muscles in this shortened position.

Submaximal isometric exercises generally are well tolerated once the acute phase of healing has ended. The PTA may instruct the patient to perform gluteal sets (possibly while pain control modalities are applied), quadriceps sets, hamstring sets, and abdominal sets. The quality (intensity) of the muscle contraction is increased as the patient develops tolerance. The use of gentle lumbar stretching exercises must be approached cautiously. Although improved low back flexibility may be indicated after muscle strains, if stretching is attempted too soon, initial healing and scarring of the muscle may be delayed. Gentle low back stretching usually can proceed once the patient can tolerate increased intensity isometric exercises. With the patient supine, single knee-to-chest and double knee-to-chest motions can be performed. Pelvic tilt exercises are considered appropriate early motion, stretching (lower back), and strengthening (isometric abdominal set with simultaneous gluteal set) exercises.

Prone extension exercises are added once the patient can perform pain-free isometric and flexibility exercises, and after the acute phase has been achieved. The progression of prone extension exercises can be viewed in three phases or positions. Prone lumbar extension necessarily involves thoracic extension and scapular retraction. By strengthening the lumbar extensors (thoracic and scapular muscles as well) with prone active extension exercises, functional strength is restored to the affected muscle groups.

The first position of prone lumbar extension requires the patient to be prone with the arms resting at the sides of the body. The head and neck must be maintained in a midline position to reduce the risk of torquing the cervical spine. In addition, some therapists advocate the

use of an abdominal bolster or support when the patient is in a prone position. This issue depends largely on the specific nature of the injury, the comfort of the patient, and the wishes of the PT. An abdominal bolster is used in this chapter's figures. Lumbar extension exercises in the first position (with arms at the sides) involve limited pain-free extension with an emphasis on slow, controlled motion, both concentrically and eccentrically (Fig. 21-7). Greater motion is allowed as the patient's condition improves.

The second position increases the intensity of effort for the back extensors. While the patient is prone, his or her hands are placed palm open on the back of the head. The patient must not push the hands hard on the back of the head, but rather let the open hands gently rest on the head. Again, the back is extended while pulling the scapulae together (retraction). Nonballistic, controlled concentric and eccentric motions are encouraged (Fig. 21-8).

The third position involves even greater intensity than the second. The patient extends both arms overhead (elbows straight) while extending the trunk in a prone position (Fig. 21-9).

Although this series of prone extension exercises is employed safely to strengthen lumbar and thoracic extension, other, more demanding exercises can be used judiciously if the patient is an active athlete. For example, prone bilateral leg lifts can be incorporated at the discretion of the PT to further strengthen the low back, gluteals, and hamstrings. Initially, the patient is prone with the arms and trunk stabilized. First, he or she performs a single-leg lift, alternating between legs. Then the patient performs bilateral elevation of the legs throughout a pain-free range of motion (ROM). Finally, the legs are lifted from a flexed knee position up to a neutral position.

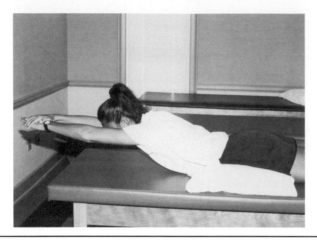

Fig. 21-9 Prone lumbar and thoracic extension in the arms-extended position.

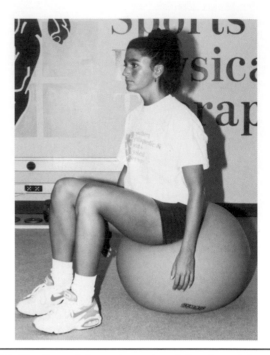

Fig. 21-10 Seated dynamic trunk stabilization while seated on a physioball.

A strong word of caution: Other symptoms may develop during the treatment of muscle strains. For example, if a patient complains of radicular pain into one or both lower extremities during or after the performance of any trunk flexion exercise (recall that trunk flexion produces posterior movement of the nucleus that can involve nerve root irritation), the exercise must be terminated and the PT notified.

Generally, local muscle soreness[11] and postexercise stiffness are anticipated consequences, and the patient must be reassured that these are normal. However, burning, numbness, tingling, and radiating pain are not normal responses and must be recognized early.

A general conditioning program should be encouraged as soon as possible after the acute phase of muscle strain has passed. Addressing functional gait mechanics early in the recovery phase, by advocating walking as both exercise and treatment, is highly effective.[10] As articulated by Edgelow,[10] walking has a rather broad impact on recovery from low back dysfunction. Walking:

■ Stimulates circulation
■ Enhances cardiovascular and cardiorespiratory fitness
■ Stimulates the mechanoreceptor system
■ Improves the coordination and strength of the muscles needed to control the movement of the mobile segment

All this is accomplished through the reciprocal contraction and relaxation of muscles engaged in walking.[10] Walking can be initiated on a treadmill to control cadence, stride length, and speed of gait. Usually patients can adapt more easily to a treadmill because the hand rails provide added support and comfort when beginning a walking program. Also, although stationary bicycle ergometers can be used as a form of aerobic fitness after acute lumbar muscle strain, a standard saddle seat may be uncomfortable for many patients. A semirecumbent cycle with a large bucket seat, where a lumbar extension roll can be used, generally is well tolerated.

The general conditioning program also must focus attention on abdominal muscle support during dynamic functional activities. Abdominal isometrics can be encouraged along with partial direct and oblique sit-ups. With all abdominal exercises after low back muscle strain, emphasis must be placed on limited flexion during the performance of the partial sit-ups. Limited ROM trunk flexion during sit-ups (with knees flexed) is effective and minimizes excessive flexion of the trunk, which can aggravate an underlying disk condition.

Throughout the course of recovery from lumbar muscle strain, patients must be directed to perform functional, dynamic back strengthening and abdominal exercises to protect the low back during ADLs. Dynamic back strengthening exercises can be viewed as end-stage or functional recovery exercises initiated once the patient can demonstrate improved static or isometric strength, increased walking without complaints of pain, improved lumbar motion, increased lumbar extension strength (through the three positions of prone lumbar and thoracic extension exercises), and improved awareness and demonstration of appropriate, safe lifting mechanics to protect the spine.

Watkins and Dillon[37] strongly advocate trunk strengthening and dynamic support exercises in the treatment and prevention of muscle strains of the lumbar spine. The concept of isometrically holding a neutral lumbar spine position during all functional activities is the cornerstone for recovery from and prevention of low back muscle strains. Watkins and Dillon[37] report: "The key to safe strengthening is the ability to maintain the

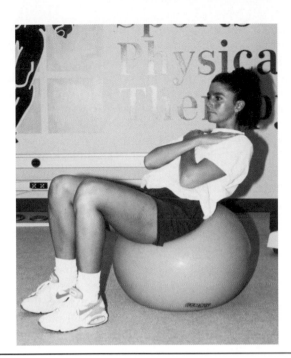

Fig. 21-11 Seated partial direct sit-ups on a physioball. This is a challenging exercise to maintain balance while performing dynamic exercise.

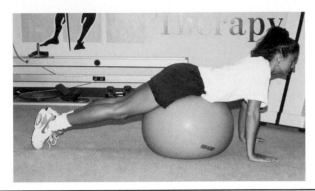

Fig. 21-12 Lying prone across a physioball with foot and arm support.

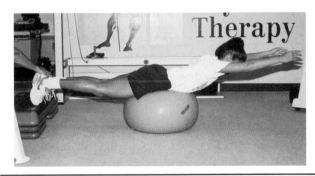

Fig. 21-13 Progressively more challenging dynamic prone extension on the physioball. The patient attempts to maintain balance while elevating one arm then both arms as the clinician provides support at the feet.

spine in a safe, neutral position during the strengthening exercises." In addition, "Trunk strength also prevents back injuries and is an important treatment method for back pain." Therefore dynamic functional strengthening of the lumbar spine after muscle strain focuses on isometric cocontractions of the abdominals, erector spinae, and gluteals, as well as challenging the lumbar and abdominal muscles to contract synergistically during functional exercises.[32]

A physioball is an extremely effective and efficient tool to use in developing dynamic lumbar and abdominal strength. A physioball is a large (3 to 4 feet in diameter) sturdy rubber ball that is safe to sit on. Dynamic strengthening using the physioball can proceed in sequential fashion progressing from a seated position to the prone and supine extension positions. Seated trunk stabilization is initiated by simply sitting on the ball while maintaining correct back extension posture and equilibrium (Fig. 21-10). The patient can be effectively challenged to maintain support by gently rolling the ball slightly from side to side, front to back, and diagonally. The patient's abdominal and back extensor muscles must quickly contract to stabilize the spine and maintain proper balance. As the patient demonstrates improved trunk control, partial sit-ups while seated on the physioball can be added for most patients (Fig. 21-11). This progression effectively challenges the patient to maintain support during dynamic muscle activity. Prone extension exercises can begin once the patient demonstrates good balance, trunk control, and strength in the

seated position. The patient maintains trunk support and balance in a neutral position while lying prone across the ball (Fig. 21-12). Initially the patient perhaps should use hand support. Gradually as control improves, the hands are lifted while the PTA supports the legs (Fig. 21-13).

Ligament Sprains

The spinal ligaments[41] (anterior longitudinal ligament, posterior longitudinal ligament, interspinous ligament, ligamentum flavum, and supraspinous ligament) can be injured by a sudden violent force or from repeated stress. The PT conducts a comprehensive evaluation of the patient to confirm or deny the presence of segmental instability (hypermobility resulting from ligament sprain) and evaluate the degree of pain with or without active or passive movement of the lumbar spine in general or in individual segments.[1,2] In addition to isolated ligament sprains, muscle strains can be superimposed, making the identification of specific single-ligament sprains exceedingly difficult.

The management of lumbar ligament sprains essentially parallels the care of muscle strains. In general terms, recovery from muscle strains, ligamentous sprains, and various degrees of disk herniations can be divided into four phases.[5] In each phase, the cornerstone of care is patient education and pain-free appropriate lifting, posture, sitting, standing, and bending body mechanics.

Phase I focuses on healing and pain control. During this phase, rest, restricted activity, pain medications, physical agents to control swelling and pain (i.e., ultrasound, ice packs, moist heat, electrical stimulation, massage), and patient education principles about body mechanics are introduced.

Phase II of recovery is characterized by the initiation of mobilization involving early active and passive motion. Therefore attention is centered on increasing the patient's activity level without undue complaints of pain, initiating motion and flexibility exercises (defined by Chappuis, Johnson, and Gines[5] as "nondestructive movement") consistent with and conducive to tissue healing, performing specific muscle-strengthening exercises (isometrics, **spine stabilization,** neutral spine strengthening, lumbar extension strengthening, and abdominal strengthening), and continuing education and reinforcement of body mechanics information.

Phase III focuses on the prevention of reinjury. A total body-conditioning program is encouraged that emphasizes overall strength, flexibility, aerobic fitness (weight management, body composition, and endurance), proprioception exercises, and advanced, more challenging neutral spine stabilization exercises.

The return to normalized activity is characteristic of phase IV. During this phase, the patient is gradually introduced to work site activities, ADLs, and sports activities, with particular attention paid to movements, loads, positions, and frequency of activity.[5]

The four-phase recovery program just outlined is offered only as a general guide and is not intended to describe a comprehensive rehabilitation plan for all spinal dysfunction. Each patient has specific, identified needs and goals that must be addressed individually through the initial evaluation performed by the PT.

Immediate attention is directed at alleviating pain and inflammation with the use of physician-prescribed NSAIDs, oral analgesics, muscle relaxants, and various agents (i.e., heat, ice, electrical stimuli, ultrasound, massage). Protection of the affected area must coincide with pain-relieving physical agents. The PTA, under the direction of the PT, must identify which specific positions are contraindicated by carefully reviewing the initial evaluation data. Both the short- and the long-range goals for recovery from lumbar strains and sprains emphasize protecting the spine from unwanted forces and positions. As with other ligament sprains, those positions that stretch the affected ligaments must be avoided. Therefore neutral spine stabilization (maintenance of pain-free posture with a normal lordotic curve during exercise) is particularly important during all phases of recovery from ligament sprains. Once the pain-free position is identified, the course of recovery focuses on isometrically strengthening the abdominals, gluteals, and lumbar extensors throughout functional activities. This does not mean that specific lumbar extension strengthening exercises (three-position prone extension) should be strictly avoided. On the contrary, these exercises, if well tolerated after the acute stage of healing, should be introduced to specifically isolate the lumbar and thoracic extension muscles. In many cases, trunk flexion stretches the affected ligaments, so flexion should be minimized.

The abdominal muscles can be conditioned effectively with isometric sets while the lordotic curve is maintained. Paris[30] identifies sitting as a characteristically uncomfortable position for many patients suffering from lumbar sprains. The sitting posture may be enhanced and the flexed lumbar posture while seated minimized using a lumbar extension roll placed in the small of the back. While maintaining a pain-free neutral spine, the patient is encouraged to walk; perform isotonic strengthening exercises that do not compromise lumbar flexion, rotation, torque, or vertical compressive loads; and do flexibility exercises, carefully avoiding all unwanted lumbar spine motions. Muscle and ligament tissues heal and repair at different rates; whereas some mild muscle strains heal quickly, a prolonged period may be necessary with ligament injuries. To avoid further injury, the patient must be educated thoroughly about lifting mechanics that do not reproduce pain, protective sitting postures, and maintenance of a general conditioning program to increase strength, flexibility, and endurance while maintaining a neutral, pain-free lumbar spine.

Injuries to the Lumbar Intervertebral Disk

The PTA is strongly encouraged to thoroughly review the anatomic relationships among the lumbar vertebral bodies, disk, spinal canal, and nerve roots. DeRosa and Porterfield[7] state, "The intervertebral disk is the largest avascular structure in the human body." Without an intense vascular response to injury, the disk has a limited capacity to heal and repair. The vascular supply to the disk is provided by diffusion from the vertebral bodies above and below the disk.[7,14,25,30] Neurologic innervation is reserved for the outer fibers of the annulus,[14] whereas the remainder of the disk is aneural. Also, the disk itself is wedge shaped, with a thick anterior portion and a thin posterior portion.[7] Understanding this relationship helps in understanding specific disk injuries and choosing the best therapeutic maneuvers.

Various terms are used to describe injuries to the disk. Although "slipped disk" is a common expression used to describe various ailments of the low back among the general population, a disk does not "slip" from within

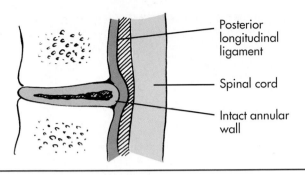

Fig. 21-14   Disk protrusion. The nucleus bulges against an intact annulus.

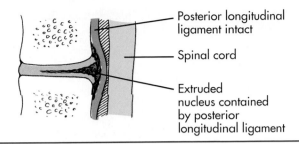

Fig. 21-15   Extruded disk. The nucleus extends through the annulus; however, the nuclear material remains confined by the posterior longitudinal ligament.

its confines between the vertebral bodies. The generally accepted term, **herniated nucleus pulposus (HNP),** is broad and should be clarified by specific nomenclature to more precisely describe the injury. Miller[27] describes the three categories of HNP as protrusion, extruded, and sequestrated. In a **disk protrusion,** the nucleus bulges against an intact annulus (Fig. 21-14). An **extruded disk** is characterized by the nucleus extending through the annulus, but the nuclear material remains confined by the posterior longitudinal ligament (Fig. 21-15). Finally, in a **sequestrated disk,** the nucleus is free within the canal (Fig. 21-16).

Macnab[24] offers a variation of this classification model:

Disk protrusion:

Type I: Peripheral annular bulge

Type II: Localized annular bulge

Disk herniation:

Type I: Prolapsed intervertebral disk

Type II: Extruded intervertebral disk

Type III: Sequestrated intervertebral disk

Thus in a disk protrusion the annular fibers are intact, although the annulus bulges. A prolapsed disk has the nucleus contained only by the outer fibers of the bulging annulus.

Regardless of the exact nature of the injury, HNP remains primarily a disease of young to middle-aged adults.[27] Age-related changes include decreased hydration, with a decreased water content from 70% to 88% by the third decade; biochemical changes in the glycosaminoglycans of the nucleus; and increases in collagen. These changes make disk herniations rare in elderly people.[27,30] Burkus[3] has identified five separate categories of low back pain that clarify the complex and interrelated nature of various organs and systems affecting it. The five categories are defined as follows:

1. *Viscerogenic pain:* Pain that originates from the kidneys, pelvisacral lesions, and retroperitoneal tumors. "This type of pain is neither aggravated by activity nor relieved by rest. This differentiates it from back pain which is a result of spinal disorders."[3]

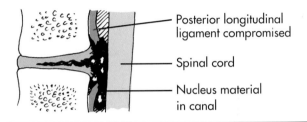

Fig. 21-16   Sequestrated disk. The nucleus is free within the spinal canal.

2. *Neurogenic pain:* Pain commonly caused by neurofibromas, cysts, and tumors of the nerve roots in the lumbar spine.

3. *Vascular pain:* Pain characterized by intermittent claudication from aneurysms and peripheral vascular disease.

4. *Psychogenic pain:* Pain that is uncommon and ascribed to inorganic causes. The physician must completely rule out all organic factors before considering psychogenic pain as the primary cause of low back dysfunction.

5. *Spondylogenic pain:* Pain directly related to the pain originating from soft tissues of the spine and sacroiliac joint. This type of pain is classically characterized as aggravated by activity and relieved by rest.

Although there are many causes of low back pain, the PTA directs attention at spondylogenic pain as it relates to the orthopedic conditions outlined in this chapter. However, other causes of back pain always must be considered and a high degree of suspicion maintained for all low back pain patients who do not demonstrate consistent objective changes after therapeutic interventions. For the PTA, pain originating from any classification model of a herniated disk is defined as spondylogenic pain.

The criteria-based rehabilitation program used to treat HNP is directly and profoundly related to the precise data gained during the initial physical therapy assessment. Not all herniated discs are treated in the

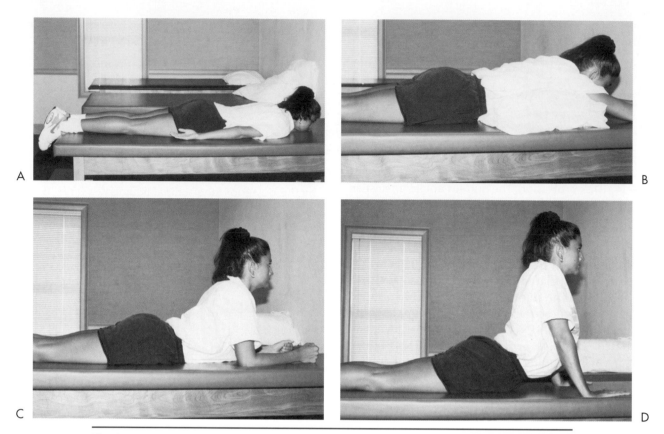

Fig. 21-17 Passive prone extension sequence. **A,** Patient lying prone without pillow for support. **B,** Patient prone with pillow under the chest for mild thoracic and lumbar extension. **C,** Patient propped up on elbows for improved extension. **D,** Prone, elbows extended for maximum extension.

same manner. Depending on the extent of the herniation, the patient may demonstrate **radicular signs,** such as pain radiating into the buttocks or legs (sciatica), posterior thigh pain, and paresthesias (numbness or tingling radiating distally below the knee as a result of nerve root impingement).

When evaluating radicular signs during the initial evaluation process, the PT confirms or denies the presence of **peripheralization** or **centralization** phenomena.[22,25] These conditions identified during the initial evaluation are defined by Kisner and Colby[22] as follows: "When repeating the forward-bending test, the symptoms increase or peripheralize. Peripheralization means the symptoms are experienced further down the leg." Centralization is defined by McKenzie[25] as, "the phenomenon whereby, as a result of the performance of certain repeated movements or the adoption of certain positions, radiating pain originating from the spine and referred distally, is made to move away from the periphery and toward the mid-line of the spine." The motion of the nucleus during lumbar spine flexion (nucleus moves posteriorly) and extension (nucleus moves anteriorly) must be abundantly clear because of three important exceptions to the centralization and peripheralization phenomenon identified by Kisner and Colby,[22] as follows:

1. If there is a lateral shift of the spinal column, backward bending increases the pain. Note that with posterolateral disk herniations and nerve root impingement, the patient may list or shift away from the painful side in an attempt to reduce pain by decreasing impingement. If the lateral shift is first corrected, then repeated backward bending lessens or centralizes the pain.
2. If the protrusion cannot be mechanically reduced, backward bending peripheralizes or increases the symptoms.
3. If there is an anterior protrusion, backward bending increases the pain and forward bending relieves the pain.

Therefore the evaluation data obtained by the PT from the patient are essential to determining treatment.

The keys to managing HNP involve the following four basic objectives:[7]

1. Reduce pain via physician-prescribed analgesics and a combination of thermal or electrical modalities.
2. Protect the affected area from unwanted stress and forces (determined from the initial evaluation) while encouraging and promoting movement.

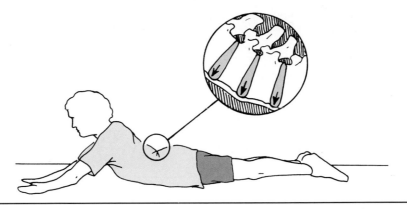

Fig. 21-18 Passive prone extension. The nucleus moves in an anterior direction.

3. Increase muscle strength, endurance, and flexibility.
4. Counsel the patient concerning correct body mechanics.

Chappuis, Johnson, and Gines[5] elaborate on these goals by specifically identifying nine essential steps:

1. Reduce pain.
2. Increase flexibility.
3. Increase strength.
4. Educate.
5. Increase cardiovascular fitness.
6. Decrease stress.
7. Improve posture.
8. Improve body mechanics.
9. Improve the sense of personal responsibility.

In addition, the nine components of a comprehensive nonsurgical rehabilitation regimen are as follows:[5]

1. Restrictions: Identify specific limitations that preclude involvement in all areas of recovery.
2. Education: Anatomy and body mechanics
3. Symptomatic treatment: Thermal or electrical agents, medications, and posture
4. Posture adjustment: Body mechanics
5. Flexibility
6. Cardiovascular training
7. Balance training
8. Strengthening
9. Ergonomics instruction: Work site evaluation, ADLs, and sports activities.

The PT determines if lumbar flexion or extension should be encouraged during recovery from HNP. Initial management generally can proceed with the patient prone on a mat or table while applying thermal or electrical agents. If the PT has determined that lumbar extension reduces radicular symptoms (centralization), initially a small pillow can be placed under the patient's chest to achieve a small, pain-free degree of passive lumbar extension. McKenzie[25] advocates that after the patient has rested a short while in this position, he or she should be encouraged to prop up on the elbows to further enhance the lordotic curve (Fig. 21-17). The PT attempts to reduce or relocate the herniated nucleus to a more anterior location and away from the impingement (Fig. 21-18). From this intermediate position, the patient now performs press-ups, which further enhance lumbar extension. Press-ups can be modified to be performed repeatedly (slow, continuous, reciprocal up-and-down motions) or held statically (maintained in a pain-free extended position) for short periods of time.

In many cases of true disk herniation with radicular signs, passive and active extension effectively relieves symptoms and provides a mechanical foundation for healing. The nucleus is reduced to a more anterior location and away from the impingement. However, for long-term care the patient must be counseled concerning proper lifting mechanics and sitting postures (using a lumbar extension roll while seated to maintain an appropriate anatomic lordotic curve) and to avoid positions that contribute to lumbar spine flexion and posterior translation of the nucleus. Occupational risks (lifting and prolonged sitting), as well as all ADLs, must be modified to enhance appropriate mechanics and minimize the potential for repeated stress to the disk.

The physician or PT may prescribe pelvic or lumbar traction to stretch muscles, enhance vertebral segment separation, reduce nerve root impingement, and decrease pain.[22] The clinical application of mechanical lumbar-pelvic traction is beyond the scope and intent of this text.

In addition to the use of passive extension procedures to relocate a posterior bulge of the disk, active prone extension exercises can be employed (three-position thoracic and lumbar active extension) once the acute phase has resolved as documented by centralization of radicular signs and control of pain. Some patients may be unable to perform various prone position exercises; standing back extension with hand support or the use of a supine back extension apparatus may prove more comfortable. During the early recovery phase, more challenging and functional exercises that also enhance normal lordotic posture while strengthening the posterior lumbar muscles should be added gradually.

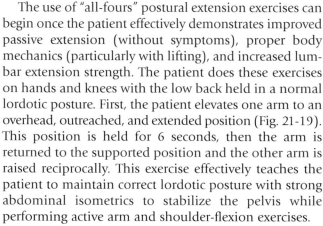

Fig. 21-19 All-fours postural extension. One arm elevated and extended while the patient maintains proper lordotic posture.

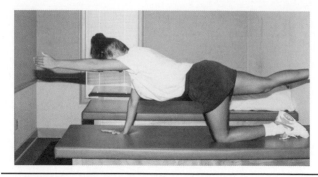

Fig. 21-20 All-fours postural extension. With one arm elevated and extended, the patient is instructed to extend the contralateral lower limb.

The use of "all-fours" postural extension exercises can begin once the patient effectively demonstrates improved passive extension (without symptoms), proper body mechanics (particularly with lifting), and increased lumbar extension strength. The patient does these exercises on hands and knees with the low back held in a normal lordotic posture. First, the patient elevates one arm to an overhead, outreached, and extended position (Fig. 21-19). This position is held for 6 seconds, then the arm is returned to the supported position and the other arm is raised reciprocally. This exercise effectively teaches the patient to maintain correct lordotic posture with strong abdominal isometrics to stabilize the pelvis while performing active arm and shoulder-flexion exercises.

The next progression on all fours requires the patient to elevate one arm while extending the contralateral lower limb (Fig. 21-20). Correct lumbar extension posture must be maintained. This exercise is intended to encourage shoulder flexion, lumbar extension, and hip extension (gluteals and hamstrings) while maintaining proper balance and posture on all fours.

Once the patient is comfortably demonstrating improved posture and control of pain, a general fitness program can begin. The goal in exercising is to improve overall body strength, aerobic fitness, and flexibility without compromising lumbar spine flexion.

Conservative management of HNP involves the introduction and continuous reinforcement of proper body mechanics (lifting, sitting, and sleeping) to control unwanted forces and stresses that are not conducive to long-term healing. The PTA educates patients as to the virtues of physical conditioning (with the use of protective postures) and the daily application of safe lifting principles to protect the spine from further injury.

Invasive Management of Lumbar Disk Herniation

When conservative physical therapy (including rest, medications, exercise, and postural counseling) fails to bring significant relief from symptoms, the physician may offer several invasive procedures designed to relieve pain and remove its cause, which is presumed to be the disk.

For some patients whose persistent radicular pain (sciatica) cannot be controlled by conservative measures, the physician may prescribe an epidural steroid injection to relieve pain.[11,27] These injections are given only to relieve pain and reduce inflammation, and are not intended as a curative procedure to correct any neurologic deficits.

When surgery is necessary to correct a herniated disk, the physician determines the exact nature of the herniation (protruded, extruded, or sequestrated) and selects the appropriate surgical procedure. As described by Miller[27] and Eismont and Kitchel,[11] the most common procedure is a laminotomy with a decompression diskectomy. In this procedure the physician gains exposure to the herniated disk by cutting into the lamina and then removing all nonviable disk material, thereby decompressing the affected nerve root (Fig. 21-21). Miller[27] reports that 95% of patients demonstrate good or excellent results with this particular surgical procedure. However, as many as 30% of these patients may have significant back pain at long-term follow-up.[8,27] Other procedures, such as microsurgical diskectomy and automated percutaneous diskectomy, also remove the cause of the nerve root impingement (disk).

Rehabilitation after any surgical procedure is highly patient-specific and directly related to the data obtained at the initial postoperative physical therapy evaluation. Generally, recovery closely parallels the criteria established with conservative management of a herniated disk. However, extensive surgical exposure is necessary to perform a laminotomy with diskectomy, and tissue-healing constraints influence recovery.

After surgery, the patient is taught bed mobility and transfer training using the log-roll technique to move from a supine to sitting position. Ambulation with a walker or crutches is allowed 1 day after surgery. Ambulation distance and endurance activities are increased according to each patient's ability. Rudimentary bed

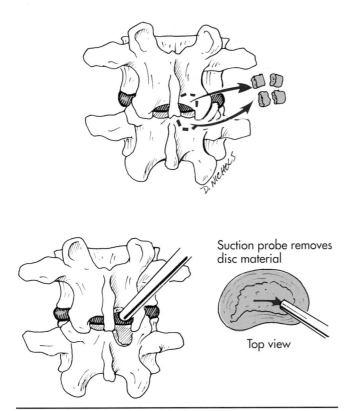

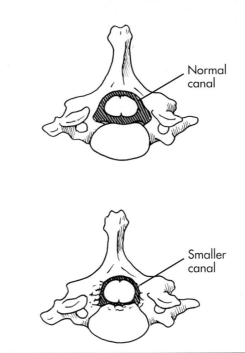

Fig. 21-22 Lumbar spinal stenosis. Narrow diameter of the spinal canal can lead to constriction and compression of nerve roots.

Fig. 21-21 Laminotomy with decompression diskectomy.

exercises can be performed the day after surgery and include active ankle pumps, gentle hip and knee flexion, and isometric exercises (quadriceps and gluteals). The PT guides the PTA concerning whether or not the postoperative patient will perform any isometric exercises. The PTA must instruct the patient in and reinforce proper breathing techniques if isometric exercises are done. The Valsalva maneuver is strictly avoided during all exercises.

For the first 3 days after surgery the patient is limited to sitting for no more than 1 hour at a time and must maintain proper spinal position with no flexion.[5] The PTA continually reinforces and encourages proper posture during the first week of recovery. The patient should be cautioned to avoid forward bending and trunk rotation.

More demanding and functionally relevant activities that do not stress the surgical site are added gradually. Transfers from supine to sitting and from sitting to standing must be demonstrated by the patient and observed by the clinician to be safe, efficient, and free from all unwanted stress. Throughout the first week, exercises can progress to include partial squats, which focus on functional closed-chain strengthening while maintaining proper neutral spine stabilization throughout the squat.

When initial wound healing is complete and pain is decreased, a more accelerated program of strengthening can begin. Extension is encouraged gradually, progress-

ing to active lumbar and thoracic extension strengthening while avoiding lumbar flexion. ROM exercises for the spine are encouraged as soon as the patient can tolerate these motions. Gentle active extension exercises and pelvic tilts (which promote pelvic motion, control, as well as limited-motion lumbar spine flexion and extension) begin early in the recovery phase.

The patient must achieve increased motion, controlled pain, improved endurance, and sufficient strength before beginning a general conditioning program after surgery. The longer recovery period is needed to allow for proper soft-tissue healing, bone healing, and control of inflammation and pain before subjecting the affected area to stress. From 3 to 5 weeks after surgery, the goals of recovery are identified as restored lumbar motion, normalized upper and lower extremity strength, improved aerobic fitness, and decreased pain and swelling.[5] Progressive functional exercises can be added as the patient achieves these criteria. These include treadmill walking, balance activities, isotonic strengthening exercises, general flexibility exercises, and cardiovascular conditioning (via upper body ergometer, recumbent cycle ergometer, treadmill, stair-stepper, and cross-country ski machine).

Spinal Stenosis

Lumbar spinal stenosis is defined as a narrowing of the spinal canal, which constricts and compresses nerve roots (Fig. 21-22).[27] This gives rise to symptoms of neurogenic or spinal claudication, as follows:

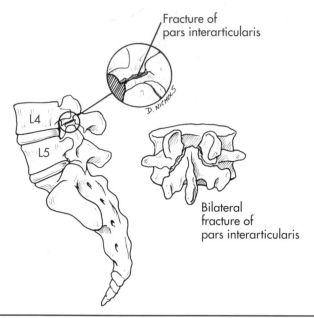

Fracture of
pars interarticularis

L4

L5

Bilateral
fracture of
pars interarticularis

Fig. 21-23 Spondylolysis. Fracture of pars interarticularis of the posterior elements of the spine.

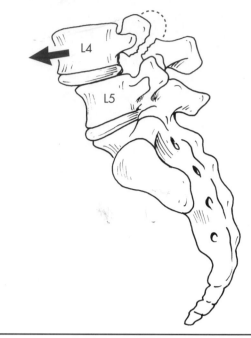

L4

L5

Fig. 21-24 Spondylolisthesis. The resultant forward slippage of a superior vertebra over an inferior vertebra.

1. Radicular ache into the thigh and less frequently into the calf[3]
2. Paresthesias into the lower extremity[13]
3. Disturbances in motor function[13]

This condition occurs in men "twice as often as females"[27] and typically is observed during late middle age and older.[13,27]

Lumbar **spinal stenosis** is most commonly acquired as a result of degenerative arthritic changes that encroach on the diameter of the canal, producing nerve root compression.[27] The patient with stenosis frequently complains of pain and increased symptoms with lumbar extension. Extension of the lumbar spine in a patient with stenosis further compresses the spinal canal, thereby increasing pain and paresthesias.[7,13,27]

During ambulation and gait training, an elderly patient typically demonstrates a forward-flexed trunk posture when using a walker. Under careful observation and questioning, the patient may suggest that leaning forward feels better and reduces back and leg pain. Unless this position is recognized as being appropriate for relieving pain in patients with stenosis, the clinician may encourage a less appropriate, erect extended trunk posture that may exacerbate the pain.

Management of spinal stenosis focuses on flexion exercises (Williams's flexion exercises, including pelvic tilts, knee-to-chest exercises, and partial direct and oblique sit-ups) and avoiding lumbar extension. The PTA also educates the patient and reinforces appropriate posture (flexed, in this case), body mechanics, lifting techniques, and sitting and sleeping changes, as well as a general physical conditioning program and a weight management program, which Miller[27]

identifies as an important adjunct in the care of spinal stenosis.

Spondylolysis and Spondylolisthesis

Spondylolysis is a bony defect (stress fracture or fracture) in the pars interarticularis of the posterior elements of the spine (Fig. 21-23).[3,4,7,11,27,30,37] **Spondylolisthesis,** on the other hand, describes a forward slippage of one superior vertebra over an inferior vertebra (usually L4-L5 and L5-S1)[8,11] as a result of instability caused by the bilateral defect in the pars interarticularis (Fig. 21-24).[3,4,7,11,27,30,37] There are specific classification types, as well as degrees of slippage or "migration" of the vertebrae in the disease process of spondylolisthesis.[11] Five types, or classifications, have been identified, as follows:[3,11,27]

Type I: Congenital or dysplastic. Results from a "congenital malformation of the sacrum or neural arch of L5, which allows forward slippage of L5 on the sacrum."[3] Most common in children.

Type II: Isthmic spondylolisthesis. The most common type, affecting persons 5 to 50 years of age.[27] Usually a result of mechanical stress that causes a stress fracture at the pars interarticularis.[11,27]

Type III: Degenerative spondylolisthesis. Most commonly affects the older population. Characterized by a loss of ligament integrity (or stability) that results in forward slippage of the vertebrae. Generally associated with the normal aging process.[3]

Type IV: Traumatic spondylolisthesis. Caused by trauma that produces an acute fracture of the pars interarticularis. Casting is the most appropriate form of treatment.[3] Because of their generally high levels of physical activity, this type usually affects young patients.[27]

Type V: Pathologic spondylolisthesis. Characterized by bone tumors that affect the pars interarticularis.

The degree or grade of slippage is determined radiographically by the examining physician and is defined as the amount of forward displacement of the superior vertebrae over the inferior vertebrae, as outlined in the following:[3,7,27]

Grade I: 0 to 25%
Grade II: 25% to 50%
Grade III: 50% to 75%
Grade IV: 75% to 100%

The cause of the defect in the pars interarticularis is in part a congenital weakness in this area. In addition, the pars interarticularis is subjected to high levels of mechanical stress.[38,39] Authorities also suggest that the primary initial cause of the most common type of spondylolisthesis (isthmic) is fatigue fracture of the pars interarticularis.[39]

Patients primarily report pain with extremes of lumbar motion, especially extension. The pain generally follows the belt line.[19] During examination, the PT also may identify a palpable step-off between the affected lumbar vertebrae (usually L4-L5) because of the forward slippage.[7]

The management of spondylolisthesis is dictated by symptoms, as well as the degree of vertebral slippage (grades I to IV). For example, an adult with isthmic spondylolisthesis of radiographically determined grade I (0 to 25% slippage) may not experience significant symptoms with activity or extremes of lumbar extension. Thus treatment is aimed at preventing any progression to grade II (25% to 50% slippage). This usually is accomplished by instructing the patient to avoid ballistic lumbar extension, as well as vertical loading while seated or standing, so as to minimize anteriorly directed shearing forces on the spine. In addition, abdominal strengthening exercises, neutral spine stabilization exercises (controlled lumbar extension strengthening, isometrics, and rectus and oblique abdominal strengthening while in the neutral spine position), and stretching exercises for the trunk and lower extremities are encouraged.

The patient may require more specific attention when there is a greater degree of slippage with significant symptoms. Generally, pain and muscle spasm are addressed with physician-prescribed analgesics, muscle relaxants, NSAIDs, and agents (heat, ice, ultrasound, and electrical stimulation) to alleviate acute pain and swelling. If the pain is related to a fatigue fracture of the pars interarticularis, initial treatment focuses on managing stress to the fracture site using a lumbosacral corset or orthosis positioned to create a slight amount of lumbar flexion, which reduces anterior shearing forces through the fracture site and allows for bone healing.[11,19]

The cornerstone in the care of spondylolisthesis is avoidance of extreme lumbar extension and application of abdominal muscle strengthening exercises to provide dynamic support for the spine during activity. A young athletic patient must modify activities that directly influence the course of this disease. For example, weight lifting contributes significantly to the occurrence of spondylolysis.[9] The young athlete must modify or avoid dynamic overhead lifting, which contributes to vertical compressive loads and anterior shearing forces of the lumbar spine, and he or she must critically examine other weight lifting activities.

Surgery is rare and usually is reserved for patients with radicular symptoms and high-grade slippage (grades III or IV), which compresses the nerve roots and causes neurologic signs.[3,27] The type of surgery advocated in these cases is a decompression laminectomy (to reduce compression of the nerve roots) with fusion to stabilize the vertebral segments.[3,27]

Rehabilitation after surgery for spondylolisthesis is deferred until solid bony union is determined radiographically. The patient is usually in a lumbosacral orthosis that does not permit lumbar extension. During immobilization, the patient can ambulate as tolerated and perform rudimentary ROM and strengthening exercises for the upper and lower extremities (ankle pumps, quadriceps sets, and knee ROM). Once bone healing is confirmed, a gradually progressive program of abdominal strengthening (from isometrics to concentric and eccentric abdominal contractions), lumbar ROM (avoiding dynamic, ballistic, and extreme lumbar extension), general conditioning, and a progressive return to function is advocated.[3,27]

Lumbar Spine Fractures

Fractures of the lumbar vertebrae generally occur after a profound traumatic event and can be classified according to the forces that produce the fracture. For example, compression, flexion, extension, flexion-distraction, flexion-rotation, and lateral flexion are forces that produce fractures.[27] Lumbar spine fractures also can be described in terms that graphically depict a specific fracture deformity, including crush, wedge, burst, shear, slice, and teardrop fractures.[27]

Perhaps the most clinically relevant spine fracture for the PTA to consider is the vertebral compression fracture. These fractures occur at a rate of approximately 530,000 annually,[17] with many lower thoracic and high-level lumbar fractures caused by osteoporosis.[7,13,23] Many benign activities can produce compression fractures in an elderly population of patients with osteoporosis.[3,23] Care must be taken to ensure that no rapid deceleration occurs when an elderly patient transfers to a bedside commode or any other hard surface. This seemingly trivial activity frequently causes multilevel compression fractures in patients with osteoporosis.

Compression fractures produce symptoms ranging from acute local pain to essentially no signs at all.[23] Thus subtle complaints of pain caused by typical daily activities, such as bending, lifting, or rising from a chair, must be viewed with a high level of suspicion in elderly patients.[23]

Treatment of compression fractures focuses on relief of pain; authorities[13,23] advocate bed rest, physician-prescribed analgesics, NSAIDs, heat, ice, massage, and electrical stimulation to control pain, swelling, and associated muscle spasm. During the acute and subacute phases of recovery, the patient with compression fractures must avoid thoracic or lumbar flexion activities.[13] Trunk flexion is contraindicated because it creates an anterior wedging of the vertebral bodies, producing greater stress and compression at the fracture site.[13]

As the symptoms of pain and swelling subside, the patient may be allowed out of bed for a few minutes each hour.[13,23] During this time, the patient performs isometric lumbar stabilization exercises (isometric abdominal sets, gluteal sets, and scapular retraction) in a comfortable position. Extension activities also are allowed to reduce vertebral body compression and build up thoracic and lumbar extension strength. Walking short distances and sitting tolerance must be closely followed and progressed according to the individual. Endurance-type activities that do not create lumbar flexion are advocated as soon as the patient can tolerate prolonged periods of ambulation. Local muscular endurance activities help with the adaptation and preparation for ADLs that use the postural muscles.

If the patient is allowed adequate rest for healing and performs lumbar stabilization exercises while avoiding lumbar flexion, the return to function and normal activities can be expected 6 to 8 weeks after injury.[13] The identification and management of acute lumbar fractures is dictated by the physician, who must determine if the fracture is stable or unstable. The most common lumbar fracture is the compression fracture, and it is treated as described in the preceding.[26] Unstable fractures may be accompanied by neurologic involvement that necessitates open reduction and internal fixation of the unstable spine segments and possible fusion of the segments.[26] McRae has outlined the goals of treatment of unstable lumbar spine fractures as follows:[26]

■ To reduce displacement of the fracture segment
■ To prevent any recurrence of displacement that may lead to catastrophic neurologic involvement

Stability can be achieved either by allowing the unstable segments to heal spontaneously through long-term conservative care (which facilitates the healing of bone and posterior longitudinal ligaments), or open reduction and internal fixation with fusion of the unstable segments.[26] In either case, any detailed discussion of recovery after spine surgery with neurologic involvement is beyond the scope of this text. Generally, recovery time parallels the time necessary for healing of bone, muscle, and ligament. A lengthy period of convalescence

is needed with a gradual, progressive sequence of active lower-extremity ROM, isometric exercises, bed mobility, transfer training, sitting tolerance, gait training, endurance activities, upper-extremity strengthening, and a slow return to function once the spine is stable.

Prevention and Education for Back Dysfunction: The Back School Model

Although understanding and managing low back dysfunction is the focus of this section, prevention of lumbar spine injuries also is pertinent to this discussion, because the PTA is frequently directed to participate in and to carry out community-based back injury prevention programs under the supervision and direction of a PT. These education programs are commonly referred to as **"back schools"** and are designed to provide an understanding of anatomy, causes of back pain, lifting mechanics, posture, self-care for back pain, exercise, nutrition (weight management), ergonomics (which involves lifting, posture, general body mechanics, job modifications, and work site protection and redesign to minimize back injury), and stress reduction for high-risk patients and the population at large.

Often patients with a history of back pain are identified as ideal candidates to participate in these programs. Also, persons at risk (identified by job responsibilities, repetitive lifting, overweight condition, poor posture, poor body mechanics, relative weakness, and poor general physical conditioning) may be referred to these programs.

Many back schools involve a 1- or 2-hour class (consisting of lectures, slides, demonstration, and participation) each week for 4 to 6 weeks. Each session or class builds on the previous lecture to convey the principles seen in spinal anatomy, causes of back dysfunction, risk factors, posture, body mechanics, and treatment approaches.[1] Back schools can be based in outpatient physical therapy clinics, hospitals, industrial health clinics, wellness programs at work, or community fitness centers. In every case, the program is under the direction and supervision of a physician and PT.

Allman[1] has identified the outline in Box 21-1 as an appropriate general back school program.

The general back school curriculum described in Box 21-1 clarifies the rudimentary concepts of education and prevention for a wide variety of back-related problems. The PTA who presents this information must be given specific information, evaluation data, indications, and contraindications for each patient participating in the back school program. In this way all phases of recovery and prevention can be individualized for each patient.

Ergonomics and Functional Capacity Evaluations

In concert with back injury prevention through education and in accordance with the back school model is

---

BOX 21-1

Appropriate General Back School Program

INTRODUCTION TO BACK DYSFUNCTION

The primary purpose is to increase the patient's awareness of back care, posture, and body mechanics.

BASIC SPINAL ANATOMY AND PHYSIOLOGY

Causes of back pain and dysfunction

1. Sprains and strains
2. Disk injuries (HNP)
3. Spinal stenosis
4. Spondylolisthesis

RISK FACTORS ASSOCIATED WITH BACK INJURY

1. Poor general conditioning
2. Poor posture
3. Poor body mechanics and poor lifting style
4. Repetitive heavy lifting
5. Long-term sitting and driving
6. Stress (emotional)

POSTURE POSITIONING AND GENERAL BODY MECHANICS

1. Sitting
2. Sleeping
3. Standing
4. Lifting
5. Activities of daily living, job assessment, and recreational activities

TREATMENT APPROACHES

1. Ice or heat
2. Stretching
3. Posture changes
4. Back support
5. Conditioning

GENERAL PHYSICAL CONDITIONING

1. *Warm-up.* Patients are introduced to the concept of a general warm-up preceding any physical activity.
2. *Aerobic fitness.* Patients are introduced to the methods, equipment, and implementation of general and specific endurance activities to improve cardiovascular fitness and control body weight.
3. *Anaerobic power.* Activities are outlined that develop intense physical effort of short duration
4. *Strength.* Patients are instructed in methods to improve general body strength and specific lumbar extension strength exercises.
5. *Flexibility.* Patients are introduced to the philosophy, design, and implementation of daily, full-body stretching exercises with specific emphasis on the trunk and lower extremities.
6. *Nutrition.* Direct attention is focused on reducing the number of calories consumed by overweight individuals. Usually this education is conducted by a registered dietitian.
7. *Relaxation techniques, stress reduction, and recreational activities.*

From Allman FL: Back school program. In Introduction to Back Injuries. Atlanta, GA, The Atlanta Sports Medicine Clinic, 1990.

---

the concept of **ergonomics** and the implementation of **functional capacity evaluations (FCEs),** which are also referred to as physical capacity assessments (PCAs), related to physical stress job analysis. The term ergonomics refers to a quantifiable system of job or ADL modification (or redesign) that allows for continued productivity while reducing work-related physical stress. As with the back school model, an FCE may require the PTA to prepare the evaluation area, set up all necessary testing equipment (see section "Quantifying Back Strength"), and assist the PT with the collection, documentation, and storage of data. The implementation of an FCE is highly specific to the individual's job task. Its goal is to identify risk factors associated with a particular job or activity and then quantify the physical capacity of the individual being asked to perform the specific task to reduce the risk of back injury. In most cases an FCE is administered to a patient recovering

from a back injury before he or she returns to the job. An FCE also can be used as a screening tool to acquire data related to preemployment risk assessment and management of back injuries. Certain job or activity risk factors have been identified[16] that directly relate to the FCE. A few ergonomic risk factors are outlined by Hebert as follows:[16]

■ How much weight is lifted
■ How often you lift
■ How low you bend to lift the load
■ How high you lift the load
■ How far you carry the load
■ How far you twist with the load
■ How far you reach with the load
■ How long you sit at your job
■ What the specific design of your seat is
■ If there is sustained or repeated bending, twisting, or reaching

---

BOX 21-2

Testing Procedure that Identifies the Various Components of a Functional Capacity Evaluation

MUSCULOSKELETAL PROFILE

1. Blood pressure
2. Posture
3. Gait
4. Balance
5. Range of motion
6. Neurologic (reflexes)
7. Sensory
8. Muscle strength

FUNCTIONAL ABILITIES SCREENING

1. Push-pull
2. Dynamic lifting
3. Gross mobility
4. Hand strength (grip dynamometer)
5. Sitting and standing

From Work Site Partners, Functional Capacity Evaluation System, Industrial Rehabilitation Solutions. U.S. Physical Therapy System Manual. Houston, TX, U.S.P.T. System Manual, 1994.

Hundreds of factors may be related to job tasks. Each item to be tested in the FCE must be quantifiable and reproducible to enable the PT to make recommendations for reducing the risk of back injury. General testing parameters may be divided into categories that attempt to duplicate the requirements of the task to be performed while evaluating the patient's physiologic responses and assessing his or her physical abilities to carry out the task.

Authorities[36] advocate a multiphase testing procedure that identifies the various components of an FCE, as shown in Box 21-2.

Within each FCE the aerobic end point (heart rate exceeds 85% of maximum heart rate) and biomechanical analysis of the patient's lifting-risk posture is assessed. In each section of the test, the parameters evaluated are performed directly as they relate to the specific job or task in question.

THE THORACIC SPINE
Thoracic Spine Muscle Injuries

Soft-tissue injuries of the thoracic spine usually involve some type of direct contact (contusion during athletic activities) or indirect overstretching or contraction of the thoracic muscles. Muscle contusions and strains of the thoracic spine occur primarily in younger active patients. The primary focus of management for these self-limiting injuries is the control of pain and swelling. Generally, ice is applied directly over the involved area during the acute stage of injury. Physician-prescribed analgesics, NSAIDs, moist heat applications, ultrasound, electrical stimulation, and massage are used judiciously to help control pain. Once pain has been effectively limited, the patient is allowed to participate in active ROM activities and strengthening exercises. The PTA may instruct the patient to perform seated, postural-awareness exercises that focus on thoracic extension and scapular retraction.

Prone thoracic and lumbar extension strengthening exercises are employed as early as the patient can tolerate. These involve a three-position progression from hands at the sides, to hands behind the head, and finally to arms fully extended while performing prone thoracic and lumbar extension. As pain is reduced and strength increases, the patient can begin isotonic strengthening exercises that focus on the scapular and thoracic spine muscles (Fig. 21-25).

Thoracic Disk Injuries

Thoracic disk herniations are rare (less than 0.3% of the population) and affect both men and women equally from the fourth through the sixth decades of life.[3] The most common segments affected are between the ninth and twelfth thoracic vertebrae.[3]

The type of treatment employed for thoracic disk herniations depends on whether the disk is herniated laterally or centrally.[3,11] Central disk prolapse generally produces symptoms of "spastic paraparesis, increased deep tendon reflexes, and a positive Babinski response."[11] However, lateral thoracic disk protrusions produce signs more consistent with nerve root compression.

The PTA is exposed to both conservative care and postsurgical recovery after thoracic spine disk herniations. Less severe lateral disk herniations can be treated effectively with periods of bed rest, analgesics, modalities to control pain and swelling, and epidural injections. More severe central disk herniations, which involve neurologic deficits, must be treated surgically to decompress the neurologic impingement and with fusion to help stabilize the affected segment.[3,11] Recovery after thoracic decompression and fusion closely follows the time necessary for healing of bone and soft tissue with extensive periods of recumbency, bracing to protect the affected spine from unwanted forces, and a progressive regimen of active motion, strengthening, and endurance activities, and a return to function with specific limitations caused by the fusion.

Kyphosis

Kyphosis is defined as an increase in the thoracic posterior convexity that is manifested by a rounded-back (and protracted scapulae) posture. Kyphosis can be subdivided

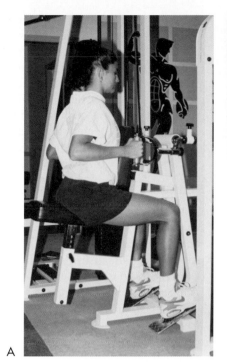
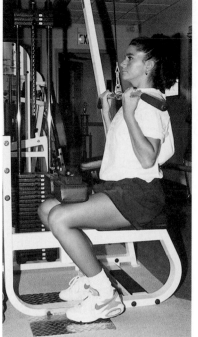

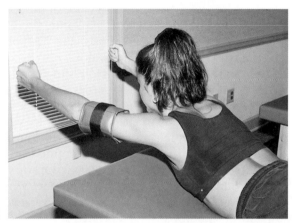

Fig. 21-25 Scapular and thoracic extension strengthening. **A,** Seated rowing machine to encourage scapular retraction; **B,** lat bar pull-down in front; **C,** prone lumbar and thoracic extension with scapular retraction using cuff weights. Notice the proximal placement of the resistance. As strength increases, the resistance can be moved to the patient's hands.

into congenital, neuromuscular, and postural categories.[11] Osteoporosis, which can lead to multilevel thoracic compression fractures, causes anterior wedging of the involved segments and creates the kyphotic curvature.

The causes of pain associated with an increased thoracic convexity have been identified as stress originating from the posterior longitudinal ligaments, muscle fatigue resulting from stretched and weakened erector spinae and rhomboid muscle groups, and various postural and neurologic syndromes.[22]

The treatment of kyphosis depends on the degree of curvature, which is determined radiographically by the treating physician; any associated disk involvement; and

the severity of symptoms.[2] In advanced cases of postural kyphosis with profound curvature and significant symptoms, the patient may require bracing of the thorax to minimize the compression associated with anterior wedging of the vertebral bodies. With less severe kyphosis, the PTA plays a critical role in patient education, postural awareness, and the application of specific exercises to simultaneously stretch the anterior shoulder and pectorals and strengthen the thoracic extension muscles.

To effectively strengthen the scapular retractors, rhomboids, middle trapezius, and erector spinae of the thoracic region, a sufficient degree of freedom of movement in these areas is needed. Generally the anterior shoulder muscles and pectorals are shortened and relatively weak in response to the increased thoracic convexity. Therefore to provide the needed stimulus for full ROM strengthening, the anterior aspect of the thorax also must be addressed. Stretching the anterior shoulder muscles can be done both actively by the patient and passively, where the clinician provides the stretching. An effective active assisted stretch can be performed with the patient facing the corner of a room or standing in an open doorway. Both of the patient's hands are placed in a comfortable position on either side of the doorway. Then the patient slowly leans forward, providing a slow, static stretch to the pectorals and anterior shoulder. This position can be held for a prolonged stretch and usually is performed for multiple sets.

A passive stretch also can be employed with the patient in a seated position. With both of the patient's hands placed behind his or her head, the PTA stands behind the patient and grasps both elbows. The PTA delivers a slow posteriorly directed stretch to the pectorals and anterior shoulder muscles. To be effective, stretching must be performed consistently each day. Therefore the patient must perform stretches two or three times daily as part of a home exercise program. In addition to stretching the thorax, posterior thoracic strengthening must be addressed. The patient performs seated active scapular retraction exercises with an emphasis on maintaining an isometric contraction or "set" of the scapular muscles with each repetition.

As described, the patient does the three-progression prone thoracic extension exercises. In addition, the patient performs scapular adduction while lying prone with both arms held straight at 90 degrees from the shoulder. Both arms are elevated while adducting the scapulae and holding the contracted position isometrically for 10 seconds.[22] This position can be modified slightly by having the patient hold weights while performing scapular adduction with both elbows flexed, creating more of a prone rowing motion.

The patient must perform both stretching and strengthening exercises daily as part of a home program. As the patient's motion improves and where posterior scapular strength increases, isotonic resistance exercises should be encouraged to a greater degree to provide increased stimulus for strengthening. In the home program, latex tubing or Thera-Band can be used in a seated rowing position to enhance scapular adduction. Commercially available isotonic rowing machines effectively provide greater resistance for the scapular muscles.

When treating postural kyphosis, the home exercise program must be carried out faithfully and the patient must develop an acute postural awareness at home and work. If the patient performs tasks at work that contribute to a rounded-shoulder position, modifications of these tasks is necessary. In many cases, the cause of poor thoracic posture is an inefficient work station

arrangement in which the patient must maintain poor posture to perform tasks such as typing, writing, assembly work, or computer data entry. A simple adjustment in the height of the workstation so that it is closer to and centered midline with the patient encourages a more erect thoracic spine. Therefore the total care of the patient focuses on symptomatic pain relief using physician-prescribed analgesics, thermal agents, massage, and a comprehensive program of stretching, strengthening, education, and work site modifications.

Scoliosis

Scoliosis can be identified as any lateral curvature of the cervical, thoracic, or lumbar spine.[21] Scoliosis usually is idiopathic (cause unknown), but it also can result from neuromuscular causes or can be related to degenerative disease, osteoporosis, trauma, and postsurgical factors.[27] Kisner and Colby[21] identify the incidence of idiopathic scoliosis as being as high as 75% to 85% of all recognized types of scoliosis. Generally scoliosis can be recognized as either structural or nonstructural.[21]

Structural scoliosis is defined as an "irreversible lateral curve of the spine with fixed rotation of the vertebrae."[21] During the PT's initial evaluation of structural scoliosis, the PTA observes that the identified lateral curve does not decrease with forward trunk flexion. Therefore structural idiopathic scoliosis is not corrected by changes in the patient's position or during active voluntary activities.[21] Nonstructural scoliosis is classified as reversible, wherein the lateral curve dissipates with positional changes. In either case, pain is the foremost presenting feature of scoliosis,[27] although cosmesis is a great concern. Other complaints involve decreased cardiopulmonary function (usually with thoracic curves greater than 65 degrees) and neurologic symptoms associated with spinal stenosis.[27]

The nonoperative management of idiopathic scoliosis primarily involves the assistant in instructing the patient about therapeutic exercises outlined and prescribed by the PT. Scoliosis treatment involves both stretching and strengthening, much like kyphosis. Exercise by itself does not halt the progression or correct scoliosis.[21] The effective use of therapeutic exercise is intended primarily to improve spinal motion, increase muscle strength, and reduce back pain.[21]

In addition to exercises, bracing also has been advocated in the treatment of scoliosis.[21,27] However, bracing is intended to halt progression of the curve and not correct cosmetic deformity.[27] Perhaps the most commonly used brace for scoliosis is the Milwaukee brace.[21,27] Generally this brace is worn 23 or 24 hours a day.[21] However, Miller[27] suggests that part-time brace wearing is as effective as the traditional long-term application.

A fundamental principle in managing idiopathic scoliosis is stretching of the tight muscles on the concave side of the curve, while strengthening the

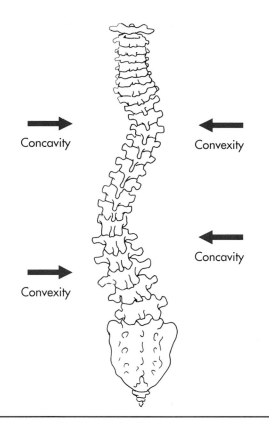

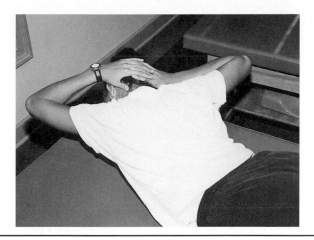

Fig. 21-27 Prone lateral trunk tilt. The patient is instructed to tilt (stretch) away from the concave side of the curve and toward the convexity.

Fig. 21-26 Scoliosis. A right thoracic convexity results in a left lower thoracic concavity and an associated right lumbar concavity with left lumbar convexity.

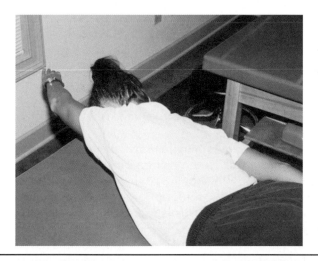

Fig. 21-28 Prone lateral trunk tilt with arm stretch. While prone the patient stretches (tilts) toward the convex side of the curve while extending the arm on the concave side, thereby effectively enhancing the thoracic stretch toward the concavity.

muscles on the convex side of the curve. In addition, trunk axial elongation (stretching vertically) is important throughout exercise. As stated in the section on kyphosis, some freedom of motion must be available for strengthening exercises to be effective.

Stretching exercises directed toward the concavity must address all of the spinal muscles. Note that a right thoracic convexity results in a left lower thoracic concavity and associated right lumbar concavity with left lumbar convexity (Fig. 21-26). Strengthening exercises are performed for all of the muscles affected on the convex side of each lateral curve.

Various stretching exercises can be performed in prone, side-lying, or heel-sitting position (21). While prone, the patient places both hands behind his or her head while tilting the thorax away from the concave side of the curve (Fig. 21-27). In another prone stretching exercise, the patient reaches overhead and extends the arm on the concave side, thereby effectively stretching the thoracic concavity (Fig. 21-28). In the heel-sitting position, the patient places both hands forward and flat while emphasizing long-axis stretching. The lateral stretching component of this exercise is accomplished by having the patient slowly stretch both arms laterally away from the concave side of the curve (Fig. 21-29).

Static stretching also can be performed with the patient lying on the side. Place a small, soft rolled pillow or towel directly under the apex of the thoracic convex curve and support and stabilize the pelvis. For an advanced progression of side-lying stretching, the patient lies over the apex bolster toward the end of a treatment table (Fig. 21-30).

As alluded to in the preceding, trunk elongation (axial stretching) also is an effective stretching procedure used to treat scoliosis. Standing, the patient faces a wall and attempts to "walk up the wall" with both hands. The patient must reach as high as possible with both hands. A more progressive form of trunk elongation

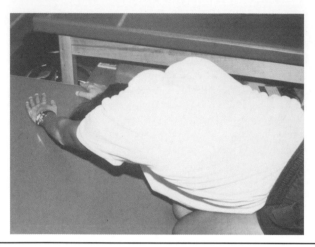

Fig. 21-29 Heel-sitting lateral trunk stretch with long-axis stretch and lateral stretch of both arms.

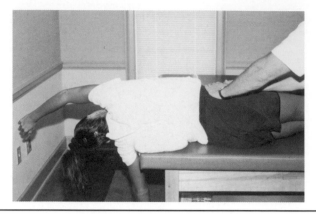

Fig. 21-30 Side-lying apex stretch over the end of a table. A pillow is placed directly under the apex of the convex curve. With the patient's pelvis stabilized, the patient slowly stretches over the end of the table. Note the patient's arm position to enhance the stretch.

is to have the patient hang by both arms from an overhead bar.

Strengthening the thoracic and lumbar spine toward the convex side focuses on thoracic and lumbar extension strength and specific lateral strengthening maneuvers. Prone thoracic and lumbar spine active exercises were outlined and described in the preceding. These are effective when used early to enhance the strength of the thorax.

Specific lateral strengthening can proceed with the patient in a side-lying position on the concave side of the curve. The PTA should stabilize the trunk, then have the patient lift the trunk up toward the convex side of the curve (Fig. 21-31). This exercise can be viewed as a side-lying sit-up.

While this brief discussion has focused on a few rudimentary stretching and strengthening exercises for mild to moderate idiopathic scoliosis, an outline of surgical procedures to correct severe scoliosis is warranted. Surgery is reserved for severe symptomatic curves—those more than 50 to 60 degrees.[27] With surgery, curves of this magnitude can be improved by approximately 50%.[21] The exact surgery performed depends on many factors. However, a spinal fusion with or without Harrington rod instrumentation[21] is designed to elongate and stabilize the spine and thereby reduce pain and improve appearance.

Physical therapy after spine fusion for advanced, severe scoliosis requires extensive convalescence, the application of a postoperative brace, and very limited activity for up to several months after surgery.[21]

THE CERVICAL SPINE

Without question, the most profound and catastrophic cervical spine injury is a fracture dislocation resulting in quadriplegia. The description of these spinal injuries is

beyond the scope of this chapter. This section identifies various soft-tissue and bony injuries of the cervical spine common to orthopedic physical therapy.

Acute Sprains and Strains

Muscular strains of the cervical spine are common among young athletes and in association with flexion-extension, lateral flexion, and acceleration-deceleration "whiplash" type automobile injuries.[34,40] The muscles involved in cervical strains appear to be the sternocleidomastoid, trapezius, scalenes, erectors, rhomboids, and levator scapulae.[40] The mechanism of injury producing cervical strains and sprains varies but includes hyperflexion, rotation, and lateral flexion of the head and cervical spine.[34]

Forces usually are great enough with automobile accidents that ligament injuries occur in conjunction with muscle strains. In fact, Stratton and Bryan's experimental studies have demonstrated a wide range of tissue damage with hyperextension type automobile injuries:[34]

1. Tearing of sternocleidomastoid muscle
2. Tearing of longissimus coli muscle
3. Pharyngeal edema
4. Tearing of anterior longitudinal ligament
5. Separation of cartilaginous end plate of the intervertebral disk

Similar types of injuries occur with hyperflexion injuries as a result of automobile accidents:[34]

1. Tears of the posterior cervical muscles
2. Tears of the ligamentum nuchae
3. Tears of the posterior longitudinal ligament
4. Intervertebral disk injury

The treatment of traumatic cervical spine sprains and strains is symptomatic during the acute stage of recovery. The treating physician usually prescribes a course of analgesics, NSAIDs, or muscle relaxants; rest; and agents

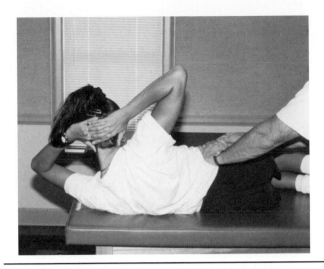

Fig. 21-31 Side-lying lateral trunk sit-up. With the patient's pelvis supported, the patient is instructed to lift the trunk toward the convex side of the curve.

to control pain and swelling (heat, cold, ultrasound, and electrical stimulation). The healing constraints of muscle and ligament tissues differ; both must be addressed throughout recovery.

After the initial pain and swelling are controlled, the patient may be introduced to a series of active ROM exercises, cervical isometric strengthening exercises, and education in cervical posture mechanics. Initial ROM exercises must be approached cautiously to avoid reproducing the motion that caused the injury. As with all soft-tissue injuries, attention must be focused on protection of the affected area while striving to prevent further injury. If, for example, the mechanism of cervical sprain and strain was hyperflexion, care must be directed at avoiding the end range of head and neck flexion. Gentle active ROM exercises can proceed after moist heat application for 20 minutes to enhance muscle relaxation, relieve pain, and stimulate greater mobility.

An important practical matter to consider when instructing patients to perform cervical ROM exercises is how to stabilize the trunk and shoulders. With both muscle and ligament damage, the long-term effect of healing is fibrous tissue contraction, which results in stiffness, restriction, and limitation of motion.[40] Therefore to effectively direct the stretch to the affected area, the surrounding structures must be supported and stabilized. For example, if a patient with a lateral flexion injury that results in muscle and ligament damage is instructed to gently stretch laterally away from the side of the injury, the opposite shoulder would elevate (because of the shortened tissues) if the shoulders are not stabilized, rendering the stretch ineffective. To stabilize the shoulder, the patient should perform the stretch while seated and use both hands to grasp under the seat. No shoulder elevation occurs when the patient

attempts to stretch the head and neck laterally with the arms fully extended and secured under the seat.

Initial strengthening of the cervical spine after a muscle-tendon strain or ligamentous sprain usually is accompanied by isometric stabilization exercises. Submaximal contractions and precise techniques are important and must be carefully explained and demonstrated to the patient. Before applying isometric exercises, the full cervical ROM must be achieved and pain controlled. For isometric stabilization exercises, the patient performs a series of four-way isometrics in an anatomically neutral cervical spine position. The four-position isometric exercises are forward flexion, lateral flexion (right and left), and extension. In preparing to perform these exercises, the patient must demonstrate the ability to hold his or her head and neck in midline without excessive rotation, lateral flexion, forward flexion, or extension malalignment.

To begin, the patient should sit before a mirror to get visual feedback while maintaining proper head and neck alignment. The proper execution of the first isometric position of forward flexion should be explained and demonstrated. With one hand placed on the midline of the forehead (the patient must bring the hand into the described position and not rotate the head toward the hand), the patient should direct a posterior force to the forehead with the hand while resisting head and neck flexion, thereby stimulating isometric strengthening of the anterior cervical muscles. The patient should gradually and slowly "build" the resistance using the rule of 10s (gradually initiate isometrics with 2-second submaximal contraction, then hold for 6 seconds, then slowly reduce for 2 seconds) rather than suddenly applying maximal force (Fig. 21-32).

The patient should use both hands to support the occiput for the second position. The patient should maintain the head and neck in the anatomic midline position and not allow the head to flex forward. The patient should be encouraged to gradually apply an anteriorly directed force with both hands while resisting extension of the head. This position effectively strengthens the head and neck extensor group (Fig. 21-33).

The next position is lateral flexion. While the PTA observes proper head and neck alignment in the mirror, the patient should bring one hand to the side of the head but not allow the head to rotate or laterally flex to meet the hand. The patient should then apply lateral pressure while resisting this force. This position is repeated on the opposite side. No head or neck motion must occur in each position. Usually the patient carries out a series of two to three sets of 10-second isometric exercises two to three times daily. As strength improves, the patient gradually increases the intensity, but avoids sudden or ballistic contractions (Fig 21-34).

Educating the patient about cervical spine postural mechanics is as important as the actual management of

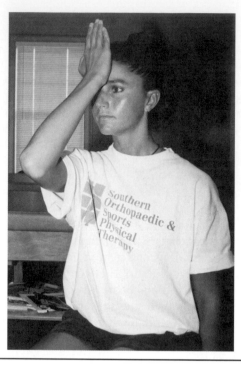

Fig. 21-32 Cervical isometrics for forward flexion. Notice the head must remain in midline and not be allowed to rotate.

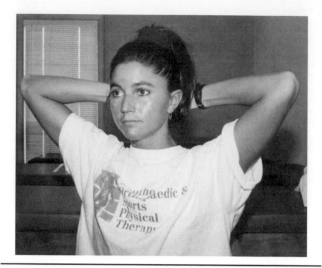

Fig. 21-33 Cervical isometrics for head and neck extension.

any physical dysfunction. One of the most commonly recognized postural malalignment syndromes affecting the cervical spine is a forward head posture. Typically, this posture is characterized by a loss of flexion in the upper cervical spine region and a loss of extension in the lower cervical spine. The patient should perform axial extension or cervical retraction exercises. The PT determines which exercises are appropriate for each patient and identifies which patients are candidates for specific axial-extension exercises.

Retraction exercises require the patient to be able to demonstrate a midline neutral position. The patient should sit in front of a mirror initially to perform this exercise correctly. Have the patient imagine that his or her head is resting on a conveyor belt. The patient must be able to align the ears with the shoulders and move the head straight back on the conveyor belt (Fig. 21-35). If done correctly, a "double chin" is produced as the patient moves the head back. If done incorrectly, the head and neck move into extension. The patient should be encouraged to perform this exercise at home for multiple sets throughout the day or as prescribed by the PT. Because this is a stretching exercise to improve motion restriction, each retraction of the head should be held for 10 seconds.

Full recovery from acute sprains and strains of the cervical spine involves the elimination of pain and swelling initially, appropriate rest from any aggravating positions, protection from unwanted stress, the return

of normal cervical spine ROM, enhanced muscle strength through isometric stabilization exercises, work site modifications, and postural-awareness activities (axial extension-retraction exercises).

Cervical Disk Injuries

The symptoms of peripheral pain, radicular signs, local cervical pain, and scapular pain are consistent with the symptoms of disk herniations observed in the lumbar spine.[34]

Iglarsh and Snyder-Mackler[18] define two types or positions of cervical spine motion that help alleviate the symptoms of disk herniations. In the first group, flexion activities improve the symptoms. In the second type, extension activities reduce symptoms.[18] As with lumbar disk herniations, the initial goals are to relieve symptoms, reduce pain and swelling, control muscle spasm, and work toward centralizing the symptoms. Iglarsh and Snyder-Mackler[18] define improvement in both categories as "a decrease in the extent or intensity of the peripheral symptoms."

The specific exercises for cervical disk herniation patients must be identified carefully by the physician and PT. Once the appropriate category of relief is recognized,[18] the PT organizes a comprehensive plan of pain relief, motion, strength, and postural education activities for the PTA to follow and apply. In the flexion group, motion is slowly developed into flexion, with close observation and documentation of any changes in radicular signs. In the extension group, the initial activities focus on axial extension and retraction. In either case, the aim is to accurately identify which motions and positions exacerbate the pain. Once these are recognized, the patient is taught to avoid these positions. As the signs and symptoms of radicular pain begin to centralize, the PT may initiate isometric stabilization

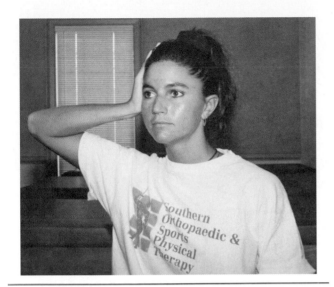

Fig. 21-34 Cervical isometrics for lateral flexion.

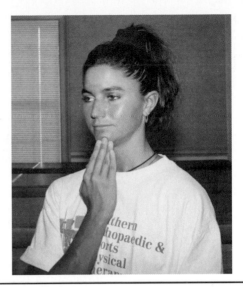

Fig. 21-35 Axial extension-cervical retraction. The head of the patient should move directly posterior. No head or cervical extension should occur. Attempt to produce a double chin without head or neck flexion.

exercises, with extreme caution to avoid positions or intensity of contractions that increase symptoms.

Cervical Spondylosis

In contrast to cervical disk herniations, **cervical spondylosis** involves chronic rather than acute degenerative disk, which results from "wear and tear on the weight-bearing structures of the cervical spine."[34] The symptoms are characteristic of spinal cord compression (myelopathy) or nerve root compression with radicular signs.[27] Cervical spondylosis is seen most often during the fourth and fifth decades of life and characteristically affects men more than women at the C5-C6 and C6-C7 segments.[27]

Sustained impact loading and repetitive microtrauma[34] are causative factors that can produce cervical cord impingement, nerve root impingement, osteophytes, bone sclerosis, loss of cervical lordosis, and central or posterolateral disk herniations.[27,34]

Initial physical therapy interventions focus on pain relief with thermal and electrical agents, physician-prescribed analgesics, and rest from aggravating positions. A semirigid cervical collar may be of some use in select cases. As with other disk conditions, the PT provides a comprehensive evaluation to accurately determine which motions cause pain and radicular symptoms and which relieve pain. From this detailed initial evaluation, the PT outlines and describes specific exercises consistent with these findings. Axial extension-retraction exercises are effective for patients who derive pain relief from extension. Flexion-type activities are reserved for patients who obtain relief from cervical flexion. In either case, traction is an effective tool to minimize joint compressive loads and reduce cord compression or nerve root irritation.[27] The PT deter-

mines if mechanical traction or manual cervical traction is more appropriate. Isometric cervical spine stabilization exercises (four-way isometrics) and ROM exercises are initiated once pain has been reduced and the appropriateness of these activities is determined by the PT.

When cord compression (myelopathy) progresses and radicular pain persists, the physician can use various surgical interventions. Miller[27] describes an anterior cervical spine approach to accomplish a diskectomy and fusion or a posterior approach for a foraminotomy or multilevel laminectomy to relieve cord or root compression.

Because cervical spondylosis is a chronic degenerative condition, long-term care involves protection from inappropriate and unwanted forces and instruction in cervical posture mechanics, flexibility exercises, and strengthening activities.

Thoracic Outlet Syndrome

Some texts cover **thoracic outlet (inlet) syndrome** within the subject matter affecting the shoulder.[41] Because of the anatomic proximity of the structures involved, this condition is discussed within the context of the cervical spine. Authorities point out that the term thoracic inlet syndrome is a more precise and anatomically accurate term used to describe compression of vascular or neurologic tissues as they exit the "superior triangle opening of the thorax" (Fig. 21-36).[34,41] Specifically, proximal compression of the subclavian artery and vein, as well as the brachial plexus, are the most probable neurovascular factors involved with thoracic inlet syndrome.[34] Many structures can cause compression of

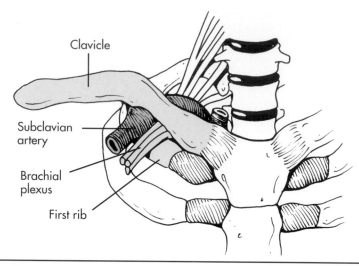

Clavicle

Subclavian
artery

Brachial
plexus

First rib

Fig. 21-36 Thoracic outlet syndrome. Note proximal compression of the subclavian artery and vein and the brachial plexus.

these tissues. Foremost is the presence of a cervical rib, a shortened or hypertrophied anterior scalene muscle, or malunion of the clavicle and subluxed first thoracic rib.[15,34,41] Symptoms of this condition include radicular signs of pain, numbness, tingling, weakness, and skin and temperature changes consistent with neurovascular tissue compression.[15,34,41]

Typically, physical therapy management addresses specifically defined limitations of movement and affected bony or soft tissues during the initial evaluation performed by the PT. An individualized comprehensive program of stretching, strengthening, and education can commence once the PT has determined which specific tissues are affected and identified any underlying causes of postural variations.

Soft-tissue stretching focuses on the anterior scalene muscles. The patient is instructed to laterally flex and extend the head to the opposite side of the shortened muscle (Fig. 21-37). Thoracic kyphosis tends to accentuate the symptoms of thoracic inlet syndrome, so pectoral stretching (facing an open doorway with hands on either side and leaning forward) and thoracic extension mobility and strengthening exercises are used to specifically address muscle weakness and soft-tissue restrictions. A host of clinically applicable thoracic extension mobility exercises can be used. Examples include seated scapular retraction, prone scapular and thoracic extension, and seated rowing activities with elastic tubing.

In addition to stretching and strengthening exercises, cervical posture correction is needed; poor cervical posture is a common problem in the workplace.[15] To address the forward head posture and tight anterior neck muscles, the patient can perform axial extension or cervical retraction stretching exercises, as described.

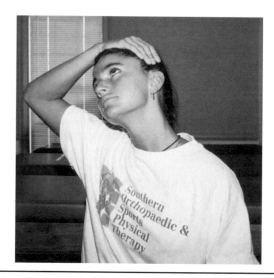

Fig. 21-37 Stretching of the anterior scalene muscles by laterally flexing and extending the head toward the opposite side of the shortened muscle. Note the gentle overpressure provided by the hand.

The effective management of thoracic inlet syndrome focuses on specific stretching of affected muscles, thoracic mobility, and extension strengthening, as well as education concerning proper cervical spine alignment and the performance of cervical retraction exercises.

MOBILIZATION OF THE LUMBAR, THORACIC, AND CERVICAL SPINE

Although peripheral joint mobilization is covered in this text, axial skeleton mobilization techniques for the lumbar, thoracic, and cervical spine are not addressed.

The extraordinarily complex arrangement and intimate anatomic relationship between vertebral segments and surrounding neurovascular structures require intense, exhaustive study and precise application of techniques after detailed training and clinical practice to be safe, effective, and efficient. The scope of the PTA's training is not consistent with the demanding working knowledge of neurovascular anatomy, biomechanics, and pathophysiology of the lumbar, thoracic, and cervical spine needed to provide mobilization techniques to these areas.

✤ ADDITIONAL FEATURES

Central Canal Stenosis: Acquired or congenital insidious onset with pain and paresthesias with neurogenic claudication.

Cervical Spine: Compression test—axial load increases symptoms and radiating pain. Distraction test—traction decreases or centralizes radiating pain.

Classification of Disk Displacement: Degenerated disk, protrusion of disk, extrusion of disk, sequestered disk.

Disk Displacement: Most commonly involves L4 to L5.

Foraminal Stenosis: Also referred to as lateral recess stenosis. Osteophytes (bone spurs) narrow the intervertebral foramen.

Muscle Weakness: L4 nerve root—tibialis anterior; L5 nerve root—extensor hallucis longus.

Neurogenic Claudication: Generally bilateral pain and weakness in thighs and calves.

Vascular Claudication: Muscle pain without paresthesias.

REFERENCES

1. Allman FL: Back School Program. The Atlanta Sports Medicine Clinic, 1990.
2. Brashear HR, Raney RB: Affections of the spine and thorax. In Handbook of Orthopaedic Surgery, 10th ed. St Louis, Mosby, 1986.
3. Burkus JK: Spine. In Loth T, ed. Orthopaedic Boards Review. St Louis, Mosby, 1993.
4. Cailliet R: Low Back Pain Syndrome, 3rd ed. Philadelphia, FA Davis, 1981.
5. Chappuis JL, Johnson GD, Gines AM: A Source Guide for Spine Care. Atlanta, GA, Greater Atlanta Spine Center, 1994.
6. DeLee JC, et al: Therapeutic exercise modalities. In Drez D, ed. Therapeutic Modalities for Sports Injuries. St Louis, Mosby, 1989.
7. DeRosa C, Porterfield JA: Lumbar spine and pelvis. In Richardson JK, Iglarsh ZA, eds. Clinical Orthopaedic Physical Therapy. Philadelphia, WB Saunders, 1994.
8. Dietrich N, Kurowski P: The importance of mechanical factors in the etiology of spondylolysis: a model analysis of loads and stresses in the human lumbar spine. *Spine* 1985;10:541–632.
9. Duda M: Elite lifters at risk of spondylolysis. *Phys Sports* Med 1987;15:107–158.
10. Edgelow PI: Dysfunction, evaluation, and treatment of the lumbar spine. In Donatelli R, Wooden MJ, eds. Orthopaedic Physical Therapy. New York, Churchill Livingstone, 1989.
11. Eismont FJ, Kitchel SH: Thoracolumbar spine. In DeLee JC, Drez D, eds. Orthopaedic Sports Medicine: Principles and Practice, vol 2. Philadelphia, WB Saunders, 1994.
12. Fulton M: Lower-Back Pain: A New Solution for an Old Problem. Rolling Meadows, IL, MedX Inc., 1992.
13. Goldstein TS: Treatment of common problems of the spine. In Lewis CB, ed. Geriatric Orthopaedics, Rehabilitative Management of Common Problems. Gaithersburg, MD, Aspen Publishers, 1991.
14. Gould JA: The spine. In Gould JA, ed. Orthopaedic and Sports Physical Therapy, 2nd ed. St Louis, Mosby, 1990.
15. Hebert LA: The Neck-Arm-Hand Book. Greenville, MA, IMPACC, 1989.
16. Hebert LA: Your Back for Life. Greenville, MA, IMPACC, 1993.
17. Holley TR: Biology of aging: the musculoskeletal system. Geriatric Physical Therapy Course Notes. Reno, NV, 1995.
18. Iglarsh ZA, Snyder-Mackler L: Temporomandibular joint and the cervical spine. In Richardson JK, Iglarsh ZA, eds. Clinical Orthopaedic Physical Therapy. Philadelphia, WB Saunders, 1994.
19. Jackson DW: Low back pain in young athletes: evaluation of stress reaction and discogenic problems. *Am J Sports Med* 1979;7:366–664.
20. Kaiser RK, Rose SJ, Apts DW: An electromyographic analysis of two techniques for squat lifting. Washington University School of Medicine, Applied Kinesiology Laboratory, Program in Physical Therapy.
21. Kisner C, Colby LA, eds. Scoliosis. In Therapeutic Exercise Foundations and Techniques, 2nd ed. Philadelphia, FA Davis, 1989.
22. Kisner C, Colby LA. eds. The spine: treatment of acute problems. In Therapeutic Exercise Foundations and Techniques, 2nd ed. Philadelphia, FA Davis, 1989.
23. Lewis CB, Bottomley JM, eds. Orthopaedic treatment considerations. In Geriatric Physical Therapy: A Clinical Approach. New York, Appleton & Lange, 1994.
24. Macnab I: Backache. Baltimore, Williams & Wilkins, 1977.
25. McKenzie RA: The Lumbar Spine: Mechanical Diagnosis and Therapy. Waikanae, New Zealand, 1981.
26. McRae R: Practical Fracture Treatment, 3rd ed. New York, Churchill-Livingstone, 1994.
27. Miller MD, ed. Spine. In Review of Orthopaedics. Philadelphia, WB Saunders, 1992.
28. O'Sullivan JJ, Ellis JJ, Makofsky HW: The five "L's" of lifting. *Phys Ther Forum* 1991;10:14.
29. Panjabi M, Abumi K, Duranceau J, et al: Spinal stability and intersegmental muscle forces. A biochemical model. *Spine* 1989; 14(2):194–200.
30. Paris SV: The spine: etiology and treatment of dysfunction including joint manipulation. Atlanta, GA, Course Notes, 1979.
31. Sawyer M, Zbieraneck CK: The treatment of soft tissue after spinal injury. *Clin Sports Med* 1986;5:2.
32. Shankman GA: Strengthening the lumbar spine in athletics. *NSCA J* 1993;15:22–45.
33. Spengler DM, Szpalski M: Newer assessment approaches for the patient with low back pain. *Contemp Orthop* 199021:4.
34. Stratton SA, Bryan JM: Dysfunction, evaluation and treatment of the cervical spine and thoracic inlet. In Donatelli R, Wooden MJ, eds. Orthopaedic Physical Therapy. New York, Churchill-Livingstone, 1989.
35. Tan JC: Understanding lumbar strength testing. In Advance for Physical Therapists. Merion Publications, 1992.
36. U.S. Physical Therapy: Work Site Partners, Functional Capacity Evaluation System, Industrial Rehabilitation Solutions. Houston, TX, U.S.P.T. System Manual, 1994.
37. Watkins RG, Dillin WH: Lumbar spine injury in the athlete. *Clin Sports Med* 1990;9:2.
38. Wiltse LL: Spondylolisthesis in children. *Clin Orthop* 1957; 21:156–163.
39. Wiltse LL, Widell EH, Jackson DW: Fatigue fracture: the basic lesion in isthmic spondylolisthesis. *J Bone Joint Surg* 1975; 57A:17–22.
40. Wroble RR, Albright JP: Neck and low back injuries in wrestling. In Clinics in Sports Medicine: Injuries to the Spine, vol 5. Philadelphia, WB Saunders, 1986.
41. Yahara ML: Shoulder. In Richardson JK, Iglarsh ZA, eds. Clinical Orthopaedic Physical Therapy. Philadelphia, WB Saunders, 1994.

REVIEW QUESTIONS

Multiple Choice

1. The second leading cause of all physician visits in the United States is:
   A. The common cold
   B. Knee sprains
   C. Ankle sprains
   D. Lumbar spine injuries

2. When the lumbar spine moves from a position of flexion into extension, the nucleus tends to displace in which direction?
   A. Anteriorly
   B. Posteriorly
   C. Laterally
   D. Diagonally

3. When the lumbar spine moves from a position of extension into flexion, the nucleus tends to displace in which direction?
   A. Laterally
   B. Diagonally
   C. Posteriorly
   D. Anteriorly

4. Which of the following accurately describe(s) key features of basic lifting mechanics? (Circle any that apply.)
   A. Keep a wide base of support.
   B. Keep the object lifted away from the body.
   C. Maintain a lordotic posture.
   D. Use the legs to lift.
   E. Exhale on the lift phase.

5. Muscular strains of the lumbar spine are common and occur from which of the following?
   A. Sudden muscular contractions
   B. Rapid stretching
   C. Torque
   D. Eccentric loading
   E. All of the above

6. Walking has been shown to be an effective exercise for the treatment of lumbar muscle strain because walking does which of the following?
   A. Stimulates circulation
   B. Enhances cardiovascular and cardiorespiratory fitness
   C. Stimulates the mechanoreceptor system
   D. Improves coordination and strength
   E. All of the above

7. A generalized phase I or acute management of lumbar sprains or strains focuses on which of the following? (Circle any that apply.)
   A. Immediate functional activities
   B. Pain control
   C. Swelling management
   D. Restricted motions
   E. Combined flexion and rotation motions

8. If the posterior longitudinal ligament of the lumbar spine is sprained, which position(s) should be avoided during the maximum-protection phase?
   A. Lateral flexion
   B. Extension
   C. Flexion
   D. Rotation
   E. All of the above

9. Which of the following describes an extruded disk?
   A. The nucleus is free in the canal.
   B. The nucleus bulges against annulus.

C. The nucleus extends through the annulus, but the nuclear material is contained by the posterior longitudinal ligament.
D. The nucleus is intact, but the annulus is ruptured.

10. Herniated nucleus pulposus (HNP) is a disease that primarily affects which age group?
    A. Young adults only
    B. Adults more than 50 years old only
    C. Elderly people more than 70 years old
    D. Young to middle-aged adults

11. Which of the following describes back pain that is aggravated by activity and relieved by rest?
    A. Neurogenic pain
    B. Vascular pain
    C. Spondylogenic pain
    D. Viscerogenic pain

12. Which of the following describes radicular signs related to HNP?
    A. Numbness
    B. Radiating pain
    C. Posterior thigh pain
    D. Paresthesias radiating distally below the knee
    E. All of the above

13. Which of the following is (are) the objective(s) for management of HNP?
    A. Protection from unwanted forces
    B. Increased muscular strength, flexibility, and endurance
    C. Enhanced awareness and performance of proper body mechanics
    D. Pain and swelling relief
    E. All of the above

14. Which of the following describes the most common surgical procedure used to treat HNP?
    A. Laminotomy with decompression diskectomy
    B. Microsurgical diskectomy
    C. Percutaneous diskectomy
    D. Multisegment fusion

15. Which of the following describe(s) Williams's exercises? (Circle any that apply.)
    A. Pelvic tilt
    B. Single knee to chest
    C. Prone extension
    D. Partial direct sit-ups
    E. Lateral trunk flexion

16. Studies have shown that isometric lumbar training and testing can produce increases of up to _____ in strength. (Circle any that apply.)
    A. 50%
    B. 80%
    C. 100%
    D. Several thousand percent
    E. 20% to 30%

17. Which of the following describes potential uses for lumbar spine testing procedures?
    A. Measure progress objectively
    B. Medicolegal use
    C. Research
    D. Job screening and work site evaluations
    E. All of the above

18. Which of the following describe(s) contraindications for static or dynamic lumbar strength testing? (Circle any that apply.)
    A. Chronic pain
    B. Unstable fractures
    C. Acute injury

D. Sequestrated disk
E. Fatigue

19. Which of the following is an ergonomic risk factor identified in the administration of a functional capacity evaluation (FCE)?
    A. Height
    B. Amount of weight that can be lifted
    C. How often load is lifted
    D. How high load is lifted
    E. All of the above

20. A narrowing of the spinal canal constricting and compressing nerve roots that produces symptoms of neurogenic or spinal claudication is called which of the following?
    A. HNP
    B. Sequestrated disk
    C. Spondylolysis
    D. Spinal stenosis

21. Spinal stenosis occurs in which of the following?
    A. Men twice as often as women
    B. Women more often than men
    C. Young men
    D. Older women more often than older men

22. Through what means is spinal stenosis most commonly acquired?
    A. By overt trauma
    B. By repetitive motion
    C. By degenerative arthritic changes
    D. Because of weakness of the paraspinal musculature

23. The patient with spinal stenosis frequently complains of increased symptoms with which of the following?
    A. Lumbar extension
    B. Lumbar flexion
    C. Ambulating in flexed lumbar posture
    D. Pelvic tilts
    E. All of the above

24. A forward slippage of one superior vertebra over an inferior vertebra (usually L4-L5 or L5-S1) is called which of the following?
    A. Spondylolysis
    B. Stenosis
    C. Spinal claudication
    D. Spondylolisthesis

25. The most common type or classification of spondylolisthesis is which of the following?
    A. Congenital
    B. Isthmic
    C. Degenerative
    D. Traumatic

26. A grade III spondylolisthesis is defined as forward slippage of which of the following?
    A. 25% to 50%
    B. 0% to 25%
    C. 50% to 75%
    D. 75% to 100%

27. Compression fractures of the spine can commonly occur in elderly persons with osteoporosis from which of the following?
    A. High force flexion
    B. Ballistic extension
    C. Benign daily activities
    D. High force rotation
    E. All of the above

28. Which of the following motions should be avoided during the acute and subacute phases after compression fractures?
    A. Flexion
    B. Extension

C. Rotation
D. Lateral flexion
E. All of the above

29. What is the incidence (percentage of the population) of thoracic disk herniations?
    A. 7%
    B. 10%
    C. 0.3%
    D. 2%

30. The segments most commonly involved with thoracic disk herniations are which of the following?
    A. Between the first and fifth vertebrae
    B. Between the ninth and twelfth vertebrae
    C. Between the second and fourth vertebrae
    D. All segments equally

31. An increase in the thoracic posterior convexity is defined as which of the following?
    A. Lordosis
    B. Kyphosis
    C. Scoliosis
    D. Osteoporosis

32. In general, the treatment of kyphosis focuses on which of the following?
    A. Postural awareness
    B. Stretching the pectorals
    C. Thoracic extension strengthening
    D. Strengthening the scapular retractors
    E. All of the above

33. With structural scoliosis the PTA notes which of the following?
    A. The identified curve does not decrease with extension.
    B. The curve dissipates with lateral flexion.
    C. The curve does not decrease with trunk flexion.
    D. The curve dissipates with trunk flexion.

34. Which of the following represents significant clinical features of scoliosis with thoracic curves greater than 65 degrees?
    A. Pain
    B. Neurologic symptoms
    C. Decreased cardiopulmonary function
    D. Cosmetic
    E. All of the above

35. The effective use of therapeutic exercise for the treatment of scoliosis is designed to do which of the following?
    A. Reduce pain
    B. Increase motion
    C. Enhance strength
    D. Promote function
    E. All of the above

36. Which of the following is a fundamental principle in the care of idiopathic scoliosis?
    A. Develop anaerobic power.
    B. Develop thoracic and lumbar extension strength.
    C. Stretch the concave side of the curve, while strengthening the convex side of the curve.
    D. Develop trunk flexion strength.

37. In experimental studies, which of the following structures have been identified as being involved with cervical hyperextension-type automobile accidents?
    A. Sternocleidomastoid
    B. Anterior longitudinal ligament
    C. Longissimus coli muscle
    D. Separation of cartilaginous end plate of the intervertebral disk
    E. All of the above

38. Similarly, hyperflexion injuries of the cervical spine can result in which of the follwing? (Circle any that apply.)
    A. Tears of the anterior longitudinal ligaments
    B. Tears of the ligamentum nuchae
    C. Intervertebral disk injury
    D. Tears of the posterior longitudinal ligament
    E. Tears of the anterior deltoid

39. Initial strengthening of the cervical spine after a strain or sprain usually is accomplished by introducing which of the following?
    A. Manually applied eccentric contractions
    B. Submaximal concentric muscle contractions
    C. Submaximal isometric contractions
    D. Maximal, multiangle isometrics

40. Which of the following represents one of the more commonly recognized malalignment syndromes of the cervical spine?
    A. Lateral flexion malalignment
    B. Cervical extension malalignment
    C. Forward head posture
    D. Cervical rotation malalignment

41. To correct for a forward head posture, a commonly applied series of exercises is which of the following? (Circle any that apply.)
    A. Cervical flexion isometrics
    B. Axial extension exercises
    C. Head extension isometrics
    D. Cervical retraction exercises
    E. All of the above

42. Proximal compression of the subclavian artery and vein, as well as the brachial plexus, are probable neurovascular structures involved with which of the following?
    A. Volkmann's ischemic contracture
    B. Carpal tunnel syndrome
    C. Thoracic outlet syndrome
    D. De Quervain's tenosynovitis

43. Which of the following is a symptom of neurovascular tissue compression?
    A. Radicular pain
    B. Weakness
    C. Numbness
    D. Tingling
    E. All of the above

44. Which of the following exercises are most appropriate for the care of thoracic outlet syndrome?
    A. Thoracic flexion exercises
    B. Lateral cervical flexion exercises
    C. Thoracic extension, scapular retraction, and pectoral stretching
    D. Cervical flexion exercises

Short Answer

45. Match the following list of percentages relating to intradiscal pressure with the appropriate and corresponding body position.

100%	supine (knees flexed)
75%	standing
35%	bending forward
25%	side-lying
275%	supine

46. List the five *Ls* of lifting, as described by O'Sullivan, Ellis, and Makofsky.

47. Identify the category of lumbar disk injury in the following figure.

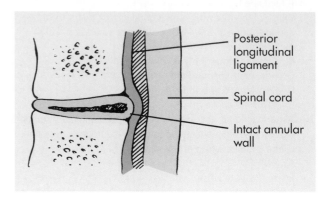

48. Identify the category of lumbar disk injury in the following figure.

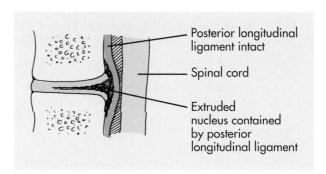

True/False

49. The intervertebral lumbar disk is essentially avascular and aneural except for the periphery of the annulus, which is innervated.

50. Ligamentous sprains of the lumbar spine can occur from sudden violent force or repeated stress.

51. It is essential that all cases of HNP be treated with lumbar extension postures.

52. Manual muscle testing is the most effective way to quantify lumbar muscle strength and performance.

53. Lumbar extension exercises are advocated for spondylolisthesis.

54. Osteoporosis, which can lead to multilevel thoracic compression fractures, can cause anterior wedging of the segments, which in turn creates the kyphotic curve.

55. Scoliosis refers to a lateral curvature of the lumbar vertebrae.

56. Generally scoliosis can be categorized as structural or nonstructural.

57. With nonstructural scoliosis, positional changes result in a decrease in the curvature.

58. Therapeutic exercise (by itself) is intended to halt the progression of scoliosis and correct resultant deformity.

59. The use of bracing in the treatment of scoliosis is intended to halt the progression of the curve and is not identified as effective in correcting cosmetic deformity.

60. Axial stretching (trunk elongation) is not advocated for the treatment of scoliosis.

61. Cervical spondylosis is an acute cervical disk disorder.

Essay Questions

Answer on a separate sheet of paper.

62. Outline and describe the basic mechanics of the lumbar spine.
63. Discuss and apply the principles of the fundamental mechanics of lifting.
64. Identify common sprains and strains of the lumbar spine.
65. Discuss common methods of management and rehabilitation of lumbar spine sprains and strains.
66. Identify and describe injuries to the lumbar intervertebral disk.
67. Discuss methods of management and rehabilitation for injuries to the lumbar intervertebral disk.
68. Define and describe methods of quantifying back strength.
69. Define and describe components of the back school model.
70. Define ergonomic and functional capacity evaluations.
71. Define spinal stenosis and describe methods of management and rehabilitation.
72. Define and contrast the terms *spondylosis* and *spondylolisthesis*.
73. Describe methods of management and rehabilitation for spondylolysis and spondylolisthesis.
74. Identify common lumbar and thoracic spine fractures.
75. Define kyphosis, lordosis, and scoliosis.
76. Identify and describe methods of management and rehabilitation for kyphosis and scoliosis.
77. Identify and describe common cervical spine injuries and discuss methods of management and rehabilitation.

Critical Thinking Application

Based on your knowledge and understanding of the mechanisms of the lumbar spine and the healing mechanisms of soft tissue and bone, develop a comprehensive rehabilitation program (critical pathway, criterion-based rehab program) for a patient with an extruded disk at L4-L5. Which activities would you recommend during the acute phase of recovery? Which positions would you encourage and discourage? Identify and list four general objectives for the care of a patient with an HNP. During each phase of recovery, recommend specific restrictions, agents to aid in pain and swelling management, alterations in body mechanics, flexibility exercises, aerobic fitness, strength training, and balance and proprioception drills. Assuming this patient is a manual laborer who is required to lift boxes from the floor and place them on a truck, what specific ergonomic modifications would you recommend? Is back school an option? If so, list the components of a comprehensive back school program. If this patient sits at a desk all day, what ergonomic design modifications would you recommend?

22

Orthopedic Management of the Shoulder*

LEARNING OBJECTIVES

1. Identify and describe methods, management, and rehabilitation for subacromial rotator cuff impingement.
2. Identify and describe methods of management and rehabilitation for tears of the rotator cuff.
3. Describe methods of management and rehabilitation for glenohumeral instability.
4. Discuss methods of management and rehabilitation for adhesive capsulitis.
5. Identify and describe common injuries of the acromioclavicular (A-C) joint.
6. Describe common methods of management and rehabilitation for injuries of the A-C joint.
7. Identify and describe common fractures of the scapula, clavicle, and proximal humerus.
8. Outline and describe methods of management and rehabilitation of fractures about the shoulder.
9. Describe methods of management and rehabilitation after shoulder arthroplasty.
10. Describe common mobilization techniques for the shoulder.

KEY TERMS

Subacromial rotator cuff impingement
Scapular stabilization exercises
Codman's pendulum exercises

Dislocation
Subluxation
Bankart lesion
Hill-Sachs lesion
TUBS
AMBRI

Capsulitis
Acromioclavicular (A-C) joint
Open reduction and internal fixation (ORIF)

CHAPTER OUTLINE

Subacromial Rotator Cuff Impingement
  Rehabilitation of Primary and Secondary Rotator Cuff Impingement
  Surgical Management of Shoulder Impingement and Rotator Cuff Tears
Glenohumeral Joint Instability and Dislocation
  Nonoperative Management
  Operative Management and Rehabilitation

Adhesive Capsulitis
Acromioclavicular Sprains and Dislocations
Scapular Fractures
Clavicle Fractures
Proximal Humerus Fractures
  Total Shoulder Arthroplasty
Mobilization of the Shoulder
  Mobilization of the Scapulothoracic Joint
  Mobilization of the Glenohumeral Joint

*Refer to orthopedic anatomy figures on the Evolve website.

This chapter introduces common injuries, treatment, and rehabilitation procedures related to the glenohumeral joint, acromioclavicular joint, scapula, and proximal humerus. To fully understand the rationale for specific rehabilitation programs after injury or disease of the shoulder complex and surrounding tissues, the physical therapist assistant (PTA) is strongly encouraged to review pertinent anatomy and kinesiology of the glenohumeral, acromioclavicular, and scapulothoracic joints. Furthermore, the PTA should review the mechanisms of tissue healing because these principles clarify tissue-healing concepts and reinforce the need for early protected motion after injury, immobilization, and recovery of strength and function after injury to the shoulder complex. This section focuses on the recognition of certain orthopedic injuries and rehabilitation procedures used to reduce pain and swelling, improve motion, restore strength and power, and return the patient to normal function.

SUBACROMIAL ROTATOR CUFF IMPINGEMENT

A common cause of shoulder pain and dysfunction in laborers, athletes, and persons who do repetitive overhead lifting is **subacromial rotator cuff impingement.** In this disorder, the tendons of the rotator cuff are crowded, buttressed, or compressed under the coracoacromial arch, resulting in mechanical wear, stress, and friction (Fig. 22-1).[7,9] Clinically, distinction must be made between primary and secondary impingement because there are important differences in treatment related to the cause of the impingement:[7,9]

1. Primary shoulder impingement refers to mechanical compression of the rotator cuff tendons, primarily the supraspinatus tendon,[21] as they pass under the coracoacromial ligament between the acromion and coracoid process.[7,13,21]
2. Secondary shoulder impingement is related to glenohumeral instability that creates a reduced subacromial space because the humeral head elevates and minimizes the area under the coracoacromial ligament.[7,9,13]

Age-related degenerative changes also can result in a decreased subacromial margin between the rotator cuff and coracoacromial arch. Bony osteophyte formation can occupy space under the anteroinferior surface of the acromion, which consequently reduces the available space.[21] The supraspinatus tendon is the most common structure involved with rotator cuff impingement; the vascularity of the supraspinatus tendon is causative.[7,9,21] An area just proximal to the insertion on the greater tuberosity is hypovascular and is commonly referred to as a "watershed zone," "critical zone," or "critical portion."[7,21,25] This area of relative transient hypovascularity occurs with repeated arm motions from abduction to adduction, which compromises the blood supply to the area.[7,25] The combination of reduced blood supply to the supraspinatus tendon and mechanical wear, stress, and friction as a result of repeated overhead motions can lead to primary impingement, supraspinatus tendinitis, and ultimately tears within the rotator cuff.[7,9,21]

The various stages of rotator cuff impingement are related to age and degenerative changes in the cuff itself. Neer has identified three specific stages of impingement (tendinitis):[7,9,17,21,25]

Stage I: Occurs in younger patients (usually under 25 years of age), but can occur at any age. Clinical features are edema and hemorrhage. Pain is worse with shoulder abduction greater than 90 degrees.[2-5] Essentially a reversible lesion that responds to conservative physical therapy interventions.[4]

Stage II: The fibrosis and tendinitis stage, which usually affects patients between the ages of 25 and 40 years.[3,4] Classified as irreversible because of long-term repeated stress wherein the supraspinatus tendon, biceps tendon, and subacromial bursa become fibrotic.[21] Pain is the predominant feature and occurs with daily activities; it frequently causes the patient difficulty at night.[21,25]

Stage III: Affects patients more than 40 years of age. Is characterized by tendon degeneration, rotator cuff tears, and rotator cuff ruptures.[13,21] Usually associated with a long history of repeated shoulder pain and dysfunction, as well as significant muscle weakness and atrophy.[21]

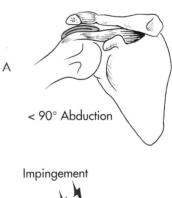

A

< 90° Abduction

Impingement

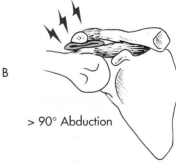

B

> 90° Abduction

Fig. 22-1 Subacromial rotator cuff impingement. **A,** Less than 90 degrees of abduction, no impingement occurs. **B,** Greater than 90 degrees of abduction results in subacromial soft-tissue impingement under the coracoacromial arch.

Various clinical tests can be used to identify the presence of pain related to specific maneuvers of the shoulder. During the initial evaluation performed by the physical therapist (PT), tests are used to elicit impingement signs. Pain signifies impingement with an arc of shoulder abduction between 60 and 120 degrees, pain with forward shoulder flexion, and pain with forced internal rotation with the affected arm abducted to 90 degrees.[7] In most cases flexion or abduction more than 80 or 90 degrees elicits pain. Therefore exercise and all activities that require the shoulder to flex or abduct past 80 or 90 degrees must be strictly avoided until all symptoms of pain have been eliminated.

Rehabilitation of Primary and Secondary Rotator Cuff Impingement

Kamkar, Irrgang, and Whitney have identified scapular weakness as leading to "function scapular instability," which affects scapular position during activities that cause a "relative decrease in the subacromial space."[9] This secondary impingement requires the scapulothoracic muscles to be strengthened and stabilized before specific rotator cuff weakness can be addressed. To effectively stabilize the humeral head so that it does not migrate superiorly, causing "winging" or "tipping," the scapular muscles (serratus anterior, upper, middle, and lower trapezius, levator scapulae, and rhomboid muscles) must be strengthened.[9] Thein[22] describes the clinical features of humeral head migration (secondary impingement) as possibly confusing the typical impingement picture. She reports:

> If the supraspinatus is overworked trying to stabilize the humeral head, then it is unable to effectively function to depress the humeral head. The resultant upward movement decreases the subacromial space and irritates the subacromial soft tissues, thus perpetuating the impingement process.[22]

The initial evaluation performed by the PT is crucial in determining which exercises are to be performed to help stabilize the scapula and which should be avoided initially to reduce rotator cuff irritation with glenohumeral instability or superior migration of the humeral head.

Scapular stabilization exercises are only one component of a successful rehabilitation program. In general a comprehensive rehabilitation program to address rotator cuff impingement, rotator cuff tendinitis (supraspinatus tendinitis), and degenerative tears of the rotator cuff tendons include modification of activities, local and systemic methods to control pain and swelling (nonsteroidal antiinflammatory drugs [NSAIDs], corticosteroid injections, ice, ultrasound, iontophoresis, phonophoresis), stretching and strengthening exercises, and a return to normal function after reevaluation by the PT and with continued maintenance of protective positions and general conditioning.[7,25]

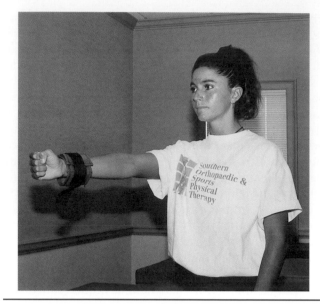

Fig. 22-2 Arm elevation in the sagittal plane.

The nonoperative treatment of impingement and symptomatic rotator cuff tears focuses on a three-phase criterion-based rehabilitation program advocated by Voight.[25] Phase I, the acute stage, concentrates on relief of symptoms and initiating exercises to improve or maintain motion. Because impingement symptoms usually are made worse with overhead activities, the patient must modify activities of daily living (ADLs) and all other motions that may place the shoulder at or above 80 to 90 degrees of abduction or forward flexion. Home activities that require modification include cleaning hard-to-reach places and painting overhead. Work site tasks that must be adapted include heavy overhead lifting, manual labor, reaching, and climbing. Sporting activities such as tennis, golf, swimming, and baseball also must be modified to avoid impingement. The key to remember in each case is *modification*, not elimination, of compromising activities. For example, for a recreational tennis player, overhead serving should be avoided but all other ground strokes can be maintained. For household activities and work site modifications, rearrangement and advanced planning of overhead tasks may be all that is needed to minimize the aggravating position of forward flexion or abduction past 80 or 90 degrees. The PTA must constantly reinforce the concept of protective positioning and should encourage compliance throughout the course of rehabilitation.

In addition to activity modification, management of pain and swelling can be achieved with various physician-prescribed oral NSAIDs and physical therapy agents. Usually ice packs, ultrasound, and some type of pharmacophoresis (iontophoresis and phonophoresis)[25] help control symptoms.

Throughout phase I, stretching exercises are performed to increase blood flow and contractility[7] and improve

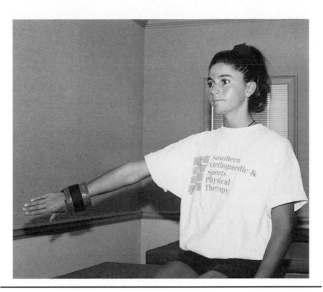

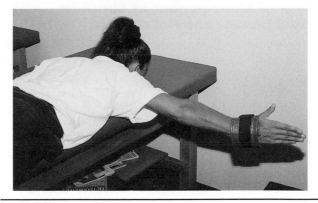

Fig. 22-4 Prone horizontal shoulder abduction with external rotation.

Fig. 22-3 Scaption. Shoulder elevation with internal rotation in the plane of the scapula.

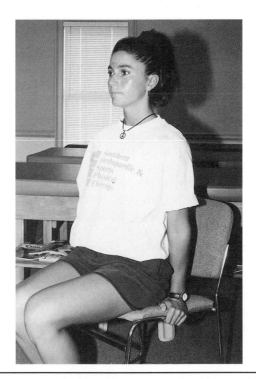

Fig. 22-5 Seated press-up.

motion. The PTA must pay particular attention to performing all stretching activities because many generalized shoulder stretches involve full forward shoulder flexion and abduction maneuvers. All phase I stretching should encourage nonballistic, slow, controlled, pain-free motion at less than 80 to 90 degrees of flexion and abduction. However, once symptoms are managed, the patient can perform all stretches involving flexion and abduction if these stretches do not produce symptoms. Depending on the initial evaluation data gathered by the PT, the patient may be instructed in two specific stretches that authorities[7,25] suggest are effective in addressing posterior capsular tightness. Shoulder adduction across the chest (cross-body stretching) and internal shoulder rotation are used cautiously to improve posterior capsular tightness and overcome the limitations on motion of internal rotation of the shoulder.

Initial strengthening activities can begin during phase I but generally are reserved for phase II, the recovery stage. Once the patient demonstrates improved motion without pain and can do ADLs without pain, phase II can begin. It emphasizes regaining the strength of the rotator cuff and scapular stabilizers, improving motion, and maintaining activity modifications. Specific rotator cuff strengthening exercises focus on the supraspinatus muscle. Studies[4,23] demonstrate that the supraspinatus, infraspinatus, subscapularis, deltoid, latissimus dorsi, and pectoral muscles are effectively strengthened by arm elevation in the sagittal plane (Fig. 22-2), shoulder elevation with internal rotation in the plane of the scapula (Fig. 22-3), prone horizontal shoulder abduction with external rotation (Fig. 22-4), and seated press-ups (Fig. 22-5).[4,22,23]

Scapular stabilization exercises also are encouraged as part of a comprehensive glenohumeral and scapulothoracic strengthening program. Electromyographic studies[16] have identified four basic scapular stabilization exercises that strengthen the upper, middle, and lower trapezius; the levator scapula; the rhomboid major; the pectoralis minor; and the middle and lower serratus anterior muscles.[16] The exercises are rowing, scapular plane elevation (scaption), press-ups, and push-ups followed by scapular protraction.[16] As strength improves and when motion increases, a gradual return to normal function signifies the beginning of phase III.

The process of functional recovery is slow and must be done cautiously. Overhead activities are introduced incrementally as the patient is able to demonstrate pain-free motion and the ability to perform strengthening activities.

Surgical Management of Shoulder Impingement and Rotator Cuff Tears

When physical therapy interventions fail to provide long-lasting relief and in cases of rotator cuff tears (Neer's stage III impingement, tendon degeneration, and cuff tears), various surgical procedures can be used to correct the underlying pathologic condition. With subacromial impingement not involving a specific rotator cuff tear, subacromial decompression can be used to "eliminate or diminish the abnormality causing the impingement between the humeral head and the undersurface of the acromion, allowing freer movement of the tendons without irritation."[25] Miller[14] has outlined surgical options that comprise subacromial decompression. These options include coracoacromial ligament resection (Fig. 22-6), anterior acromioplasty, excision of the outer end of the clavicle, osteotomies of the glenoid or acromion, acromionectomy, and combinations of these procedures.[14,25] If there is an associated rotator cuff tear (small tear less than 1 cm, medium tear less than 3 cm, large tear greater than 5 cm),[14] a subacromial decompression procedure is used in conjunction with direct repair of the rotator cuff defect.[14] The subacromial decompression procedure can be performed as an open arthrotomy or as an arthroscopic procedure.[7]

Rehabilitation after subacromial decompression or rotator cuff repair closely parallels nonoperative rehabilitation of rotator cuff impingement. However, time must be allowed for healing of the soft tissues and bone after surgery.

Some clearly identified differences exist between rehabilitation procedures used for decompression and small cuff tears (less than 1 cm) and repairs of medium (less than 3 cm) and large (greater than 5 cm) cuff tears with subacromial decompression.[7,14,25] With a small cuff tear repaired in conjunction with a decompression procedure, active motion and pain-free exercise can begin as soon as the patient can tolerate these activities.[7,14,25] However, if the rotator cuff tear is between 1 and 5 cm, tissue protection must be longer to allow for extensive soft-tissue healing. If full active range of motion (ROM) is allowed too early, healing of the rotator cuff may be compromised because of the stresses placed on the repaired tissues. Wilk and Mangine[28] state that "rehabilitation must match the surgical procedure"; therefore the PT must choose procedures to parallel the size of the cuff defect, "the adequacy of the repair,"[25] the type of surgical procedure used (open procedure-anterior deltoid fiber resection; mini–open procedure-lateral deltoid fiber splitting and arthroscopic decompression),[28] as well as the healing constraints necessary for a secure repair. Thus larger cuff tears require longer periods of time for recovery to achieve improved healing.

Generally, recovery after subacromial decompression with or without rotator cuff repair follows a prescribed

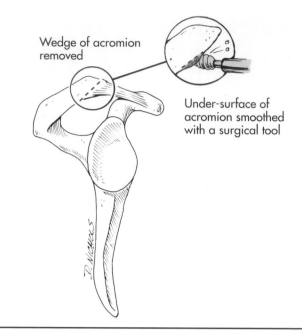

Wedge of acromion removed

Under-surface of acromion smoothed with a surgical tool

Fig. 22-6 Subacromial decompression for impingement.

three-phase rehabilitation program.[7,12,14,22,25,28] Phase I, the early recovery period (acute stage) or maximum-protection phase, lasts approximately 6 weeks[28] and focuses on control of pain and swelling with NSAIDs, oral analgesics, ice packs, ultrasound, phonophoresis, iontophoresis, transcutaneous electrical nerve stimulation (TENS), and various degrees and durations of immobilization, depending on the extent of tissue injury. The concept of early protected motion applies depending on the precise nature of the injury and which surgical procedure is used (if any). **Codman's pendulum exercises** can be used within the first few weeks to restore mobility and influence the mechanoreceptor system.

With small rotator cuff repairs (less than 1 cm),[28] isometric submaximal muscle sets of the shoulder abductors, external rotators, internal rotators, elbow flexors, and shoulder flexors can begin as early as pain allows. Active assisted ROM activities using a wall-pulley system begin during the first 3 weeks of recovery[28] and must be performed pain free. ROM and strength gradually increase as pain and swelling are controlled.

With increased strength and motion, phase II, the intermediate or fibroblastic phase, can begin.[25] It generally lasts from weeks 7 through 12 after surgery. During this moderate-protection phase, progressive motion can be used, although with caution for repetitive shoulder abduction and forward flexion above 90 degrees. Strength is increased using elastic tubing. In addition, dumbbell isotonic concentric and eccentric exercises, humeral head stabilization exercises (scapular stabilization exercises),[16] and the maintenance of pain and swelling control procedures are components of phase II management. Reinforcement of shoulder protection is then addressed, specifically avoiding repetitive motions that may slow the healing process. During phase II, local muscle resistance exercises are carried out in a pain-free, noncompromising position (above 90 degrees of shoulder abduction or flexion).

Phase III, the minimum-protection or maturation and tissue remodeling phase,[25] can begin once the patient can demonstrate increased motion without symptoms and with improved strength. This phase lasts approximately from week 13 to week 21[28] and is characterized by a gradual return to normal activities.

During each phase of recovery (maximum, moderate, and minimum protection), core rotator cuff strengthening exercises of forward flexion, scaption, prone horizontal abduction with external rotation, and press-ups, as well as scapular (humeral head) stabilization exercises of rowing, scaption, press-ups, and scapular protraction (push-ups with a plus),[9,16,23,25] form the foundation of improving strength that eventually leads to full functional recovery.

The recovery phases and periods of passive motion are extensive for rehabilitation after surgical repair of massive rotator cuff tears. Generally, no active shoulder motion or active concentric or eccentric strengthening is allowed for 3 to 4 months after surgery.[13,25] Extensive soft-tissue healing must proceed unabated to foster the recovery of functional motion and strength.

Initially the patient is placed in a brace, splint (airplane splint), sling, or abduction pillow after surgery to allow the repaired tissues of the rotator cuff and deltoid to be shortened. Early active muscle strengthening and active motion are avoided to allow for appropriate healing. Generally, passive ROM with full motion restriction is allowed during the first several weeks of recovery. Codman's pendulum exercises, as well as very gentle active assistive ROM activities, can begin 3 months after surgery.[13,25]

Submaximal isometrics and scapular stabilization exercises must be added cautiously 8 to 16 weeks after surgery.[13,25] Specific rotator cuff strengthening exercises[23] performed isotonically with dumbbells, Thera-Band, and similar devices are reserved until 3 to 4 months after surgery to accommodate the healing constraints of the tendons and muscles of the rotator cuff and deltoid. Full functional recovery of motion and strength may take up to 10 months after the repair of massive rotator cuff tears.[25]

GLENOHUMERAL JOINT INSTABILITY AND DISLOCATION

Dislocations and **subluxations** (partial dislocation) of the glenohumeral joint (the articulation between the humeral head and the glenoid fossa of the scapula) frequently occur after indirect trauma with the arm abducted, extended, and externally rotated (anterior dislocation) and with the arm abducted, flexed, and

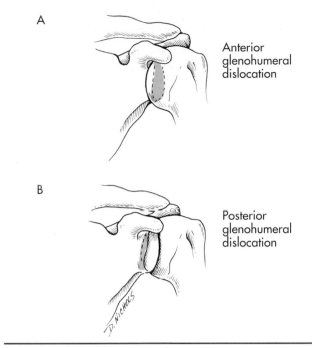

Fig. 22-7 Anterior and posterior glenohumeral dislocations. **A,** Anterior glenohumeral dislocation; **B,** posterior glenohumeral dislocation.

internally rotated (posterior dislocation) (Fig. 22-7).[21] The shoulder is the most commonly dislocated joint in the body,[13] and dislocation occurs in men more often than in women. Anterior dislocations occur more frequently than posterior dislocations.[13,21] Authorities classify shoulder instability based on frequency, cause, direction, and degree of instability.[13,19] Also rotator cuff tears of various dimensions (small, less than 1 cm; medium, less than 3 cm; and large, greater than 5 cm) occur with relative frequency.[21] Strege reports that rotator cuff tears occur 30% of the time with acute anterior dislocations in patients more than 40 years of age and 80% of the time in patients more than 60 years of age.[21]

Two associated injuries may occur as a result of acute glenohumeral dislocation and instability. Because the shoulder is the most mobile joint in the body, bony restrictions do not provide substantial restraint.[19] Rather, the fibrocartilaginous glenoid labrum deepens the articulation between the humeral head and bony glenoid fossa (Fig. 22-8). Injury to the labrum can occur if forces are great enough to dislocate the humerus from its confines within the glenoid. This injury is referred to as a **Bankart lesion**[7,13,19,21,22] and is defined as "an avulsion of the capsule and glenoid labrum off of the anterior rim of the glenoid resulting from traumatic anterior dislocation of the shoulder" (Fig. 22-9).[21]

The head of the humerus is subject to injury as a result of anterior shoulder instability. A **Hill-Sachs lesion** is a compression or "impaction fracture"[19] of the posterolateral aspect of the humeral head as a result of anterior

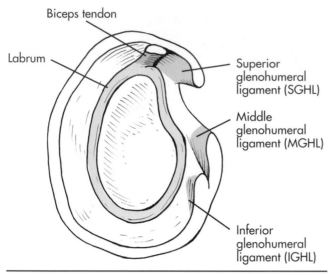

Fig. 22-8 Anatomy of glenoid labrum.

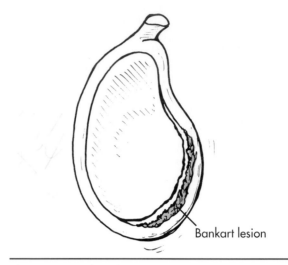

Fig. 22-9 Bankart lesion.

shoulder instability (Fig. 22-10).[7,13,14,19,21,22] This lesion results from instability and is not the essential cause of glenohumeral instability.[19]

As stated, anterior dislocations are more prevalent than posterior dislocations. However, shoulder instability can be defined as multidirectional, wherein the humeral head may sublux or dislocate anteriorly, interiorly, and posteriorly.[14,19,21]

Nonoperative Management

The initial management of acute shoulder dislocations (anterior and posterior) calls for a period of immobilization lasting for up to 6 weeks.[19,27] All positions that may reproduce the mechanism of dislocation are avoided.

Management of pain and swelling is addressed with physician-prescribed NSAIDs, analgesics, ice packs, electrical stimulation, or other physical agents. While the patient is immobilized, the hand, wrist, and elbow of the affected shoulder must receive active motion and rudimentary strengthening exercises that do not compromise the shoulder. Also a general conditioning program of strength, flexibility, and endurance activities can begin during immobilization. With an anterior shoulder subluxation (spontaneous reduction of the humeral head) or dislocation, the patient must avoid shoulder abduction and external rotation to allow proper capsular scarring and soft-tissue healing to occur. It is interesting to note that patients over age 40 who are not at significant risk of recurrent dislocation because of a relatively sedentary lifestyle may only need immobilization for a couple of weeks before rehabilitation can begin and motion can be regained.[19] Generally, ROM exercises are employed as the patient tolerates after immobilization.

Codman's pendulum exercises, active assistive stretching for flexion, and cable pulleys help the patient regain

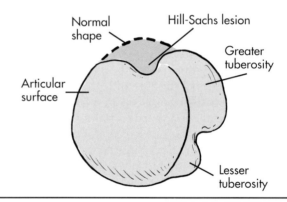

Fig. 22-10 Hill-Sachs lesion.

lost motion after relatively lengthy immobilization while protecting the shoulder from excessive abduction and external rotation.

Initial strengthening begins while the patient is immobilized and pain is controlled. Submaximal isometric exercises can be safely started while the patient's shoulder and arm are adducted and internally rotated in the shoulder sling and immobilizer. Isometric shoulder adduction and abduction, internal and external rotation, and flexion and extension can be performed at a pain-free level while immobilized. Once the patient can demonstrate an increase from submaximal isometric contractions to near-maximal contractions, progressive internal and external rotation can begin using latex rubber tubing with the affected shoulder in zero degrees of abduction.[27]

When the symptoms of pain are reduced and the intensity and quality of muscle contractions are improved, the patient may increase ROM activities to

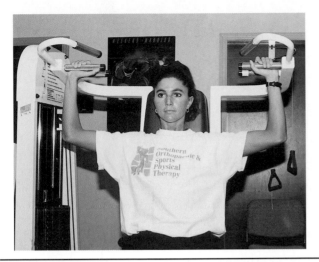

Fig. 22-11 Typical position for the performance of a seated overhead shoulder press. Notice the arms are held in an abducted and slightly externally rotated position.

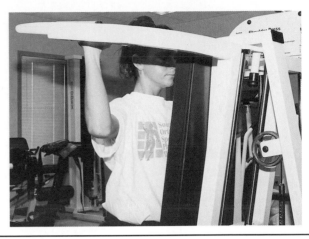

Fig. 22-12 If the patient faces the apparatus, the shoulder can be placed in a more protected position. Notice the upper arm is in a more adducted position, thereby reducing shoulder abduction and external rotation.

forward flexion, extension, scapular mobility, and internal and external rotation and abduction. As the patient progresses through the moderate-protection phase, combined shoulder abduction and external rotation are avoided. In fact, some authorities recommend avoiding extremes of shoulder abduction and external rotation for 3 months after removal of the sling.[19] The hallmark of the moderate- and minimum-protection phases of recovery after anterior shoulder dislocation or subluxation is progressive strengthening of the rotator cuff, anterior shoulder muscles, and scapular stabilizers, with particular attention given to eccentric strengthening of the posterior rotator cuff (infraspinatus and teres minor).[22] Latex rubber tubing and cuff weights are effective because of the wide variety of motions that can be addressed and can carry over to home exercises.

Synchronous shoulder motion, or scapulohumeral rhythm, must be addressed before and throughout recovery from a shoulder dislocation. The 2:1 ratio of motion between the scapula and glenohumeral joint (meaning that for every 2 degrees of glenohumeral flexion or abduction after the first 30 degrees of shoulder motion, the scapula must rotate upwardly 1 degree)[10] must be addressed early to prevent the facilitation of abnormal motions between the scapula and glenohumeral joint during strengthening activities. This can be accomplished adequately by focusing on normalized scapular motion and stabilization exercises during the early or maximum-protection phase as long as symptoms of pain and harmful glenohumeral joint positions are avoided.

Throughout each phase of recovery, various tissues that contain the humeral head in the glenoid fossa (glenoid labrum, capsule, and ligaments; superior, middle, and inferior glenohumeral ligaments; and musculotendinous rotator cuff) can be stressed or torn.

By definition, glenohumeral instability identifies ligamentous and capsular restraints as being "attenuated";[15] therefore the appropriate progressive application of strengthening activities for the rotator cuff and scapulothoracic muscles becomes central to the recovery of motion and function.

The criteria established by Wilk[27] to progress to the minimum-protection phase are described as follows:

- Full, nonpainful ROM
- No palpable tenderness
- Continued progression of shoulder strength

Thus the assistant must address functional motions and stimulate the afferent neural input system through closed kinetic chain activities. These enhance proprioception and promote dynamic joint stability.[25]

Initiating isotonic resistance exercises is quite challenging and stressful to the glenohumeral joint; consequently, many appropriate exercises must be modified to accommodate limitations of motion, pain, and the provocative positions of abduction and external rotation. For example, the overhead seated shoulder press can place the shoulder in a compromised position (Fig. 22-11), so the patient should consider turning and facing the apparatus, thereby reducing shoulder abduction and creating a more adducted shoulder posture (Fig. 22-12). The seated or supine chest press is another example of isotonic exercise that promotes anterior shoulder strength. However, this particular exercise can place the shoulder in a horizontally abducted position that stresses the anterior shoulder capsule, causing the head of the humerus to rock forward within the glenoid (Fig. 22-13). This exercise can be modified by adjusting the starting ROM to a more adducted shoulder posture and changing the hand position to a more neutral location (Fig. 22-14).

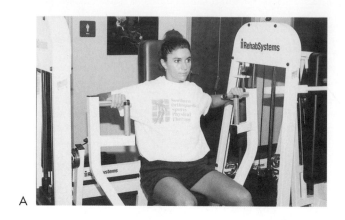

A

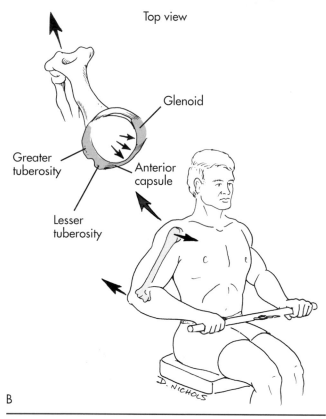

Top view

Glenoid

Greater
tuberosity

Anterior
capsule

Lesser
tuberosity

B

Fig. 22-13 A, Seated chest press. This initial position can place stress on the anterior shoulder capsule. **B,** In this figure, notice how the head of the humerus can rock forward within the glenoid, causing stress to the anterior shoulder capsule.

Cable systems offer various exercises and positions that duplicate functional activities. Wall pulleys and cable systems are particularly useful in athletic patients, because sport-specific tasks can be reproduced with this equipment.

Local muscle endurance activities are done using an upper body ergometer, closed kinetic chain "stepping" on a stair-stepper, or "walking" on a treadmill (Fig. 22-15). Weight bearing closed-chain exercises can be introduced gradually once the patient has regained sufficient

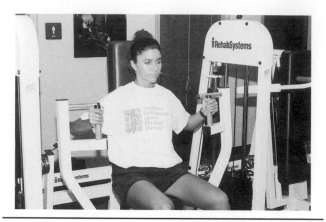

Fig. 22-14 Modification of the seated shoulder press can include adjusting the initial starting range of motion while also changing the hand position to avoid or limit horizontal abduction.

strength and motion to tolerate these challenging activities. The PT must identify the appropriate timetable for each patient with regard to advanced closed-chain resistance exercises. Initially, simple wall push-ups can provide needed proprioceptive stimulation to the mechanoreceptor system. Gradually, more challenging weight bearing activities that demand progressive control of the glenohumeral joint in multiplane and diagonal motions are added (Fig. 22-16). A balance board also can help train the shoulder muscles to respond and "fire" quickly for sufficient stabilization (Fig. 22-17). In addition, a Plyoball can be used as part of a closed-chain proprioception exercise program during the minimum-protection phase. The Plyoball can be used in a seated, weight bearing, or standing position (Fig. 22-18).

The process of recovery after shoulder dislocation matches the degree of injury (dislocation vs. subluxation), duration of immobilization (10 days to 6 weeks),[19] and any associated tissue damage (Bankart or Hill-Sachs lesion). Full functional recovery is not always possible. In some cases, minor stress causes the shoulder to dislocate again after acute traumatic dislocation. With repeated episodes of shoulder dislocation or subluxation, recurrent anterior instability can result.[20] If patients fail to respond to an aggressive physical therapy program, the physician may choose one of several operative procedures to correct the instability.[7,10,13,14,19–22,25] Miller[13] reports that most surgical candidates have recurrent traumatic anterior dislocations. Two distinct factors have been identified as helping to guide treatment decisions about anterior shoulder dislocations.[13,19,22] Patients with a *T*raumatic *U*nidirectional injury and a *B*ankart lesion frequently require *S*urgery **(TUBS).** Patients with *A*traumatic *M*ultidirectional *B*ilateral instability respond well to *R*ehabilitation, but occasionally require an *I*nferior capsular shift surgical procedure **(AMBRI).**[13,22]

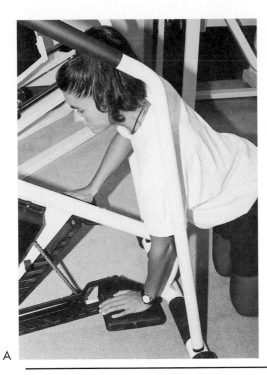

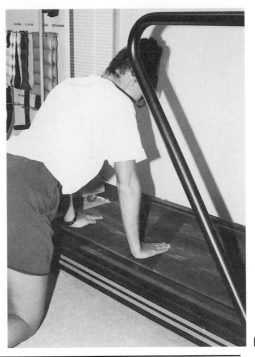

Fig. 22-15 **A,** Closed-chain stair-stepping activity; **B,** side stepping on a treadmill for upper extremity reciprocal opened- and closed-chain "walking."

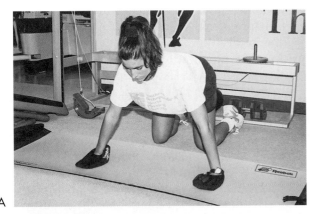

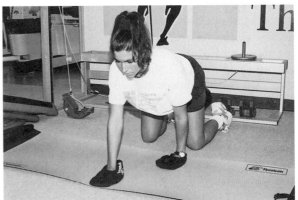

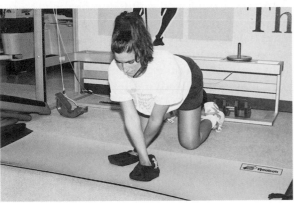

Fig. 22-16 Multiplane and diagonal closed-chain weight bearing activities. **A,** Shoulder abduction and adduction on a slide board in a kneeling position. Extreme caution must be taken to ensure that a limited range of abduction be allowed when initiating this activity. **B,** Shoulder flexion and extension in a kneeling position. When beginning all slide board activities the patient must be able to eccentrically and concentrically control the affected shoulder globally. **C,** Diagonal patterns on the slide board.

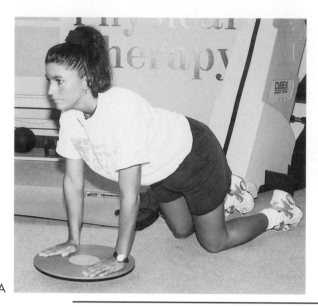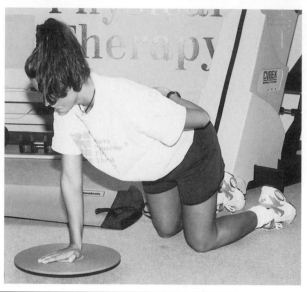

A   B

Fig. 22-17 Closed kinetic chain wobble board activity for stimulating shoulder stability. **A,** Initially, both arms are used when introducing this exercise. **B,** When strength, control, and confidence improve, the patient can progress to one arm.

Operative Management and Rehabilitation

Because *posterior* shoulder dislocations account for only 2% to 4% of all shoulder dislocations,[19] this discussion focuses on repairs and rehabilitation procedures to enhance joint stability and promote function in patients with *anterior* glenohumeral instability. Surgical procedures for shoulder instability can be classified as open or arthroscopic techniques.[19] The three general categories of open stabilization techniques are as follows:[13,19]

- Surgical repairs of Bankart lesions
- Procedures used to limit external rotation of the shoulder
- Bone block procedures and coracoid process transfers

The Bankart procedure essentially reattaches the torn capsule to the glenoid.[13] Anterior shoulder staple capsulorrhaphy (staple or repair of a joint capsule) can be used to reattach and tighten the torn capsule. A potential complication of this particular procedure is migration of the staple used to secure the torn capsule.[13] In the Magnusen-Stack procedure, the surgeon moves the subscapularis from the lesser to the greater tuberosity.[13,22] The primary disadvantage with this procedure is that the patient may be left with some residual decreased external rotation.[13,22]

An example of a coracoid transfer to increase anterior glenohumeral stability is the Bristow procedure.[13,22] This technique calls for the surgical repositioning of the coracoid process, the attached coracobrachialis, and the short head of the biceps to the glenohumeral neck[13,22] (Fig. 22-19). As with other transfer-type procedures that use bone and soft-tissue stabilization hardware

(e.g., screws or staples), a common complication is the potential for migration of the fixation devices and possible nonunion at the bone transfer site.[13] The capsular shift procedure transposes the capsule from an inferior position to a superior position and from superior to inferior position[13] (Fig. 22-20).

Anterior shoulder instability also can be corrected arthroscopically.[13,19,22] Interestingly, although arthroscopic techniques afford certain advantages over open surgical repairs (e.g., less postoperative pain and reduced soft-tissue damage), there appears to be a higher risk for recurrent dislocations as compared with open surgical procedures.[19]

Rehabilitation after open or arthroscopic stabilization for anterior glenohumeral instability varies and must specifically match the procedure.[27,28] Although postoperative rehabilitation closely parallels nonoperative rehabilitation, specific limitations result from the process of bone and soft-tissue healing. Each patient and surgical procedure must be addressed differently, and the following rehabilitation plan represents general principles only. It is not meant to demonstrate precise physical therapy interventions for all surgical cases.

Initial postoperative care begins with a period of immobilization in a sling or shoulder immobilizer to allow for appropriate soft-tissue healing.[7,14,19,20,22,25,27] During this period, medications for pain and swelling may be prescribed by the physician. Frequently, ice packs are applied to the shoulder for 15 to 20 minutes, three to five times daily, as part of the home program to control postoperative pain and swelling. Also the patient can actively perform finger, hand, wrist, and elbow mobility exercises. In addition, submaximal isometric

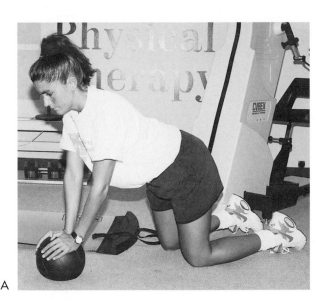

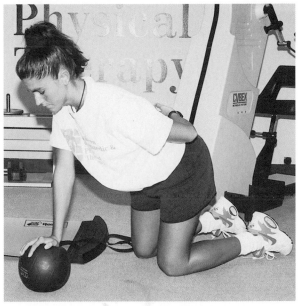

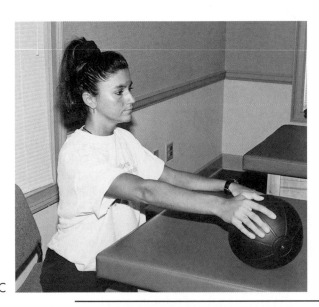

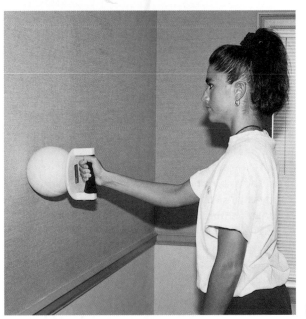

Fig. 22-18 Plyoball closed-chain proprioception exercises. **A,** The patient is introduced to this activity by using both arms. **B,** As strength, balance, and confidence improve, the patient can progress to one arm. **C,** If the patient is unable to perform vertical loading on the Plyoball, the patient may be started on this exercise in a seated position without vertical-compression loads. **D,** Standing wall pushes with the use of a Plyoball. Multiplanar stability is essential to perform any of these activities.

exercises can be initiated while the arm is still in the sling. These must be performed pain free.

The degree and direction of shoulder motion allowed are specific to the surgical procedure, the wishes of the physician, and the direction of the PT. Generally, shoulder shrugs; scapular protraction and retraction; Codman's pendulum exercises; various active assisted ROM exercises using a rope and pulley system, cane, or wand; and wall walking exercises can be used to

increase motion. The initiation of motion exercises is important because faulty scapulothoracic and glenohumeral mobility can be affected early. Care must be taken to encourage scapular motion, as well as glenohumeral mobility, and to identify any limitations affecting normal scapulohumeral rhythm. With certain procedures (e.g., coracoid transfers, muscle transfers, and bone block procedures), avoiding shoulder abduction and external rotation (in various degrees) early is

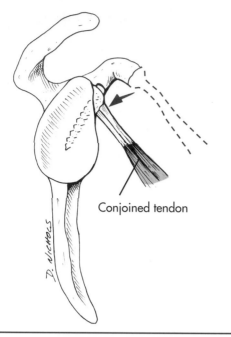

Fig. 22-19 Bristow procedure. Coracoid transfer to increase anterior glenohumeral stability.

Conjoined tendon

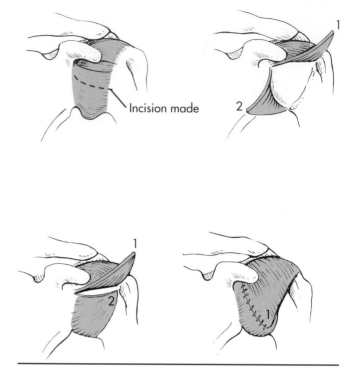

Incision made

Fig. 22-20 Capsular shift surgical procedure.

essential to allow bone and soft tissues to heal and not be overloaded. Therefore the assistant must be aware of the exact procedure used to understand the rationale behind limiting early active or passive shoulder abduction and external rotation.

Progressive motion and strengthening exercises are allowed as the patient is gradually weaned from the sling. Progressive shoulder strengthening must address both the glenohumeral and scapulothoracic joints. To recover functional mobility of the shoulder, a program of "proximal stability for distal mobility" is suggested.[24] Because the scapula forms the base of support for glenohumeral motion, stabilization exercises must be initiated.[16] However, with some muscle transfer procedures, the initiation of strengthening for a specific muscle group (transferred muscle group) may be deferred for longer periods of time for secure healing to take place. As the patient demonstrates improved mobility without complaints of pain, the quality of muscle contraction (from submaximal to maximal) must be encouraged gradually. Progressive resistive exercises using surgical tubing or dumbbells within an active, pain-free ROM can begin, along with more challenging flexibility exercises, between 6 and 8 weeks after surgery.[20]

The eccentric contraction phase of each exercise must be encouraged. Hisamoto[8] reports, "Rehabilitation must incorporate eccentric loading to be successful with overhead activities." Applying this concept during the early recovery phase involves emphasizing the eccentric loading phase of all internal rotation, abduction, external rotation, adduction, and shoulder flexion exercises. Local muscle endurance also must be considered once

the patient has achieved improved motion and strength. Usually an upper body ergometer or some other form of low-intensity, high-repetition shoulder-specific activity is appropriate. Functional activities, proprioception, and closed kinetic chain exercises, although necessary for functional recovery, may be delayed to allow for secure healing. However, weight bearing, closed-chain resistance exercises, and proprioception activities are necessary during the moderate- to minimum-protection phases of recovery to stimulate the mechanoreceptor system and encourage purposeful, functional motion that duplicates ADLs.

Generally the total length of rehabilitation after surgical stabilization of the glenohumeral joint ranges from 3 to 6 months, depending on the exact procedure used.[2]

ADHESIVE CAPSULITIS

Adhesive **capsulitis,** which is also referred to as "frozen shoulder," is characterized by decreased shoulder ROM, pain, capsular inflammation, fibrous synovial adhesions, and reduction of the joint cavity (Fig. 22-21).[3,13,26,32] Adhesive capsulitis occurs more commonly in females and affects patients between 40 and 60 years of age.[3,13,32] The two distinct classifications of "frozen shoulder" are primary and secondary adhesive capsulitis. Primary idiopathic frozen shoulder is the most common lesion and occurs spontaneously from unknown causes. Secondary adhesive capsulitis generally occurs after trauma or immobilization.[26,32]

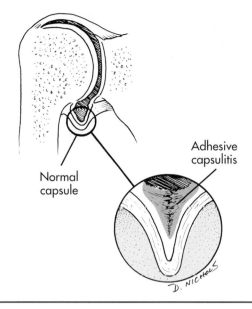

Normal capsule

Adhesive capsulitis

D. NICHOLS

Fig. 22-21 Adhesive capsulitis, or "frozen shoulder."

Among older patients, secondary adhesive capsulitis can develop because of limited immobilization for as little as 1 or 2 days.[5] In the early stages of this disabling condition, pain occurs both at rest and during activity.[5,26] However, as the condition progresses, pain gradually subsides, then spontaneously disappears. Severely restricted motion and profound loss of function remain.[5,26,32] During the acute painful phase, treatment is focused on controlling inflammation and symptoms of pain. Physician-prescribed analgesics, NSAIDs, and intraarticular steroid injections can provide some pain relief.[26]

Physical therapy interventions during this acute painful stage include the judicious use of ice, heat, ultrasound, iontophoresis, phonophoresis, and TENS.[3] Also, central to this initial management phase is the stimulation of pain-free motion and relaxation of muscle guarding of the glenohumeral joint, cervical area, and scapulothoracic muscles.[3] Passive, active, and active assisted motion exercises must occur within a pain-free ROM to stimulate removal of metabolic waste, increase local blood flow, and assist in the reduction of edema in the local tissues.[3,26] Codman's pendulum exercises must be performed during this acute stage within a pain-free range. These exercises can be preceded by the use of thermal agents (ice, moist heat, ultrasound, phonophoresis, and iontophoresis) to minimize spasm and pain. Both wand and rope and pulley systems can be used early if they are performed in a slow, controlled, pain-free ROM. For severely restricted glenohumeral motion, the PT may prescribe the application of specific joint mobilization techniques to help modulate pain and reduce muscle guarding.[3,5,26,32] As addressed, grades I and II low-amplitude physiologic and accessory oscil-

lations can help encourage relaxation while reducing pain.[3,5,26]

If the scapula is not stable and free from restriction while the patient attempts to regain shoulder motion and function, normal scapulohumeral rhythm cannot be obtained. Therefore early scapular stabilization exercises[16] can be employed as long as pain does not inhibit the correct performance of the exercise.[16] Normalized motion must precede specific strengthening activities to avoid developing faulty shoulder mechanics.

The complete restoration of glenohumeral joint mobility is the goal of treatment for the late stage of adhesive capsulitis.[3,26] The PT must identify the appropriate application of increased joint mobilization techniques to address specific capsular restrictions and initiate more challenging progressive resistance exercises. When the patient demonstrates improved glenohumeral motion and appropriate scapulohumeral rhythm, strengthening exercises can begin for the deltoid, scapular muscles, rotator cuff, and upper-arm muscles.[5]

Although control of pain and inflammation is the primary feature of early physical therapy management, submaximal isometric exercise can be used to initiate strengthening if pain is not increased with exercise. Progressing from submaximal isometrics to maximal isometrics usually precedes the use of latex rubber tubing, cuff weights, or dumbbells for concentric and eccentric exercises. A comprehensive series of rotator cuff exercises[23] and scapular stabilization exercises[16] can be encouraged as early as pain and motion allow. To address normalized function, the patient does closed-chain resistance exercises and overhead loading along with proprioception exercises (e.g., balance board, slide board, and Plyoball) in a sequential, orderly fashion once sufficient strength, improved motion, and scapulohumeral rhythm have been established. Local muscle endurance activities focus on purposeful, functional movements that duplicate ADLs.

Again, pain control, restoration of motion, and improved function must be reinforced continually to encourage compliance with a home exercise program and the avoidance of positions that may exacerbate pain and muscle guarding.

ACROMIOCLAVICULAR SPRAINS AND DISLOCATIONS

Ligamentous sprains of the **acromioclavicular (A-C) joint** usually result from a fall on the acromion (direct force)[1] or when force is transmitted from a fall on an outstretched arm proximally to the A-C joint (indirect force).[1,30] A-C joint sprains and dislocations are graded according to the degree of injury to specific ligamentous structures (A-C and coracoclavicular ligaments), as well as the position of the clavicle in complete rupture of both the A-C and coracoclavicular ligaments, as follows:[1,13,30,32]

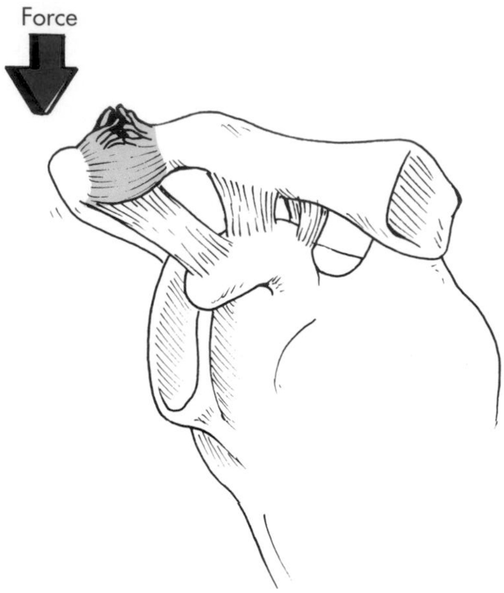

Force

Force

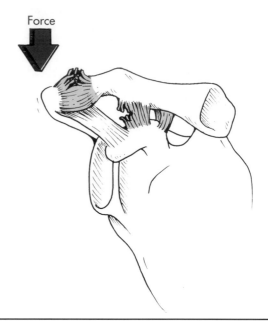

Fig. 22-22 Grade I acromioclavicular (A-C) joint sprain. Partial tear of the A-C ligaments.

Fig. 22-23 Grade II acromioclavicular (A-C) sprain. Rupture of the A-C ligaments and partial tearing of the coracoacromial ligaments.

First-degree, grade I A-C joint sprain: Characterized by partial tearing of the A-C ligaments, with resultant joint tenderness over the A-C joint, no joint instability or laxity of the ligament, and minimal loss of function (Fig. 22-22).[1,13,30,32]

Second-degree, grade II A-C sprain: Complete rupture of the A-C ligaments with partial tearing of the coracoacromial ligaments.[1,13,30,32] The patient has moderate pain, some dysfunction (reduction in shoulder abduction and adduction), and a palpable gap between the acromion and the clavicle (Fig. 22-23).[1,13,30,32]

Third-degree, grade III A-C ligament injury: Dislocation between the acromion and clavicle where both the A-C and coracoclavicular ligaments are ruptured and the distal clavicle becomes displaced superiorly (Fig. 22-24). Patients demonstrate marked pain and severe limitation of shoulder motion.[1]

Three additional classifications have been proposed that describe the degree of vertical, posterior, and inferior separation of the clavicle in a grade III A-C dislocation.[1,13,30,32]

Rehabilitation and management of grade I A-C sprains focus on symptomatic relief. Typically, pain is controlled with the use of ice packs, NSAIDs, analgesics, and rest. Because the A-C ligaments have been partially torn, the A-C joint must be protected from further direct or indirect forces that may stress the A-C ligaments. The patient may be allowed to resume activities within 2 weeks and usually does not require a rehabilitation program of significant duration.[1]

Grade II A-C sprains require more direct attention to approximate the torn A-C ligaments and allow for secure ligament healing. Usually this injury is managed nonoperatively using a shoulder harness or sling, which

depresses the clavicle and supports the arm to provide close approximation of the torn ligaments. For A-C ligaments to heal, authorities advocate 3 to 6 weeks of "continuous uninterrupted pressure on the superior aspect of the clavicle"[30] after a grade II A-C sprain.

As noted, there is usually a palpable step-off between the acromion process and distal clavicle with grade II A-C sprains. This deformity represents a permanent loss of joint continuity because of lost ligamentous support between the acromion and clavicle.[1]

The rehabilitation program for a grade II A-C sprain commences during immobilization. Symptomatic relief includes ice packs, NSAIDs, analgesics, ultrasound, phonophoresis, iontophoresis, and TENS to help minimize pain and inflammation. Immobilization is used in the maximum-protection phase, with patient education focusing on the avoidance of both direct and indirect forces that stress the A-C ligaments. During immobilization, submaximal isometrics can be performed for all muscles of the shoulder girdle. However, care must be taken to avoid contractions that stress the A-C joint in the sling or shoulder harness. Active shoulder motion can begin after the immobilization device is removed. Even after immobilization, the torn ligaments are not fully recovered and still must be protected from inappropriate stress.

The moderate-protection phase begins with active shoulder motions and active assisted rope and pulley activities. The patient is encouraged to perform active shoulder flexion, abduction to tolerance, and shrugs, which promote activation of the trapezius and levator scapula muscles. The patient must avoid downward dis-

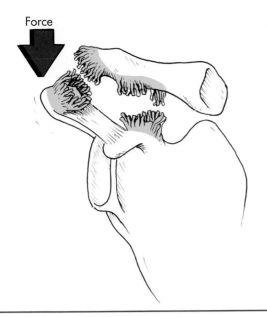

Fig. 22-24 Grade III acromioclavicular (A-C) sprain. Both the A-C and coracoacromial ligaments are ruptured.

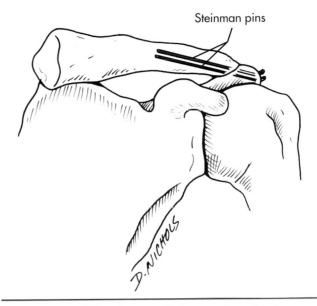

Fig. 22-25 Stabilization surgical procedure for the acromioclavicular (A-C) joint. Steinman pins are inserted to stabilize and approximate the A-C joint.

placement of the scapula or distraction of the humerus, both of which stress the A-C joint.

Progressive-resistive exercises are initiated during the moderate-protection phase and include scapular stabilization exercises, deltoid strengthening, and specific rotator cuff exercises. Latex rubber tubing, cuff weights, and dumbbells are effective and versatile for compliance and carryover to a prescribed home exercise program. As mentioned, the performance of scapular and humerus elevation exercises helps approximate the torn ligaments and provides dynamic muscular support to the torn structures. However, with both active and resistance exercises the downward or "relaxation" phase of shoulder shrugs can create unwanted traction on the A-C joint. Therefore the patient must perform the contraction or elevation phase of the shoulder shrug to tolerance but limit the eccentric lowering phase to avoid distraction of the A-C joint. As with all other injuries, the whole person should be addressed during each phase of recovery. For example, during the maximum-protection phase of recovery, while the patient is immobilized, it is appropriate to encourage active and resistive exercises for the hand, wrist, and elbow of the affected arm if no excessive stress is directed to the A-C joint. In addition, a general conditioning program is warranted to improve or maintain aerobic fitness, strength, and flexibility.

The treatment of grade III A-C sprains (dislocation of the distal clavicle and acromion process) is controversial.[1,30] Although many surgeons advocate open surgical repair, others favor closed reduction, immobilization, and progressive rehabilitation. The nonoperative treatment of grade III A-C sprains is centered on reducing

the dislocation and maintaining the reduction in immobilization for up to 6 weeks.[1,30] The goals of the initial course of treatment in physical therapy is to minimize pain and swelling, with the judicious use of ice, iontophoresis, phonophoresis, ultrasound, physician-prescribed NSAIDs, analgesics, and protection of the A-C joint from unwanted stress. To ensure proper healing of the ligaments, the rehabilitation team must continuously reinforce compliance using the immobilizer for the entire period prescribed by the treating physician.

While the patient is immobilized, submaximal isometric exercises can be initiated for the shoulder and scapula if no stress is applied to the healing ligaments. As with grade II A-C sprains, the hand, wrist, and elbow of the affected arm can be safely and effectively strengthened during immobilization. Generally the nonoperative treatment of grade III sprains parallels the treatment plan for grade II sprains. The primary differences are the longer duration of immobilization and the more cautious and delayed application of motion and resistance exercises so as not to adversely affect ligament healing. In some cases, nonoperative treatment is ineffective and surgical correction must be addressed.

Four general categories of grade III A-C repairs have been reported.[26] The surgeon may elect to insert pins directly through the A-C joint to stabilize and approximate the joint (Fig. 22-25). Another procedure calls for the surgeon to place sutures around the distal clavicle and the coracoid process to stabilize the joint (Fig. 22-26). The surgeon also may place a screw between the clavicle and coracoid process to provide more rigid stability to the A-C joint (Fig. 22-27). In addition, the distal clavicle may be excised.[30]

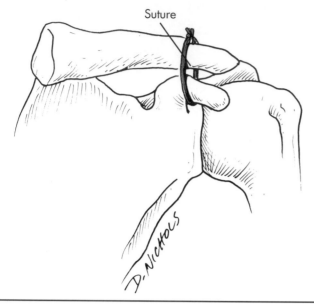

Fig. 22-26 Stabilization of the acromioclavicular joint by suturing the distal clavicle and the coracoid process.

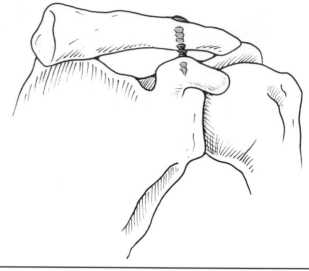

Fig. 22-27 A screw can be inserted between the clavicle and the coracoid process to stabilize the acromioclavicular joint.

Active motion and light resistance exercises for the hand, wrist, and elbow of the affected limb are encouraged in the early- or maximum-protection phase. Isometric exercises focus on the shoulder and scapular muscles once the A-C joint is stabilized and protected from unwanted forces. Progressive-active and active-assisted shoulder motion is allowed as pain and soft-tissue healing progress. Bergfeld[1] advocates light resistive exercises after 3 weeks and more progressive weight-lifting exercises 8 to 10 weeks postoperatively. Once the sling is removed, a progressive return to function closely follows the patient's level of motion and strength. As stated, heavy, intense resistance exercises must be delayed for 8 weeks until secure union has occurred, pain is abolished, and active shoulder motion returns.

SCAPULAR FRACTURES

Most scapular fractures result from direct, severe trauma.[11,29] Therefore there is a high incidence of significant associated injuries, including other fractures, glenohumeral dislocations, pneumothorax, and neurovascular injuries.[11,13,21,29] Interestingly fractures of the scapular body (Fig. 22-28) are the most common (49% to 89%)[29] and demonstrate the highest incidence of associated injuries (35% to 98%).[21] However, the treatment of fractures to the scapular body is conservative if associated injuries have not occurred, using ice and immobilization with a sling for 2 to 3 weeks.[11,21,29] During the immobilization period, hand, wrist, and elbow exercises can be initiated for the affected arm along with a general conditioning program. Early passive ROM exercises for the shoulder begin as the pain and swelling subside.

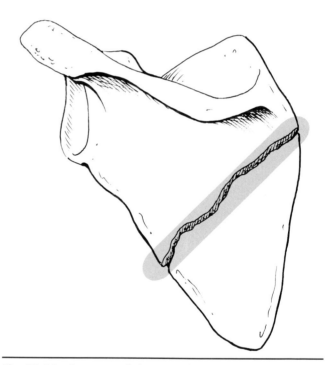

Fig. 22-28 Fracture of the scapular body.

Isometric exercises performed submaximally also can be initiated early if the patient remains pain free. As pain and swelling subside, strengthening exercises can be added within a pain-free ROM. Nonunion and malunion of this fracture are rare and usually are not associated with a loss of function or clinical symptoms.[21,29]

The second most common scapular fracture occurs to the glenoid neck (Fig. 22-29). If the fracture is extraarticular, Williams and Rockwood[29] suggest that healing can occur at 6 weeks and that management involves

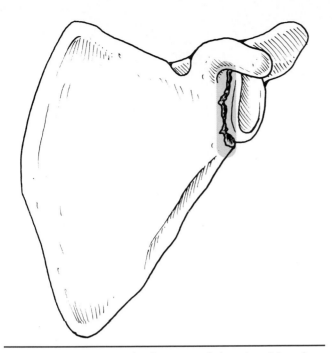

Fig. 22-29 Extraarticular fracture of the glenoid neck.

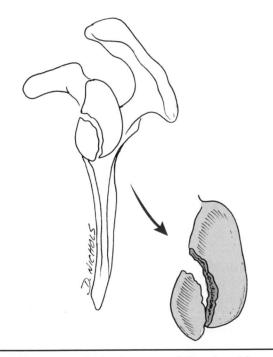

Fig. 22-30 Intraarticular fracture of the glenoid.

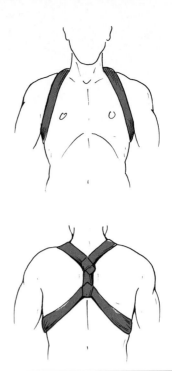

Fig. 22-31 Figure-of-eight bandage for alignment and stabilization of clavicle fractures.

needed to stabilize the fragments.[29] Usually a screw is inserted into the fracture fragments; therefore immobilization is needed to minimize stress at the fracture site. Pendulum exercises can be initiated soon after surgery to minimize postoperative joint stiffness. Although gentle passive shoulder flexion and external rotation are initiated 2 to 3 weeks postoperatively, active stretching and resistance exercises must be deferred for up to 6 to 8 weeks to allow for secure bone healing.[29]

CLAVICLE FRACTURES

Fractures of the clavicle occur as a result of direct or indirect trauma. These injuries are common and primarily affect men under 25 years of age.[33]

Care is focused on achieving reduction of the fracture fragments, maintaining the reduction, and minimizing the immobilization of the glenohumeral joint of the affected arm.[33] Usually the patient is placed in a commercially available figure-of-eight bandage (Fig. 22-31) to maintain proper alignment of the area. The duration of immobilization varies, but authorities suggest that healing takes 4 to 6 weeks or longer.[33]

During the initial period of immobilization, with the figure-of-eight bandage, the hand, wrist, and elbow of the affected arm are exercised with active motion and resistance exercises. Unwanted stress to the fracture site is avoided during this period. In addition, the patient may perform gentle pendulum exercises and submaximal isometrics for the shoulder and scapula once pain has been controlled.

conservative symptomatic care. Glenoid fractures also can be intraarticular, where the fracture extends through the glenoid fossa (Fig. 22-30). The treatment of these fractures depends on whether or not there is associated glenohumeral instability. If no instability is present, then these fractures are treated with sling immobilization and a return to motion and strength.[29] However, if there is glenohumeral instability associated with an intraarticular glenoid fracture, then surgical repair is

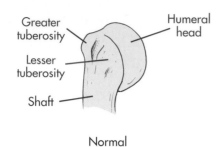

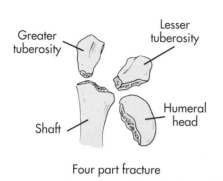

Fig. 22-32 **A,** Normal anatomy of proximal humerus. **B,** Four-part fracture of the proximal humerus.

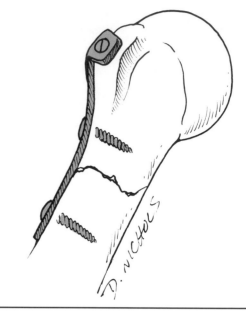

Fig. 22-33 Open reduction with internal fixation procedure for transverse proximal humerus fracture. Fracture site fixation with side plate and screws.

Active shoulder flexion must not be greater than 40 to 50 degrees until after 4 to 6 weeks[29] (although patients may be encouraged to perform gentle active shoulder motion no greater than 40 degrees when pain free). As the healing process continues and when bone healing is confirmed radiographically (approximately 4 to 6 weeks), greater degrees of shoulder motion are allowed, with progressive resistive exercises added as tolerated.

If the fracture is located at the distal end of the clavicle, open reduction and internal fixation may be more appropriate, because these fractures tend to be unstable and do not maintain proper alignment with a figure-of-eight bandage.[21] The fracture fragments of a displaced distal clavicle fracture usually are secured with an intramedullary fixation pin.[21]

PROXIMAL HUMERUS FRACTURES

Proximal humerus fractures usually are classified according to a four-part classification.[11,13,18,21] The four parts are the humeral head, lesser tuberosity, greater tuberosity, and humeral shaft (Fig. 22-32).[13,18,21]

Physical therapy management of humerus fractures depends on the severity and complexity of the fracture, as well as the means used to secure fixation of the fracture site. Generally with nondisplaced one-part fractures (the most common type), the affected arm is placed in a sling for a period of time and the patient is given analgesics and encouraged to apply ice liberally to minimize pain and swelling. Within the first 2 or 3 weeks, gentle active motion is allowed, as well as active motion of the elbow, wrist, and hand of the affected arm.[11] In fact, the patient may be allowed to remove the sling for active motion exercises a few times each day.[11,13]

Submaximal shoulder isometrics are initiated as early as pain allows. Perhaps the most salient aspect of physical therapy care in proximal humerus fracture is the functional restoration of glenohumeral motion and strength after protracted periods of immobility to allow for appropriate bone healing. Early scapular motion exercises minimize the restriction of scapular mobility. Submaximal scapular stabilization exercises[16] also can be encouraged early, as pain allows, to provide a stable base for glenohumeral motion exercises. Progressive motion and resistance exercises for the deltoid, rotator cuff, and upper arm muscles closely parallel bone healing and the patient's ability to demonstrate improved motion without pain.

Other more complex fractures can require **open reduction and internal fixation (ORIF)** with screws and a plate (Fig. 22-33), as well as prolonged periods of immobilization. As with all fractures, during immobility the patient can participate in a total body-conditioning program that does not compromise the healing of the fracture. In addition, the hand, wrist, and elbow of the affected limb must be exercised without stressing the fracture site.

The ultimate task after the healing of humerus fractures is regaining purposeful, functional strength and motion of the glenohumeral joint. Indeed, the time necessary to heal significant fractures may cause serious glenohumeral and scapular restrictions. The long-term healing restraints of bone form the primary guide for the physician and PT in deciding when to employ progressive motion activities and when to initiate strengthening tasks without compromising the fracture site.

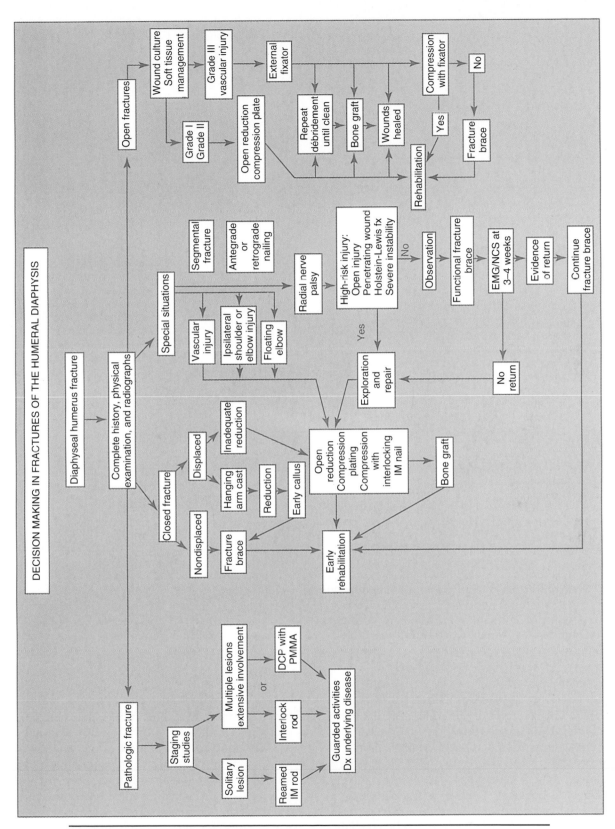

Algorithm for management of humeral shaft fractures.
IM, Intramedullary; *DCP,* dynamic compression plate; *PMMA,* polymethyl methacrylate; *Dx,* diagnosis; *fx,* fracture; *EMG/NCS,* electromyography/nerve conduction study. (From Browner BD, Jupiter J, Levine A, et al: Skeletal Trauma, 3rd ed, vol 2. Philadephia, WB Saunders, 2003.)

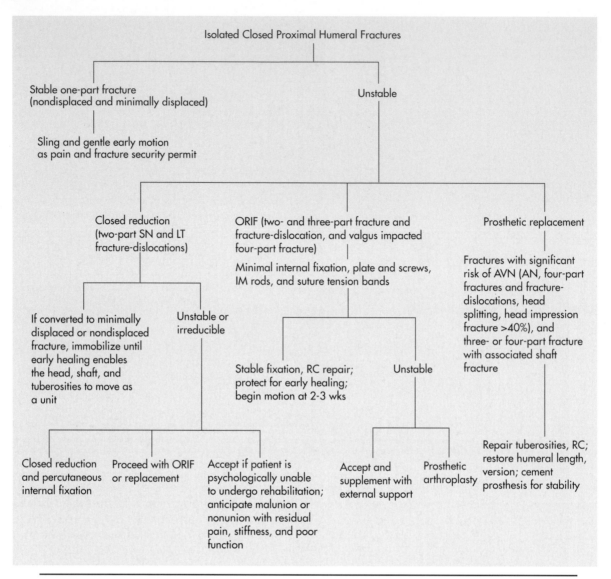

Algorithm for isolated proximal humerus fractures.
AN, Anatomic neck; *AVN,* avascular necrosis; *IM,* intramedullary; *LT,* lesser tuberosity; *ORIF,* open reduction and internal fixation; *RC,* rotator cuff; *SN,* surgical neck. (From Browner BD, Levine A, Jupiter J, et al, eds: Skeletal Trauma, 3rd ed, vol 2. Philadelphia, 2003, WB Saunders.)

Avascular necrosis (AVN) may be a risk with some significant fractures (displaced fractures of the anatomical neck).[11] For example, in an older population of patients with advancing osteoporosis who have a four-part proximal humerus fracture, internal fixation may be poor because of the osteopenic bone. A prosthetic humeral head may be more appropriate in this case.[21]

As the fracture begins to stabilize, and under the direction and supervision of the PT, some patients begin closed kinetic chain exercises to stimulate the mechanoreceptor system (afferent neural input system) of the elbow, shoulder, and wrist and to effect proper bone healing (Wolff's law) by providing submaximal intermittent stress to the healing bone.

The PTA participates in the rehabilitation process of proximal humerus fractures by following and supervising a comprehensive program of early protected limited ROM, submaximal isometrics for the scapular stabilizers,[16] rotator cuff, and upper arm muscles, and by providing continued protection for the injured site. As pain, motion, and bone healing progress, the PTA must carefully observe the scapulothoracic and glenohumeral motion. If scapulohumeral rhythm is adversely affected, specific attention must be addressed to regain a stable scapula and proper glenohumeral motion. In many cases if a restriction is noted, the PT may use scapular and glenohumeral mobilization techniques to modulate pain and encourage improved motion. However, the fracture site must be secure and stable, with radiographic confirmation of this, and the physician must order this protocol before mobilization can commence.

Functional shoulder activities and resistance exercises are added gradually as bone healing advances and the patient demonstrates greater confidence, motion, and strength without pain. Proprioception and closed kinetic chain activities also may be added during the minimum-protection phase of recovery in preparation for normalized purposeful motion and strength of the involved limb.

Total Shoulder Arthroplasty

With severe four-part fractures of the proximal humerus, avascular necrosis of the humeral head, osteoporosis, rheumatoid arthritis, and advanced osteoarthritis, the proximal humerus may be replaced with a prosthesis, or a total shoulder arthroplasty may be indicated (Fig. 22-34).[5,6,21] The condition of the rotator cuff is a significant feature in patients receiving a hemiarthroplasty or total shoulder arthroplasty. Goldstein[5] reports that in patients suffering from rheumatoid arthritis, as many as 38% have a torn rotator cuff. If a rotator cuff tear is repaired in addition to the arthroplasty, postoperative immobilization may be as long as 6 to 8 weeks, with the affected arm held in an abduction splint to allow for healing of the repaired cuff.[5,6]

Thus a rotator cuff repair added to shoulder arthroplasty guides the course of rehabilitation and dictates the need for a protracted period of immobility in addition to a longer program of rehabilitation.[5] In addition, in terms of restoration of shoulder motion, if the rotator cuff is not repaired, postoperative abduction averages 143 degrees, whereas patients requiring rotator cuff repair may achieve an average of only 63 degrees of shoulder abduction.[6]

The course of rehabilitation after shoulder arthroplasty usually allows for early (day 1 or 2) gentle active assisted ROM and isometric exercises. Muscle contractions of the deltoid are contraindicated in cases of rotator cuff repair. In these cases, isometric exercise must be deferred until soft-tissue healing has occurred to the repaired deltoid and cuff.[6] Usually during the first postoperative week, the patient is allowed active exercise of the wrist, hand, and elbow of the affected shoulder. The postoperative immobilizer also is frequently removed for hygiene and exercises.[5,6] By the end of the first week, the sling may be removed and Codman's pendulum exercises initiated while active assisted ROM exercises are continued.[5] At the end of the second postoperative week, the patient is introduced to scapular motion and stabilization exercises while the quantity and quality of isometric exercises and motion exercises are progressed.[5] The assistant must encourage compliance with a comprehensive home exercise program of motion and strength. The use of wand exercises and rope and pulley systems at home is appropriate. By week 6 the use of light resistance exercise can begin.[5] Latex rubber tubing is an effective tool for the home exercise program.

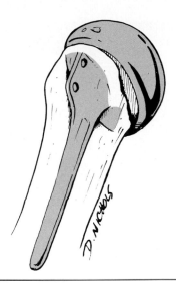

Fig. 22-34 Proximal humerus prosthesis.

If the patient has received a rotator cuff repair, the sequence of care and initiation of resistance exercise and active shoulder motion are delayed.[6] Functional use of the affected arm can be expected around 6 months postoperatively. However, Goldstein suggests that for optimal results, the patient should participate in an active home exercise program for up to 2 years after surgery.[5]

MOBILIZATION OF THE SHOULDER

The precise application of specific peripheral joint mobilization techniques is extremely effective for pain reduction and restoration of normalized joint motion. In addition to various soft-tissue injures and fractures, immobilization frequently causes limitations in scapulothoracic and glenohumeral mobility. For a normalized scapulohumeral rhythm to be restored, any limitations in motion must be identified early in the rehabilitation period.

During the initial immobilization, the PT documents all limitations of specific joint motion. Each limitation is addressed as part of the rehabilitation program. However, if the PTA recognizes delayed restoration of motion, reduced motion, or increased pain during the rehabilitation program, then he or she immediately must communicate this to the PT.

The following scapular and glenohumeral mobilization techniques represent only a few of the many techniques available. The PT decides which specific technique is to be used, when to apply the technique, in which direction, and with what amplitude, grade, or oscillation.

Before the PTA uses any mobilization technique, the position and comfort of the patient must be assessed. The use of oral physician-prescribed analgesics, thermal agents (e.g., heat, ultrasound, and ice), and proper body and limb positioning enhance relaxation and compliance during treatment.

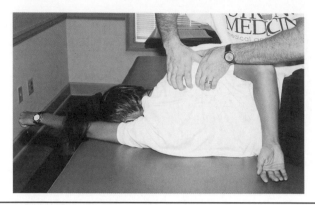

Fig. 22-35 Vertebral border scapular distraction.

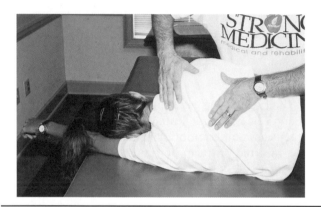

Fig. 22-36 Superior and inferior glide of the scapula.

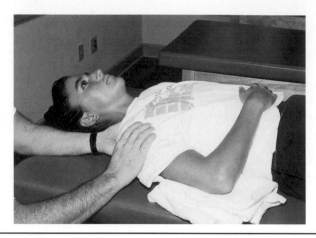

Fig. 22-37 Anterior and posterior glide of the gleno-humeral joint.

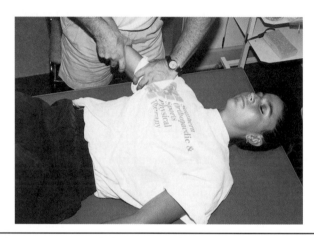

Fig. 22-38 Lateral distraction of the humeral head.

Mobilization of the Scapulothoracic Joint

While the patient is in a side-lying position on the unaffected side, the scapula can be effectively mobilized in a superior and inferior direction, as well as distracted from the thorax.[31] To distract the scapula, the PTA should stand facing the patient. The PTA should firmly grasp the medial or vertebral border of the affected scapula and purposefully distract the scapula away from the thorax (Fig. 22-35).[31] To glide the scapula superiorly and inferiorly, the PTA should assume the same position and support the inferior border of the scapula with one hand while placing the opposite hand on the superior border of the scapula. The PTA should use the hand on the inferior border to direct a force to glide the scapula in a superior direction, then use the hand on the superior border to direct a force to glide the scapula in an inferior direction (Fig. 22-36).[31]

Mobilization of the Glenohumeral Joint

Anteroposterior glide of the glenohumeral joint can be accomplished with the patient supine. The PTA should sit near the affected shoulder. In this position, Wooden recommends putting towels under the elbow of the affected shoulder to place the humerus in a more horizontal position.[31] The humeral head should be grasped firmly with the thumb and fingers of one hand while the scapula is actively stabilized with the other hand. If

the glenohumeral joint is stiff and motion is applied to the joint without stabilizing the scapula, the glenohumeral joint and scapula will move as a single unit. While stabilizing the scapula with one hand, the other hand is used on the humeral head to provide an anteriorly or posteriorly directed force (Fig. 22-37).

Lateral distraction of the humeral head can also be achieved while the patient is supine. The PTA should sit near the affected shoulder; then abduct the affected shoulder to 45 degrees and flex the elbow of the affected shoulder to 90 degrees. The flexed elbow should rest on and be supported by the PTA's shoulder. Both of the PTA's open hands should firmly grasp the proximal humerus and direct a straight lateral force, effectively translating the humeral head from the glenoid (Fig. 22-38).

The motion of humeral head depression (inferior glide) can be accomplished while the patient is supine and the PTA is standing near the affected shoulder. The arm of the affected shoulder should be abducted as close to 90 degrees as possible. The distal humerus should be firmly grasped with one hand, and a straight axial force should be directed to distract the humeral head from the glenoid. The open palm of the other

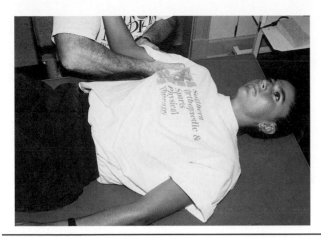

Fig. 22-39 Inferior glide of the glenohumeral joint.

hand should be placed on the superior aspect of the humeral head, and an inferior force should be directed simultaneously to the humerus (Fig. 22-39).

❖ ADDITIONAL FEATURES

Bankart's Lesion: Dislocation of glenohumeral joint or repetitive subluxation may lead to fractures of the anteroinferior aspect of the glenoid rim.

Glenohumeral Joint: Greatest range of motion and least stable of any joint.

Hill-Sachs Lesion: Glenohumeral joint dislocation or repetitive subluxation, may lead to bone defect on posterolateral aspect of humeral head. Also called impression fracture.

Instability Patterns: Traumatic, unilateral Bankart's lesion (TUBS), which is treated surgically. Atraumatic, multidirectional, bilateral, rehabilitation, occasionally inferior capsular shift surgery (AMBRI).

Joints of the Shoulder Complex: Glenohumeral, sternoclavicular, acromioclavicular, and scapulothoracic.

Mumford Procedure: Resection of distal clavicle-subacromial spur resection for decompression of impingement.

Neer's Stage I Impingement: Edema, hemorrhage, generally reversible, typically presented when the patient is at a young age.

Neer's Stage II Impingement: Fibrosis, tendinitis, pain influenced by activity.

Neer's Stage III Impingement: Cuff tear with subacromial osteophyte (spur), progressively disabling. This lesion requires surgery.

Rotator Cuff "SITS": Supraspinatus, infraspinatus, teres minor, and subscapularis.

SLAP Lesion: Superior labrum—anterior to posterior defect in glenoid labrum and possibly long head of biceps.

REFERENCES

1. Bergfeld JA: Acromioclavicular complex. In Nicholas JA, Hershman EB, eds. The Upper Extremity in Sports Medicine. St Louis, Mosby, 1990.
2. Blackburn TA, Voight ML: Rehabilitation of the unstable shoulder. In Advances in Clinical Education. Course Notes. Mobile, AL, 1994.
3. Boissonnault WG, Janos SC: Dysfunction, evaluation and treatment of the shoulder. In Donatelli R, Wooden MJ, eds. Orthopaedic Physical Therapy. New York, Churchill Livingstone, 1989.
4. Chandler TJ, Kibler WB, Stracener EC, et al: Shoulder strength, power and endurance in college tennis players. *Am J Sports Med* 1992;20(4):455–458.
5. Goldstein TS, ed. Treatment of common problems of the shoulder complex. In Geriatric Orthopaedics: Rehabilitative Management of Common Problems. Gaithersburg, MD, Aspen Publishers, 1991.
6. Halbach JW, Tank RT: The shoulder. In Gould JA, ed. Orthopaedic and Sports Physical Therapy, 2nd ed. St Louis, Mosby, 1990.
7. Hawkins RJ, Mohtadi N: Rotator cuff problems in athletes. In DeLee JC, Drez D, eds. Orthopaedic Sports Medicine: Principles and Practice, vol 1. Philadelphia, WB Saunders, 1994.
8. Hisamoto J: Eccentric training: myth vs. reality in functional loading of the shoulder complex. Course Notes. Atlanta, GA, 1995.
9. Kamkar A, Irrgang J, Whitney SL: Nonoperative management of secondary shoulder impingement syndrome. *J Orthop Sports Phys Ther* 1993;17:212–224.
10. Lippert L: Shoulder girdle. In Clinical Kinesiology for the Physical Therapist Assistant, 2nd ed. Philadelphia, FA Davis, 1994.
11. McRae R: Practical Fracture Treatment, 3rd ed. New York, Churchill Livingstone, 1994.
12. Mendoza FX, Nicholas JA, Sands A: Principles of shoulder rehabilitation in the athlete. In Nicholas JA, Hershman EB, eds. The Upper Extremity in Sports Medicine. St Louis, Mosby, 1990.
13. Miller MD: Review of Orthopaedics. Philadelphia, WB Saunders, 1992.
14. Miller RH: Rotator cuff survey. In Shoulder Rehabilitation. Course Notes. Nashville, TN, 1990.
15. Morrison DS: The shoulder. In Shoulder Rehabilitation. Course Notes. Nashville, TN, 1990.
16. Moseley JB Jr, Jobe FW, Pink M, et al: EMG analysis of the scapular muscles during a shoulder rehabilitation program. *Am J Sports Med* 1992;20(2):128–134.
17. Neer CS: Impingement lesions. *Clin Orthop* 1983;173:70–77.
18. Neer CS, Rockwood CA: Fractures and dislocations of the shoulder. In Rockwood CA, Green DR, eds. Fractures in Adults, 2nd ed. Philadelphia, JB Lippincott, 1984.
19. Pagnani MJ, Galinat BJ, Warren RF: Glenohumeral instability. In DeLee JC, Drez D, eds. Orthopaedic Sports Medicine: Principles and Practice, vol 1. Philadelphia, WB Saunders, 1994.
20. Skyhar MJ, Warren RF, Altchek DW: Instability of the shoulder. In Nicholas JA, Hershman EB, eds. The Upper Extremity in Sports Medicine. St Louis, Mosby, 1990.
21. Strege D: Upper extremity. In Loth T, ed. Orthopaedic Boards Review. St Louis, Mosby, 1993.
22. Thein LA: Rehabilitation of shoulder injuries. In Prentice WE, ed. Rehabilitation Techniques in Sports Medicine, 2nd ed. St Louis, Mosby, 1994.
23. Townsend H, et al: Electromyographic analysis of the glenohumeral muscles during a baseball rehabilitation program. *Am J Sports Med* 1991;19:264–272.
24. Voight ML: Overview of shoulder rehabilitation: a scientific biomechanical approach to the problem. In Advances in Clinical Education. Course Notes. Mobile, AL, 1994.
25. Voight ML: Rotator cuff disorders. In Advances in Clinical Education. Course Notes. Mobile, AL, 1994.
26. Wadsworth CT: Frozen shoulder, *Phys Ther* 1986;66:12878–1883.
27. Wilk KE: Conservative treatment for the unstable shoulder. In Advances in the Knee and Shoulder. Course Notes. Hilton Head, SC, 1993.
28. Wilk KE, Mangine R: Post-operative rehabilitation of rotator cuff repairs. In Advances in the Knee and Shoulder. Course Notes. Hilton Head, SC, 1993.
29. Williams GR, Rockwood CA: Fractures of the scapula. In DeLee JC, Drez D, eds. Orthopaedic Sports Medicine: Principles and Practice, vol 1. Philadelphia, WB Saunders, 1994.
30. Williams GR, Rockwood CA: Injuries to the acromioclavicular joint. In DeLee JC, Drez D, eds. Orthopaedic Sports Medicine: Principles and Practice, vol 1. Philadelphia, WB Saunders, 1994.

31. Wooden MJ: Mobilization of the upper extremity. In Donatelli R, Wooden MJ, eds. Orthopaedic Physical Therapy. New York, Churchill Livingstone, 1989.

32. Yahara ML: Shoulder. In Richardson JK, Iglarsh ZA, eds. Clinical Orthopaedic Physical Therapy. Philadelphia, WB Saunders, 1994.

33. Young DC, Rockwood CA: Fractures of the clavicle. In DeLee JC, Drez D, eds. Orthopaedic Sports Medicine: Principles and Practice, vol 1. Philadelphia, WB Saunders, 1994.

REVIEW QUESTIONS

Multiple Choice

1. Mechanical compression of the rotator cuff tendons, primarily the supraspinatus tendon, as they pass under the coracoacromial ligament between the coracoid and acromion process is termed which of the following?
   A. Secondary impingement
   B. Thoracic outlet syndrome
   C. Primary impingement
   D. Bicipital tendinitis

2. Which of the following is the most common structure involved with impingement of the shoulder?
   A. Subscapularis tendon
   B. Infraspinatus tendon
   C. Supraspinatus tendon
   D. Biceps tendon

3. An area just proximal to the insertion of the supraspinatus on the greater tuberosity is (are) which of the following? (Circle any that apply.)
   A. Hypervascular
   B. The watershed zone
   C. Hypovascular
   D. The critical zone
   E. Neer's zone

4. Which of the following describe(s) Neer's stage II impingement? (Circle any that apply.)
   A. Is a reversible lesion
   B. Occurs to persons 25 to 40 years of age
   C. Is characterized by tendon degeneration
   D. Is fibrosis of the subacromial tissues
   E. Is an irreversible lesion

5. Which of the following describe(s) rotator cuff impingement signs? (Circle any that apply.)
   A. Pain with shoulder abduction between 60 and 120 degrees
   B. Pain with forward flexion
   C. Pain with shoulder extension
   D. Pain with forced internal rotation with the affected arm abducted to 90 degrees
   E. Pain with elbow flexion

6. Which of the following muscles must be strengthened before addressing specific rotator cuff weakness in the presence of secondary rotator cuff impingement? (Circle any that apply.)
   A. Pectorals
   B. Serratus anterior
   C. Latissimus dorsi
   D. Rhomboids
   E. Middle deltoid

7. A general, comprehensive rehabilitation plan for treatment of rotator cuff impingement during the early recovery stage includes which of the following?
   A. Scapular stabilization exercises
   B. Repetitive overhead lifting
   C. Specific rotator cuff strengthening
   D. Pectoral strengthening
   E. None of the above

8. Activities of daily living modifications and exercise modifications in the presence of subacromial rotator cuff impingement include which of the following?
   A. Avoid forward flexion above 30 degrees.
   B. Limit abduction below 80 or 90 degrees.
   C. Avoid abduction entirely.
   D. Avoid internal rotation.
   E. All of the above

9. Studies demonstrate the highest electromyographic activity for strengthening the supraspinatus, infraspinatus, subscapularis, deltoid, latissimus dorsi, and pectorals involves which of the following? (Circle any that apply.)
   A. Scaption
   B. Prone horizontal abduction with external rotation
   C. Elbow extension
   D. Arm elevation in sagittal plane
   E. Scapular elevation

10. Rowing exercises, scapular plane elevation (scaption), press-ups, and push-ups with a plus define which of the following?
    A. Specific rotator cuff exercise
    B. Specific throwing exercises
    C. Scapular stabilization exercises
    D. Specific exercises for scoliosis

11. Which of the following describe(s) the most common positions that may induce anterior glenohumeral subluxation or dislocation? (Circle any that apply.)
    A. Arm abducted
    B. Internal rotation
    C. Shoulder extension
    D. External rotation
    E. Shoulder adduction

12. Which is the most commonly dislocated joint in the body?
    A. Knee
    B. Elbow
    C. Shoulder
    D. Hip

13. This injury occurs as a result of glenohumeral dislocation and is defined as an avulsion of the capsule and glenoid labrum off of the anterior rim of the glenoid.
    A. Rotator cuff tear
    B. Bankart lesion
    C. Hill-Sachs lesion
    D. Subacromial impingement

14. The initial nonoperative management of glenohumeral instability calls for a period of immobilization lasting how long?
    A. 2 weeks
    B. More than 8 weeks
    C. Up to 6 weeks
    D. 3 weeks

15. Which of the following exercises are prescribed for the affected immobilized shoulder with acute anterior glenohumeral dislocation?
    A. Full range-of-motion (ROM) concentric exercise
    B. Limited ROM eccentric exercises
    C. Submaximal isometrics
    D. Isokinetic exercise
    E. All of the above

16. For up to 3 months or longer after removal of the sling, which motions should be limited after anterior glenohumeral dislocation?

A. Flexion and extension
B. Internal and external rotation
C. Abduction and external rotation
D. Extension and internal rotation

17. Which of the following is the appropriate ratio of motion between the scapula and glenohumeral joint after the first 30 degrees of glenohumeral flexion or abduction?
    A. 3:1
    B. 2:2
    C. 2:1
    D. 1:1

18. Which of the following represent(s) general categories of surgical stabilization procedures used for glenohumeral instability? (Circle any that apply.)
    A. Surgical repairs of Bankart lesions
    B. Surgical repairs of Hill-Sachs lesions
    C. Bone block and coracoid process transfers
    D. Procedures to limit external rotation
    E. Surgical procedures to limit internal rotation

19. Which of the following describes adhesive capsulitis, or "frozen shoulder"?
    A. Pain
    B. Reduced range of motion
    C. Inflamed capsule
    D. Fibrous synovial adhesions
    E. All of the above

20. Adhesive capsulitis commonly affects which of the following?
    A. Men 40 to 60 years old
    B. Women 20 to 30 years old
    C. Women 40 to 60 years old
    D. Men 60 years and older

21. Which of the following is (are) the classifications of adhesive capsulitis? (Circle any that apply.)
    A. Tertiary
    B. Resistant
    C. Secondary
    D. Primary
    E. Profound

22. Adhesive capsulitis, which occurs spontaneously from unknown causes, is referred to as which of the following?
    A. Tertiary
    B. Primary adhesive capsulitis
    C. Secondary adhesive capsulitis
    D. Resistant capsulitis

23. Which of the following are most appropriate to utilize during the acute phase of adhesive capsulitis?
    A. Closed-chain exercises
    B. Active full ROM exercises
    C. Iontophoresis
    D. Eccentric resistance exercises

24. In the presence of adhesive capsulitis with restricted glenohumeral motion, it is also essential to address which of the following during each phase of recovery?
    A. Active assistive full glenohumeral ROM
    B. Scapular stabilization and motion exercises
    C. Plyometrics
    D. Closed kinetic chain exercises
    E. All of the above

25. After a grade II A-C sprain, which of the following is the most common method of treatment?
    A. Surgery: open reduction with internal fixation (ORIF)
    B. Cast immobilization
    C. Shoulder harness and sling for 3 to 6 weeks
    D. Early active motion

26. During periods of immobilization after a grade II A-C sprain, which of the following can be prescribed?
    A. Isokinetic exercise
    B. Submaximal isometrics
    C. Eccentric exercise
    D. Closed-chain exercise
    E. All of the above

27. Which of the following are associated injuries that occur in conjunction with scapular fractures?
    A. Other fractures
    B. Neurovascular injuries
    C. Glenohumeral dislocations
    D. Pneumothorax
    E. All of the above

28. Which of the following is a treatment for isolated fractures of the scapular body?
    A. ORIF procedure
    B. Immobilization for 8 to 12 weeks
    C. Immobilization for 2 to 3 weeks
    D. Complete bed rest for 6 weeks

29. Which of the following is the most common fracture of the scapula?
    A. Extraarticular glenoid neck
    B. Scapular body
    C. Intraarticular glenoid neck
    D. All glenoid neck fractures

30. If an intraarticular glenoid neck fracture is associated with glenohumeral instability, what is the treatment of choice?
    A. Ice, sling, and immobilization for 6 to 8 weeks
    B. Sling immobilization for 20 weeks
    C. Bed rest
    D. ORIF

31. Clavicular fractures occur commonly to which of the following?
    A. Women 20 to 30 years of age
    B. Men younger than 25 years of age
    C. Men between 30 and 45 years of age
    D. Women 25 years of age and younger

32. Which of the following should be employed during immobilization of a proximal humerus fracture treated with an ORIF procedure? (Circle any that apply.)
    A. Active shoulder flexion
    B. General conditioning program
    C. Active forward flexion
    D. Active hand, wrist, and elbow exercises for the arm of the affected shoulder
    E. Eccentric exercise

33. Which of the following is a potential significant clinical complication in an elderly person with a four-part proximal humerus fracture?
    A. Muscular atrophy
    B. Avascular necrosis
    C. Weakness
    D. Reduced ROM

34. Which of the following may be most appropriate with significant displaced four-part proximal humerus fractures in an elderly patient?
    A. ORIF procedure
    B. Immobilization for 6 to 10 weeks
    C. Prosthetic humeral head
    D. Fusion

35. Which of the following is an indication for a proximal humerus prosthesis or total shoulder arthroplasty?
    A. Avascular necrosis
    B. Rheumatoid arthritis
    C. Severe osteoarthritis
    D. Displaced Neer's four-part proximal humerus fractures
    E. All of the above

36. In terms of restoration of shoulder motion after a shoulder arthroplasty, if the rotator cuff is not repaired, the postoperative shoulder abduction average is how much?
    A. 90 degrees
    B. 110 degrees
    C. 143 degrees
    D. 160 degrees

37. Those patients requiring rotator cuff repair in addition to shoulder arthroplasty may achieve an average abduction of how much?
    A. 63 degrees
    B. 78 degrees
    C. 90 degrees
    D. 110 degrees

38. Which of the following exercises should be initiated by the end of the first postoperative week of rehabilitation after shoulder arthroplasty without rotator cuff repair?
    A. Isokinetic
    B. Closed-chain resistance
    C. Codman's pendulum
    D. Eccentric loading

39. In general, when can light resistance exercises begin after shoulder arthroplasty?
    A. End of the third week
    B. By the sixth week
    C. By the eighth week
    D. By the twelfth week

Short Answer

40. Identify the pathology and the structures involved in the following figure.

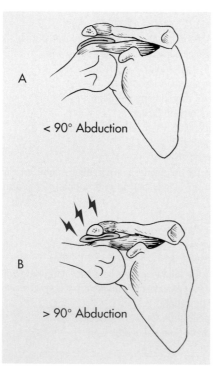

41. Identify the lesion in the following figure.

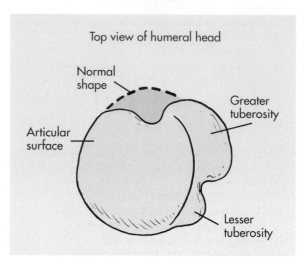

42. What does *TUBS* refer to in regard to shoulder instability?

43. What does *AMBRI* refer to in regard to shoulder instability?

44. In the following figure, identify the injury and the structures involved.

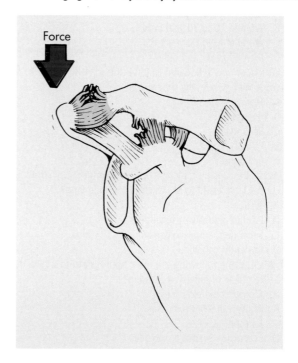

45. In the following figure, identify the injury and the structures involved.

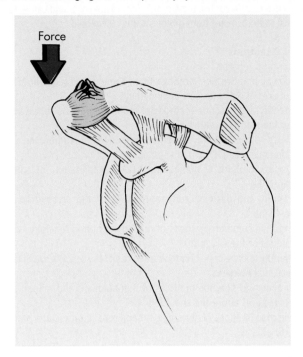

46. In the following figure, identify the technique or procedure and describe when it is used.

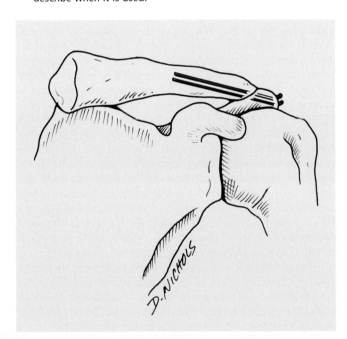

47. In the following figure, identify the specific type and location of this injury.

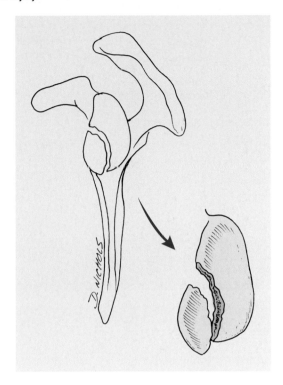

48. In the following figure, identify the device shown and describe for what it is used.

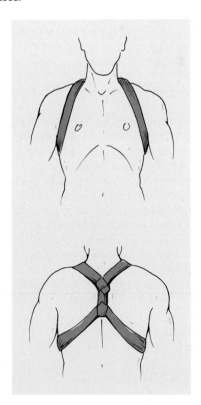

49. In the following figure, identify each of Neer's four-part proximal humerus fracture classification.

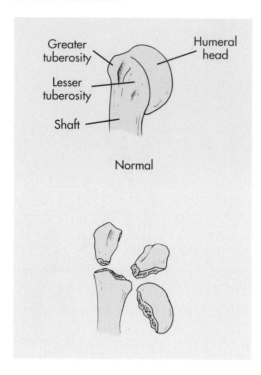

Normal

True/False

50. Secondary subacromial impingement is related to glenohumeral instability, which creates a reduced subacromial space, because the humeral head migrates upward and minimizes the area under the coracoacromial ligament.
51. Age-related arthritic changes and bony osteophyte formation have no effect on subacromial impingement of the shoulder.
52. Posterior shoulder dislocations occur more often than anterior dislocations.
53. It is not uncommon for rotator cuff tears to occur with shoulder dislocations.
54. During immobilization for anterior glenohumeral dislocation, it is necessary to provide ROM and strengthening exercises for the hand, wrist, and elbow, as well as of the affected shoulder.
55. Using the stair-stepper and treadmill is an appropriate closed kinetic chain exercise to employ after shoulder dislocations during the minimum-protection stage of recovery.
56. Transfer-type procedures that utilize bone and soft-tissue stabilization hardware occasionally demonstrate complications of the fixation devices, as well as at the bone transfer site.
57. Secondary adhesive capsulitis generally occurs after trauma or immobilization.
58. Rehabilitation after a grade II A-C sprain must commence once the period of immobilization has ended.

59. Scapular fractures occur from indirect and insignificant trauma.
60. Active muscle contractions of the deltoid are contraindicated during the early recovery from direct rotator cuff repair.

Essay Questions
Answer on a separate sheet of paper.
61. Identify and describe methods, management, and rehabilitation for subacromial rotator cuff impingement.
62. Identify and describe methods of management and rehabilitation for tears of the rotator cuff.
63. Describe methods of management and rehabilitation for glenohumeral instability.
64. Discuss methods of management and rehabilitation for adhesive capsulitis.
65. Identify and describe common injuries of the acromioclavicular (A-C) joint.
66. Describe common methods of management and rehabilitation for injuries of the A-C joint.
67. Identify and describe common fractures of the scapula, clavicle, and proximal humerus.
68. Outline and describe methods of management and rehabilitation of fractures about the shoulder.
69. Describe methods of management and rehabilitation after shoulder arthroplasty.
70. Describe common mobilization techniques for the shoulder.

Critical Thinking Application
As a role-playing activity, one student plays the part of a patient with a postoperative repair of recurrent traumatic anterior glenohumeral dislocation (coracoid transfer), while another student plays the role of a practicing PTA. For the "PTA": Based on your knowledge and understanding of bone and soft-tissue healing, instruct the patient and demonstrate for a comprehensive initial postoperative care program. Is immobilization necessary? For how long? Why is this necessary? Specifically instruct your patient in the use of agents he or she can use at home for pain and swelling management. Discuss the rationale for the use of other agents you might use in the clinic for pain and swelling reduction. Which precautions would you outline for your patient? Clearly identify these and demonstrate. Which specific motion activities would you recommend? Have the patient demonstrate the correct performance of these exercises. What specific muscle contraction types are employed while the patient is immobilized? Describe these in detail and then have the patient demonstrate. List and demonstrate exercises for all other noninvolved joints that are appropriate. Thoroughly describe the rationale for scapulothoracic stability and strength related to this case. Have the patient demonstrate the correct performance of all scapulothoracic exercises you would recommend. During the minimum-protection phase, what role does eccentric loading play in the rehabilitation of anterior glenohumeral instability? Are closed kinetic chain proprioception exercises encouraged for this case? If so, describe three examples and have your patient demonstrate.

23

Orthopedic Management of the Elbow*

LEARNING OBJECTIVES

1. Identify and describe common overuse, soft-tissue injuries of the elbow.
2. Discuss common methods of management and rehabilitation of overuse, soft-tissue injuries of the elbow.
3. Identify and describe intercondylar fractures, radial head fractures, olecranon fractures, and fracture-dislocations of the elbow.
4. Describe methods of management and rehabilitation of various fractures and fracture-dislocations of the elbow.
5. Describe common mobilization techniques for the elbow.

KEY TERMS

"Tennis elbow"
Overuse
Epicondylitis
"Overload forces"

Valgus stress overload
Olecranon
Supracondylar fracture
Volkmann's ischemic contracture

Intercondylar fractures
"Bag of bones technique"
"Carrying angle"

CHAPTER OUTLINE

Lateral Epicondylitis
Medial Epicondylitis
Medial Valgus Stress Overload
Fractures of the Distal Humerus
    (Supracondylar Fractures)

Intercondylar "T" or "Y" Fractures
Radial Head Fractures
Olecranon Fractures
    Fracture-Dislocations
Mobilization of the Elbow

*Refer to orthopedic anatomy figures on the Evolve website.

This chapter introduces the physical therapist assistant (PTA) to common soft-tissue injuries and fractures of the distal humerus and elbow. Specific attention is directed at identifying treatment programs used to control pain and swelling, and improve motion, strength, and function of the elbow after injury or immobilization.

LATERAL EPICONDYLITIS

Commonly referred to as **"tennis elbow,"** lateral epicondylitis affects the common wrist extensor origin of the extensor carpi radialis longus, extensor carpi radialis brevis, extensor digitorum, and extensor digiti minimi.[4,15] The repetitive **overuse** of this area leads to tendinitis of the origin of the extensor carpi radialis brevis tendon (Fig. 23-1).[5,15]

Interestingly, lateral **epicondylitis** (tennis elbow) can affect anyone involved with repetitive activities of the wrist extensors.[14] Thus persons involved with the use of hand tools (e.g., hammer, screwdriver, or pliers) and various activities involving wrist twisting, pulling, extending, and hand grasping can be affected by lateral epicondylitis.[14]

Generally the patient suffering from lateral epicondylitis has pain with palpation of the lateral epicondyle, with active or resisted wrist extension, and occasionally with grasping of the affected hand.[4,12,14] Because this is a chronic overuse tendinitis, the intense inflammatory response in the affected area of the lateral epicondyle is "an attempt to increase the rate of tissue production to compensate for the increased rate of tissue microdamage."[14]

Initial acute management focuses on resolving pain and swelling with the judicious use of ice massage directly over the affected area, phonophoresis or iontophoresis, physician-prescribed analgesics and nonsteroidal antiinflammatory drugs (NSAIDs), rest, and protection of the area from unwanted stress to allow for healing.[4,12,14]

"Relative rest" rather than strict immobilization is used. A wrist cock-up splint can be used in severe cases to minimize stress on the inflamed wrist extensor tendons. The patient is allowed to remove the splint as needed to participate in controlled motion exercises that do not produce pain. Long-term, rigid immobilization is *not* indicated, because treatment goals are to not only reduce pain and swelling but also to encourage proper collagen alignment and scar tissue maturation.[14] Without early protected motion, excessive tissue scarring and random collagen fiber alignment would severely limit normalized motion and function of the elbow and wrist.

During the initial healing stage, the PTA must encourage the patient to avoid any and all motions that may adversely affect healing. Short-term modifications in activities of daily living (ADLs), sports, and job-related activities must be addressed to provide a pain-free environment for healing. When this initial program fails to bring significant relief of symptoms, some physicians elect to inject the area with a steroid to reduce the inflammation.[10,12]

In addition, active gentle static stretching is advised for the wrist extensors to produce normalized, pain-free wrist flexion and extension (Fig. 23-2). Although specifically addressing treatment for the elbow, active motion and resistance exercises for the elbow and shoulder can be initiated if no wrist motion occurs to increase symptoms.

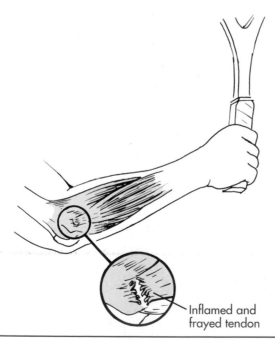

Fig. 23-1 Lateral epicondylitis, "tennis elbow," affects the common wrist-extensor origin.

Inflamed and frayed tendon

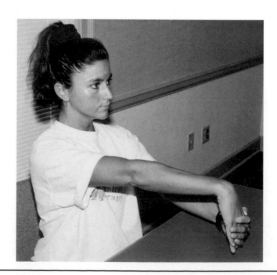

Fig. 23-2 Stretching of the wrist extensors.

The PTA can enhance the effectiveness of low-load, long-duration static stretching by applying moist heat packs (provided the acute inflammatory process has ended) or ultrasound to the lateral epicondyle to stimulate local circulation and relieve congestion caused by metabolic waste products and relax soft tissues in preparation for stretching.

Resistance exercise can begin as pain is reduced with active motion exercises. Generally, submaximal isometrics are used for wrist extension, flexion, forearm pronation and supination, and radial and ulnar deviation.

The PTA must carefully instruct the patient to perform all exercises within a pain-free range of motion (ROM). Throughout all phases of recovery, the patient must avoid stressful, pain-producing activities to prevent the continuation of the inflammatory condition. Progressive motion exercises and increased resistance exercise is the foundation for a return to functional activities. Concentric and eccentric muscle contractions are added once the patient can demonstrate increased quality of multiangle isometric contractions. Care must be taken when initiating both concentric and eccentric resistance exercises because frequently these contractions produce symptoms. Light resistance is advocated when having patients perform these exercises for the first time. An important component for all resistance exercises used with lateral epicondylitis is the performance of slow, controlled eccentric contractions. As noted in Chapter 5, eccentric muscle contractions produce greater tension than either concentric or isometric exercise. In addition, energy use involving adenosine triphosphate (ATP) is less for eccentric exercise than for either concentric or isometric exercise. Eccentric muscle contractions are, in fact, advocated by Curwin and Stanish[4] for the treatment of "tennis elbow," and the rationale for the performance of eccentric exercise is described by Reid and Kushner as, "Exercising the muscle eccentrically allows it to withstand greater resistance and prevent injury, which occurs by eccentrically loading an inflexible muscle."[13]

Resistive exercises emphasizing the eccentric phase are described in Figure 23-3. A hammer is an effective strengthening tool for the treatment of lateral epicondylitis. However, when instructing the patient to perform pronation and supination of the forearm for the first time, the PTA should have the patient hold the hammer close to its head (Fig. 23-4). As the patient gains strength and can control the resistance of the hammer eccentrically, the patient should gradually hold the hammer at the midshaft. As strength improves further, the patient should be allowed to hold the hammer at the end of the shaft, which requires greater eccentric muscle control, strength, and torque. In the same manner, strength can be gained for radial and ulnar deviation through use of the hammer. With a gradual return to functional activities, some physicians and therapists advocate the use of a counterforce brace to help dissipate the **"overload forces"** on the common origin of the wrist extensors (Fig. 23-5).[4,10,14]

Surgery is rarely necessary for this condition because physical therapy management frequently is effective. In

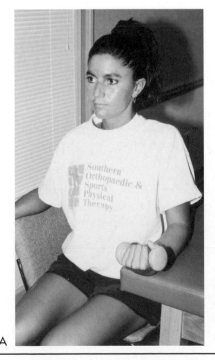
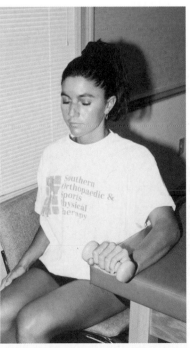

Fig. 23-3 Common wrist and forearm strengthening exercises. **A,** Wrist flexion; **B,** wrist extension. Encourage slow, controlled, nonballistic concentric and eccentric contractions.

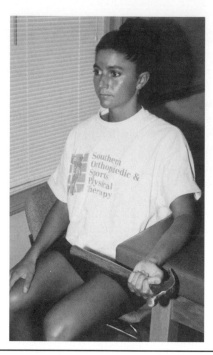

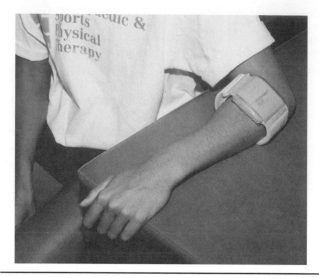

Fig. 23-5 Counterforce brace may help spread or dissipate overload force on the common wrist extensor origin.

Fig. 23-4 Pronation exercise with a hammer. Notice that the grip is held close to the head of the hammer when first introducing this exercise.

rare instances when conservative means fail to reduce pain and improve function, the surgeon may elect to surgically excise the "angiofibroblastic tissue at the origin of the extensor carpi radialis brevis muscle."[15]

MEDIAL EPICONDYLITIS

This overuse condition affects the origin of the pronator teres, flexor carpi radialis, flexor digitorum sublimis, and flexor carpi ulnaris at the medial epicondyle of the elbow.[12] Although it occurs less often than lateral epicondylitis (the lateral epicondylitis-to-medial epicondylitis ratio is 7:1),[14] it is no less incapacitating to the patient. Again the dominant feature is pain with palpation over the medial epicondyle, active motion, and particularly with resisted wrist flexion and full passive wrist extension (Fig. 23-6).[12,13]

The acute management phase of this inflammatory overuse condition, also referred to as "golfer's elbow," concentrates on the management of pain and swelling. Usually the physician prescribes NSAIDs, ice (to protect the ulnar nerve), phonophoresis or iontophoresis, rest (not immobilization), protection, and gentle active motion exercises. The criteria-based treatment plan parallels that for lateral epicondylitis, although it obviously focuses on the wrist flexors. Static low-load, long-duration stretching can proceed as pain allows. The PTA must encourage the patient to avoid repetitive flexing of the wrist and pronating of the forearm if these motions produce pain. Modifications in lifting, twisting, pulling, or turning of

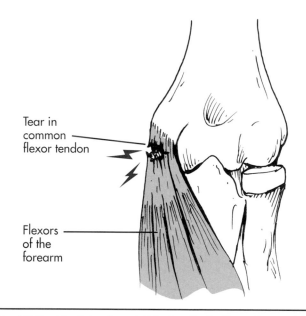

Fig. 23-6 Medial epicondylitis, "golfer's elbow." Repetitive overuse injury.

the wrist and forearm must accompany each phase of recovery to avoid stress on the medial structures. Moist heat and ultrasound can be applied to the medial epicondyle before stretching once motion has improved without pain. Resistance training can then begin with submaximal isometrics, progressing to higher-quality isometric multiangle contractions, and ultimately to concentric and eccentric isotonic and isokinetic resistance exercises. The patient is instructed in the active use of the shoulder of the affected limb and strongly encouraged to follow a conditioning program to maintain or enhance cardiovascular fitness, strength, and flexibility throughout the rehabilitation process.

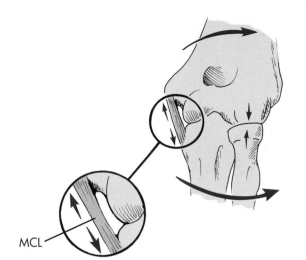

Fig. 23-7 Medial valgus stress overload. Repetitive valgus stress to the elbow may stress the capsuloligamentous structures of the elbow.

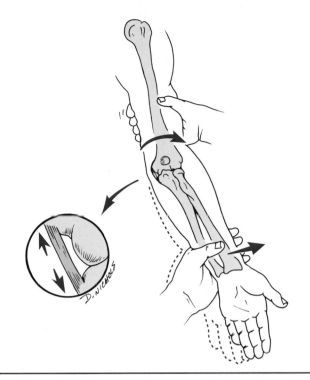

Fig. 23-8 Clinical valgus stress examination to test the stability of the medial (ulnar) collateral ligament.

Although the resolution of pain and swelling is paramount for active use of the wrist and forearm, regaining lost motion caused by pain and muscular dysfunction is critical for function and a return to normal daily activities. The normal ROM of the elbow is 0 degrees to approximately 145 degrees of flexion.[15] However, most daily activities can be carried out within a functional ROM of 30 to 130 degrees of flexion.[15] In addition, normal pronation of 75 degrees and supination of 85 degrees exceeds the functional arc of motion of 50 degrees needed to carry out most ADLs. Therefore the PTA must encourage pain-free early protected motion to facilitate the collagen fiber alignment needed for both functional scar maturation and purposeful motion to perform ADLs.

MEDIAL VALGUS STRESS OVERLOAD

Medial **valgus stress overload** occurs commonly among patients who participate in repetitive throwing and racquet sports such as javelin throwing, baseball, racquetball, and tennis.[5,11,12] Clinical differences exist between medial valgus stress overload and medial epicondylitis. Although medial epicondylitis represents a chronic overuse syndrome affecting the soft-tissue musculotendinous origin of the wrist flexors and pronators, medial valgus stress overload occurs to the capsuloligamentous structures (medial [ulnar] collateral ligament) as a result of repetitive valgus stress to the elbow (Fig. 23-7).[5,11,12]

Patients usually complain of pain over the medial aspect of the elbow and the posterior aspect of the **olecranon.**[11,12] During the physical therapist's (PT) initial evaluation the PTA may observe the performance of ligament stability tests to confirm the presence of

ulnar collateral ligament laxity. The affected arm is held in 10 to 30 degrees of flexion while the humerus is held in full external rotation. A medial or valgus stress then is applied to the elbow to assess the stability of the medial (ulnar) collateral ligament (Fig. 23-8).[11,12]

Management of valgus stress injuries must take into account the healing constraints of ligaments. The patient may receive physician-prescribed NSAIDs, analgesics, ice massage, phonophoresis, or iontophoresis to reduce pain and swelling. Rest and protection of the injured medial ligamentous structures, while avoiding valgus stress, are the hallmarks of management. Because most of these injuries occur to active sports enthusiasts, the patient must omit activities that produce medial valgus stress. To ensure compliance, it may be necessary to suggest short-term rest from the activity, during which the patient should participate in running, cycling, and strength training and should perform flexibility exercises as long as no valgus load is applied to the elbow joint. In addition, the wrist, hand, and shoulder of the affected limb must be exercised during each phase of recovery.

Gentle low-load static stretching begins as soon as pain allows. All valgus stress must be eliminated for spontaneous ligamentous healing to occur. Therefore the stretching regimen focuses on all wrist motions, forearm pronation and supination, and elbow flexion and extension as long as no symptoms of pain occur with these activities.

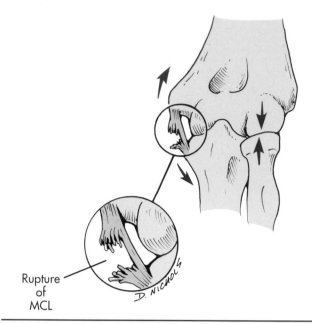

Fig. 23-9 Sudden valgus force applied to a skeletally mature adult may result in rupture of the medial collateral ligament.

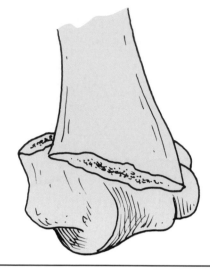

Fig. 23-10 Supracondylar fracture type I or extension-type fracture in which the distal humeral fragment is displaced posteriorly.

The strengthening component of recovery must be modified to prevent any valgus stress. Full ROM (flexion-extension) concentric and eccentric resistance exercise is allowed with light weights as motion and pain dictate. Wrist and hand exercises are encouraged early and pose no threat to the healing ligament. In addition, forearm pronation and supination with use of a hammer (as outlined) is employed as the patient is able to demonstrate improved motion without pain.

With time, the PT reassesses the stability of the medial collateral ligaments. If these structures demonstrate improved stability without pain, a gradual return to throwing can begin.

Surgery is considered if conservative treatment fails to restore function and eliminate pain. Degenerative changes, which are usually present in the adult, *must* be addressed surgically.[11,13] In general, an osteotomy is performed to remove osteophytes (bone spurs) and fibrotic, degenerated tissue.[11,13]

Acute rupture (grade III ligament rupture) of the medial (ulnar) collateral ligament can occur in skeletally mature adults if valgus stress is applied suddenly with sufficient force (Fig. 23-9).

First, these patients are managed conservatively with ice, NSAIDs, analgesics, and, most important, rest and protection. The progression from the acute, maximum-protection phase to return-to-normal function parallels treatment outlined for valgus stress injuries. However, because the ligament has been ruptured, a longer period of recovery is needed and rest and joint protection from valgus stress will last longer. Normal elbow function, which means flexion, extension, pronation, and supination, should be encouraged as early as pain and motion allow.

If early active protected joint motion and progressive resistance exercise have been used, authorities suggest that the injured patient can resume throwing activities approximately 3 months after injury.[11] However, surgery may be necessary to stabilize the joint if the patient does not demonstrate improved valgus stability and continues to have dysfunction.

Generally if the ulnar collateral ligament is ruptured midsubstance, either a direct repair is carried out or a reconstructive procedure is used wherein a free tendon graft of the palmaris longus is routed through drill holes to reconstruct the medial stabilizers of the elbow.[11,12]

Postoperative rehabilitation begins immediately, with the patient's affected limb immobilized in a brace to protect against valgus stress. Instructions are given to perform hand, wrist, and shoulder exercises to maintain motion. Usually by the third week postoperatively, ROM should approach 20 to 110 degrees.[5] The continuous use of ice and therapeutic agents (e.g., ultrasound, transcutaneous electrical nerve stimulation, and galvanic stimulation)[13] are prescribed as necessary. Progressive resistance concentric and eccentric contractions are used for the wrist of the involved limb, whereas submaximal isometrics can begin for elbow flexion and extension.

Shoulder strengthening and flexibility exercises also can begin during the third week of recovery.[5] However, care must be taken to avoid external shoulder rotation exercises because this motion produces valgus stress on the elbow.[5]

Usually by 4 to 6 weeks after surgery, ROM should be 0 to 130 degrees.[5] In addition, concentric and eccentric resistance exercises for elbow flexion and extension are added progressively as tolerated. Gentle forearm prona-

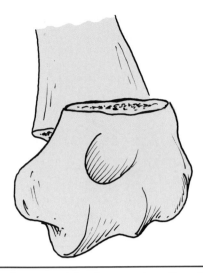

Fig. 23-11 Supracondylar fracture type II, or flexion-type in which the distal humeral fragment is displaced anteriorly.

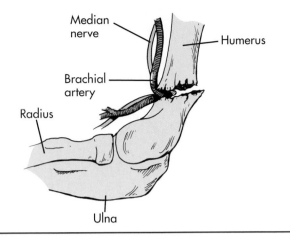

Fig. 23-12 Volkmann's ischemic contracture.

tion and supination exercises also can be made more challenging. From 2 to 4 months after surgery, functional training can begin with an emphasis on shoulder, elbow, and wrist strengthening, motion exercises, and gentle throwing for the athlete. Ultimately, it takes 12 months after elbow reconstruction and rehabilitation for valgus instability before a functional return to competitive sports is allowed.[11]

FRACTURES OF THE DISTAL HUMERUS (SUPRACONDYLAR FRACTURES)

By definition a **supracondylar fracture** is a transverse fracture of the distal third of the humerus.[7] These frequent injuries usually occur in children.[7,11,14] Supracondylar fractures generally are of two types.[3,7,15] Type I is the most common and refers to an injury that occurs as a result of a fall on an extended, outstretched arm in which the distal humerus fragment is displaced posteriorly and is maintained in that position because of the strong pull of the triceps (Fig. 23-10).[3,15] Type II is considered a flexion injury and occurs after direct trauma to the posterior aspect of the elbow in which the distal humeral fragment lies anterior to the humerus (Fig. 23-11).[3,15]

The most common treatment of these fractures is by closed reduction and immobilization for 4 to 6 weeks. The affected arm is held in a flexed position to allow the triceps to help maintain the fracture in a stable position.[7,15]

As with all other fractures, the initial phase of recovery focuses on motion and strengthening exercises for the contralateral limb, general body conditioning, and active motion of the hand, wrist, and shoulder of the injured limb, as along as no undue stress is directed at the fracture site.

Physical therapy treatment after immobilization focuses on gentle active motion exercises, which can be preceded by the use of moist heat or a warm whirlpool to encourage relaxation, removal of wastes, and improved local circulation. In most cases, progressive active motion of the elbow and resistance exercises proceed as radiographic evidence confirms solid union, a minimum of 6 weeks has elapsed since surgery (consistent with the healing constraints of bone tissue), and the patient demonstrates improved motion without pain.

Complications arising from supracondylar fractures[8] include nonunion, malunion, and joint contracture. Perhaps the most disastrous complication results from vascular compromise.[3,7,8,15] As the fracture fragments are displaced, hemorrhage beneath the deep fascia produces an ischemic injury that creates an arterial and venous obstruction (usually affecting the brachial artery), leading to **Volkmann's ischemic contracture** (Fig. 23-12).[3,8,14] What is most important is that the clinical signs and symptoms of ischemic obstruction may not be noticed until the end of immobilization.[3] The symptoms of Volkmann's ischemic contracture can occur throughout each phase of recovery after a supracondylar fracture.

Stralka and Brasel[14] outline six symptoms authorities define as indicating vascular obstruction:
- Severe pain in the forearm muscles
- Limited and extremely painful finger movement
- Purple discoloration of the hand with prominent veins
- Initial paresthesia followed by loss of sensation
- Loss of radial pulse and later loss of capillary return
- Pallor, anesthesia, and paralysis

Restoration of elbow function (e.g., flexion, extension, pronation, and supination of the forearm) after supracondylar fractures initially focuses on motion exercises that do not stress the fracture site. Therefore passive stretching is contraindicated during the early healing phase.[7] Gentle active exercises for the upper arm, wrist, and shoulder, of course, should be performed to the patient's tolerance. Resistance exercises consisting of

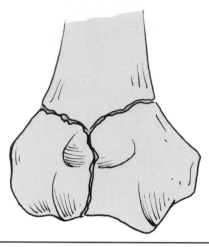

Fig. 23-13   Intercondylar fracture, type I-nondisplaced.

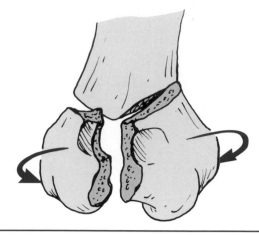

Fig. 23-15   Intercondylar fracture, type III-displaced with rotation of fragments.

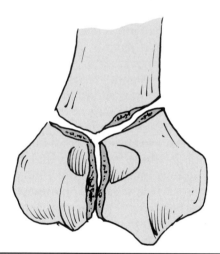

Fig. 23-14   Intercondylar fracture, type II-displaced without rotation.

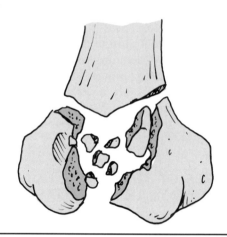

Fig. 23-16   Severely comminuted type IV intercondylar fracture with significant displacement.

submaximal isometrics and progressing to concentric and eccentric muscle contractions are allowed, pending confirmation of secure union of the fracture fragments.

INTERCONDYLAR "T" OR "Y" FRACTURES

In addition to nondisplaced or displaced transverse supracondylar fractures, potentially more significant fracture patterns can occur with falls or direct trauma to the elbow. **Intercondylar fractures** describe injuries that extend between the condyles of the humerus and involve the articular surfaces of the elbow joint.[3,7,8,15] According to Strege and Miller, there are four classifications of intercondylar fractures that display a T or Y configuration:[3,7,8,11,15]

Type I: A nondisplaced fracture that extends between the two condyles (Fig. 23-13)

Type II: A displaced fracture without rotation of the fracture fragments (Fig. 23-14)

Type III: A displaced fracture with a rotational deformity (Fig. 23-15)

Type IV: A severely comminuted fracture with significant separation between the two condyles (Fig. 23-16)

The type of fracture dictates a course of treatment that parallels the significance of the injury. With a type I nondisplaced fracture, treatment can be immobilization for approximately 3 weeks, followed by progressive, gentle active motion. Resistance exercises are deferred until secure bone union has been confirmed radiographically. With types II and III displaced fractures, the treatment is open reduction and internal fixation (ORIF) with the use of Kirschner wires, side plates, and lag screws to secure and stabilize the displaced fracture fragments (Fig. 23-17).[7,8,15] Type IV comminuted intercondylar fractures are treated differently for adults

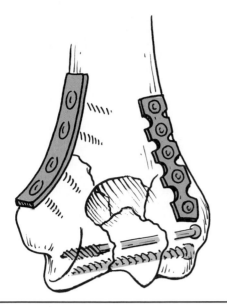

Fig. 23-17   Displaced intercondylar fracture open reduction with internal fixation.

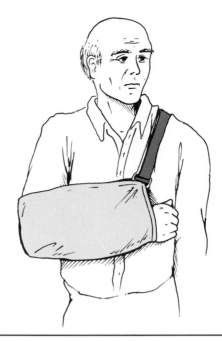

Fig. 23-18   In cases where elderly patients with osteoporosis suffer a severely comminuted intercondylar fracture, a treatment referred to as the "bag of bones" technique is used.

and elderly patients with poor bone quality (osteoporosis).[8,15] Adult patients are usually treated with an ORIF procedure to stabilize the fragments. However, in elderly patients with generally poor bone quality (osteopenic bone), a treatment procedure referred to as the **"bag of bones technique"** is used.[7,8,15] This technique calls for the use of a "collar and cuff" sling, with the affected elbow flexed as far as the limits of swelling and circulatory compromise allow.[15] With the elbow flexed and able to hang freely within the sling, gravity is used to help obtain possible reduction of the fracture fragments (Fig. 23-18).[8,15]

With intercondylar fractures of the elbow, the patient is instructed in a general conditioning program during immobilization while close attention is paid to avoiding all stress to the affected arm. In addition, the wrist, hand, and shoulder of the affected limb may be exercised with active motion if prescribed by the physician and PT. With intercondylar fractures, the anatomic relationship of the elbow (being extremely compact, with significant bony stability) dictates that the restoration of purposeful, functional motion becomes paramount during recovery. Soft-tissue scarring and bone callus formation can lead to early joint stiffness, arthrosis, and contractures.

During the early postimmobilization period, no passive manipulation or passive stretching can be performed.[15] Strege reports an appreciable risk of joint ankylosis when passive stretching and manipulation are performed during early postinjury elbow rehabilitation.[15]

Once wound closure has occurred after an ORIF procedure, the use of a whirlpool bath may aid local circulation, removal of waste, reduction in soft-tissue congestion, and enhancement of soft-tissue relaxation

in preparation for protected active motion. Elbow flexion and extension, as well as forearm pronation and supination, are encouraged as prescribed by the physician and directed by the PT. Stable union of the fracture signifies more active involvement with progressive motion exercises and the initiation of resistance exercise training to regain strength. If the patient demonstrates loss of motion, the physician and PT may decide to perform specific joint mobilization techniques once bone union is secure. This does not conflict with the mentioned contraindication for passive manipulation and stretching immediately after immobilization. Some patients ultimately may have residual loss of motion. However, functional activities can be performed with flexion and extension of 30 to 130 degrees and pronation and supination of 50 degrees.[15]

RADIAL HEAD FRACTURES

Another common fracture that occurs as a result of a fall on an outstretched arm is a radial head fracture. These fractures represent approximately one third of all elbow fractures and nearly 20% of all elbow trauma.[6]

The definition of the **"carrying angle"** of the elbow and the difference noted between men and women are important in understanding radial head fractures. The carrying angle is formed between the intersection of the long axis of the humerus and the axis of the ulna, with the elbow joint in full extension.[15] A normal carrying angle for men is 10 degrees of valgus; in women, it is

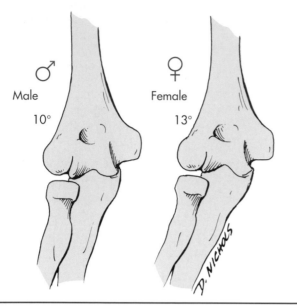

Fig. 23-19 Elbow carrying angles.

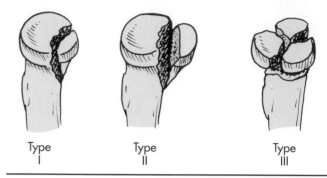

Fig. 23-20 Radial head fractures: type I-nondisplaced, type II-displaced, and type III-comminuted.

13 degrees of valgus (Fig. 23-19).[15] The clinical relevance is that a fractured radial head can lead to an increased valgus deformity and the varus elbow malalignment called a "gunstock deformity."[6]

Radial head fractures generally are classified into four types, as follows:

Type I: A nondisplaced fracture

Type II: A marginal fracture with displacement

Type III: A comminuted fracture of the entire radial head

Type IV: Any radial head fracture with elbow dislocation[15] (Fig. 23-20)

Treatment options parallel the significance of the injury and dictate the course of rehabilitation. Patients with type I nondisplaced radial head fractures usually need a period of immobilization ranging from 5 to 7 days up to 3 to 4 weeks.[7,15] Usually, early active motion is allowed as soon as pain subsides. Because these fractures generally are stable (nondisplaced), healing occurs with very good results.[7] Terminal elbow extension may be recovered many months after type I radial head fractures.[7]

With a type II displaced fracture, the radial head can be excised or stabilized with an ORIF procedure. With a type III comminuted radial head fracture, the fractured area is excised.[6-8,15]

Rehabilitation after an ORIF or radial head excision usually calls for immobilization in a hinged splint to protect the healing bone (ORIF procedure) and soft tissues (excision). As noted, excision of the radial head can lead to increased varus or valgus deformity. In either case, migration of the radial shaft may occur after excision and place stress on the distal ligamentous radioulnar articulation.[6-8] Therefore any discomfort expressed by the patient at the distal radioulnar joint after excision of the radial head usually results from added stress on

this area created by the disrupted proximal radial segment.[6-8] When the patient is immobilized, the hand, wrist, and shoulder of the affected limb are exercised as tolerated. The patient also is encouraged to participate in a general conditioning program of aerobic exercise, strength training, and flexibility exercises. Pain and swelling usually are managed satisfactorily by placing ice packs directly over the painful area. Early active ROM exercises are advocated 3 to 5 days postoperatively by some or deferred for up to 3 weeks by others.[6,15] Restoration of motion is the cornerstone for recovery after radial head fractures. As noted, joint restrictions secondary to arthrofibrosis and contractures can occur, with pronation and supination most commonly affected after radial head fractures.

The PT may elect to perform specific joint mobilization techniques to enhance pronation and supination if secure fixation has occurred after an ORIF procedure. Once wound closure has occurred, a whirlpool bath can be an effective adjunct preceding motion exercises. After excision of the radial head, resistance exercises of elbow flexion and extension and forearm pronation and supination can begin as soon as pain and motion allow. These exercises may be deferred for longer periods if an ORIF procedure was used so that stable bone union and soft-tissue healing can occur.

OLECRANON FRACTURES

Olecranon fractures commonly result after a fall on the point of the elbow (olecranon process) or indirectly from forceful contraction of the triceps.[7] Generally, they are classified as either nondisplaced or displaced fractures. Displaced fractures of the olecranon have four subclassifications:[8]

■ Avulsion fracture, displaced

■ Oblique or transverse fracture

■ Comminuted fracture

■ Fracture-dislocation

The treatment for nondisplaced olecranon fractures requires immobilization for 6 to 8 weeks,[3,7] although as little as 3 weeks or less is used in some cases (particularly in elderly patients).[8,15] The position in which nondisplaced olecranon fractures are immobilized is somewhat controversial, in that some authorities advocate placing the affected arm in extension or slight flexion,[1,3,6,7] whereas others recommend placing the affected arm in 45 to 90 degrees of flexion.[8,15] The rationale for placing the elbow in 45 degrees of flexion is the likelihood of the loss of flexion after immobilization.[15] In addition, Strege suggests that immobilization should not exceed 45 degrees because of the risk of displacing fracture fragments.[15]

Usually, nondisplaced olecranon fractures are allowed gentle active ROM exercises after 3 weeks of immobilization. Flexion of the affected arm should not exceed 90 degrees for the first 6 to 8 weeks after injury so that fracture fragments can heal.[6,15]

Displaced or comminuted fractures of the olecranon can be treated with an ORIF procedure to secure the fragments. With severely comminuted fractures, excision of as much as 80% of the olecranon can occur without loss of joint stability.[8,15]

Physical therapy can begin during the initial stages of immobilization. Active motion of the ipsilateral hand, wrist, forearm (pronation and supination), and shoulder can commence once acute pain has subsided. A general physical conditioning program is allowed as soon as tolerated by the patient. Active elbow flexion must not exceed 90 degrees for the first 2 months after injury. Active resistance exercises for elbow extension must be minimized because the forceful contraction of the triceps can displace the fracture fragments before secure bone healing at 8 weeks. Resistance exercises for elbow flexion can begin earlier if motion is limited and the muscle contractions are submaximal. Submaximal isometric triceps extensions can proceed once bony union has been verified. Progressive concentric and eccentric loading is added as motion increases and secure fixation of the fragments has occurred.

Progressive flexion and extension movements must proceed cautiously and slowly to prevent displacement of the fragments. In addition, the patient must be carefully instructed to initially perform resistance exercises well within the limits of pain and motion restrictions to allow for proper bone healing. The strong contractions of the biceps during flexion and the triceps during extension activities are effective to gradually overcome most motion limitations observed early after injury or surgery. Full recovery after olecranon fractures may take 6 months to 1 year.[6]

Fracture-Dislocations

A fall on an extended outreaching arm causes isolated elbow dislocations and combined fracture-dislocations (Fig. 23-21).[5,7,9,13,14] Conwell[3] reports that "with the exception of the shoulder, the elbow is the most fre-quently dislocated joint in the body." This injury occurs most often in men, with the nondominant arm representing about 60% of these injuries.[9]

Posterior elbow dislocations are the most common, whereas anterior dislocations represent 1% to 2% of all elbow dislocations.[9] Associated fractures of the radial head occur in approximately 10% of elbow dislocations.[9,14] In addition, associated neurovascular injuries can occur with either isolated elbow dislocations or with fracture-dislocations.[7,9,14,15] Injuries involve the median, radial, and ulnar nerves, as well as the brachial artery with elbow dislocations.[9,15]

Isolated posterior elbow dislocations are managed with closed reduction and immobilization.[3,5,7-9,14] The elbow is placed in 90 degrees of flexion in a splint for 3 to 6 weeks.[3,7,15] During this period, hand and shoulder motion is allowed if no offensive stress is applied to the elbow. Early active ROM exercises can begin during the first week after reduction.[15] However, no passive ROM or stretching is allowed because of the risk of myositis ossificans,[7,14] which results from aggressive passive stretching and mobilization. Active motion is not believed to cause this condition.[14] Therefore gentle active flexion and extension exercises are added as pain, swelling, and soft-tissue healing dictate. Because this injury represents a hyperextension trauma that significantly affects the joint capsule, muscle, tendon, and frequently ligamentous restraints, extensive soft-tissue healing is necessary for a stable, functional joint. The joint capsule of the elbow may require 8 to 10 weeks to heal satisfactorily.[5] Restoration of elbow extension

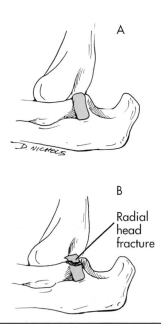

Fig. 23-21 **A,** Posterior elbow dislocation without radial head fracture; **B,** posterior elbow dislocation with radial head fracture.

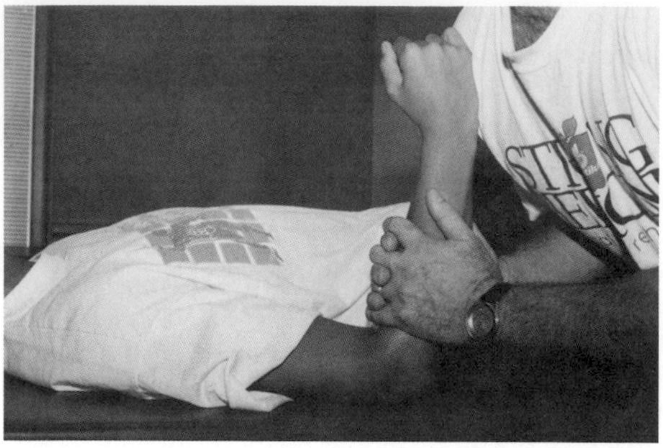

Fig. 23-22 Elbow distraction.

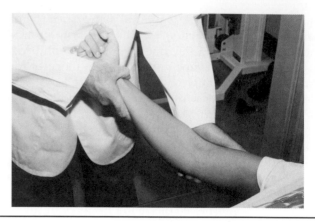

Fig. 23-23 Valgus or humeral-ulna abduction.

therefore must proceed cautiously because the mechanism of injury is usually elbow hyperextension. Resistance exercises can begin as soft-tissue healing progresses. Eccentric and concentric resistance exercises for the biceps can be emphasized to reduce hyperextension forces.[5] Resistance-type exercises are deferred for at least 3 weeks to allow for acute symptoms to subside. However, aggressive elbow extension must be prevented until 8 to 10 weeks have elapsed.[5,9]

The most common complication after elbow dislocation is loss of extension.[9,14,15] Ten weeks after dislocation, a 30-degree flexion contracture is common, and a 10-degree flexion contracture is typically observed 2 years after injury.[9] However unacceptable this loss of motion may be, it does not represent an "overwhelming functional deficit."[15]

The treatment of fracture-dislocations centers on the appropriate management of the fracture (most commonly the radial head) and reduction of the elbow. In most cases, radial head excision is performed to minimize the development of myositis ossificans.[14] Therefore with radial head excision, proximal migration of the radius can result in stress and pain to the distal radioulnar ligamentous articulation.[7,8,15]

Rehabilitation after fracture-dislocation of the elbow gains focus on early protected active motion. Passive stretching again is strictly avoided during the early recovery phases of healing. With radial head excision, a loss of 25 to 30 degrees of pronation and supination can be expected if postoperative immobilization lasts longer than 4 weeks.[14] As with isolated dislocation, loss of full elbow extension is not uncommon.

MOBILIZATION OF THE ELBOW

The rationale for specific joint mobilization is to avoid joint restrictions or hypomobility.[2] In many instances, arthrofibrosis occurs as a result of immobilization and internal fixation methods used to stabilize fracture fragments.

The PT determines if mobilization is indicated after injury, surgery, or immobilization based on tissue healing constraints; the nature of the joint restriction (hypomobility of noncontractile tissue or articular surface dysfunction);[2] and whether passive motion is indicated for the treatment of joint limitations (see Chapter 16). The PT must clearly define the specific indications for mobilization with reference to the exact technique to be employed, rate of movement, amplitude of force, and direction of the force applied to the elbow. To obtain relaxation, the PTA must place the patient in a comfortable position, with specific attention paid to the support and stability of the shoulder, elbow, and arm of the patient. Before joint mobilization is applied, thermal agents are employed to reduce tissue congestion, aid in the removal of wastes, and enhance relaxation of the patient and the affected joint.

Injuries to the elbow that require mobilization should increase in flexion, extension, or both. Wooden outlines three techniques used to enhance general motion, flexion, and extension of the elbow.[16]

To enhance general mobility of the elbow, the patient should be supine with the affected elbow flexed to 90 degrees. The shoulder of the affected limb is held at the patient's side or in an abducted position. The PTA places both hands at the proximal aspect of the forearm, and directs a straight lateral distraction force that directs the forearm away from the humerus (Fig. 23-22).

Humeral-ulnar abduction is employed to promote elbow extension.[16] The patient should be supine with the affected arm abducted and the elbow slightly flexed. The PT sits to the patient's affected side with one hand stabilizing the distal lateral humerus and the other hand firmly grasping the ulnar aspect of the distal forearm. In this position, the PT directs a valgus or abduction force to the elbow (Fig. 23-23).[16]

An adduction technique is applied to increase elbow flexion.[16] The patient remains supine with the affected arm abducted. The PT sits to the patient's affected side and stabilizes the distal humerus on the medial aspect

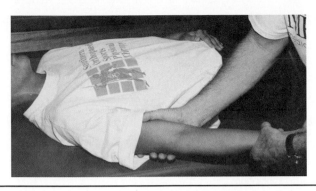

Fig. 23-24 Varus or humeral-ulna adduction.

with one hand, while placing the opposite hand on the distal radial aspect of the forearm. In this position, the PT directs a varus or adduction force to the elbow (Fig. 23-24).

Although these few techniques are representative of the more common motions requiring mobilization, other positions and techniques can be used to enhance elbow motion.

✢ ADDITIONAL FEATURES

Cubital Tunnel Syndrome: Ulnar nerve entrapment at the medial aspect of the elbow.

Galeazzi's Fracture: Radial shaft fracture at the distal metaphysis-diaphysis with radioulnar dislocation.

Ligament Stability: Anterior band of the medial ulnar collateral ligament is the main ligamentous stabilizer.

Mobile WAD of Henry—Descriptive Eponym of Common Origin of Wrist Extensors: Brachioradialis, extensor carpi radialis brevis, and extensor carpi radialis longus.

Monteggia's Fracture: Ulnar shaft-proximal aspect with radial head dislocation.

Pronator Syndrome: Median nerve compression at the pronator teres muscle, bicipital aponeurosis (lacertus fibrosis), flexor digitorum superficialis, or other sites in the forearm.

REFERENCES

1. Bennett JB, Tullos HS: Acute injuries to the elbow. In Nicholas JA, Hershman EB, eds. The Upper Extremity in Sports Medicine. St Louis, Mosby, 1990.
2. Bowling RW, Rockar PA: The elbow complex. In Gould JA, ed. Orthopaedic and Sports Physical Therapy, 2nd ed. St Louis, Mosby, 1990.
3. Conwell HE: Injuries to the elbow. Ciba-Geigy, 1969, Clinical Symposia.
4. Curwin S, Stanish WD: Tendinitis: Its Etiology and Treatment. Lexington, MA, DC Heath, 1984.
5. Dickoff-Hoffman S, Foster D: Rehabilitation of elbow injuries. In Prentice WE, ed. Rehabilitation Techniques in Sports Medicine, 2nd ed. St Louis, Mosby, 1994.
6. LaCroix E: Treatment of common problems of the elbow, forearm, and wrist joints. In Goldstein TS, ed. Geriatric Orthopaedics: Rehabilitative Management of Common Problems. Gaithersburg, MD, Aspen Publishers, 1991.
7. McRae R, ed. Injuries about the elbow. In Practical Fracture Treatment, 3rd ed. New York, Churchill Livingstone, 1994.
8. Miller MD: Review of Orthopaedics. Philadelphia, WB Saunders, 1992.
9. Morrey BF: Elbow dislocation in the athlete. In DeLee JC, Drez D, eds. Orthopaedic Sports Medicine: Principles and Practices, vol 1. Philadelphia, WB Saunders, 1994.
10. Morrey BF, Regan WD: Tendinopathies about the elbow. In DeLee JC, Drez D, eds. Orthopaedic Sports Medicine: Principles and Practices, vol 1. Philadelphia, WB Saunders, 1994.1
11. Morrey BF, Regan WD: Throwing injuries. In DeLee JC, Drez D, eds. Orthopaedic Sports Medicine: Principles and Practices, vol 1. Philadelphia, WB Saunders, 1994.
12. Parks JC: Overuse injuries of the elbow. In Nicholas JA, Hershman EB, eds. The Upper Extremity in Sports Medicine. St Louis, Mosby, 1990.
13. Reid DC, Kushner S: The elbow region. In Donatelli R, Wooden MJ, eds. Orthopaedic Physical Therapy. New York, Churchill Livingstone, 1989.
14. Stralka SW, Brasel JG: Elbow. In Richardson JK, Iglarsh ZA, eds. Clinical Orthopaedic Physical Therapy. Philadelphia, WB Saunders, 1994.
15. Strege D: Upper extremity. In Loth TS, ed. Orthopaedic Boards Review. St Louis, Mosby, 1993.
16. Wooden MJ: Mobilization of the upper extremity. In Donatelli R, Wooden MJ, eds. Orthopaedic Physical Therapy. New York, Churchill Livingstone, 1989.

REVIEW QUESTIONS

Multiple Choice

1. Lateral epicondylitis is caused by which of the following?
   A. Acute direct trauma
   B. Concentric contraction of wrist flexors
   C. Overuse, repetitive motion disorder, cumulative trauma
   D. Eccentric loading of the biceps
   E. All of the above
2. Which of the following describe(s) the muscles of the common wrist extensor origin? (Circle any that apply.)
   A. Biceps brachii
   B. Extensor carpi radialis longus
   C. Extensor carpi radialis brevis
   D. Extensor digitorum
   E. Brachioradialis
3. Which of the following is not advocated during the early recovery phase of rehabilitation for lateral epicondylitis?
   A. Ice
   B. Phonophoresis
   C. Functional activities
   D. Nonsteroidal antiinflammatory drugs (NSAIDs)
4. Lateral epicondylitis occurs at what ratio to medial epicondylitis?
   A. 2:1
   B. 1:1
   C. 7:1
   D. 4:1
5. Which muscles make up the common flexor tendon of the medial epicondyle? (Circle any that apply.)
   A. Pronator teres
   B. Flexor carpi radialis
   C. Brachioradialis
   D. Flexor carpi ulnaris
   E. Biceps brachii
6. Supracondylar fractures occur most often to which of the following?
   A. Adults 25 to 40 years of age
   B. Older adults 55 to 75 years of age
   C. Younger women 20 to 30 years of age
   D. Children

7. Which of the following describes the types of supracondylar fractures?
   A. Type II
   B. Extension type
   C. Type I
   D. Flexion type
   E. All of the above

8. What is the most common treatment for supracondylar fractures?
   A. Open reduction with internal fixation (ORIF)
   B. Rigid cast immobilization for 8 to 10 weeks
   C. Closed reduction and immobilization for 4 to 6 weeks
   D. Early active motion

9. Which of the following is considered the most significant complication after supracondylar fracture?
   A. Joint contracture
   B. Malunion
   C. Vascular compromise
   D. Nonunion

10. Which of the following is not a symptom of vascular obstruction after supracondylar fracture?
    A. Paresthesia
    B. Pain in forearm muscles
    C. Crepitus at fracture site
    D. Painful and reduced finger motion

11. A type I nondisplaced intercondylar fracture is treated with which of the following?
    A. ORIF
    B. Active motion
    C. Immobilization for approximately 3 weeks
    D. Passive motion

12. Because of general bone quality (osteoporosis), which of the following can be used for treatment in an elderly patient with a type IV intercondylar fracture?
    A. ORIF
    B. "Bag of bones" procedure
    C. Early active motion
    D. Fusion

13. What is the average normal carrying angle for men?
    A. 15 degrees
    B. 8 degrees
    C. 10 degrees
    D. 5 degrees

14. What is the normal carrying angle for women?
    A. 13 degrees
    B. 20 degrees
    C. 10 degrees
    D. 8 degrees

15. Radial head fractures are generally classified into four types. Type I is defined as which of the following?
    A. Any radial head fracture with elbow dislocation
    B. A comminuted fracture
    C. A nondisplaced fracture
    D. A marginal fracture with displacement

16. Treatment of type I radial head fractures involves which of the following?
    A. An ORIF procedure
    B. Immobilization for up to 4 weeks
    C. An excision
    D. Active motion

17. Type II radial head fractures always are treated with which of the following? (Circle any that apply.)
    A. ORIF
    B. Immobilization
    C. Excision
    D. Fusion
    E. Closed kinetic chain resistance

18. Which motion is most commonly affected (restricted) after radial head fractures? (Circle any that apply.)
    A. Flexion of the elbow
    B. Extension of the elbow
    C. Supination
    D. Pronation
    E. Radial deviation

19. Nondisplaced olecranon fractures generally are treated with which of the following?
    A. ORIF
    B. Percutaneous pinning
    C. Immobilization for up to 8 weeks
    D. Excision

20. It is clinically important that flexion of the elbow after nondisplaced olecranon fractures not exceed _____ for the first 6 to 8 weeks after injury.
    A. 45 degrees
    B. 30 degrees
    C. 90 degrees
    D. 15 degrees

21. For secure bone healing to occur, active elbow flexion past 90 degrees and resistance exercises for elbow extension after olecranon fractures must be deferred for how many weeks after injury?
    A. 3 to 6 weeks
    B. 12 weeks or longer
    C. 8 weeks
    D. 3 to 4 weeks

22. What percentage of elbow dislocations are anterior?
    A. 10%
    B. 15%
    C. 1% to 2%
    D. 7%

23. Which of the following represents structures that can be injured as a result of elbow dislocation?
    A. Ulnar nerve
    B. Radial nerve
    C. Brachial artery
    D. Median nerve
    E. All of the above

24. Isolated posterior elbow dislocations are managed by which of the following?
    A. Immobilization in an extension
    B. ORIF
    C. Fusion
    D. Immobilization in flexion

25. Early active motion usually can begin after the first week after immobilization for a dislocated elbow; however, passive stretching is related to the development of which of the following?
    A. Flexion contractures
    B. Vascular injury
    C. Myositis ossificans
    D. Extension contractures

26. What is the most common complication after elbow dislocation?
    A. Myositis ossificans
    B. Volkmann's ischemic contracture
    C. Loss of elbow extension
    D. Neurovascular compromise
27. Which of the following is the most common fracture that occurs with elbow dislocation?
    A. Supracondylar fractures
    B. Radial head fractures
    C. Radius fractures
    D. Ulnar fractures

Short Answer

28. In the following figure, identify the injury, mechanism of injury, and structure involved.

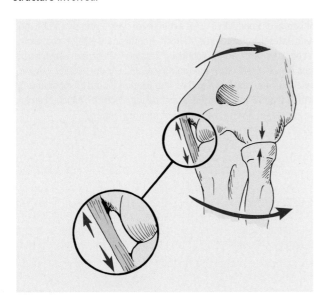

29. Name the most common type of supracondylar fracture.

30. In the following figure, identify the fracture type:

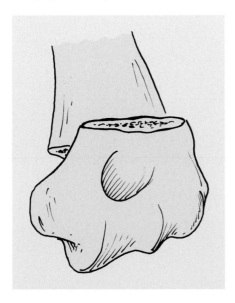

31. In the following figure, identify the general fracture, label the structure(s) that may be compromised, and identify the potential injury that may ensue.

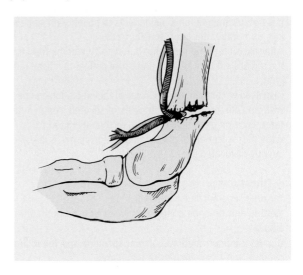

32. In the figure shown, identify the type and classification of fracture:

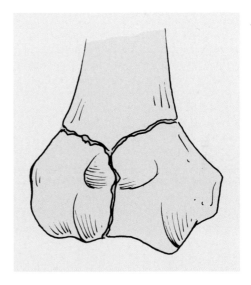

33. What is the most common direction of elbow dislocation?

True/False

34. In severe cases of "tennis elbow," the use of a wrist cock-up splint is advocated for the management of inflamed wrist extensor tendons.
35. During the subacute recovery phase of rehabilitation for lateral epicondylitis, initial instruction for patients to perform forearm pronation and supination must include the use of a hammer while holding the end of the shaft away from the head of the hammer.
36. Medial valgus stress overload is synonymous with medial epicondylitis.
37. The signs and symptoms of ischemic obstruction are always immediately evident after injury.

38. Passive stretching is advocated during the early recovery phase of healing after supracondylar fractures.
39. A type IV intercondylar fracture, which is severely comminuted with significant separation, always is treated with an ORIF procedure.
40. It is not uncommon for some patients to be left with some residual loss of motion after intercondylar fractures.
41. After excision of the radial head in type IV comminuted fractures, the radial shaft may migrate and cause pain at the distal radioulnar joint.
42. Displaced or comminuted fractures of the olecranon can be treated with an ORIF procedure or, in cases of severely comminuted fractures, excision of as much as 80% of the olecranon.
43. With the exception of the shoulder, the elbow is the most frequently dislocated joint in the body.

Essay Questions

Answer on a separate sheet of paper.

44. Identify and describe common overuse, soft-tissue injuries of the elbow.
45. Discuss common methods of management and rehabilitation of overuse, soft-tissue injuries of the elbow.
46. Identify and describe intercondylar fractures, radial head fractures, olecranon fractures, and fracture-dislocations of the elbow.
47. Describe methods of management and rehabilitation of various fractures and fracture-dislocations of the elbow.
48. Describe common mobilization techniques for the elbow.

Critical Thinking Application

Develop two case studies, one concerning a patient with a diagnosis of lateral epicondylitis, the other an elderly woman with a type IV severely comminuted intercondylar fracture. In each case, outline and describe a comprehensive critical pathway (criterion-based rehabilitation program) concerning pain and swelling management, restoration of motion, muscle contraction types, cardiovascular fitness, general physical conditioning and open- and closed-chain proprioception activities. Your progressive recommendations should parallel the stages of bone and soft-tissue healing and should be organized within the maximum protection phase, moderate protection phase, and minimum-protection phase of recovery. What role does eccentric loading play in the recovery of lateral epicondylitis? What activities of daily living should be modified with lateral epicondylitis? Which significant vascular compromise is recognized with a supracondylar fracture? Describe which structures can be affected with this complication. For an elderly person with osteoporosis, which method of stabilization would be most appropriate with a type IV comminuted intercondylar fracture? Which exercises can be employed during the period of immobilization?

24

Orthopedic Management of the Wrist and Hand*

LEARNING OBJECTIVES

1. Identify and describe common compression neuropathies of the wrist.
2. Discuss methods of management and rehabilitation of compression neuropathies of the wrist.
3. Identify and describe common ligament injuries of the wrist.
4. Describe and discuss methods of management and rehabilitation of ligament injuries of the wrist.
5. Describe methods of management and rehabilitation for distal radial and ulnar fractures.
6. Identify methods of management and rehabilitation for scaphoid fractures.
7. Identify and describe common metacarpal fractures and methods of management and rehabilitation.
8. Describe methods of management and rehabilitation of Dupuytren's contracture.
9. Identify and describe common extensor and flexor tendon injuries.
10. Discuss methods of management and rehabilitation of extensor tendon and flexor tendon injuries.
11. Identify methods of management and rehabilitation for reflex sympathetic dystrophy.
12. Describe common mobilization techniques for the wrist and hand.

KEY TERMS

Carpal tunnel syndrome
Compression neuropathy
Nerve entrapment
De Quervain's
  tenosynovitis
Cumulative trauma
  disorder
Colles' fracture

Smith's fracture
Dinner fork deformity
Scaphoid fracture
Anatomic "snuffbox"
Avascular necrosis (AVN)
Nonunion
Skier's thumb
Boxer's fracture

"Fighter's fracture"
Bennett's fracture
Dupuytren's contracture
Mallet finger
Boutonnière deformity
Flexor tendon
Reflex sympathetic
  dystrophy (RSD)

CHAPTER OUTLINE

Carpal Tunnel Syndrome
De Quervain's Tenosynovitis
Ligament Injuries of the Wrist
Distal Radial and Ulnar Fractures
  Radius
  Ulna
Scaphoid Fractures
Skier's Thumb
Metacarpal Fractures

Dupuytren's Contracture
Mallet Finger
Boutonnière Deformity
Flexor Tendon Injuries
Reflex Sympathetic Dystrophy
Mobilization of the Wrist and Hand
  Mobilization of the Wrist
  Mobilization of the Hand

*Refer to orthopedic anatomy figures on the Evolve website.

This chapter introduces common soft-tissue injuries and fractures affecting the wrist and hand. The focus is on general therapeutic interventions to control pain and swelling and specific techniques to enhance motion, strength, and functional restoration of the wrist and hand after injury, surgery, and immobilization. The study of hand and wrist anatomy, kinesiology, and pathomechanics of injury is a difficult task. The physical therapist assistant (PTA) must understand the interrelationships among the foundations of basic science (anatomy, kinesiology, injury, immobilization, and tissue healing) of the wrist and hand to effectively carry out and supervise rehabilitation programs prescribed by the physical therapist (PT). Therefore before reading this chapter, the PTA is strongly urged to thoroughly review pertinent anatomy and kinesiology of the wrist and hand to more fully appreciate the rationale for immobilization, surgery, and rehabilitation after injuries to these areas.

CARPAL TUNNEL SYNDROME

Carpal tunnel syndrome refers to an entrapment **compression neuropathy** of the median nerve within the wrist (Fig. 24-1).[4-6,9,15] This syndrome represents the most common compression neuropathy of the wrist.[4-6,9,15] It is caused by repetitive motions of the wrist (e.g., flexion, ulnar deviation, supination, gripping, and pinching),[4] as well as specific job tasks, occupations, and various leisure and sporting activities that place great repetitive demand on the wrist.[4-6,9,15] With repetitive motions, the carpal tunnel (formed by the transverse carpal ligament

and the carpal bones, through which neurovascular structures pass) may become swollen and irritated, thereby "entrapping" and "compressing" the median nerve, which is located between the transverse carpal ligament and the carpal bones. There are many clinical symptoms of carpal tunnel syndrome. Some of the more common ones include numbness; tingling; pain; clumsiness in hand activity; weakness of grip, pinch, and thumb actions; swelling in the hand and forearm; atrophy of the thenar muscles; and symptoms that become worse at night.[4,5] The effect of this overuse injury (also referred to as cumulative trauma disorder or repetitive motion injury) is rather startling, with estimates that overuse injuries, in general, occur in approximately 4% of the entire United States's work force.[4]

Physical therapy management of carpal tunnel syndrome focuses on eliminating the motions that produce symptoms, using physician-prescribed nonsteroidal antiinflammatory drugs (NSAIDs), and splinting the affected wrist in 0 to 20 degrees of extension.[5,9,15] Wrist cock-up splints are commonly advocated nocturnally and as needed during the day.[5,9,15] Obviously occupational tasks must be modified and those activities of daily living (ADLs), jobs, and recreational activities that call for repetitive motions of the wrist identified. In many cases, the use of NSAIDs and splinting is enough to minimize the inflammatory condition and reduce symptoms of pain, swelling, and tingling. However, if symptoms do not respond to this initial course of action, the physician may elect to inject the area with a corticosteroid to reduce pain and swelling. Furthermore, if a history of constant sensory loss, atrophy, and weakness of the thenar muscles is present, surgery may be indicated.[7] In general, the transverse carpal ligament is cut using an open technique or with endoscopic instrumentation.[5,9]

Physical therapy management during nonoperative splinting, rest, and antiinflammatory medications usually calls for active motion and resistance exercises for the elbow and shoulder of the affected limb, as well as a general conditioning program. Usually a course of specific motion and resistance exercises for the affected wrist is deferred for 4 to 5 weeks to allow the acute inflammation to subside.[5] Finger, hand (gripping), and wrist range of motion (ROM) and gentle resistance exercise must proceed cautiously once the patient can tolerate active motion of the wrist and hand without pain. All aggravating motions that produce symptoms must be avoided.

If a surgical release is performed, the affected wrist is immobilized for as long as 10 to 14 days or as little as 2 to 7 days.[5,9] During wrist immobilization, the patient is encouraged to actively use the elbow and shoulder of the affected limb and to participate in a general physical conditioning program. In addition, the patient should flex and extend the fingers and use the hand of

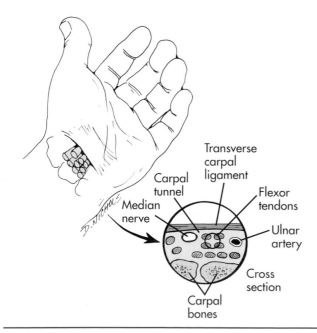

Fig. 24-1 Carpal tunnel syndrome. Compression neuropathy of the median nerve.

the affected wrist.[9] As the surgical wound heals (sutures removed in 10 to 14 days), active wrist motion exercises are initiated, along with motion and resistance exercises for the fingers and hand.[9] Because a decompression surgical procedure was employed to reduce **nerve entrapment** and compression, the prevention of postoperative scarring to the wrist area is of paramount concern. Therefore the patient should be instructed in active motion exercises and massage of the tissues around and through the incision (scar management).[5,9] A program of functional activities begins once the sutures are removed, the wound is closed, and the patient is able to tolerate massage to the area, along with wrist motion and strengthening. In some instances, a full return to activities (particularly those duties that caused the problem in the first place) may be restricted or modified to accommodate the healing of the soft tissue.

DE QUERVAIN'S TENOSYNOVITIS

De Quervain's tenosynovitis is a repetitive motion injury or a **cumulative trauma disorder** that affects the tendons of the abductor pollicis longus and extensor pollicis brevis as they pass within the first dorsal compartment (Fig. 24-2).[5,6,9,15] Generally, motions that produce repetitive ulnar deviations can create tenosynovitis at the first dorsal compartment of the wrist. This condition is characterized by pain and swelling at the radial styloid, as well as reduced motion of the thumb.[5,9,15]

This overuse syndrome is managed conservatively at first with the use of NSAIDs and wrist and thumb immobilization. Any motions that produce pain must

be eliminated for appropriate soft-tissue inflammation to subside. The elbow and shoulder of the affected limb must be exercised with active ROM and resistance exercises from the time immobilization begins. In addition, ice and iontophoresis or phonophoresis may be effective adjuncts to reduce pain and swelling during the acute phase of recovery.[6] Active motion of the wrist and thumb can commence if pain and swelling are much improved after a few weeks of immobilization. Resistance exercises must focus on slow, controlled concentric and eccentric muscle contractions that do not produce symptoms. Usually all motions of the wrist and forearm are addressed, including flexion, extension, radial and ulnar deviation, pronation, and supination. Limited ulnar deviation motion may be needed when ROM and resistance exercises are initiated. The volume and rate of activity involving radial and ulnar deviation also may require modification to accommodate soft-tissue healing.

When conservative care fails to relieve symptoms, the physician may elect to inject the first dorsal compartment with a corticosteroid to reduce pain and inflammation.[5,9,15] Chronic cases of De Quervain's disease also may require surgical decompression of the affected area.[9] The postoperative care closely parallels care for carpal tunnel syndrome. The affected wrist is immobilized for approximately 1 week with a compression bandage.[5,9]

Some authorities recommend immediate ROM exercises, whereas others suggest that active ROM exercises of the thumb and wrist begin after 3 to 5 days.[5,9] The important common denominator remains the management of normalized, pain-free motion (ulnar deviation) without undue scar formation, which would congest and occlude the surgically released and decompressed first dorsal compartment. Therefore motion exercises must be encouraged as directed by the PT, with specific attention directed at scar management once the sutures are removed and wound closure occurs. Pain-free resistance exercises can commence once the patient demonstrates improved wrist and thumb motion without pain.

LIGAMENT INJURIES OF THE WRIST

Stability of the wrist depends primarily on intracapsular ligaments and not on intrinsic dynamic support from musculotendinous tissue.[15] Ligament sprains with varying degrees of carpal instability usually result from a fall with the wrist hyperextended (Fig. 24-3).[5,6,9,15]

With partial ligament sprains not involving carpal instability, the wrist should be immobilized to allow for proper alignment, stability, and healing of the partially torn ligament. Concurrent with immobilization, oral NSAIDs and ice packs may be prescribed to control pain and swelling. Without question, a major factor in healing is the elimination of motions that stress the torn ligaments (usually the end ROM of wrist extension).

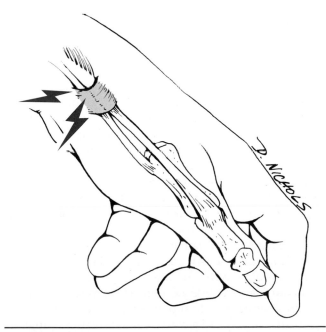

Fig. 24-2 De Quervain's tenosynovitis.

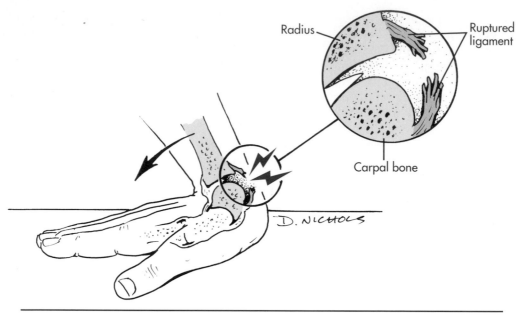

Radius

Ruptured ligament

Carpal bone

D. NICHOLS

Fig. 24-3 Hyperextension ligament sprain of the wrist.

During immobilization, the elbow and shoulder of the affected limb are exercised with active motion and resistance exercises if no stress is applied to the healing ligaments of the wrist. To maintain or enhance fitness, a general conditioning program is encouraged throughout each phase of recovery. The hand and fingers of the ipsilateral limb also should be exercised during immobilization. Once the splint is removed, gentle active, pain-free motion can begin, with specific attention paid to avoiding full wrist extension. As motion improves and pain subsides, resistance exercises are employed to promote a gradual return to function. Both concentric and especially eccentric muscle contractions contribute to strengthening of the wrist flexors. To encourage eccentric control and dynamic support of wrist flexion and enhance muscle control of wrist extension (usually the mechanism of wrist ligament injuries), a progressive resistance exercise program focusing on the eccentric phase of wrist flexion is added gradually.

The restoration of functional motion and strength after incomplete or partial ligament sprains (grades I and II) of the wrist generally follows the course of ligament healing constraints (see Chapter 9).

With more significant ligament injuries accompanied by carpal instability, the treatment is more complex. Options include rigid cast immobilization, closed reduction with percutaneous pinning, and open reduction and internal fixation (ORIF).[9,15] If cast immobilization is used to stabilize the joint, the patient is placed in a cast for approximately 6 to 12 weeks.[15] However, authorities question the ability of rigid immobilization to maintain the reduction satisfactorily to effect functional stability.[9,15] With closed reduction and pinning with wires, the wrist is immobilized for about 2 months,

the pins are removed, and the arm is placed in a cast for an additional 4 weeks (Fig. 24-4).[15] With an ORIF procedure, the ligaments are directly repaired and the unstable carpal articulations are stabilized with wires or pins. The duration of immobilization is similar to that for closed reduction with percutaneous pinning.[15] Rehabilitation after cast immobilization or surgical repair begins during immobilization. The fingers and hand of the affected wrist, the elbow, and the shoulder all should be exercised with active pain-free motion (cautiously avoiding unwanted stress to the wrist) and resistance exercises. A general body-conditioning program is encouraged universally.

Immediately after removal of the cast, splint, or immobilizer, active pain-free protected (limited ROM) activities are begun. If wound closure is complete, the use of a whirlpool before active mobility exercises can effectively reduce tissue congestion and aid in soft-tissue extensibility. Initially the injured or surgically repaired wrist should be protected from unwanted pressure, motions, and from extremes of active motion, consistent with long-term ligament healing constraints. Active assisted ROM exercises gradually can be added once active motion has increased and pain is controlled. Resistance exercises can be initiated once active motion has improved and pain is reduced. Submaximal isometric contractions can be used initially, gradually progressing to maximal multiangle isometric contractions and concentric and eccentric contractions. Protection of the wrist continues well into the final recovery stages of rehabilitation. The use of functional, protective wrist splints is encouraged to protect the repaired and healing ligaments. A generalized wrist rehabilitation program after ligament injury or repair is shown in Box 24-1.

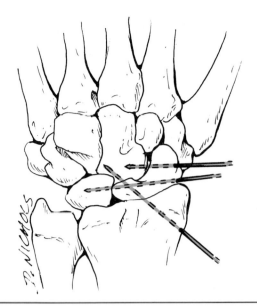

Fig. 24-4 Insertion of pins for stabilization after ligament sprain with carpal instability.

DISTAL RADIAL AND ULNAR FRACTURES

Radius

The most common distal radius fractures are extra-articular **Colles' fractures** and **Smith's fractures.**[5,10,11] A Colles' fracture is defined as a radius fracture within 2.5 cm of the wrist in which the distal radius is displaced in a dorsal direction (Fig. 24-5).[5,10,11] This fracture is recognized as the most common of all fractures, affecting mainly middle-aged and elderly women, with the mechanism of injury being a fall on an outstretched arm.[5,10] As with other types of fractures, the various treatment options generally parallel the degree of significance of the fracture type. Generally, Colles' fractures can be managed with closed reduction and rigid immobilization if the fracture is minimally displaced and stable.[10,12] However, if the fracture is comminuted and unstable, an ORIF procedure or an external fixator (for severely comminuted fractures) can be used to stabilize the fracture (Fig. 24-6).[5,10,12]

Rehabilitation after a Colles' fracture begins immediately, during immobilization. The hand, elbow, and shoulder of the ipsilateral wrist undergo active motion and resistance exercises as directed by the PT. The contralateral limb is allowed to exercise freely, and a general conditioning program is employed, provided no undue stress is allowed to the affected wrist. Restoration of purposeful, functional motion is the foundation of the rehabilitation program during each phase of recovery. Therefore gentle active pain-free motion is encouraged after immobilization, with radiographic confirmation of secure bone healing, and under the direction of the PT. However, extreme caution is urged

---

BOX 24-1

General Wrist Rehabilitation Program after Ligament Injury

MAXIMUM-PROTECTION PHASE—ACUTE
1. Immobilization, protection, rest
2. Nonsteroidal antiinflammatory drugs, analgesics
3. Ice packs
4. Active, gentle finger, hand, elbow, shoulder motion, and resistance exercise
5. General conditioning

MODERATE-PROTECTION PHASE—SUBACUTE
1. Continue protection, slowly reduce immobilization
2. If no inflammation, then use whirlpool before active, gentle protected, range of motion
3. Active-assisted range of motion
4. Resistance exercise for the hand and fingers
5. Submax isometric wrist exercises
6. Continue elbow and shoulder exercises and general conditioning program

MINIMUM-PROTECTION PHASE—MATURATION
1. Functional splint for protection
2. Active motion, whirlpool before exercise
3. Active assisted motion
4. Concentric, eccentric resistance
5. Hand and finger resistance exercise

---

to ensure that the patient perform the active motion exercises in a pain-free manner.

Once the sutures are removed (after an ORIF procedure), a whirlpool can be effective to reduce edema and encourage soft-tissue extensibility before the performance of active motion exercises. Resistance exercise is deferred until secure bone union has occurred, which is reported to take 5 to 8 weeks.[5]

Colles' fractures can result in a loss of reduction of the fracture fragments, nonunion, malunion, tendon adhesions, median nerve compression, instability, Volkmann's ischemic contracture, and reflex sympathetic dystrophy.[5,12] Therefore the PTA must be able to identify the need to advance patients' exercises gradually without increasing symptoms and immediately communicate slow progress, reduced motion, and signs of neurovascular compromise to the PT. Recovery may take up to 1 year.[5]

Smith's fracture is also referred to as a "reverse Colles' fracture."[10] The fracture usually occurs from a fall on the dorsum of the hand, with resultant distal radial fragment displaced in a palmar direction (Fig. 24-7). The

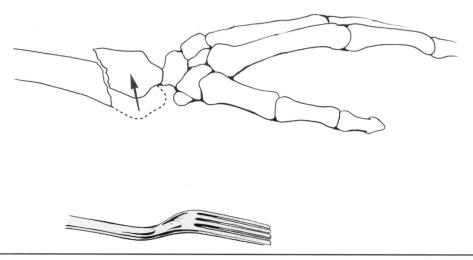

Fig. 24-5 Colles' fracture with resultant **dinner fork deformity.**

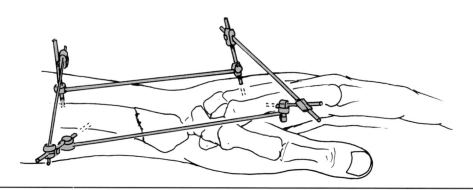

Fig. 24-6 External fixator for stabilization of severely displaced, unstable comminuted fractures.

course of treatment is either closed reduction with rigid cast immobilization or ORIF in cases of unstable, displaced, or comminuted fractures. The rehabilitation program after these injuries is similar to that of Colles' fracture.[5,10–12]

Ulna

Fractures of the distal ulna rarely occur as isolated injuries.[11] Usually, distal ulnar fractures occur in combination with distal radius fractures.[11] In fact, Melone reports that avulsion fracture of the ulnar styloid occurs in nearly 90% of unstable distal radius fractures.[11] In general, "successful treatment of the fractured radius results in accurate reduction and uncomplicated healing of the ulnar component with a favorable recovery of radioulnar and ulnocarpal joint function."[11] Therefore rehabilitation of distal ulnar fractures closely parallels treatment for fractures of the radius.

SCAPHOID FRACTURES

Before discussing treatment for fractures of the scaphoid, the PTA should outline the vascular anatomy of the scaphoid because the location and degree of fragment displacement profoundly affects treatment and rehabilitation. Usually fractures of the scaphoid occur within the proximal pole, midportion, or distal pole of the bone.[5] The distal portion and midportion of the scaphoid are vascular, whereas the proximal pole, because of the distal-to-proximal direction of blood flow, if fractured is more likely to result in nonunion and avascular necrosis (Fig. 24-8).[5,7] Therefore the intrinsic ability of the scaphoid to heal is directly related to the location of the fracture and the resultant impact on the blood supply to the fractured area.

Scaphoid fractures are recognized universally as the most common fracture that occurs to the carpal bones,

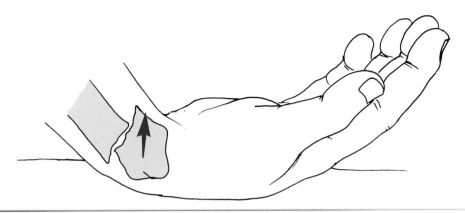

Fig. 24-7 Smith's fracture, also referred to as a reverse Colles' fracture. The mechanism of injury is usually a fall on the dorsum of the hand.

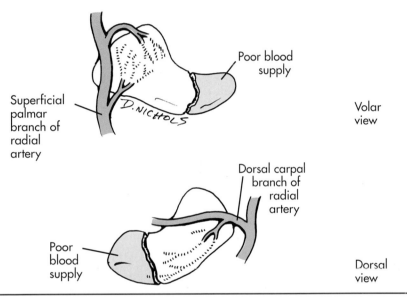

Fig. 24-8 Vascular anatomy of the scaphoid. The proximal pole of the scaphoid has a poor blood supply. If fractured in the proximal pole, there is the likelihood of avascular necrosis and resultant nonunion.

affecting nearly 60% of all carpal fractures.[5,9] It is interesting to note that the initial injury is frequently minor, with the mechanism of injury being wrist hyperextension with ulnar deviation.[9] Perhaps the most significant clinical feature of this fracture is pain localized to the **anatomic "snuffbox."**[9] When the fracture is stable and nondisplaced, treatment is usually with closed reduction and rigid cast immobilization for approximately 6 weeks, whereas proximal pole nondisplaced fractures may require immobilization for 12 to 24 weeks.[5,9]

Generally, displaced fractures require ORIF with wires and rigid immobilization.[5,9,11] Because of the increased risk of **avascular necrosis (AVN)** and **nonunion** occurring with proximal pole fractures, immobilization lasts

quite long. Fracture site protection and immobilization form the cornerstone of recovery after fracture of the scaphoid. When nonunion and avascular necrosis ensue, bone grafts from the distal radius may be necessary as an osteogenic stimulus.[11] Noninvasive, pulsed electrical stimulation is used to expedite recovery after bone graft surgery.[11] When used in conjunction with bone grafting, electrical stimulation can reduce the time to union and eventual healing "regardless of fracture location or the presence of avascular necrosis."[11]

Rehabilitation must proceed cautiously during immobilization and on removal of the cast. Finger, elbow, and shoulder motion is encouraged during immobilization, as is a general conditioning program. Early pain-free

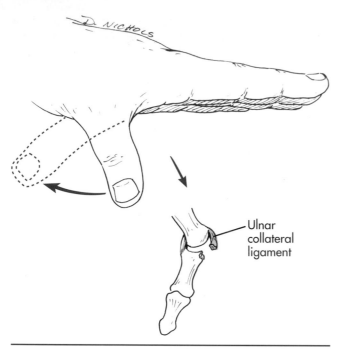

Fig. 24-9 Gamekeeper's thumb, also referred to as skier's thumb. Sudden valgus stress and hyperextension can result in partial or complete rupture of the ulnar collateral ligament of the thumb.

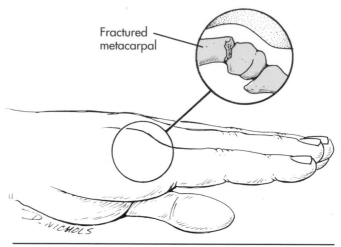

Fig. 24-10 Boxer's fracture, or "fighter's fracture."

active thumb and wrist motion is allowed once immobilization has ended. However, caution is needed so that no undue stress or extremes of motion that produce pain occur during recovery. The full return to functional motion is affected by the protracted period of immobility and methods of bone fixation. After wound closure, the use of a whirlpool may aid in soft-tissue extensibility. Passive stretching or mobilization exercises are contraindicated after immobilization. Passive exercise and joint mobilization techniques must be deferred until solid bone union has been confirmed radiographically. Resistance exercises for the wrist can begin gradually as pain allows, as motion increases, and when bone union occurs. As a general rule, every effort should be made to eliminate undue forces that may negatively affect bone healing.

SKIER'S THUMB

Skier's thumb is an acute sprain of the ulnar collateral ligament of the thumb. The mechanism of injury is usually sudden valgus stress and hyperextension of the thumb, which results in either a partial ligament tear (grade I or II) or a complete rupture (grade III) (Fig. 24-9).[3,5,6]

Partially torn ligaments can be treated nonsurgically with a thumb spica cast or rigid immobilization. Usually, immobility lasts 3 to 6 weeks.[3] On removal of the splint, gentle active thumb motion, while avoiding extremes of abduction (valgus) and hyperextension, can proceed

cautiously. Resistance exercises for the elbow and shoulder of the involved limb are prescribed throughout each phase of recovery. The initiation of progressive resistance exercises for the involved thumb must be deferred for approximately 2 months after injury for appropriate ligament healing to occur.[5] Generally, a series of submaximal isometrics is used to encourage adduction of the thumb. As motion and pain improve, more demanding exercises are added that include the use of putty for resistance. If the ulnar collateral ligament is ruptured, gross instability occurs that profoundly affects function. Surgical stabilization may be indicated in this case. Generally, an ORIF procedure is used where wires and pins help approximate and stabilize the joint for ligament healing to proceed. A short arm, thumb spica cast is applied for approximately 4 to 6 weeks.[3,5] On removal of the cast, active, pain-free motion of the fingers, wrist, and thumb is advocated, with caution taken to avoid thumb abduction (valgus stress) and hyperextension. With complete ligament sprains, the patient must avoid harmful stress to the healing ligaments. After cast removal, the injured thumb is placed in a protective splint that is removed only for active, protected motion exercises for about 10 weeks.[5] Once active motion is increased and pain does not affect activity, gentle resistance exercises are used to enhance purposeful, functional use of the thumb.

METACARPAL FRACTURES

Two of the more common metacarpal fractures are **boxer's fractures ("fighter's fracture")**[3] and **Bennett's fracture.** A boxer's fracture is a fracture to the neck of the second, third, fourth, or fifth metacarpal.[12] It is aptly named because of the incidence of this fracture among fighters (Fig. 24-10).[3,5] Treatment can be with closed reduction and rigid immobilization or with an ORIF procedure to rigidly fix and stabilize the fracture site.

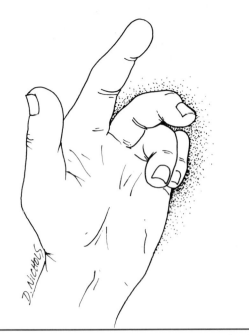

Fig. 24-11 Dupuytren's contracture most commonly affects the ulnar digits, with flexion contracture of the ulnar metacarpal phalangeal joint.

Generally the following indications are recognized to pursue ORIF procedures with metacarpal fractures:[17]

- Unstable fractures
- Inadequately reduced fractures
- Open fractures
- Associated soft-tissue problems
- Multiple fractures
- Articular fractures
- Bone loss

However, with a boxer's fracture, the physician may elect closed reduction and immobilization rather than an ORIF procedure, depending on the degree of angulation demonstrated at the fracture site.[3,5,12] If closed reduction is used, fracture consolidation is noted between 3 and 5 weeks after injury.[17] Throughout immobilization, the digits, elbow, and shoulder of the involved limb are exercised. On removal of the cast, active motion of the hand is encouraged if radiographic evidence confirms solid union and active motion poses no threat to displace the fracture segments. Progressive resistance exercises must be added gradually as pain, motion, and stable bone union dictate. Putty exercises, pinching, and sand can be used to encourage functional strength of the hand after fractures.

A Bennett fracture is a "fracture-subluxation" of the proximal first metacarpal.[3,5,12] As with a boxer's fracture, treatment can be with closed reduction and rigid cast immobilization or with an ORIF procedure, depending on the severity of the fracture. In either case, there must be nondisplaced solid union at the fracture site before active motion. If closed reduction is used, immobiliza-

tion lasts 6 to 8 weeks to promote stable union.[5] If an ORIF procedure is used, immobilization is slightly shorter because of the rigid internal fixation. Rehabilitation closely parallels the treatment for a boxer's fracture and depends on the degree of bone healing, presence of pain, and amount of active motion demonstrated by the patient.

DUPUYTREN'S CONTRACTURE

Dupuytren's contracture is a disease process that affects the palmar fascia.[5] Miller describes this disease as "proliferative fibrodysplasia of the palmar connective tissue; (this) can lead to contractures from nodules and cords that progressively develop."[12] A common characteristic of this disease is the development of immature type III collagen (normal fascia is composed of type I collagen); it is associated with myofibroblast proliferation (Fig. 24-11).[5,7,12] Usually this disease affects men 40 years or older; it is bilateral in 45% of cases and most frequently involves the ulnar digits.[12] Although tender nodules occasionally are present, this disease generally is not painful.[5,7] Therefore treatment is centered on the correction of deformity and restoration of function rather than resolution of pain. Loth notes that a 20- to 30-degree flexion contracture of the ulnar metacarpophalangeal (MCP) joint is an indication for surgery because this degree of flexion contracture is associated with an inability to lay the hand flat.[7] Even a small degree of contracture of the proximal interphalangeal (PIP) joint necessitates surgical correction.[7]

The treatment of contractures and functional limitation secondary to Dupuytren's contracture is to surgically excise the palmar fascia or perform a fasciectomy (Fig. 24-12).[1,5] In many cases, the surgical incision is left open rather than sutured together.[1,5] Historically, procedures that closed the tissue after excision of the palmar fascia resulted in scar tissue formation, tendon adhesions, tissue necrosis, and infection.[1,5] Leaving the surgical wound open means that skin care, wound cleansing, and infection control become central to the initial course of physical therapy management. The open incision may require 4 to 6 weeks to close completely.[1]

Maintenance of motion (extension) after palmar fascia release is essential for a good functional outcome. Fietti and Mackin[1] recommend the use of a whirlpool on the fifth day postoperatively to promote healing through removal of surface eschar and bacteria, enhance circulation, and provide for greater soft-tissue extensibility.[1,5] During the whirlpool treatment, the patient performs active hand and finger extension ROM exercises to maintain freedom of motion gained through surgical release. During each phase of recovery, the wrist, elbow, and shoulder of the affected hand must be exercised actively, and a general physical conditioning program is encouraged.

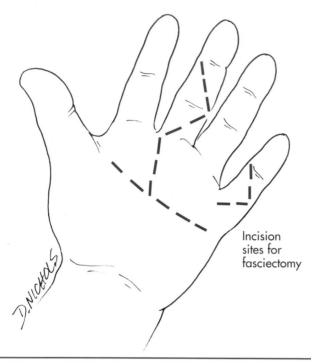

Fig. 24-12 Fasciectomy for Dupuytren's contracture. The dotted lines represent the surgical incision that is usually left open and not sutured together.

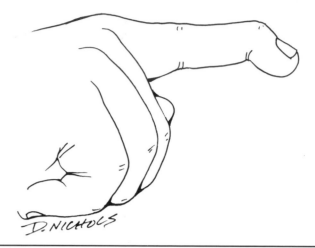

Fig. 24-13 Mallet finger. Avulsion fracture or tendon rupture results in distal interphalangeal joint flexion contracture.

Along with the concept of maintaining or increasing function and motion of the hand and digits after surgical release, the fabrication, application, and close daily supervision and possible revision of a static resting splint is used to provide stretching of the palmar fascia and affected digits. Usually the occupational therapy rehabilitation team designs and fabricates the static and dynamic splints necessary to enhance function, but PTs with specific experience and training in splint fabrication for hand and finger injuries also can initially design and apply static and dynamic splints.

In conjunction with daily whirlpool treatments, active ROM movements, and static splinting, the following general exercises can be used to enhance early motion and a return to function:[1]

- Thumb opposition to all fingers
- Flexion of each finger to distal palmar crease
- Full flexion of the PIP joints
- Making a fist
- Abduction and adduction of the fingers
- Finger extension
- Full wrist and thumb motion
- Crossing the fingers

The application of scar tissue massage is appropriate once the surgical wound is healed. Retrograde massage and specific cross-fiber scar massage can be performed as soon as pain, swelling, and wound healing allow.[1,5] The patient is instructed to perform automassage techniques a few times daily to enhance tissue extensibility, prevent adhesions, and reduce edema.

The ultimate restoration of function after surgical care of Dupuytren's contracture is achieved by maintaining and enhancing hand and finger extension, controlling swelling and edema, reducing scar tissue proliferation, and promoting active motion while enhancing static soft-tissue stretching using splints.

MALLET FINGER

Mallet finger is a tendon injury (rupture) or avulsion fracture (tendon-bone) of the extensor tendon that results in a distal interphalangeal (DIP) joint flexion contracture (Fig. 24-13). This injury usually occurs as a result of direct trauma to the distal end of the phalanx, causing the terminal tendon or digit to rupture or fracture.[5] With either tendon rupture or avulsion fracture, the treatment is essentially the same. Continuous, uninterrupted splinting of the DIP joint for 6 to 10 weeks in zero degrees of extension allows for appropriate tendon or bone healing.[3,5] Throughout immobilization, the patient actively exercises all noninvolved joints of the upper extremity. The affected joint begins active exercise at the sixth to eighth week. Passive flexion exercises of the DIP are contraindicated to protect the healing tendon and bone from extremes of motion and unwanted forces. Instead the patient performs only gentle active DIP flexion to 20 degrees to avoid excessive stretch of the healing tendon.[5] Extension lag may develop. If the patient is unable to actively extend the DIP when the splint is removed, active flexion exercises are terminated and continuous splinting in 0 degrees of extension to 10 degrees of hyperextension resumed for an additional 2 to 4 weeks before active exercises are reinitiated.[3,5] Extension lag may recur.[3] If no extension lag is noted during early (6 to 8 weeks) active flexion of the DIP, during the following weeks, active flexion gradually is allowed with progressions in 5- to 10-degree incre-

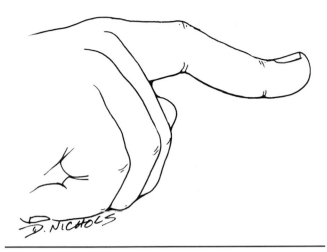

Fig. 24-14 Boutonnière deformity, proximal interphalangeal flexion with distal interphalangeal extension.

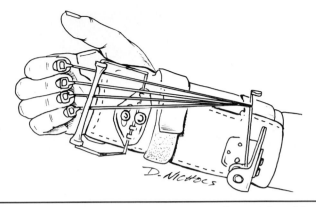

Fig. 24-15 Postoperative protective splint with rubber band traction after flexor tendon repair.

ments. The PTA must continue to observe for any extension lag of the DIP.

The strength of the involved digit must be increased as motion gradually improves. Tendon or bone healing must not be overstressed before secure union occurs; therefore active resistance exercises are deferred for up to 12 weeks after injury and are begun only in the absence of extension lag.[5]

BOUTONNIÈRE DEFORMITY

Direct trauma to the terminal phalanx can also result in a rupture or stretch of the central extensor tendon at the PIP joint, which creates PIP flexion with DIP extension and the recognizable **boutonnière deformity** (Fig. 24-14).[3,16] When the tendon is ruptured and no associated avulsion fracture is present, the treatment is to immobilize the PIP joint in full extension for a minimum of 6 to 8 weeks.[3,16] The DIP joint is not immobilized; the patient performs both active and passive DIP flexion with the PIP in extension.[3] As with DIP extensor tendon injuries (mallet finger), the course of recovery follows the course of tendon or bone healing.

FLEXOR TENDON INJURIES

Although extensor tendon injuries occur approximately five times more often than flexor tendon injuries, **flexor tendon** injuries, repair, and rehabilitation are universally considered more complicated and challenging.[3,5,16] To apply appropriate motion and stress after flexor tendon injuries and subsequent surgical repair, the PTA must be aware of the dynamic nature of tendon healing while focusing on the desired outcome of functional motion and strength via normal tendon glide and excursion as a result of inhibition by adhesions.[2,5,13]

Adhesions generally form early in the recovery stage of tendon healing and affect both motion and function.

Without appropriate stress and directed motion, scar tissue forms in a random pattern and does not attain normal intact tendon strength.[2] Therefore to preferentially develop mature collagen fibers, which align in the direction of applied forces, mechanical stimuli are necessary during remodeling, similar to Wolff's law for bone healing.[2] Specifically, intermittent purposeful stress and motion enhance tendon healing and collagen fiber alignment. Because the ultimate goal of recovery after flexor tendon injury and repair is to achieve motion and strength of the involved tendon, early, controlled passive motion and stress are used to influence the organization, maturation, and remodeling of collagen fibers.[2,5,13]

The most salient features of rehabilitation after flexor tendon repair involve the interrelationship between immobilization and the application of early, protected, limited passive motion.[2,5,13] After flexor tendon repair, "carefully applied early protected motion can produce a consistent range of gliding in the early postoperative period that is not associated with significant repair site deformation."[2]

Although a detailed description of the various tendon repair procedures is beyond the scope and intent of this discussion, general rehabilitation procedures parallel tendon healing and motion influences appropriate cellular response in the injured tendon tissue.[2] Gentle motion is allowed 2 to 3 days after repair.[5] Progressive motion is encouraged within the limits of postoperative protective plaster splinting and rubber band traction (Fig. 24-15). The purpose of this postoperative immobilization arrangement is to maintain the interphalangeal (IP) joint in 30 to 50 degrees of passive flexion while encouraging active IP extension within the limits of the plaster splint.[5] This is consistent with the "concept that a limited, immediate mobilization program improves the quality of the biologic repair response after flexor tendon repair within the digital sheath by effectively eliminating the associated adhesion formation."[2]

Jacobs advocates that more "aggressive" flexion and extension exercises can begin around 6 weeks and that

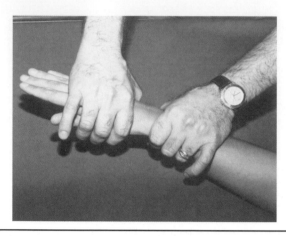

Fig. 24-16 Anterior-posterior, medial, and lateral glides of the wrist.

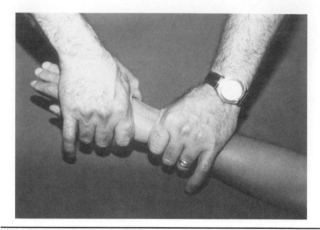

Fig. 24-17 Long axis or longitudinal distraction of the wrist.

manual resistance exercise can be initiated at 8 weeks.[5] As motion and strength improve, more challenging resistance exercises using incremental degrees of putty tension, rubber balls, and spring and cable hand exercises are employed. At approximately 12 weeks, functional ADLs and specific job tasks requiring repetitive hand motions are begun, with all motion restrictions eliminated.[5]

REFLEX SYMPATHETIC DYSTROPHY

Reflex sympathetic dystrophy (RSD) is a vasomotor dysfunction or reflex vasomotor response to a chronic sensory stimulus.[5,8,14] Perhaps one of the most complex and challenging conditions to treat, RSD is characterized by pain (predominant feature), hyperesthesia, edema, discoloration, and loss of motion and function.[8] This pain syndrome develops gradually after various fractures, soft-tissue injuries, and surgery.[8,14] It is interesting to note that there is no direct relationship between the injury and the degree of pain experienced by persons suffering from RSD.[5,8,14] Generally, persons who are susceptible to RSD demonstrate a low pain threshold and dependent personality.[14] The mechanism of RSD is not completely clear, but it has been proposed that the vasoconstriction occurring after an injury becomes severe and prolonged, developing into a painful stimulus that perpetuates abnormal vasomotor reflexes.[14]

Jacobs identifies three stages of RSD.[5] Stage I represents the acute episode, which may last as long as 3 months. Pain and edema are the dominant clinical symptoms during the acute stage. Discoloration and excessive sweating (hyperhydrosis) are obvious, as are temperature changes.[5] Stage II lasts from the third month to approximately 1 year after injury.[5] Classically, pain and edema increase during this period, and skin coloration changes from red to a "pale cyanosis."[5] In addition, the skin becomes dry (changing from hyperhidrosis) and tissue atrophy becomes more apparent. Radiographic exami-

nation frequently reveals the development of osteoporosis.[5,8,14] Stage III involves increasing trophic changes, severe motion restrictions, atrophy, and the production of inelastic fibrous tissue.[5,14]

Treatment focuses on controlling pain and swelling and completely eliminating all pain-producing activities. Treatment must be initiated as soon as a diagnosis is confirmed. Initially, medical management focuses on using sympathetic nerve blocks that do not affect numbness, weakness, or paralysis, but significantly reduce hypersensitivity and pain.[8] Moist heat, gentle massage, transcutaneous electrical nerve stimulation, and electrical stimulation are effective tools to use for pain and swelling control. Protection of the involved extremity from activities that produce pain is critical to successful treatment. Aggressive exercise or passive motions that produce pain are strictly avoided during each phase of recovery. Splints can be used to modify motions and allow for intermittent gentle active pain-free motion. The management of swelling can be enhanced if the patient elevates the involved extremity, uses compression wraps or garments, and applies therapeutic gentle retrograde massage and electrical stimulation.[5,8,14] Unfortunately for persons suffering from RSD, many therapeutic exercises perpetuate the pain. Therefore use of active exercises is determined by the patient's tolerance of pain with passive motion and control of edema, as well as the ability to demonstrate continued pain relief with splints to eliminate unwanted motions. At no point in the course of recovery from RSD is aggressive, active motion prescribed in the presence of pain.

MOBILIZATION OF THE WRIST AND HAND

The use of peripheral joint mobilization techniques can be quite effective to modulate pain and increase motion of the wrist and hand. The specific applications of these techniques are determined by the PT, and the appropri-

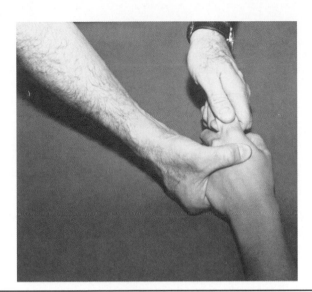

Fig. 24-18 Anterior-posterior, medial, and lateral glides of the metacarpal phalangeal joint.

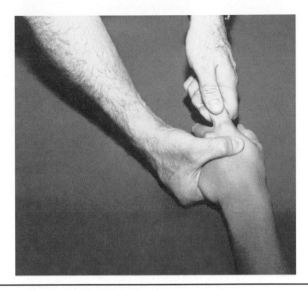

Fig. 24-19 Long axis or longitudinal distraction of the metacarpal phalangeal joint.

ate direction and amplitude of force are dictated by the specific injury and degree of soft-tissue and bone healing (see Chapter 16).

Moist heat, paraffin baths, whirlpools, electrical stimulation, and gentle active exercise can be used immediately before mobilization to encourage soft-tissue relaxation and evacuation of waste from the injured area. In addition, physician-prescribed analgesics, muscle relaxants, and NSAIDs may be effective before beginning mobilization techniques.

The position of the patient is a critical feature of effective mobilization. The injured extremity must be positioned to provide comfort, relaxation, and support while affording the clinician access to the extremity.

As with other joints, many different techniques are used. This discussion introduces only a few of the more common and easily performed techniques. The intricate and complex nature of the wrist and hand demands mastery of anatomy, kinesiology, pathomechanics of injury, and biomechanics to effectively perform the more difficult techniques described in orthopedic texts.[18]

Mobilization of the Wrist

Anterior, posterior, medial, and lateral glides of the wrist are performed with the patient either sitting with the affected arm supported or supine. The PTA uses one hand to stabilize the distal radius and ulna on the dorsal aspect while firmly grasping the proximal row of carpal bones with the other hand.[18] Using the hand supporting the carpal bones, the PTA directs an anterior and posterior force or a medial and lateral force to "glide" the carpal bones from the stabilized distal radius and ulna (Fig. 24-16).[18]

Distraction of the carpals is done with the patient either sitting or supine. The hand position is exactly the same as described in the preceding, but the direction of

force is distal or longitudinal to the radius and ulna. This direction of force distracts or displaces the carpal bones from the stabilized radius and ulna (Fig. 24-17).[18]

Mobilization of the Hand

Anterior, posterior, medial, and lateral glides of the MCP joint can be performed with the patient supine or sitting. The PTA uses one hand to stabilize the shaft of the affected metacarpal while firmly grasping the proximal phalanx with the other hand. With the metacarpal firmly stabilized, the PTA uses the hand contacting the phalanx to direct an anterior, posterior, or medial and lateral force that glides the MCP joint (Fig. 24-18).[18]

Distraction of the MCP joint occurs with the patient in the same position as described in the preceding. With the hand placement the same, the direction of force is applied to distract the phalanx from the stabilized metacarpal (Fig. 24-19).[18]

✤ ADDITIONAL FEATURES

Anatomic "Snuffbox": Area between the extensor pollicis longus and extensor pollicis brevis. Significant anatomy within snuffbox, radial artery, and scaphoid.

Guyon's Canal: Area between the volar carpal ligament and the transverse carpal ligament.

Kienböck's Disease: Osteonecrosis of the lunate.

Scapholunate Advanced Collapse: Arthritis from scaphoid nonunion from avascular necrosis.

Stener's Lesion: Interposition of adductor pollicis aponeurosis between torn section (ends) of the ulnar collateral ligament.

Triangular Fibrocartilage Complex: Important stabilizing complex of ligaments that support the distal radioulnar joint.

Triangular Fibrocartilage Complex Ligaments: Articular disk, ulnocarpal ligament, dorsal radioulnar ligament, volar radioulnar ligament, and tendon of the extensor carpi ulnaris.

Ulnar Tunnel Syndrome: Ulnar nerve compression within Guyon's canal.

REFERENCES

1. Fietti VG, Mackin EJ: Dupuytren's disease. In Hunter JM, Schneider LH, Mackin EJ, et al, eds. Rehabilitation of the Hand. St Louis, Mosby, 1978.
2. Gelberman R, et al: Tendon. In Woo SL-Y, Buckwalter JA, eds. Injury and Repair of the Musculoskeletal Soft Tissues. Rosemont, IL, American Academy of Orthopaedic Surgeons, 1988.
3. Green DP, Strickland JW: The hand. In DeLee JC, Drez D, eds. Orthopaedic Sports Medicine: Principles and Practice, vol 1. Philadelphia, WB Saunders, 1994.
4. Hebert LA: The Neck-Arm-Hand Book. Greenville, ME, IMPACC, 1989.
5. Jacobs JL: Hand and wrist. In Richardson JK, Iglarsh ZA, eds. Clinical Orthopaedic Physical Therapy. Philadelphia, WB Saunders, 1994.
6. Lephart S: Injuries to the hand and wrist. In Prentice WE, ed. Rehabilitation Techniques in Sports Medicine, 2nd ed. St Louis, Mosby, 1994.
7. Loth TS: Hand and wrist. In Loth TS, ed. Orthopaedic Boards Review. St Louis, Mosby, 1993.
8. Mayer AV, McCue FC: Rehabilitation and protection of the wrist and hand. In Posner MA, ed. The Upper Extremity in Sports Medicine, Hand Section. St Louis, Mosby, 1990.
9. McCue FC, Bruce JF: The wrist. In DeLee JC, Drez D, eds. Orthopaedic Sports Medicine: Principles and Practice, vol 1. Philadelphia, WB Saunders, 1994.
10. McRae R, ed. Practical Fracture Treatment, 3rd ed. New York, Churchill Livingstone, 1994.
11. Melone CP: Fractures of the wrist. In Nicholas JA, Hershman EB, eds. The Upper Extremity in Sports Medicine. St Louis, Mosby, 1990.
12. Miller MD: Review of Orthopaedics. Philadelphia, WB Saunders, 1992.
13. Nissenbaum M: Early care of flexor tendon injuries: application of principles of tendon healing and early motion. In Hunter JM, Schneider LH, Mackin EJ, et al, eds. Rehabilitation of the Hand. St Louis, Mosby, 1978.
14. Omer GE: Management of pain syndromes in the upper extremity. In Hunter JM, Schneider LH, Mackin EJ, et al, eds. Rehabilitation of the Hand. St Louis, Mosby, 1978.
15. Wilgis EFS, Yates AY: Wrist pain. In Nicholas JA, Hershman EB, eds. The Upper Extremity in Sports Medicine. St Louis, Mosby, 1990.
16. Wilson RL, Carter MS: Joint injuries in the hand: preservation of proximal interphalangeal joint function. In Hunter JM, Schneider LH, Mackin EJ, et al, eds. Rehabilitation of the Hand. St Louis, Mosby, 1978.
17. Wilson RL, Carter MS: Management of hand fractures. In Hunter JM, Schneider LH, Mackin EJ, et al, eds. Rehabilitation of the Hand. St Louis, Mosby, 1978.
18. Wooden MJ: Mobilization of the upper extremity. In Donatelli R, Wooden MJ, eds. Orthopaedic Physical Therapy. New York, Churchill Livingstone, 1989.

REVIEW QUESTIONS

Multiple Choice

1. Which of the following is a clinical symptom of carpal tunnel syndrome?
   A. Pain
   B. Numbness
   C. Weakness
   D. Tingling
   E. All of the above

2. Carpal tunnel syndrome is considered which of the following? (Circle any that apply.)
   A. An acute traumatic injury
   B. A repetitive motion disorder
   C. An overuse injury
   D. A cumulative trauma injury
   E. Rare

3. After diagnosis, which of the following may have the greatest effect on reducing symptoms of carpal tunnel syndrome in the years ahead?
   A. Strengthening
   B. Stretching
   C. Identifying and modifying activities of daily living (ADL) and occupational risks
   D. Bracing

4. How long is the affected wrist immobilized if a surgical release is performed for carpal tunnel syndrome (cutting of the transverse carpal ligament, thereby decompressing the neurovascular tissues underneath)?
   A. 6 to 8 weeks
   B. 3 to 5 weeks
   C. 2 to 14 days
   D. 8 to 10 weeks

5. Which of the following is (are) treatment for De Quervain's tenosynovitis? (Circle any that apply.)
   A. Wrist and thumb immobilized
   B. Corticosteroid injection
   C. Surgical decompression
   D. Excision of the radial styloid
   E. Tendon release

6. Ligament sprains of the wrist, without carpal instability, are managed with which of the following?
   A. Percutaneous pinning
   B. Immobilization
   C. Open reduction with internal fixation (ORIF)
   D. Direct surgical repair of torn ligaments
   E. All of the above

7. Ligament sprains of the wrist with resultant carpal instability can be treated with which of the following? (Circle any that apply.)
   A. ORIF
   B. Closed reduction with percutaneous pinning
   C. Cast immobilization
   D. Fusion of carpals
   E. Early active full range of motion (ROM)

8. A Colles' fracture affects primarily which of the following?
   A. Teenage men
   B. Elderly men
   C. Middle-aged and elderly women
   D. Young women

9. If a Colles' fracture is minimally displaced and stable, the method of treatment is usually which of the following?
   A. Percutaneous pinning
   B. ORIF
   C. Closed reduction with rigid immobilization
   D. Sling immobilization

10. Which of the following are identified as possible complications after Colles' fractures?
    A. Nonunion
    B. Tendon adhesions
    C. Median nerve compression
    D. Reflex sympathetic dystrophy
    E. All of the above

11. Avulsion fractures of the ulnar styloid can occur in _____ of unstable distal radius fractures.
    A. 10%
    B. 90%
    C. 50%
    D. 60%

12. Which of the following is a major concern after proximal pole fractures of the scaphoid?
    A. Muscular weakness
    B. Avascular necrosis
    C. Arthrofibrosis
    D. Wrist flexion contracture
    E. All of the above

13. Where is pain most clinically significant in the presence of a scaphoid fracture?
    A. Volar aspect of the wrist (diffuse)
    B. Dorsal aspect of the wrist (diffuse)
    C. Anatomic "snuffbox"
    D. Ulnar styloid

14. In cases where the scaphoid fracture is nondisplaced and stable, the treatment is usually with closed reduction and rigid cast immobilization for approximately 6 weeks. However, fractures of the proximal pole require immobilization for how long?
    A. 8 weeks
    B. 12 to 24 weeks
    C. 10 weeks
    D. 9 to 11 weeks

15. If nonunion or avascular necrosis occurs after a proximal pole scaphoid fracture, which of the following can be employed to aid healing? (Circle any that apply.)
    A. Bone grafts
    B. Electrical stimulation
    C. Vascular shunts
    D. Closed kinetic chain exercises
    E. Early active motion

16. Which of the following describe(s) the cornerstone of treatment for scaphoid fractures? (Circle any that apply.)
    A. Early active motion
    B. Fracture site protection
    C. Closed kinetic chain exercises
    D. Immobilization
    E. Early proprioception exercises

17. In general, which of the following are indications that physicians should consider for an ORIF for metacarpal fractures?
    A. Articular fractures
    B. Unstable fractures
    C. Bone loss
    D. Open fractures
    E. All of the above

18. A proliferative fibrodysplasia disease that affects the palmar fascia and leads to contractures is called which of the following?
    A. De Quervain's disease
    B. Volkmann's contracture
    C. Dupuytren's contracture
    D. Palmar fasciitis

19. Dupuytren's contracture affects mainly which of the following?
    A. Women 20 to 40 years of age
    B. Young men 25 years of age and younger
    C. Men 40 years of age and older
    D. Women 45 to 60 years of age

20. Treatment of Dupuytren's contracture is centered on which of the following?
    A. Resolution of painful nodules
    B. Correction of deformity and loss of function
    C. Improving vascular supply to the palmar fascia
    D. Increasing wrist flexion motion

21. Which of the following describes a clinically significant feature after fasciectomy for Dupuytren's contracture?
    A. The sutures are left in place for only 7 to 10 days.
    B. The surgical incision is left open.
    C. There is significant sensory loss.
    D. Extreme pain is noted for many days.

22. To restore function after surgery for Dupuytren's contracture, which of the following exercises is employed to enhance early motion?
    A. Finger flexion to distal palmar crease (active)
    B. Active proximal interphalangeal (PIP) flexion
    C. Active abduction and adduction of the fingers
    D. Active finger extension
    E. All of the above

23. Which of the following are appropriate treatment measures for extensor tendon rupture or avulsion fracture of the fingers? (Circle any that apply.)
    A. Distal interphalangeal (DIP) flexion with splinting
    B. Continuous splinting for 6 to 10 weeks
    C. Active extension
    D. DIP terminal extension with splinting
    E. ORIF

24. Which of the following is contraindicated after extensor tendon rupture or avulsion fracture?
    A. Active extension of the DIP between the sixth and eighth weeks
    B. Active flexion of the DIP to 20 degrees
    C. Passive flexion of the DIP
    D. Passive extension of the DIP

25. In general, flexor tendon injuries and repairs are treated with which of the following?
    A. Rigid immobilization for 6 to 10 weeks
    B. Immobilization for 10 weeks or longer
    C. Early protected motion
    D. Immobilization for 4 to 6 weeks

26. Which of the following is characteristic of reflex sympathetic dystrophy?
    A. Edema
    B. Loss of function
    C. Pain
    D. Hyperesthesia
    E. All of the above

27. Which of the following are clinical symptoms of stage I reflex sympathetic dystrophy (RSD)?
    A. Pale cyanosis
    B. Production of inelastic fibrous tissue
    C. Increased tissue atrophy
    D. Pain and edema, discoloration, and hyperhydrosis

28. The treatment of RSD primarily is focused on which of the following?
    A. Restoration of strength
    B. Improved motion
    C. Pain and swelling management
    D. Early return to functional activities

29. Which of the following is a measure that can be employed to manage pain and swelling with RSD? (Circle any that apply.)
    A. Ice
    B. Heat
    C. Transcutaneous electrical nerve stimulation, electrical stimulation
    D. Sympathetic nerve block injections
    E. Full active range of motion
30. Which of the following is (are) strictly avoided during each stage of recovery with RSD if pain is present? (Circle any that apply.)
    A. Splint applications
    B. Plyometrics
    C. Full-range slow- and fast-speed isokinetic exercise
    D. Eccentric full-range isotonic exercise
    E. Thermal agents

Short Answer
31. Name the most common compression neuropathy of the wrist.

32. In the following figure, identify the injury and the tissues involved.

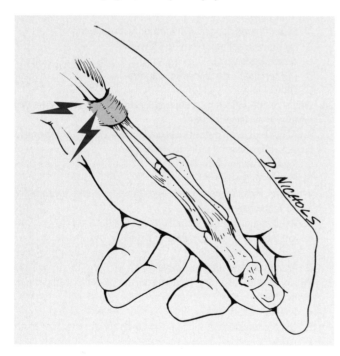

33. In the following figure, identify the injury and name the common deformity.

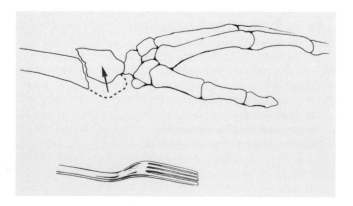

34. In the following figure, identify the injury and describe the method of fixation.

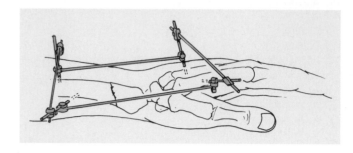

35. Name the injury in the following figure.

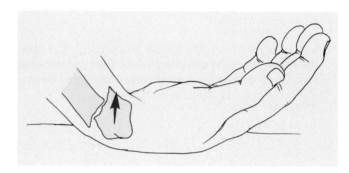

36. In the following figure, identify the injury and the structures involved. Also identify a common name for this injury.

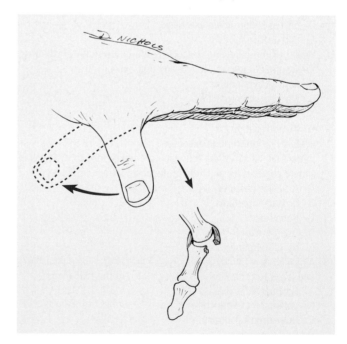

37. Identify the injury in the figure and give a common name that describes the injury.

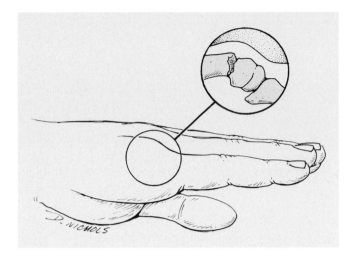

38. A fracture-subluxation of the proximal first metacarpal describes what type of fracture?

39. Identify the injuries or deformities in the following figures.

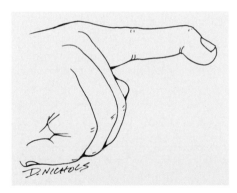

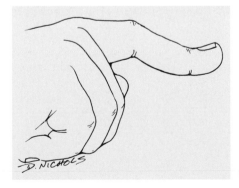

40. A rupture or avulsion fracture of the extensor tendon that results in a DIP joint flexion contracture is called _____ .

41. A rupture or stretch of the central extensor tendon at the PIP joint that creates PIP flexion with DIP extension is called a _____ .

True/False

42. Generally, motions that produce repetitive ulnar deviations can create tenosynovitis at the first dorsal compartment of the wrist.

43. The stability of the wrist is primarily dependent on musculotendinous support and intracapsular ligaments.

44. A Colles' fracture is the most common of all fractures.

45. Distal ulnar fractures commonly occur as isolated injuries.

46. Scaphoid fractures are considered the most common fractures that occur to the carpal bones.

47. Although occasionally tender nodules are present, Dupuytren's contracture is commonly not painful.

48. An open surgical procedure (fasciectomy or excision of the palmar fascia) should be performed if a 20- to 30-degree flexion contracture of the ulnar metacarpophalangeal (MCP) joint results from Dupuytren's contracture.

49. There is usually a direct relationship between the severity of injury and the degree of pain experienced by persons suffering from RSD.

50. It is true that at no point in the course of recovery from RSD is aggressive active motion prescribed in the presence of pain.

Essay Questions

Answer on a separate sheet of paper.

51. Identify and describe common compression neuropathies of the wrist.

52. Discuss methods of management and rehabilitation of compression neuropathies of the wrist.

53. Identify and describe common ligament injuries of the wrist.

54. Describe and discuss methods of management and rehabilitation of ligament injuries of the wrist.

55. Describe methods of management and rehabilitation for distal radial and ulnar fractures.

56. Identify methods of management and rehabilitation for scaphoid fractures.

57. Identify and describe common metacarpal fractures and methods of management and rehabilitation.

58. Describe methods of management and rehabilitation of Dupuytren's contracture.

59. Identify and describe common extensor and flexor tendon injuries.

60. Discuss methods of management and rehabilitation of extensor tendon and flexor tendon injuries.

61. Identify methods of management and rehabilitation for reflex sympathetic dystrophy.

62. Describe common mobilization techniques for the wrist and hand.

Critical Thinking Application

You are treating two patients, one with the diagnosis of carpal tunnel syndrome (nonoperative), the other with a stable, minimally displaced Colles' fracture. Based on your understanding of bone and soft-tissue healing, develop a comprehensive critical pathway (criterion-based rehabilitation program) for each case in which you will recommend specific therapeutic interventions for pain and swelling management, restoration of motion, muscle contraction types, cardiovascular fitness, general physical conditioning, and closed-chain proprioception functional activities. Organize your outline so that the rehabilitation program you recommend parallels the phases of soft-tissue and bone healing, which in turn coincides with the maximum-protection phase, moderate-protection phase, and minimum-protection phase of recovery. Which ergonomic and functional ADL modifications do you recommend for the patient with carpal tunnel syndrome? Which exercises and activities do you recommend for the patient with the Colles' fracture during periods of immobilization? Clearly note and identify complications that can occur after a Colles' fracture.

Answers to Review Questions

CHAPTER 1

Patient Supervision and Observation During Treatment

Multiple Choice
1. F

Short Answer
2. Refer to Chapter 1
3. Refer to Chapter 1
4. Communication
5. Understanding, sensitivity, warmth, and reassurance
6. Listening
7. Open-ended questions
8. Close-ended questions
9. Refer to Chapter 1
10. Refer to Chapter 1
11. Summary-type statements
12. Refer to Chapter 1
13. Dominance, submission, hostility, and warmth
14. See Figure

Dominance

| **Quadrant 1 (Q1)** Dominance plus hostility | **Quadrant 4 (Q4)** Dominance plus warmth |

Hostility — **Warmth**

| **Quadrant 2 (Q2)** Submission plus hostility | **Quadrant 3 (Q3)** Submission plus warmth |

Submission

15. Q4
16. Appropriately friendly, attentive, responsive, involved, exploring, analytical, and task oriented
17. Refer to Chapter 1
18. Refer to Chapter 1
19. Goniometric measurements (ROM); circumferential measurements (swelling, hypertrophy, and atrophy); manual muscle testing; endurance; heart rate, blood pressure; respiration; balance; and coordination

Essay Questions 20–27
Refer to Chapter 1 text for all essay question answers and explanations.

CHAPTER 2

The Role of the Physical Therapist Assistant in Physical Assessment

Multiple Choice
1. B
2. D
3. B
4. D
5. A
6. D
7. C
8. C
9. A
10. B

Short Answer
11. Hand washing
12. Nausea, pallor, and profuse perspiration
13. Centralization
14. Age, body size, stature, exercise, and body position
15. Crepitus
16. Scarring or granulomatosis

True/False
17. F
18. T
19. F
20. F
21. T
22. F
23. T
24. T
25. F
26. F

Essay Questions 27–30
Refer to Chapter 2 text for all essay question answers and explanations.

CHAPTER 3

Physical Agents Used in the Treatment of Common Musculoskeletal Conditions

Multiple Choice

1. A
2. D
3. B
4. D
5. A
6. D
7. D
8. C
9. A
10. D

Short Answer

11. No. The weight of the body may increase heat transfer beyond therapeutic levels and impair local circulation by compression of blood vessels.
12. Conforms to uneven body part; softens skin in preparation for soft-tissue work; wax can be used for exercise after removal.
13. Cold
14. High frequency (3 mHz) for superficial. Low frequency (1 mHz) for deep.
15. 5 minutes/2× area of sound head

True/False

16. F
17. F
18. T
19. T
20. F
21. F
22. F
23. T
24. T
25. F

Essay Questions 26–29

Refer to Chapter 3 text for all essay question answers and explanations.

CHAPTER 4

Flexibility

Multiple Choice

1. C
2. B
3. E
4. C
5. D
6. C
7. C
8. C and D
9. D
10. B
11. D

Short Answer

12. Active
13. Static, ballistic, and proprioceptive neuromuscular facilitation (PNF)
14. Golgi tendon organ (GTO)
15. Muscle spindle

True/False

16. T
17. F
18. T
19. T
20. T
21. F
22. F

Essay Questions 23–32

Refer to Chapter 4 text for all essay question answers and explanations.

CHAPTER 5

Strength

Multiple Choice

1. D
2. D
3. C and D
4. B
5. B, D, and E
6. D
7. E
8. A, C, and D
9. B, C, and D
10. A, B, and C
11. B, D, and E
12. B
13. C
14. C
15. B
16. C
17. D
18. C
19. C
20. D
21. C
22. D
23. C
24. E

Short Answer

25. Two
26. Oxidative
27. 1: Slow twitch (type I)
    2: Fast twitch (type II)
    3: Fast twitch (type II-A)
    4: Fast twitch (type II-AB)
    5: Fast twitch (type II-B)
28. Manual muscle testing, cable tensiometry, dynamometry, isotonic one-repetition maximum lift, isokinetics

29. 3: Concentrics   2: Isometrics   1: Eccentrics
30. 3: Eccentrics   2: Isometrics   1: Concentrics
31. Atrophy and hypertrophy
32. Specific Adaptions to Imposed Demands
33. Frequency, intensity, and duration
34. Refer to chart.

True/False
35. T
36. F
37. F
38. F
39. T
40. F
41. F
42. F
43. T
44. F
45. T
46. F
47. F

Essay Questions 48–62
Refer to Chapter 5 text for all essay question answers and explanations.

CHAPTER 6

Endurance

Multiple Choice
1. D
2. C
3. E
4. B and D
5. B
6. C
7. A
8. C
9. B
10. C
11. B and D
12. A, B, and C
13. B, C, and D

True/False
14. F

Essay Questions 15–22
Refer to Chapter 6 text for all essay question answers and explanations.

CHAPTER 7

Balance and Coordination

Multiple Choice
1. E
2. C
3. A
4. C
5. C
6. B
7. E
8. E
9. A, B, and C

Short Answer
10. Provide manual external resistance; ask the patient to close his or her eyes.
11. Single-leg stance test (SLST)
12. 1: Sitting balance—eyes open
    2: Standing—weight shifting
    3: Double leg standing—eyes closed
    4: Single-leg standing—eyes closed
    5: Single-leg standing—eyes closed with manual resistance
13. Refer to chapter.

True/False
14. T
15. F
16. F
17. T
18. T
19. T
20. T
21. F

Essay Questions 22–28
Refer to Chapter 7 text for all essay question answers and explanations.

CHAPTER 8

Composition and Function of Connective Tissue

Multiple Choice
1. C
2. B
3. C
4. D
5. C
6. B
7. C
8. C
9. B

Short Answer
10. Inflammation and fibroplasia
11. Fibroblast growth factor (FGF), tumor necrosis factor-β (TNF-β), and wound angiogenesis factor (WAF)

True/False
12. F
13. F
14. F
15. T
16. T
17. F
18. T

19. T
20. T
21. F
22. T
23. F
24. T
25. F

Essay Questions 26–30
Refer to Chapter 8 text for all essay question answers and explanations.

CHAPTER 9

Ligament Healing

Multiple Choice
1. B
2. A
3. D
4. D
5. A
6. B
7. D
8. C and D
9. A and B
10. B and D
11. C
12. C
13. E
14. B, C, D, and E

Short Answer
15. Phase I: inflammatory response; Phase II: repair; Phase III: remodeling
16. Redness, swelling, pain, heat, and loss of function
17. Repair phase
18. Contact, controlled stress, and excessive forces
19. Refer to chapter.

True/False
20. F
21. F
22. F
23. F
24. F
25. T

Essay Questions 26–31
Refer to Chapter 9 text for all essay question answers and explanations.

CHAPTER 10

Bone Healing

Multiple Choice
1. B, C, and D
2. C
3. D
4. D

5. E
6. B, C, and D
7. A, C, and D
8. C
9. D
10. C and D
11. C
12. A and D
13. A and C
14. C
15. A and B
16. E
17. E
18. E

Short Answer
19. Internal and external fixation
20. Pain, crepitus, and swelling

True/False
21. F
22. T
23. T

Essay Questions 24–36
Refer to Chapter 10 text for all essay question answers and explanations.

CHAPTER 11

Cartilage Healing

Multiple Choice
1. B
2. E
3. A, B, D, and E
4. C and D
5. C and D
6. B, C, and D
7. E
8. B
9. E
10. C
11. C
12. A and C
13. A, C, D, and E
14. A and B

Short Answer
15. Total meniscectomy, subtotal meniscectomy, and meniscal repair
16. Traumatic or degenerative

True/False
17. T
18. T
19. F
20. F
21. F
22. F
23. T

Essay Questions 24–31
Refer to Chapter 11 text for all essay question answers and explanations.

CHAPTER 12

Muscle and Tendon Healing

Multiple Choice
1. D
2. C and D
3. C
4. A
5. B
6. D
7. A, B, and C
8. C
9. D
10. C and D
11. C
12. B
13. C

Short Answer
14. Indirect
15. Direct

True/False
16. T
17. T
18. T
19. T
20. T
21. F

Essay Questions 22–31
Refer to Chapter 12 text for all essay question answers and explanations.

CHAPTER 13

Neurovascular Healing and Thromboembolic Disease

Multiple Choice
1. A, C, D
2. C
3. B
4. B
5. B, D
6. B
7. C
8. B, D
9. C
10. C
11. D
12. D
13. C
14. A, C, D
15. A, C, D
16. B
17. D

Short Answer
18. Epineurium, perineurium, and endoneurium
19. Neurapraxia, axonotmesis, and neurotmesis
20. Common peroneal nerve, radial nerve, median nerve, and lateral femoral cutaneous nerve
21. "Burner" and "stinger"
22. Double crush
23. Tunica intima, tunica media, and tunica adventitia
24. Hip-common or external iliac artery; and knee-popliteal artery
25. Pulselessness, pallor, paraesthesias, pain, paralysis, massive bleeding, and rapidly expanding hematoma
26. Hypercoagulability, venous stasis, and endothelial vessel wall injury
27. Total joint arthroplasty, femur fracture, pelvic fracture, obesity, older patient (>40), immobility, smoking history, varicose veins, and congestive heart failure
28. Edema, palpable warmth, skin discoloration, prominent superficial veins, and presence of Homans' sign

True/False
29. F
30. T
31. F
32. F
33. F
34. T
35. T
36. F
37. F
38. T
39. F
40. F
41. T

Essay Questions 42–47
Refer to Chapter 13 text for all essay question answers and explanations.

CHAPTER 14

Concepts of Orthopedic Pharmacology

Multiple Choice
1. D
2. C
3. D
4. C
5. B
6. C
7. C
8. D

Short Answer
9. Mouth, intramuscular, subdermal, inhalation, sublingual, buccal, rectal, topical, and intravenous
10. Bactericidal: termination of the organism; bacteriostatic: inhibits reproduction of the organism
11. *Staphylococcus aureus, Staphylococcus epidermidis,* and *Streptococcus* species

True/False

12. F
13. T
14. T
15. T
16. F
17. F
18. T
19. T
20. F
21. F
22. T
23. F

Essay Questions 24-25
Refer to Chapter 14 text for all essay question answers and explanations.

CHAPTER 15

Fundamentals of Gait

Multiple Choice

1. D
2. B
3. B
4. B
5. D
6. A
7. C
8. C
9. C
10. B
11. C
12. B
13. B
14. A
15. C
16. E
17. B
18. D
19. C
20. A
21. D
22. C
23. D
24. C
25. C

Short Answer

26. Step length
27. Stance phase and swing phase
28. Heel strike, foot flat, midstance, heel off, and toe off
29. Acceleration, midswing, and deceleration
30. Shock absorption
31. Uninvolved side

True/False

32. T
33. F
34. T

Essay Questions 35–41
Refer to Chapter 15 text for all essay question answers and explanations.

CHAPTER 16

Concepts of Joint Mobilization

Multiple Choice

1. C
2. C, D, and E
3. B
4. C and D
5. C
6. B
7. A
8. B
9. C
10. C
11. B
12. A
13. D
14. B
15. C
16. B
17. C
18. A
19. B
20. A, C, and D
21. C
22. B, D, and E
23. E

Short Answer

24. Opposite
25. Same

True/False

26. F
27. T
28. T
29. F

Essay Questions 30–38
Refer to Chapter 16 text for all essay question answers and explanations.

CHAPTER 17

Biomechanical Basis for Movement

Multiple Choice

1. B
2. A
3. B
4. B
5. C
6. A
7. C
8. D
9. B

10. D

Short Answer

11. Center of mass (gravity)
12. Rotate and translate
13. Second class
14. Newton's second law
15. Strains, sprains, and avulsion fractures

True/False

16. T
17. F
18. T
19. T
20. F
21. F
22. T
23. T
24. T
25. F

Essay Questions 26–31

Refer to Chapter 17 text for all essay question answers and explanations.

CHAPTER 18

Orthopedic Management of the Ankle, Foot, and Toes

Multiple Choice

1. C
2. C
3. B
4. E
5. B
6. C
7. B
8. D
9. D
10. A
11. B
12. C
13. B, C, D, and E
14. C
15. C
16. D
17. B
18. C and D
19. C
20. C and E
21. C and D
22. A
23. D
24. D
25. C
26. C
27. B
28. B
29. E
30. D
31. B, C, and D

32. C
33. A and B
34. E
35. B
36. E
37. C
38. D
39. C
40. D
41. B
42. A and C
43. B
44. C
45. C
46. E
47. B
48. A, B, D, and E
49. A and C
50. C

Short Answer

51. Mechanical and functional
52. Anterior talofibular, fibulocalcaneal, and posterior talofibular
53. Refer to chapter.
54. A: Mallet toe

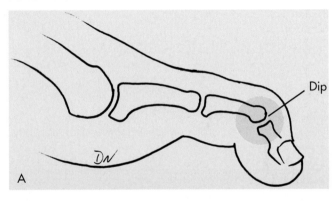

B: Claw toe

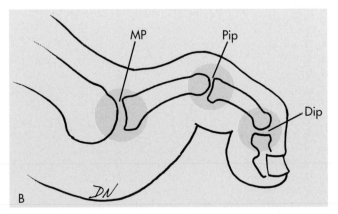

C: Hammer toe

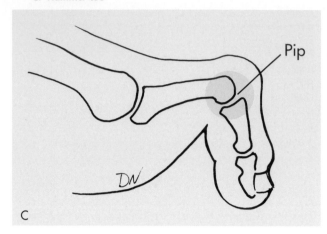

C

True/False

55. F
56. T
57. T
58. F
59. F
60. T
61. T
62. T
63. F
64. T
65. T
66. F

Essay Questions 67–74

Refer to Chapter 18 text for all essay question answers and explanations.

CHAPTER 19

Orthopedic Management of the Knee

Multiple Choice

1. B and D
2. C
3. C
4. D
5. C
6. D
7. C
8. D
9. B
10. C
11. B and C
12. A, B, C, and D
13. B
14. A and B
15. C
16. C
17. C, D, and E
18. A, B, and E
19. A and C

20. B, C, and D
21. A
22. C
23. C
24. B
25. C
26. B
27. A, B, and D
28. B
29. B
30. B
31. B
32. D
33. C
34. C
35. A, B, and E
36. A, D, and E
37. B
38. A
39. B
40. B and D
41. C
42. B
43. C
44. C
45. C
46. B, C, and D
47. A, B, C, and E
48. E
49. B
50. C
51. E
52. A, B, and C
53. C
54. C
55. D
56. E
57. A, B, and C
58. B and C
59. A
60. E
61. C and D
62. A
63. B
64. A
65. B
66. D

Short Answer

67. Anterior cruciate ligament tear
68. Ligament is posterior cruciate ligament; examination is anterior drawer test
69. Mechanism of injury is valgus force; torn structure is medial collateral ligament
70. A: Bucket handle
    B: Parrot break
    C: Longitudinal
71. A: Red-on-white zone
    B: White-on-white zone
    C: Red-on-red zone

72. A: Patella alta
    B: Normal
    C: Patella baja
73. Patellar mobility, active quad strengthening exercises, and active knee flexion
74. Transverse patella fracture; tension band wire and cerclage wire
75. Constrained and unconstrained

True/False

76. T
77. F
78. F
79. F
80. F
81. F
82. T
83. T
84. F
85. F
86. T
87. T
88. F
89. T
90. F
91. F
92. F
93. T
94. F

Essay Questions 95–104
Refer to Chapter 19 text for all essay question answers and explanations.

CHAPTER 20

Orthopedic Management of the Hip and Pelvis

Multiple Choice

1. A and C
2. C
3. B and D
4. C
5. C
6. B
7. B
8. C
9. E
10. C
11. B
12. D
13. A, C, and D
14. C, D, and E
15. C
16. A and C
17. C
18. C
19. B, C, and D
20. C
21. C
22. B, C, and E

Short Answer

23. Subtrochanteric hip fracture
24. Femoral neck fracture
25. Intertrochanteric hip fracture
26. Greater trochanteric bursitis
27. Iliopectineal bursitis
28. Ischial bursitis
29. See Figure

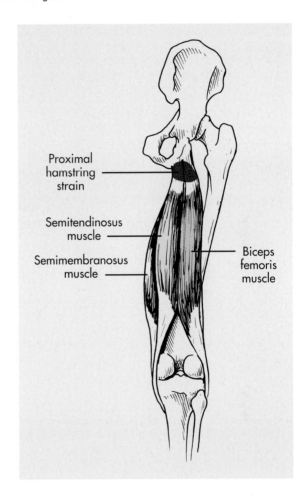

30. Avulsion fracture of iliac crest

True/False

31. T
32. T
33. F
34. T
35. T
36. T
37. T
38. F
39. T
40. F

Essay Questions 41–48
Refer to Chapter 20 text for all essay question answers and explanations.

CHAPTER 21

Orthopedic Management of the Lumbar, Thoracic, and Cervical Spine

Multiple Choice
1. D
2. A
3. C
4. A, C, D, and E
5. E
6. E
7. B, C, and D
8. C
9. C
10. D
11. C
12. E
13. E
14. A
15. A, B, and D
16. D
17. E
18. B, C, and D
19. E
20. D
21. A
22. C
23. A
24. D
25. B
26. C
27. C
28. A
29. C
30. B
31. B
32. E
33. C
34. E
35. E
36. C
37. E
38. B, C, and D
39. C
40. C
41. B and D
42. C
43. E
44. C

Short Answer
45. 100%, standing; 75%, side-lying; 35%, supine (knees flexed); 25%, supine; 275%, bending forward
46. Load, lever, lordosis, legs, and lungs
47. Disk protrusion
48. Sequestrated disk

True/False
49. T
50. T
51. F
52. F
53. F
54. T
55. F
56. T
57. T
58. F
59. T
60. F
61. F

Essay Questions 62–77
Refer to Chapter 21 text for all essay question answers and explanations.

CHAPTER 22

Orthopedic Management of the Shoulder

Multiple Choice
1. C
2. C
3. B, C, and D
4. B, D, and E
5. A, B, and D
6. B and D
7. A
8. B
9. A, B, and D
10. A
11. A, C, and D
12. C
13. B
14. C
15. C
16. C
17. C
18. A, C, and D
19. E
20. C
21. C and D
22. B
23. C
24. B
25. C
26. B
27. E
28. C
29. B
30. D
31. B
32. B and D
33. B
34. C
35. E
36. C
37. A
38. C
39. B

Short Answer

40. Subacromial rotator cuff impingement; and supraspinatus tendon
41. Hill-Sachs lesion
42. Traumatic unidirectional instability and Bankart lesion that frequently requires surgery
43. Atraumatic multidirectional bilateral instability; responds to rehabilitation; occasionally patients require inferior capsular shift
44. Grade II A-C sprain; and rupture of A-C ligament plus partial tear of coracoacromial ligament
45. Grade I A-C sprain; and partial tear of A-C ligament
46. Pin insertion to stabilize grade III A-C sprain
47. Intraarticular fracture of glenoid
48. Figure-of-eight bandage; used for clavicle fracture
49. See Figure

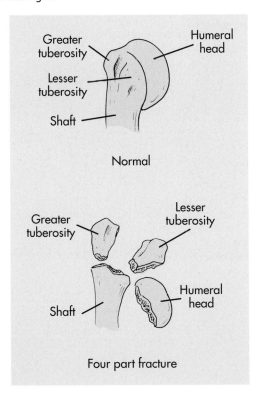

True/False

50. T
51. F
52. F
53. T
54. T
55. T
56. T
57. T
58. F
59. F
60. T

Essay Questions 61–70
Refer to Chapter 22 text for all essay question answers and explanations.

CHAPTER 23
Orthopedic Management of the Elbow

Multiple Choice

1. C
2. B, C, and D
3. C
4. C
5. A, B, and D
6. D
7. E
8. C
9. C
10. C
11. C
12. B
13. C
14. A
15. C
16. B
17. A and C
18. C and D
19. C
20. C
21. C
22. C
23. E
24. D
25. C
26. C
27. B

Short Answer

28. Medial valgus stress; repetitive valgus stress; and medial collateral ligament
29. Type I-extension
30. Type II-flexion type supracondylar fracture
31. Supracondylar fracture; brachial artery; and Volkmann's ischemic contracture
32. Type I-intercondylar nondisplaced fracture
33. Posterior dislocations

True/False

34. T
35. F
36. F
37. F
38. F
39. F
40. T
41. T
42. T
43. T

Essay Questions 44–48
Refer to Chapter 23 text for all essay question answers and explanations.

CHAPTER 24

Orthopedic Management of the Wrist and Hand

Multiple Choice
1. E
2. B, C, and D
3. C
4. C
5. A, B, C
6. B
7. A, B, C
8. C
9. C
10. E
11. B
12. B
13. C
14. B
15. A and B
16. B and D
17. E
18. C
19. C
20. B
21. B
22. E
23. B, C, and D
24. C
25. C
26. E
27. D
28. C
29. B, C, and D
30. B, C, and D

Short Answer
31. Carpal tunnel syndrome
32. De Quervain's tenosynovitis; abductor pollicis longus; and extensor pollicis brevis
33. Colles' fracture; and dinner fork deformity
34. Colles' comminuted fracture; and external fixator
35. Smith's fracture
36. Valgus hyperextension of the thumb; sprain of ulnar collateral ligament; gamekeeper's thumb; and skier's thumb
37. Fractured metacarpal; boxer's fracture; and fighter's fracture
38. Bennett's fracture

39. Mallet finger

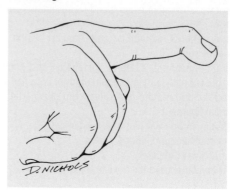

Boutonnière deformity

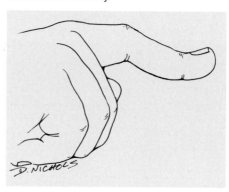

40. Mallet finger
41. Boutonnière deformity

True/False
42. T
43. F
44. T
45. F
46. T
47. T
48. T
49. F
50. T

Essay Questions 51–62
Refer to Chapter 24 text for all essay question answers and explanations.

Appendix A
Commonly Used Medications in Musculoskeletal Medicine

Type of Medication	Brand Name (Company)	Generic Name	Sizes Available	Mechanism of Action	Adult Dosage	Maximum Daily Dosage	Comments
Anti-inflammatory (oral)	Clinoril (Merck)	Sulindac	150 mg, 200 mg	Inhibition of prostaglandin synthesis	150 to 200 mg bid	400 mg per day	
	Daypro (Searle)	Oxaprozin	250 mg, 500 mg	Inhibition of prostaglandin synthesis	600 mg bid	1800 mg per day or 26 mg/kg (whichever is lower)	
	Dolobid (Merck)	Diflunisal	250 mg, 500 mg	Inhibition of prostaglandin synthesis	250 to 500 mg q 8 to 12 hours	1500 mg per day	
	Feldene (Pfizer)	Piroxicam	10 mg, 20 mg	Inhibition of prostaglandin synthesis	20 mg per day	20 mg per day	
	Indocin (Merck)	Indomethacin	25 mg, 50 mg, 75 mg (SR)	Inhibition of prostaglandin synthesis	25 to 50 mg bid to tid	150 to 200 mg per day	
	Lodine (Wyeth-Ayerst)	Etodolac	200 mg, 300 mg, 400 mg, 500 mg, 600 mg	Inhibition of prostaglandin synthesis	400 to 1000 mg per day	1000 mg per day	
	Motrin (McNeil)	Ibuprofen	400 mg, 600 mg, 800 mg	Inhibition of arachidonic acid	400 to 800 mg tid	2400 mg per day	
	Naprosyn/Anaprox (Roche)	Naproxen	250 mg, 375 mg, 500 mg	Inhibition of prostaglandin synthesis	250 to 500 mg bid	1000 mg per day	
	Orudis (Wyeth-Ayerst)	Ketoprofen	25 mg, 50 mg, 75 mg	Inhibition of prostaglandin and leukotriene synthesis	75 mg tid or 50 mg qid	300 mg per day	
	Relafen (SmithKline-Beecham)	Nabumetone	500 mg, 750 mg	Inhibition of prostaglandin synthesis	1000 to 2000 mg per day in single or divided dosages	2000 mg per day	
	Tolectin (Ortho-McNeil)	Tolmetin	200 mg, 400 mg, 600 mg	Inhibition of prostaglandin synthesis	300 mg tid	1800 mg per day	
	Toradol (Roche)	Ketorolac tromethamine	10 mg oral (also available in IV or IM 30 to 60 mg)	Inhibition of prostaglandin synthesis	20 to 40 mg orally for a maximum of 5 days or 60 to 120 mg IV/IM	40 mg orally and 120 mg IV/IM	
	Voltaren (Novartis)	Diclofenac	25 mg, 50 mg, 75 mg, 100 mg	Inhibition of prostaglandin synthesis	100 to 150 mg bid or tid	225 mg per day	

Type of Medication	Brand Name (Company)	Generic Name	Sizes Available	Mechanism of Action	Adult Dosage	Maximum Daily Dosage	Comments
Analgesic (oral)	Aspirin (Many manufacturers)	Acetylsalicylic acid	325 mg, 500 mg	Inhibition of prostaglandin synthesis and inhibition of platelet function	325 to 1000 mg q 4 to 6 hours (dosage for platelet effects for TIAs is 325 mg bid)	4000 mg per day	
	Tylenol (McNeil)	Acetaminophen	325 mg, 500 mg	Regulation of the hypothalamus	650 to 1000 mg q 4 to 6 hours as needed	4000 mg per day	
	Ultram (Ortho-McNeil)	Tramadol hydrochloride	50 mg	Central blockage of opioid receptors	50 to 100 mg q 6 hours	400 mg per day	
	Talwin Compound (Sanofi)	12.5 mg of pentazocine hydrochloride & 325 mg aspirin	—	Narcotic antagonist	2 tablets tid or qid	8 tablets per day	Schedule IV drug
	Darvocet/Darvon (Eli Lilly)	50 mg propoxyphene napsylate & 325 mg acetaminophen	—	Centrally acting narcotic	2 tablets q 4 hours as needed for pain	600 mg per day	Schedule IV drug
	Demerol (Sanofi)	Meperidine	50 mg, 100 mg	Opioid agonist	50 to 150 mg q 4 hours	600 mg per day	Schedule II drug
	Dilaudid (Knoll)	Hydromorphone hydrochloride	8 mg	Opioid agonist	8 mg q 3 to 4 hours as needed	48 mg per day	Schedule II drug
	Fiorinal with codeine (Novartis)	50 mg butalbital, 325 mg aspirin, 40 mg caffeine, & 30mg codeine	—	Barbiturate and narcotic opioid agonist	1 or 2 tablets q 4 hours	6 tablets per day	Schedule III drug
	Lortab (UCB Pharma)	Hydrocodone bitartrate & acetaminophen	2.5/500 mg or 5/500 mg	Opioid analgesic and anticonvulsant	2.5 to 5 mg q 4 to 6 hours	8 tablets per day	Schedule III drug

Type of Medication	Brand Name (Company)	Generic Name	Sizes Available	Mechanism of Action	Adult Dosage	Maximum Daily Dosage	Comments
Analgesic (oral)	MS Contin (Purdue Frederick)	Morphine sulfate	15 mg, 30 mg, 60 mg, 100 mg, 200 mg	Opioid receptors	15 to 20 mg q 4 to 6 hours as needed for severe pain	Based on tolerance	Schedule II drug
	Oramorph (Roxane)	Morphine sulfate	15 mg, 30 mg, 60 mg, 100 mg	Opioid receptors	15 to 200 mg q 4 to 6 hours as needed for severe pain	Based on tolerance	Schedule II drug
	OxyContin (Purdue Pharma)	Oxycodone hydrochloride	10 mg, 20 mg, 40 mg, 80 mg	Opioid agonist	10 to 80 mg q 4 to 6 hours as needed	Based on tolerance	Schedule II drug
	Percocet (Endo Labs)	5 mg oxycodone & 325 mg acetaminophen	—	Opioid agonist	1 to 2 tablets q 4 to 6 hours	8 to 10 tablets per day	Schedule II drug
	Tylenol with codeine (Ortho-McNeil)	30 mg codeine & 300 mg acetaminophen	—	Opioid agonist	1 to 2 tablets q 4 to 6 hours as needed for pain	8 tablets per day	Schedule III drug
	Tylox (Ortho-McNeil)	5 mg oxycodone hydrochloride & 500 mg acetaminophen	—	Opioid agonist	1 to 2 tablets q 4 to 6 hours as needed for pain	8 tablets per day	Schedule II drug
	Vicodin (Knoll Labs)	10 mg hydrocodone bitartrate & 660 mg acetaminophen	5/500 mg	—	1 to 2 tablets q 4 to 6 hours as needed for pain	8 tablets per day	Schedule III drug
	Wygesic (Wyeth-Ayerst)	65 mg proproxyphene hydrochloride & 650 mg acetaminophen	—	Centrally acting narcotic analgesic agent	1 to 2 tablets q 4 to 6 hours as needed for pain	390 mg per day or 6 tablets per day	Schedule IV drug

Type of Medication	Brand Name (Company)	Generic Name	Sizes Available	Mechanism of Action	Adult Dosage	Maximum Daily Dosage	Comments
Antibiotics (oral)—first-generation cephalosporins	Keflex (Many manufacturers)	Cephalexin monohydrate	250 mg, 500 mg	Inhibition of cell wall synthesis	250 to 500 mg q 6 hours	2000 mg per day	Gram-positive coverage
	Velosef (Lederle Standard)	Cephradine	250 mg, 500 mg	Inhibition of cell wall synthesis	250 mg, 500 mg q 6 hours	2000 mg per day	Gram-positive coverage
	Duricef (Bristol-Myers Squibb)	Cefadroxil monohydrate	500 mg, 1000 mg	Inhibition of cell wall synthesis	250 to 500 mg q 6 hours	2000 mg per day	Gram-positive coverage
Antibiotics (oral)—second-generation cephalosporins	Ceclor (Dura, Mylan, Eli Lilly)	Cefaclor	375 mg, 500 mg	Inhibition of cell wall synthesis	500 mg bid	4000 mg per day	Gram-positive coverage
	Ceftin (Glaxo Wellcome)	Cefuroxime axetil	125 mg, 250 mg, 500 mg	Inhibition of cell wall synthesis	125 to 500 mg q 12 hours	1000 mg per day	
Antibiotics (oral)—macrolides	Biaxin (Abbott)	Clarithromycin	250 mg	Inhibition of protein synthesis	500 mg q 8 to 12 hours	1500 mg per day	Aerobic and anaerobic gram-positive and gram-negative coverage and *Mycobacterium avium* coverage
	Erythromycin (Abbott/Mylan)	Erythromycin	250 mg, 500 mg	Inhibition of protein synthesis	250 mg q 6 hours or 500 mg q 12 hours	1000 mg per day	Gram-positive coverage for penicillin-insensitive organisms and patients who do not tolerate penicillin
	Zithromax (Pfizer)	Azithromycin	250 mg, 500 mg	Inhibition of protein synthesis	500 mg per day for 5 days of treatment	500 mg per day	Used primarily for respiratory infections
	Clecocin (Pharmacia, Upjohn)	Clindamycin hydrochloride	75 mg, 150 mg, 300 mg	Inhibition of protein synthesis	150 to 300 mg q 6 hours; 300 to 450 mg q 6 hours for severe infections	1800 mg per day	Used for anaerobic infections

Type of Medication	Brand Name (Company)	Generic Name	Sizes Available	Mechanism of Action	Adult Dosage	Maximum Daily Dosage	Comments
Antibiotics (oral)—penicillins	Amoxil (SmithKline-Beecham)	Amoxicillin	125 mg, 500 mg	Inhibition of cell wall synthesis	250 mg q 8 hours	1000 mg per day	Good coverage against gram-positive organisms that are not penicillinase resistant
	Augmentin (SmithKline-Beecham)	Amoxicillin/clavulanate	250 mg, 500 mg, 875 mg	Inhibition of cell wall synthesis	250 to 500 mg q 12 hours	1000 mg per day	Good coverage for respiratory infections and skin infections, especially animal bites
	Omnipen (Wyeth-Ayerst)	Ampicillin trihydrate	250 mg, 500 mg	Inhibition of cell wall synthesis	500 mg qid	2000 mg per day	Good coverage for gram-positive infections that are penicillinase sensitive
	Penicillin-VK (Wyeth-Ayerst)	Penicillin V potassium	250 mg, 500 mg	Inhibition of cell wall synthesis	250 to 500 mg q 6 to 8 hours	2000 mg per day	Good coverage for gram-positive nonpenicillinase resistant organisms
Antibiotics (oral)—tetracycline	Achromycin, Helidac, Tetracycline (Procter & Gamble, Lederle)	Tetracycline hydrochloride	500 mg	Inhibition of protein synthesis	500 mg bid to qid	2000 mg per day	Good coverage for various micro-bacteria, Pasteurella, Brucella, others
	Vibramycin (Pfizer)	Doxycycline hyclate	50 mg, 100 mg	Inhibition of protein synthesis	100 mg q 12 hours for the first day and then 100 mg qid for the following days treatment	200 mg per day	

Type of Medication	Brand Name (Company)	Generic Name	Sizes Available	Mechanism of Action	Adult Dosage	Maximum Daily Dosage	Comments
Antibiotics (oral)—quinolones	Cipro (Bayer)	Ciprofloxacin	100 mg, 250 mg, 500 mg, 750 mg	Inhibition of DNA gyrase enzymes	500 to 750 mg q 12 hours	1500 mg per day	Good coverage for aerobic gram-negative organisms and other difficult infections including chlamydia and microbacteria infections
	Floxin (Ortho-McNeil)	Ofloxacin	200 mg, 300 mg, 400 mg	Inhibition of DNA gyrase enzymes	200 to 400 mg q 12 hours	800 mg per day	Good coverage for gram-negative aerobes
Antibiotics (oral)—sulfonamides	Bactrim (Roche)	Trimethoprim-sulfamethoxazole	160 mg of trimethoprim, 100 mg of sulfamethoxazole	Sulfamethoxazole inhibits dihydrofolic acid synthesis and trimethoprim blocks dihydrofolic acid formations	1 double-strength to 2 double-strength tablets q 12 hours	4 tablets per day	Good coverage in urinary tract infection, bronchitis, and other problems
Antifungals (oral)	Fulvicin (Schering)	Griseofulvin	165 mg, 330 mg	Inhibition of cell wall synthesis	330 mg	330 mg per day	Good coverage for tinea, *Trichophyton, Microsporum* species
	Grifulvin V (Ortho Pharmaceutical)	Griseofulvin	250 mg, 500 mg	Keratin exfoliation	500 mg	500 mg per day	
	Flagyl (Searle)	Metronidazole	375 mg	Free-radical mechanism	750 mg tid	2250 mg per day	Good coverage for amebiasis and anaerobic infections

Type of Medication	Brand Name (Company)	Generic Name	Sizes Available	Mechanism of Action	Adult Dosage	Maximum Daily Dosage	Comments
DVT prophylaxis	Coumadin (DuPont)	Warfarin	1 mg, 2 mg, 2.5 mg, 4 mg, 5 mg, 7.5 mg, 10 mg	Inhibits vitamin K-dependent clotting factors	Depends on effect (oral)	Effect to INR 2-3	
	Heparin (Wyeth-Ayerst)	Heparin	1000 to 20,000 U/mL	Inhibits factor X	Depends on effect (IV)	PTT to 1.5 to 2 times normal	
	Lovenox (Rhone-Poulenc Rorer)	Enoxaparin sodium	30 mg/0.3 mL 40 mg/0.4 mL	Forms complexes between antithrombin III and factors IIa and Xa	15 to 40 mg (SC injection)	15 to 40 mg bid	
	Ecotrin (SmithKline-Beecham)	Enteric-coated aspirin	325 mg	Antiplatelet	650 mg bid (oral)	—	
Injectables—analgesics	Xylocaine (Astra)	Lidocaine	0.5%, 1%, 2%	Stabilizes neuronal membranes	1 to 5 mL	500 mg	
	Marcaine (Abbott)	Bupivacaine hydrochloride	0.25%, 0.5%, 0.75% (10, 30, 50 mL vials)	Increases threshold for nerve stimulation	1 to 5 mL	200 mg	
Injectables—steroids	Celestone (Schering)	Betamethasone	6 mg/mL (5-mL vials)	Antiinflammatory	0.5 to 2.0 mL	3 or 4 doses	
	Decadron (Merck)	Dexamethasone	4 mg/mL (5-mL vials)	Antiinflammatory	2 to 4 mg (1 mL)	3 or 4 doses	
	Hydrocortone (Merck)	Hydrocortisone	50 mg/mL (5-mL vials)	Antiinflammatory	25 to 50 mg (1 mL)	3 or 4 doses	
	Solu-Medrol (Pharmacia, Upjohn)	Methylprednisolone	125 mg/2 mL (2-mL vials)	Antiinflammatory	125 mg/1 vial	125 mg (1 vial)	
Injectables—hyaluronic acids	Hyalgan (Wyeth-Ayerst)	Hyaluronic acid	Prepackaged	Binds receptors and increases hyaluronic acid production	1 dose 4 to 5 times over 4 to 6 weeks (intra-articular)	—	
	Synvisc (Orthologic)	Hylan fluid-gel mixture	Prepackaged	Binds receptors and increases hyaluronic acid production	1 dose 4 to 5 times over 4 to 6 weeks (intra-articular)	—	

bid, twice a day; IM, intramuscular; INR, international normalized ratio; IV, intravenous; PTT, partial thromboplastin time; q, every; qid, four times a day; SC, subcutaneous; SR, substained release; TIA, transient ischemic attack; tid, three times a day. (From Brinker MR, Miller MD: Fundamentals of Orthopedics. Philadelphia, W.B. Saunders, 1999.)

Appendix B
Reference Ranges for Commonly Used Tests

Test	Conventional Units
Alanine aminotransferase (ALT, SGPT, GPT)	0–35 IU/L (laboratory-specific)
Alkaline phosphatase	41–133 IU/L (method- and age-dependent)
Angiotensin-converting enzyme (ACE)	12–35 U/L (method-dependent)
Aspartate aminotransferase (AST, SGOT, GOT)	0–35 IU/L (laboratory-specific)
Blood urea nitrogen (BUN)	8–20 mg/dL
Calcium (Ca^{2+})	8.5–10.5 mg/dL
	Panic: <6.5 or >13.5 mg/dL
Carbon dioxide (CO_2), total (bicarbonate)	22–28 mEq/L
	Panic: <15 or >40 mEq/L
Chloride (Cl^-)	98–107 mEq/L
Complement C3	64–166 mg/dL
Complement C4	15–45 mg/dL
Cortisol	8:00 A.M.: 5–20 µg/dL
Creatine kinase (CK)	32–267 IU/L (method-dependent)
Creatine (Cr)	0.6–1.2 mg/dL
Erythrocyte count (RBC count)	$4.2–5.6 \times 10^6/\mu L$
Erythrocyte sedimentation rate	Male: <10 mm/h
	Female: <15 mm/h (laboratory-specific)
Erythropoietin (EPO)	5–20 mIU/mL
Ferritin	Male: 16–300 ng/mL
	Female: 4–161 ng/mL
Fibrin D-dimers	Negative
Folic acid (red cells)	165–760 mg/mL
Gamma-glutamyl-transpeptidase (GGT)	9–85 U/L (laboratory-specific)
Glucose	60–115 mg/dL
	Panic: <40 or >500 mg/dL
Glucose-6-phosphate dehydrogenase (G6PD) screen	4–8 U/g Hb
Glutamine	6–16 mg/dL
	Panic: >40 mg/dL
Hematocrit (Hct)	Male: 39%–49%
	Female: 35%–45%
	(age-dependent)
Hemoglobin, total (Hb)	Male: 13.6–17.5 g/dL
	Female: 12.0–15.5 g/dL
	Panic: ≤7 g/dL (age-dependent)
Iron (Fe^{2+})	50–175 µg/dL
Iron-binding capacity, total (TIBC)	250–460 µg/dL
Lactate dehydrogenase (LDH)	88–230 units/L (laboratory-specific)
Lactate dehydrogenase (LDH) isoenzymes	LDH_1/LDH_2: <0.85

Continued

Test	Conventional Units
Leukocyte alkaline phosphatase (LAP)	40–130
	Based on 0 to 4+ rating of 100 PMNs stained for alkaline phosphatase
Leukocyte (white blood cell) count, total (WBC count)	$3.4–10 \times 10^3/\mu L$
	Panic: $<1.5 \times 10^3/\mu L$
Mean corpuscular hemoglobin (MCH)	26–34 pg
Mean corpuscular hemoglobin concentration (MCHC)	31–36 g/dL
Mean corpuscular volume (MCV)	80–100 fL
Osmolality	285–293 mOsm/kg H_2O
	Panic: <240 or >320 mOsm/kg H_2O
Oxygen, partial pressure (PO_2)	83–108 mm Hg
Partial thromboplastin time, activated (PTT)	25-35 seconds (range varies)
	Panic: ≥60 seconds
pH	Arterial: 7.35–7.45
	Venous: 7.31–7.41
Platelet count (Plt)	$150–450 \times 10^3/\mu L$
	Panic: $<25 \times 10^3/\mu L$
Prothrombin time (PT)	11–15 seconds
	Panic: ≥30 seconds
Sodium (Na^+)	135–145 mEq/L
	Panic: <125 or >155 mEq/L
Testosterone	Male: 3.0–10.9 ng/mL
	Female: 0.3–0.7 ng/mL

From Tierney LM, McPhee SJ, Papadakis M: Current Medical Diagnosis and Treatment 1995. Norwalk, CT, Appleton and Lange, 1995.

Appendix C
Laboratory Values as Clues

BLOOD CHEMISTRIES

alkaline phosphatase, serum.   *Pathophysiology:* This includes a number of cellular enzymes that hydrolyze phosphate esters; they are named from their optimum activity in alkaline media. High concentrations of the enzymes occur in the blood during periods of rapid growth, either physiologic or pathologic, and from cellular injury. The enzymes are normally plentiful in hepatic parenchyma, osteoblasts, intestinal mucosa, placental cells, and renal epithelium. Abnormally rapid growth or cell destruction will augment the blood concentration of these enzymes.

Normal Concentration: 30–115 U/L (0.5–1.92 µkat/L)

Increased Concentration: Physiologic (high in newborn, declining to puberty; rising every decade after 60 years of age); *bone* (osteitis fibrosa cystica, Paget's disease, osteoblastic bone tumors, metastatic carcinoma in bone, osteogenesis imperfecta, familial osteectasis, myeloma, osteomalacia, rickets, acromegaly, polyostotic fibrosis dysplasia); *muscle* (strenuous exercise, clonic and tonic seizures, tissue necrosis); *brain* (cerebral damage); *thyroid* (hyperthyroidism [effect on bone], subacute thyroiditis); *parathyroids* (sometimes hyperparathyroidism [effect on bone]); *heart* (myocardial infarction); *lungs* (sometimes pulmonary infarction); *kidneys* (renal infarction); *liver* (metastatic tumors, abscesses, cysts, parasitic infestations, amyloid, tuberculosis, sarcoid, leukemia); *biliary system* (common duct obstruction from stone or carcinoma, cholangiolar obstruction from hepatitis); *pancreas* (pancreatitis, diabetes mellitus); *stomach* (peptic ulcer); *bowel* (intestinal obstruction, ulcerative colitis, regional enteritis); *genital* (last half of pregnancy); *blood* (pernicious anemia, and other hemolytic anemias); *neoplasia* (carcinoma of prostate); *infections* (infectious mononucleosis); *chemical imbalances* (hyperphosphatasia); *intake/output* (dehydration, rapid loss of weight); *drugs* (chloropropamide, ergosterol, sometimes intravenous injection of albumin); *technical error* (dehydration of blood specimen).

Decreased Concentration: Bone (osteoporosis); *thyroid* (hypothyroidism); *bowel* (celiac disease); *intake/output* (excess ingestion of vitamin D, deficit of vitamin D, deficit of vitamin C [scurvy], malnutrition); *chemical imbalances* (uremia, hypophosphatasia, milk-alkali syndrome of Burnett); *blood* (half the patients with pernicious anemia); *technical errors* (use of oxalate in blood collection).

aspartate aminotransferase, serum (see glutamate-oxaloacetate transferase, serum SGOT, and transaminase, serum SGOT.

bicarbonate, total serum (Co₂ content).   *Pathophysiology:* Mol wt 61. A negative ion with monovalence, CO_2 is formed by cell metabolism and diffused through the body fluids as ionized bicarbonate (HCO_3). About one fifth of the total blood bicarbonate is in the form of carbaminohemoglobin. The carbonates are major buffers, along with hemoglobin, phosphates, and free amino and carbonyl groups.

Normal Concentration: 22–26 meq/L (22–26 mmol/L) [in venous blood, serum].

Increased Concentration (hypercapnia): Thyroid (severe hypothyroidism); *kidneys* (hyperaldosteronism); *adrenals* (Cushing's disease); *chemical imbalance* (respiratory acidosis, metabolic alkalosis); *drugs* (diuretics).

Decreased Concentration (hypocapnia): Kidneys (renal failure); *adrenals* (Addison's disease); *intake/output* (diarrhea, starvation); *chemical imbalance* (respiratory alkalosis, metabolic acidosis, diabetic ketosis).

bilirubin, total serum. *Pathophysiology:* Unconjugated bilirubin is manufactured in the reticuloendothelial system with four pyrrole nuclei of heme. It is insoluble in water until conjugated in the liver with glucuronic acid. Four fifths or more is derived from the catabolism of the heme from aging erythrocytes. The water-soluble conjugated bilirubin is normally excreted in the bile. It is bound to the plasma proteins; when the level exceeds 0.4 mg/dL, the water-soluble form appears in the urine.

Normal Concentration: 0.0–1.0 mg/dL (0–17 μmol/L).

Increased Concentration (hyperbilirubinemia): Lungs (pulmonary infarction); *biliary system* (diseases of the liver, acute cholecystitis, obstructive jaundice, Gilbert's disease, Dubin-Johnson's disease); *gastrointestinal tract* (bleeding into it); *blood* (intravascular hemolysis, large hematoma); *infections* (infectious mononucleosis); *poison* (alcohol).

Decreased Concentration (hypobilirubinemia): Nonhemolytic anemia and hypoalbuminemia.

calcium, serum (Ca⁺⁺). *Pathophysiology:* At wt 40. About 99% of the body calcium is in the form of insoluble phosphate and carbonate supporting the collagen matrix of the bones. It is in equilibrium with a small amount in the extracellular fluid. The amount varies with the rate of absorption of Ca^{++} from the small intestine and the resorption rate in the glomeruli. Clinically, the body Ca is present in three forms: *ionized* or *free* Ca that is physiologically active; *protein-bound* or *nondiffusible,* most of which is loosely bound to plasma albumin; and *complexed* or *complex-bound* that forms relatively soluble fractions complexed with carbonates, citrates, or phosphates. Parathormone (PTH) accelerates release of Ca^{++} and PO_4^{---} from bone with increased excretion of urinary PO_1^{---}; it also converts vitamin D to a more active form. Thyrocalcitonin inhibits bone resorption and decreases serum Ca and PO_1 in the extracellular fluids; in turn, this reduces membrane permeability.

Normal Concentration: 8.5–10.5 mg/dL (2.1–2.6 mmol/L) [varies with chemical method].

Increased Concentration (hypercalcemia): Bone (tumor metastatic to bone, lymphoma, multiple myeloma, osteoporosis, immobilization of young persons, Paget's disease); *thyroid* (sometimes hyperthyroidism, sometimes hypothyroidism); *parathyroids* (primary hyperparathyroidism [hyperplasia, adenoma, or cancer hormone]); *adrenals* (sometimes Cushing's disease, sometimes Addison's disease); *genital* (sometimes carcinoma of prostate); *blood* (lymphoma, myeloma, leukemia); *intake/output* (excessive intake of vitamin D); *chemical imbalances* (milk-alkali syndrome of Burnett, hypercalcemia in infants, infantile hypophosphatasia, hyperproteinemia [sarcoidosis, multiple myeloma]); *drugs* (thiazide diuretics); *poisons* (berylliosis); *technical error* (use of cork-stoppered tubes for collection of blood specimens).

Decreased Concentration (hypocalcemia): Bone (osteomalacia, rickets); *thyroid* (hypothyroidism); *parathyroids* (hypoparathyroidism [postthyroidectomy, idiopathic or pseudohypoparathyroidism]); *kidneys* (renal disease with uremia); *pancreas* (acute pancreatitis with much fat necrosis); *genital* (late pregnancy, prostatic carcinoma); *intake/output* (excessive fluid intake, malabsorption of calcium and vitamin D from jaundice, lack of intake of Ca and vitamin D); *chemical imbalances* (hypoproteinemia [cachexia, nephrosis, celiac disease, cystic fibrosis of the pancreas]); *drugs* (antacids, corticosteroids).

chloride, serum (Cl⁻). *Pathophysiology:* A wt 35.5. The principal anion in the extracellular fluids Cl^-, balanced by Na^+; anions present in smaller quantities are HCO_3^- and HPO_4^{--}. The cations of lesser amounts are K^+, Ca^{++}, and Mg^{++}. By contrast, in the cellular fluid the chief anions are HPO_4^{--} and SO_4^{--}, balanced by K^+ and Mg^{++}. The quantity of Cl^- is usually proportionate to Na^+, except when there is selective loss of Cl^- in the HCl of vomited gastric juice, or when HCO_3^- is retained in the breath, or when certain diuretics cause disproportionate losses of Na^+ or Cl^-.

Normal Concentration: 100–108 mEq/L (100–108 mmol/L).

Increased Concentration (hyperchloremia): Brain (cerebral damage); *parathyroids* (hyperparathyroidism); *kidneys* (renal tubular acidosis, acute renal failure); *pancreas* (diabetes mellitus); *intake/output* (diabetes insipidus, dehydration); *chemical imbalances* (respiratory alkalosis, metabolic acidosis); *drugs* (diamox, ammonium salts, salicylates); *technical error* (bromide in blood gives false test for Cl^-).

Decreased Concentration (hypochloremia): Lungs (pulmonary emphysema); *heart* (congestive cardiac failure); *stomach* (pyloric obstruction); *bowels* (steatorrhea); *pancreas* (diabetic acidosis); *kidneys* (primary aldosteronism); *adrenals* (Addison's disease); *liver* (cirrhosis); *intake/output* (sweating, diarrhea, malabsorption); *drugs* (diuretics).

cholesterol, serum. *Pathophysiology:* This is one of the plasma lipids that also include triglycerides, phospholipids, and free fatty acids. They are all insoluble in water and are carried in the circulation by four types of lipoproteins as vehicles. Of the four, the low-density lipoproteins (LDL) carry the most cholesterol. Much of the cholesterol comes from the diet, but some is synthesized by the liver, skin, and other organs. Cholesterol is essential to every body cell, and it is a precursor to adrenal steroids, gonadal steroids, and bile salts.

Desirable Concentration: <200 mg/dL (<5.18 mmol/L). [varies with method].

Increased Concentration (hypercholesterolemia): Thyroid (hypo-thyroidism); *kidneys* (nephrosis, chronic nephritis, renal vein thrombosis, amyloidosis, systemic lupus erythematosus [SLE], periarteritis, diabetic glomerulosclerosis); *liver and biliary system* (biliary obstruction [gallstone, carcinoma, cholangiolitic cirrhosis], von Gierke's disease); *pancreas* (diabetes mellitus, sometimes pancreatitis, total pancreatectomy); *intake/output* (dehydration); *chemical imbalances* (idiopathic hypercholesterolemia, lipodystrophy); *poisons* (alcohol).

Decreased Concentration (hypocholesterolemia): Thyroid (hyperthyroidism); *liver* (severe cellular damage); *intake/output* (malnutrition, starvation); *chemical imbalances* (uremia, steatorrhea, Tangier's disease); *malignant neoplasms; blood* (pernicious anemia, other hemolytic anemias, hypochromic anemias); *drugs* (cortisone, ACTH).

creatine phosphokinase, serum (CPK). *Pathophysiology:* This enzyme catalyzes the transfer of high energy phosphate between creatine and phosphocreatine, and between ADP and ATP. Principal concentrations of it are found in cardiac and skeletal muscle and in the brain. Erythrocytes lack this enzyme, so autolyzed serum specimens are acceptable for testing.

Normal Concentration: Males 5–55 mU/mL; females: 5–35 mU/mL (same).

Increased Concentration: Muscle (severe exercise, muscle spasms, clonic and tonic seizures, muscle trauma [crush syndrome, postoperatively for about 5 days, electroshock for defibrillation, muscle necrosis and atrophy, intramuscular injections for 48 h, polymyositis, progressive muscular dystrophy]); *brain* (2 days after cerebral infarction and lasting for 14 days); *thyroid* (hypothyroidism); *heart* (myocardial infarction, dissecting aneurysm); *pancreas* (pancreatitis); *genital* (parturition and last few weeks of pregnancy); *blood* (megaloblastic anemia); *drugs* (salicylates); *poison* (alcohol).

creatinine, serum. *Pathophysiology:* Mol wt 113. This is an organic acid resulting from the metabolism of creatine in the muscles. It is distributed throughout the body water. Creatine is formed in the liver and pancreas from arginine and glycine; it is taken up by muscle tissue and converted to creatine phosphate, catalyzed by the enzyme CPK. The creatine decomposes to creatinine at a rate of 1% or 2% per day. Creatinine is cleared from the blood by the glomerular filtration and is not resorbed. Urinary excretion of creatinine thus becomes an accurate indicator of renal function.

Normal Concentration: 0.6–1.5 mg/dL (53–133 µmol/L).

Increased Concentration: Skin and muscle (burns, high fevers, cachexia, acromegaly, gigantism); *kidneys* (azotemia, inadequate blood flow to the kidneys [heart failure, dehydration], ureterocolostomy with urinary resorption); *liver* (hepatic insufficiency); *pancreas* (pancreatitis with cholecystitis); *bowel* (blood in the gut); *blood* (plasma cell myeloma); *intake/output* (ingestion of roast beef with excess of creatinine, excessive intake of protein, diarrhea, steatorrhea, vomiting); *chemical imbalances* (alkali-milk syndrome of Burnett); *drugs* (corticosteroids, thiazide diuresis).

Decreased Concentration: None significant.

BUN/Creatinine Ratio Greater than 10:1: Excessive protein intake, blood in the gut, excessive tissue destruction (cachexia, burns, fever, corticosteroid therapy), postrenal obstruction, inadequate renal circulation (heart failure, dehydration, shock).

BUN/Creatinine Ratio Less than 10:1: Low protein intake, multiple dialyses, severe diarrhea or vomiting, hepatic insufficiency.

glucose, serum. *Pathophysiology:* Mol wt 180. This is the principal body sugar, a 6-carbon monosaccharide. It permeates all body water; the serum level remains fairly constant during fasting; there is a moderate rise after the ingestion of food. The liver cells transform other carbohydrates to glucose. Surpluses of this sugar are converted to glycogen for hepatic storage, or they form fat that is deposited throughout the body. Peripheral utilization of glucose by the tissues depends on having the proper amounts of insulin. After an average meal, the normal person experiences a blood sugar rise to approximately 180 mg/dL serum; this returns to normal fasting levels within 2 h. Higher glucose levels in the blood result from either failure to utilize it or the ingestion of superfluous quantities. When the blood concentration of glucose becomes high, the renal threshold is exceeded and glucose is excreted in the urine (glycosuria). The normal renal threshold occurs with a serum glucose of 160–190 mg/dL. This may be higher in a damaged kidney.

Normal Concentration: 70–110 mg/dL (3.9–6.1 mmol/L).

Increased Concentration (hyperglycemia): Bone and muscle (acromegaly, gigantism); *brain* (Wernicke's syndrome, subarachnoid hemorrhage, hypothalamic lesions, convulsions); *thyroid* (hyperthyroidism); *heart* (myocardial infarction); *lungs* (asthma, pneumonia, pulmonary embolism); *stomach* (bleeding peptic ulcer); *bowel* (regional enteritis, ulcerative colitis); *liver* (hemochromatosis, cholecystitis); *kidneys* (nephritis, renal failure; *adrenals* (Cushing's disease, increased adrenalin, ACTH, pheochromocytoma, stress); *blood* (hemolytic anemia); *genital* (toxemia of pregnancy); *malignant neoplasm; intake/output* (dehydration, malnutrition).

Decreased Concentration (hypoglycemia): Brain (hypopituitarism, hypothalamic lesions); *thyroid* (hypothyroidism); *stomach* (postgastrectomy dumping syndrome, gastroenterostomy, carcinoma); *pancreas* (pancreatitis, islet tumor, hypoplasia, sometimes diabetes mellitus); *liver* (glycogen deficiency, hepatitis, cirrhosis, primary or secondary carcinoma); *adrenals* (carcinoma, Addison's disease, medullary unresponsiveness); *neoplasms; chemical imbalances* (von Gierke's disease, galactosuria, maple syrup urine disease, fructose intolerance, leucine sensitivity); *intake/output* (malnutrition).

glutamate-oxaloacetate transminase, serum (SGOT) (synonyms: aspartate aminotransferase, serum, and transaminase, serum SGOT). *Pathophysiology:* This enzyme catalyzes the transfer of the amino groups from aspartate to glutamate and oxaloacetate, involving it in both amino acid metabolism and gluconeogenesis. It is concentrated mostly in the cells of heart, liver, muscle, and kidney; lesser amounts are in pancreas, spleen, lung, brain, and erythrocytes. Tissue injury releases the enzyme into the extracellular fluids, but not necessarily in amounts proportionate to the injury.

Normal Concentration: 9–40 U/L (0.15–0.67 µkat/L).

Increased Concentration: Muscle (severe exercise, clonic and tonic seizures, crushing or burning or necrosis of muscle, inflammation from intramuscular injections, polymyositis, muscle dystrophy, rhabdomyolysis); *bone* (neoplastic metastasis, myeloma, Paget's disease); *brain* (cerebral infarction, cerebral neoplasm); *heart* (myocardial infarction—onset after 18 h, peak in 2 days); *lungs* (pulmonary infections); *kidneys* (myoglobinemia, infarction, azotemia); *liver* (necrosis, cirrhosis, viral hepatitis, cholecystitis, administration of opiates in presence of biliary disease); *pancreas* (pancreatitis, diabetes mellitus); *stomach* (peptic ulcer); *bowel* (regional ileitis, ulcerative colitis); *blood* (hemolytic disease including pernicious anemia, rhabdomyolysis); *intake/output* (dehydration); *drugs* (salicylates); *poisons* (alcohol); *technical error* (false-positive from prostaphilin, polycillin, opiates, erythromycin, dehydration of blood specimen, dust contamination from laboratory).

Decreased Concentration: Beriberi, severe liver disease, chronic dialysis, uremia, pregnancy, pyridoxine deficiency, ketoacidosis.

iron, serum (Fe⁺⁺). *Pathophysiology:* At wt 56. The body contains about 3–4 g of this inorganic element essential for hemoglobinization of erythrocytes. Its deficiency represents one of the most common disorders in the world. Approximately 1 mg of iron is absorbed and excreted each day. Most of the iron circulates in erythrocyte hemoglobin (1.0 mg/1.0 mL packed erythrocytes), with the rest bound to ferritin in stores (approximately 1.0 g), in myoglobin, and with a small fraction incorporated into respiratory enzymes and other sites. Bound to transferrin, radioiron is cleared from the plasma in 60–120 min, with 80% to 90% incorporated into new circulating erythrocytes over subsequent 2 weeks. The serum concentration of iron decreases by 50–100 µg/dL with the diurnal acceleration of erythropoiesis in the afternoon, so the times sequential specimens are obtained should be uniform if trends are to be followed.

Normal Concentration: Males 80–180 µg/dL (14–32 µmol/L); females 60–160 µg/dL (11–29 µmol/L).

Increased Concentration (hyperferremia): Intestinal tract (excessive absorption [iron therapy, dietary excess, idiopathic hemochromatosis]); *liver* (acute hepatic necrosis, some cases of cirrhosis); *blood* (hemolytic anemia, repeated blood transfusions); *bone marrow* (aplastic anemia, thalassemia, pernicious anemia).

Decreased Concentration (hypoferremia): Blood (iron deficiency anemia, repeated phlebotomy, intravascular hemolysis with hemoglobinuria [paroxysmal nocturnal hemoglobinuria, march hemoglobinuria, prosthetic heart valves]; anemia of chronic disorders [tuberculosis, osteomyelitis, rheumatoid arthritis, cancer]); *lungs* (intrapulmonary hemorrhage in idiopathic pulmonary hemosiderosis); *gastrointestinal tract* (diminished absorption [decreased ingestion, pica, postgastrectomy], chronic bleeding [peptic ulcer disease, gastritis, polyps, ulcerative colitis, colonic carcinoma]); *genitourinary tract* (menorrhagia, iron loss to fetus during gestation, chronic hematuria, loss of transferrin in proteinuria of nephrosis).

iron-binding capacity, serum total (TIBC). The TIBC mainly reflects transferrin and, with the serum iron, may help distinguish between anemias of iron deficiency and those of chronic disorders.

Normal Capacity: 250–460 µg/dL (45–82 µmol/L).

Increased Capacity: Blood (iron deficiency anemia, acute or chronic blood loss), *liver* (hepatitis), *genitourinary tract* (late pregnancy).

Decreased Capacity: Blood (anemias of chronic disorders [infections, inflammations, and cancer], thalassemia), *gastrointestinal tract and liver* (hemochromatosis, cirrhosis), *genitourinary tract* (nephrosis).

ferritin, serum. Mol wt 680,000. As the major iron-storage protein in the body, it reflects iron stored in the reticuloendothelial system.

Normal Concentration: 18–300 ng/mL (18–300 µg/L).

Increased Concentration: Blood (excessive body iron stores from transfusion hemosiderosis, anemias of chronic disorders, leukemias, Hodgkin's disease), *gastrointestinal tract and liver* (excess dietary iron, transfusion hemosiderosis, hemochromatosis).

Decreased Concentration: Iron deficiency anemia (0–18 µg/L).

Increased Concentration: Hemochromatosis >400 ng/L (>160 nmol/L).

lactic dehydrogenase, serum (LDH). *Pathophysiology:* Mol wt 140,000. This enzyme catalyzes the oxidation of lactate to pyruvate reversibly. It is found in all tissues, so an elevation of the blood level is a nonspecific indicator of tissue damage.

Normal Concentration: 110–250 U/L (1.83–4.23 µkat/L).

Increased Concentration: Muscle (necrosis, polymyositis in 25% of cases, muscular dystrophy in 10% of cases, dermatomyositis, progressive muscular dystrophy, myotonic dystrophy [but CPK is more specific for muscle than LDH]); *bone* (carcinomatous metastasis);

brain (cerebral damage); *thyroid* (hypothyroidism); *heart* (acute myocardial infarction [begins within 10–12 h, peaks at 48–72 h, prolonged elevation for 10–14 days—long after CPK and SGOT have returned to normal]); combination myocardial infarction and congestive failure (increase in LDH and LDH_5, but LDH isoenzyme normal in cardiac failure alone); insertion of prosthetic heart valve, cardiovascular surgery; *lungs* (pulmonary embolism or infarction); *kidneys* (renal infarction), high LDH with normal or slight increase in SGOT, *liver* (hepatitis with jaundice, common bile duct obstruction); *bowel* (intestinal obstruction, sprue); *blood* (untreated pernicious anemia, also in other hemolytic anemias, 50% of cases of lymphoma and leukemia); *infections* (infectious mononucleosis); *malignant neoplasm* (50% of cases); *poisons* (alcohol).

Decreased Concentration: X-irradiation; ingestion of clofibrate.

phosphate, serum inorganic (HPO_4^{--}). *Pathophysiology:* This term includes the inorganic phosphorus of ionized HPO_4^{--} and $H_2PO_4^-$ in equilibrium in the serum; only 10% to 20% is protein bound. P furnishes the element for synthesizing nucleotides, phospholipids, and the high-energy ATP. When the energy demands are great for glycolysis, the serum inorganic P is decreased.

Normal Concentration: 2.6–4.5 mg/dL (0.84–1.45 mmol/L).

Increased Concentration (hyperphosphatemia): Bone (healing fractures, some multiple myelomas, Paget's disease, osteolytic metastases, osteomalacia, acromegaly, rickets); *muscle* (necrosis); *parathyroids* (hypoparathyroidism); *adrenals* (Addison's disease); *liver* (acute yellow atrophy); *bowel* (high intestinal obstruction); *blood* (myelocytic leukemia); *infections* (sepsis); *congenital* (Fanconi's disease); *chemical imbalances* (milk-alkali syndrome of Burnett, rickets, respiratory alkalosis, excess of vitamin D); sarcoidosis.

Decreased Concentration (hypophosphatemia): Parathyroids (hyperparathyroidism); *kidneys* (renal tubular defects [Fanconi syndrome]); *pancreas* (diabetes mellitus); *congenital* (primary hypophosphatemia); *intake/output* (anorexia, vomiting, diarrhea, lack of vitamin D, hyperalimentation in refeeding after starvation, malnutrition); *chemical imbalances* (gout, ketoacidosis, respiratory alkalosis, hypokalemia, hypomagnesemia, primary hyperphosphatemia); *drugs* (intravenous glucose, anabolic steroids, androgens, epinephrine, glucagon, insulin, salicylates, phosphorus-binding antacids, diuretic drugs); *poison* (alcohol).

potassium, serum (K^+, L, kalium). *Pathophysiology:* At wt 39. This is the predominant cation in the cellular fluid, whereas sodium predominates in the extracellular fluids. About 90% of the exchangeable K^+ is within the cells; less than 1% in the normal serum. Thus small shifts of K^+ from the cells cause relatively large changes in the smaller serum compartment. Changes in serum concentration of K^+ produce profound effects on nerve excitation, muscle contraction, and in myocardial potential. Since the concentration of K^+ in the erythrocytes is about 18 times as great as that in the serum, hemolysis raises the serum K considerably.

Normal Concentration: 3.5–5.0 mEq/L (3.5–5.0 mmol/L).

Increased Concentration (hyperkalemia) (Note: high levels of serum K^+ pose great danger of producing cardiac arrest); *Muscle* (status epilepticus, periodic paralysis, tissue necrosis); *stomach* (hemorrhage from peptic ulcer); *bowel* (hemorrhage into the gut); *kidneys* (renal failure with oliguria or anuria, aldosteronism); *adrenals* (Addison's disease, deficit in renin-angiotensin-aldosterone system); *blood* (accumulation of blood in extracellular spaces, *in vivo* clotting); *intake/output* (dehydration, urinary obstruction, excessive oral intake of K^+ as drug or in food [fruit juices, soft drinks, oranges, peaches, bananas, tomatoes, high-protein diet]); *chemical imbalances* (acidosis, inappropriate antidiuretic hormone ADH, respiratory acidosis); *drugs and therapy* (spironolactone [aldosterone antagonist], triamterene [retains K^+], hemolyzed transfused blood); *technical error* (hemolysis in performing venipuncture or intentional clotting in collecting blood specimens, especially with thrombocytosis).

Decreased Concentration (hypokalemia) (almost always associated with depletion of K^+ in total body water): *Stomach* (loss of K^+ from vomiting, gastric suction, postgastrectomy dumping syndrome, gastric atony); *bowel* (villous adenoma, colonic cancer, laxative abuse, Zollinger-Ellison syndrome, adynamic ileus); *pancreas* (diabetes mellitus); *kidneys* (polyuria, renal injury, salt-losing nephritis, ureterosigmoidostomy with urinary reabsorption); *adrenals* (Cushing's syndrome); *chemical imbalances* (metabolic alkalosis [from diuresis, primary aldosteronism, pseudoaldosteronism], metabolic acidosis [from renal tubular acidosis, diuresis, phase of tubular necrosis, chronic pyelonephritis, diuresis after release of urinary obstruction]); *intake/output* (malabsorption and malnutrition); *drugs* (diuretics, estrogens, salicylates, corticosteroids).

protein, total serum. This is determined as a fraction containing serum albumin and the serum globulins; the fibrogen was discarded in the clot that separated from the plasma to form the serum specimen. The quantity of the total serum protein, minus the albumin fraction, gives an estimate of the serum globulins.

Normal Concentration: 6–8 g/dL (60–80 g/L).

Increased Concentration (hyperproteinemia): Water depletion, multiple myeloma, macroglobulinemia, and sarcoidosis.

Decreased Concentration (hypoproteinemia): Lymph nodes (Hodgkin's disease); *heart* (congestive cardiac failure); *stomach* (peptic ulcer); *bowel* (ulcerative colitis); *biliary tract* (acute cholecystitis); *kidneys* (nephrosis, chronic glomerulonephritis); *liver* (cirrhosis, viral hepatitis).

—**albumin, serum.** *This serum fraction is determined directly by the autoanalyzer.*

Pathophysiology: Mol wt about 65,000. Normally, this fraction comprises more than half the total serum protein. Because its molecular weight is low compared with that of the globulins (between 44,000 and 435,000), its smaller molecules exert 80% of osmotic pressure of the plasma. Thus the concentration of the serum albumin controls the passage of water through the cell membranes by osmosis. In addition, (1) serum albumin serves as a protein store for the body that can be utilized when a deficit develops; (2) it serves as a solvent for fatty acids and bile salts; and (3) it serves as a transport vehicle by loosely binding hormones, amino acids, drugs, and metals.

Normal Concentration: 3.1–4.3 g/dL (31–43 g/L).

Increased Concentration (hyperalbuminemia): No significant correlation with diseases.

Decreased Concentration (hypoalbuminemia): Bone (multiple myeloma); *lymph nodes* (Hodgkin's disease); *heart* (congestive cardiac failure); *stomach* (peptic ulcer); *bowel* (ulcerative colitis, protein-losing enteropathies); *liver* (cirrhosis, viral hepatitis); *biliary tract* (acute cholecystitis); *pancreas* (diabetes mellitus); *kidneys* (nephrosis, chronic glomerulonephritis); *blood* (lymphocytic leukemia, myelocytic leukemia, macroglobulinemia, analbuminemia); *collagen diseases* (lupus erythematosus, polyarteritis, rheumatoid arthritis, rheumatic fever); stress, hypersensitivity; *drugs* (estrogens); malnutrition.

—**globulins, serum** (calculated from SMA 12/60). The difference between the values for total serum protein and for serum albumin, as measured by the autoanalyzer, is assumed to be serum globulins, the plasma fibrinogen being discarded in the clot in preparing the serum specimen. When the globulin level is increased, an analysis of the group of globulins is indicated to identify each component. This is accomplished by *electrophoresis.*

—**globulins, serum** (by electrophoresis). A solution of the serum is added to a medium that is electrified to serve as an electric field. The medium may be filter paper, certain liquids, cellulose acetate, starch block, agar gel, or acrylamide gel. In an electric field the various proteins migrate, each at its own rate, depending on its molecular weight. Each protein may be recognized by its mobility. A specimen of blood plasma subjected to electrophoresis will be found to contain proteins that migrate in several *zones* according to their mobility rates. These zones have been named with Greek small letters; the proteins are named for the zone in which they are found: *alpha-0* (α_0) (for albumin), *alpha-1* (α_1), *alpha-2* (α_2), *beta* (β), *gamma* (γ), and *phi* (ϕ) (for fibrinogen).

Alpha-1 (α_1) globulin (includes antitrypsin, oromucil, some cortisol-binding globulin). *Increased Concentration:* Lymph nodes (Hodgkin's disease); *stomach* (peptic ulcers); *bowel* (ulcerative colitis); *liver* (cirrhosis); *neoplasm* (metastatic carcinoma); *intake/output* (protein-losing enteropathy); hypersensitivity, stress. *Decreased Concentration:* viral hepatitis.

Alpha-2 (α_2) globulin (includes macroglobulins, haptoglobin, HS glycoprotein, ceruloplasmin, and some immunoglobulins). *Increased Concentration: Lymph nodes* (Hodgkin's disease); *stomach* (peptic ulcers); *bowel* (ulcerative colitis); *liver* (cirrhosis); *kidneys* (nephrosis, chronic glomerulonephritis); *collagen diseases* (systemic lupus erythematosis, polyarteritis nodosa, rheumatoid arthritis); *neoplasm* (metastatic carcinoma); *intake/output* (protein-losing enteropathies. *Decreased Concentration: Liver* (cirrhosis, viral hepatitis).

Beta (β) globulin (includes transferrin, C_3, C_1, hemopexin, some immunoglobulins). *Increased Concentration: Collagen diseases* (rheumatoid arthritis, rheumatic fever); *chemical imbalance* (analbuminemia). *Decreased Concentration: Kidneys* (nephrosis); *blood* (lymphocytic leukemia); *neoplasm* (metastatic carcinoma).

Gamma (γ) globulins (include all the immunoglobulins). *Increased Concentration: Liver* (cirrhosis); *blood* (myelocytic leukemia); *collagen diseases* (lupus erythematosus, rheumatoid arthritis); *chemical imbalance* (analbuminemia). *Decreased Concentration: Kidneys* (nephrosis); *blood* (lymphocytic leukemia, hypogammaglobulinemia); *intake/output* (protein-losing enteropathies).

Monoclonal Gamma Globulins (recognized in the electrophoresis records by a *sharp and narrow* spike in the gamma region). This is inferred to be the result of proteins of unmixed nature from a single cell line. Such a result calls for further identification in immunoelectrophoresis. *Occurrence:* Multiple myeloma, macroglobulinemia, malignant lymphoma, amyloidosis, monoclonal gammopathy of undetermined significance.

Polyclonal Gamma Globulins (recognized in the electrophoresis records by a *broad-based pattern* in the gamma zone). The inference indicates the presence of abnormal proteins from many lines of cells. *Occurrence:* Hepatic cirrhosis, diffuse skin diseases, hyerglobulinemic purpura.

—**gammopathies** (by immunoelectrophoresis). This group of disorders is characterized by the proliferation of one or more of the five human immunoglobulins—IgG, IgA, IgM, IgD, and IgE—normally present in human serum. Their molecular structures differ among them by the possession of various combination of two of five *heavy chains* (H-chains) and various coupled two *light chains* (L-chains). The heavy chains are named with small Greek letters, corresponding to the large Arabic capitals of the immunoglobulins: α, β, γ, δ, ϵ; the light chains are called κ and λ. The five immunoglobulins can be identified by *immunoelectrophoresis.* In this procedure, regular electrophoresis is modified by the addition to the medium of specific antibodies.

Immunoglobulin IgG. Mol wt 160,000. This is the smallest molecule of the immunoglobulins and the only one that can pass the placental membranes; therefore it serves as protection for the newborn until the child's own globulins can be generated. In the adult, the immunoglobulin seems to participate in all immune reactions, including the isoantibodies for antigen C, D, and E. *Normal Concentration:* 500–1200 mg/dL (5.00–12.00 g/L). *Increased Concentration: Bone* (myeloma); *lungs* (pulmonary tuberculosis); *liver* (hepatitis, cirrhosis); *collagen diseases* (systemic lupus erythematosus, rheumatoid arthritis). *Decreased Concentration: Lymph nodes* (lymphoid aplasia); *kidneys* (nephrosis); *blood* (agammaglobulinemia, dysgammaglobulinemia, heavy-chain disease, IgA myeloma, macroglobulinemia, chronic lymphocytic leukemia).

Immunoglobulin IgA. Mol wt 170,000. This globulin is especially involved in the protection against viral infections. It has the added feature of an *excretory form* with a molecular weight of 400,000, found in colostrum, saliva, tears, bronchial secretions, gastrointestinal secretions, and nasal discharges. It has a special action against viruses of influenza, poliomyelitis, adenoviral diseases, and rhinoviruses. *Normal Concentration:* 50–350 mg/dL (0.50–3.50 g/L). *Increased Concentration: Liver* (cirrhosis); *blood* (IgA myeloma); *infections; collagen diseases* (systemic lupus erythromatosus, rheumatoid arthritis); *congenital* (Wiskott-Aldrich syndrome); *sarcoidosis. Decreased Concentration:* Normal in some persons; *kidneys* (nephrosis); *congenital* (hereditary telangiectasia, lymphoid aplasia); *collagen disease* (Still's disease, systemic lupus erythematosus); *liver* (cirrhosis); *blood* (type III dysgammaglobulinemia, agammaglobulinemia, heavy-chain disease, acute lymphocytic leukemia, chronic lymphocytic leukemia, chronic myelocytic leukemia).

Immunoglobulin IgM. Mol wt 900,000. This is the largest molecule of the immunoglobulins. It is most often elicited during a primary antibody response. The rheumatoid factor and the isoantibodies anti-A and anti-B belong mostly to this class. *Normal Concentration:* 30–230 mg/dL (0.30–2.30 g/L). *Increased Concentration: Liver* (hepatitis, biliary cirrhosis); *collagen disease* (rheumatoid arthritis, systemic lupus erythematosus); *blood* (macroglobulinemia); *trypanosomiasis.*

Immunoglobulin IgD. Mol wt 185,000. There is no known specific activity for this protein. *Normal Concentration:* <6 mg/dL (<60 mg/L). *Increased Concentration:* Chronic infections, IgD myeloma.

Immunoglobulin IgE. Mol wt 200,000. This protein is involved in atopic reactions. *Normal Concentration:* 20–1000 ng/mL (20–1000 μg/L). *Increased Concentration:* Extrinsic asthma (60% of cases), hay fever (30% of cases), atopic eczema, parasitic infestations, IgE myeloma.

—**heavy-chain disease.** This is a disease characterized by excessive production of proteins with heavy chains. In the electrophoresis they occur as a sharp peak in the beta or gamma region. Immunoelectrophoresis shows marked decrease in the normal IgG, IgA, and IgM.

sodium, serum (Na⁺, L. natrium). *Pathophysiology:* At wt 23. This is the predominant cation in the extracellular fluid, including plasma. Together with Cl⁻, it makes a major contribution to the osmotic pressure of the serum. Water diffuses between the cellular compartment containing K^+ and the extracellular compartment containing Na^+. The concentration of Na^+ is in equilibrium with K^+ and total body water. Loss of Na^+ is frequently accompanied by an equivalent amount of water (as an isotonic solution), so normal levels of serum Na^+ do not exclude the possibility of water shifts. Thus, a careful history of water intake and output may be necessary to interpret the meaning of the value for serum Na^+.

Normal Concentration: 135–145 mEq/L (135–145 mmol/L).

Increased Concentration (hypernatremia): Brain (thalamic lesions); *parathyroids* (hyperparathyroidism); *kidneys* (aldosteronism); *intake/output* (water loss greater than Na loss [vomiting, sweating, hyperpnea, diarrhea], diuresis [diabetes insipidus, diabetes mellitus, diuretic drugs, diuretic phase of acute tubular necrosis, diuresis after relief of urinary obstruction], excessive Na^+ intake); *chemical imbalances* (hypercalcemia, hypokalemic nephropathy); *drugs* (corticosteroids).

Decreased Concentration (hyponatremia): Heart (serum dilution from congestive cardiac failure); *kidneys* (serum dilution from salt-losing nephritis or nephritis); *liver* (dilution from cirrhosis with ascites); *adrenals* (Addison's disease), *intake/output* (fluid loss [vomiting, sweating, diarrhea, diuresis], malnutrition), *chemical imbalance* (inappropriate antidiuretic hormone); *spuriously normal serum osmolality* (hyperlipidemia, hyperglycemia [reciprocal decrease of serum Na^+ by 3 mEq/L for every increase of glucose level of 100 mg/dL]).

transaminase, serum (synonyms: glutamate-oxaloacetate, serum SGOT, which see, and aspartate aminotransferase).

urea-nitrogen (blood urea nitrogen, BUN, Urea-N). *Pathophysiology:* Mol wt 60. Urea is the nitrogenous end product of protein metabolism. It permeates all body water and is exreted in the urine. The traditional method of expression is a urea-nitrogen that is approximately half the weight of urea. The serum level of urea-N results from a balance between the rate of amino acid substrate presented to the liver, the rate of synthesis of urea by the liver, and the rate of urinary excretion of urea. Protein breakdown is accentuated by high-protein diets, blood in the gastrointestinal tract, increased metabolism of tissue, and inhibition of anabolism by corticosteroid drugs.

Normal Concentration: 8–25 mg/dL (2.9–8.9 mmol/L).

Increased Concentration (azotemia): Thyroid (increased catabolism in hyperthyroidism); *heart* (myocardial infarction); *kidneys* (impaired renal function, reduced blood flow to the kidneys in congestive cardiac failure, postrenal obstruction); *bowel* (hemorrhage into the gut); *input/output* (salt and water loss [vomiting, sweating, diarrhea, diuresis, lack of drinking water]).

Decreased Concentration: Muscle (acromegaly); *kidneys* (sometimes nephrosis); *liver* (liver failure, hepatitis); *genital* (late pregnancy); *intake/output* (low-protein, high-carbohydrate diet, intravenous feedings exclusively, celiac disease).

Wallach: BUN 6–8 mg/dL is frequently the result of dehydration; 10–20 mg/dL usually indicates normal renal function; 50–150 mg/dL usually from seriously impaired renal function.

uric acid, serum. *Pathophysiology:* Mol wt 169. Uric acid is the end product of purine metabolism. The substrates, phosphoribosylpyrophosphate (PRPP), glutamine, glycine, and aspartic acid, are converted to inosinic acid. This latter, in turn, plus adenylic and guanylic acids, is transformed by hypoxanthine-guanine phosphoribosyl transferase (HGPRTase) to form hypoxanthine. This is further transformed to uric acid by action of xanthine oxidase. Normally uric acid is produced at the rate of 10 mg/kg/day in a healthy adult. The body pool is about 1200 mg, distributed to the body water. *Increased synthesis* of nucleic acid breakdown results in the increased uric acid production. Uric acid leaves the body by two routes: through the renal glomeruli and by bacterial catabolism of uric acid in the gut. Renal excretion of uric acid is increased by expansion of body fluids (by salt or osmotic diuresis) and by vasoconstriction (from angiotensin or norepinephrine infusions). Excretion of uric acid is decreased by dehydration or diuretics.

Normal Concentration: 3.0–7.0 mg/dL (0.18–0.42 mmol/L).

Increased Concentration (hyperuricemia) (Note: High values for uric acid are among the most common abnormalities encountered in routine testing, according to Hall and Halfman. This probably accounts for the much too frequent diagnosis of gout. The serum uric acid is elevated in 90% of the cases of gouty arthritis, but the same elevation is noted in 25% of the cases of acute nongouty arthritis and in 25% of relatives of gouty patients. The diagnosis of gout should not be made without the symptoms and signs of the disease). Skin (about half the patients with psoriasis); *thyroid* (hypothyroidism); *parathyroids* (hypoparathyroidism, primary hyperparathyroidism); *lungs* (resolving pneumonia); *kidneys* (renal failure, polycystic kidneys); *genital* (toxemia of pregnancy); *blood* (increased destruction of nucleoproteins [leukemia, multiple myeloma, polycythemia vera, lymphoma], other disseminated neoplasias, hemolytic anemias, sickle cell anemia); *neoplasms* (metastasis); *congenital or familial* (Wilson's disease, Fanconi's disease, von Gierke's disease, Down syndrome); *therapy* (irradi-ation, cancer therapy, thiazides, other diuretics, small doses of salicylates); *intake/output* (high-protein, low-calorie diet, high nuclear diet [sweetbreads, liver], starvation); *chemical imbalance* (gout, relatives of gouty patients, calcinosis universalies, diabetic ketosis); *poisons* (acute alcoholism, lead poisoning, berylliosis); certain normal *populations* (Blackfoot and Pima Indians, Filipinos, New Zealand Maoris); *sarcoidosis. Decreased concentration* (hypouricemia): *bone* (acromegaly); *kidneys* (xanthinuria, healthy adults with Dalmation-dog mutation [isolated defect in tubular transport of uric acid]; *bowel* (celiac disease); *blood* (pernicious anemia in relapse); *congenital* (Fanconi syndrome, Wilson's disease); *neoplasms* (carcinoma, Hodgkin's disease); *drugs* (ACTH, glyceryl guaicolate, x-ray contrast media).

HEMATOLOGIC DATA

blood film examination. A blood film, prepared or available in the office, nursing unit, or outclinic laboratory, provides the physician with an opportunity of immediately evaluating clues from the history and physical examination and of personally confirming results of electronic counters in central laboratories requiring hours to days for reporting. Examples of information to be obtained will be given with encouragement to consult standard textbooks of hematology for comprehensive treatment of the subject. Appreciate that cellular morphology may vary depending on the technique, stain, and location on the blood smear. Select an area for examination where the erythrocytes are close but do not touch each other.

Erythrocyte Morphology: Evaluate color, size, shape, and contents. *Macrocytes* (reticulocytosis, liver disease, megaloblastic anemia); *hypochromic microcytes* (defects in hemoglobin synthesis [iron deficiency, thalassemias, sickle cell disease, and other hemoglobinopathies]); *spherocytes* (hereditary spherocytosis); *schistocytes* (disseminated intravascular coagulation, thrombotic thrombocytopenic purpura, vasculitis, thrombotic microangiopathy, prosthetic heart valves); *tear drop or dacryocytes* (extramedullary hemopoiesis, myelophthisic anemia); *erythroblasts* (extramedullary hemopoiesis, myelophthisic anemia, severe hemolytic anemia, erythroleukemia); *Howell-Jolly bodies* (postplenectomy, megaloblastic anemia); *basophilic stippling* (lead poisoning, hemolytic disease); *malaria and Bartonella parasites.*

Leukocyte Morphology: Confirm the report of the electronic enumeration and differential leukocyte count. *Toxic granulation of neutrophils and metamyelocytes* (bacterial infections); *giant cytoplasmic granules* (Chediak-Higashi syndrome); *bilobed neutrophils* (Pelger-Huet anomaly); *hypersegmented neutrophils* (pernicious anemia, vitamin B_{12} deficiency, folate deficiency, myeloproliferative diseases); *myeloblasts, promyelocytes, myelocytes* (depending on the number and appearance of immature cells, consider [acute myeloblastic leukemia, acute promyelocytic leukemia, chronic myelocytic leukemia, myelofibrosis, polycythemia vera]); *atypical lymphocytes* (viral infections); *large granular lymphocytes* (natural killer cells of T-gamma lymphoproliferative disease); *lymphoblasts* (acute lymphoblastic leukemia, prolymphocytic leukemia, infectious mononucleosis); *plasmablasts* (multiple myeloma).

Platelet Morphology: Confirm the electronic enumeration of the platelet count. In oil immersion fields of 1000× magnification, where the erythrocytes are close but not touching, expect to count 15 to 20 platelets per field in normal blood films. Scan the sides of the smear for clumps of platelets that may have been counted inaccurately by instrument. *Megathrombocytes* (platelets greater than 2.5 micrometer μm in diameter may be increased in conditions of accelerated platelet production, compensating for increased destruction B_{12} deficiency, folate deficiency, myeloproliferative diseases, Bernard-Soulier syndrome).

erythrocyte measurements (counts, hemoglobin content, and hematocrit). *Normal values: Counts:* 4.2–6.2 × 10^6/μL. *Hematocrit:* males: 42%–52%; females: 37% to 47%; *Hemoglobin:* males: 14–18 g/dL; females: 12–16 g/dL.

erythrocytic indices. These values are all calculated from the counts, hemoglobin content, and hematocrit. The normal ranges are as follows:

$$Mean\ Corpuscular\ Volume\ (MCV) = \frac{Hct \times 10}{RBC\ in\ millions}$$
$$= 82\text{--}92\ fL$$

$$Mean\ Corpuscular\ Hemoglobin\ Concentration\ (MCHC)$$
$$= \frac{Hgb\ in\ g/dL \times 100}{Hct}$$
$$= 32\text{--}36\ g/dL$$

$$Mean\ Corpuscular\ Hemoglobin\ (MCH)$$
$$= \frac{Hgb\ in\ g/dL \times 10}{RBC\ in\ millions}$$
$$= 27\text{--}31\ pg/cell$$

high RBC counts. *Muscle* (burns [contracted blood volume]); *heart* (venous-arterial shunt [right-to-left shunt]); *lungs* (hypoxic diseases); *liver* (hepatoma); *kidney* (renal cyst or carcinoma); *blood* (contracted blood volume [dehydration, burns, shock], hemoglobinopathies [carboxyhemoglobinemia, sulfhemoglobinemia],

polycythemia vera and secondary); *genital* (third to ninth month of pregnancy and to third week postpartum, ruptured ectopic pregnancy); *intake/output* (diarrhea, profuse sweating, fluid deprivation); *chemical imbalance* (diabetic acidosis, high-altitude hypoxia); *drugs* (androgens, diuretics).

low RBC counts. *Heart* (congestive cardiac failure); *kidneys* (renal failure, oliguria); *genital* (pregnancy [expanded plasma volume]); *blood* (macrocytic anemias [pernicious anemia, folate deficiency, refractory anemia, hemolysis or bleeding], normocytic normochromic anemias [bone marrow failure, acute hemorrhage, hemolysis, chronic disease, infections, renal failure, liver disease], microcytic hypochromic anemias [Fe deficiency, thalassemia, pyridoxine-responsive anemia, hemoglobinopathies]).

erythrocyte sedimentation rate (ESR). *Normal Values: Wintrobe method:* males 1–13 mm/hour; females: 0–20 mm/hour. *Westergren method:* males: 0–13 mm/hour; females: 0–20 mm/hour.

Increased Rate: Thyroid (hyperthyroidism, hypothyroidism); *genital* (pelvic inflammation, ruptured ectopic pregnancy, normal pregnancy from third month to termination plus 3 weeks postpartum, menstruation); *blood* (hyperglobulinemia, hypoalbuminemia, dextran or polyvinyl plasma substitutes); *infections* (many, but especially tuberculosis, necrosis); *collagen disease* (rheumatoid arthritis); *neoplasm; poison* (as in lead).

Not Increased Rate: Bone and joints (osteoarthritis); *heart* (angina pectoris); *stomach* (peptic ulcer); *genital* (unruptured ectopic pregnancy, early pregnancy); *blood* (polycythemia vera, sickle cell anemia); *certain infections* (typhoid fever, undulant fever, malaria, infectious mononucleosis); *acute appendicitis* (first 24 h); *acute allergic disorders.*

leukocytes, total count. *Normal Concentration:* 4300–10,800/μL (or mm³).

—neutrophil counts. *Normal Concentration:* 1830–7250/μL (or mm³) (34%–71% of total).

Increased Concentration (leukocytosis): *Skin and muscle* (exercise, seizures, burns, inflammation, gangrene, necrosis); *heart* (myocardial infarction); *genital* (eclampsia); *blood* (acute hemorrhage, acute hemolysis, myeloproliferative diseases [polycythemia vera, chronic myelocytic leukemia, myelofibrosis, idiopathic thrombocythemia]); *neoplasms* (malignant); *infections; chemical imbalances* (uremia, diabetic acidosis, gout); *drugs* (epinephrine, corticosteroids, lithium carbonate, parenteral foreign proteins, vaccines): *poisons* (venoms, mercury, black widow spider venom).

Decreased Concentration (leukopenia or neutropenia): *Bone marrow* (failure); *kidneys* (severe renal injury); *spleen* (hypersplenism, Felty's syndrome); *liver* (cirrhosis, portal obstruction); *blood* (pernicious anemia, folate deficiency, aleukemic leukemia, aplastic anemia, acute myeloblastic leukemia, cyclic neutropenia, autoimmune neutropenia); *congenital* (Gaucher's disease); *infections* (viral [infectious mononucleosis, hepatitis, HIV, influenza, rubeola, psittacosis], bacterial [streptococcal, staphylococcal diseases, sepsis, tularemia, brucellosis, tuberculosis]); *rickettsial disease* (scrub typhus, sandfly fever); *rotozoal* (malaria, kala-azar); *intake/output* (cachexia); *drugs and therapy* (cancer chemotherapy, sulfonamides, antibiotics, analgesics, antidepressants, arsenicals, antithyroid drugs, x-radiation); *poisons* (benzene); *collagen disease* (systemic lupus erythematosus).

—**eosinophil counts.** *Normal Concentration:* 0–700/μL (or mm^3) (0%–7.8% of WBC).

Increased Concentration (eosinophilia): *Skin* (pemphigus, dermatitis berpetiformis); *bone* (metastatic carcinoma to bone); *heart* (Loeffler parietal fibroplastic endocarditis); *gastrointestinal* (eosinophilic gastroenteritis, ulcerative colitis, regional enteritis); *spleen* (postsplenectomy); *blood* (pernicious anemia, hypereosinophilic syndrome, chronic myelocytic leukemia, polycythemia vera, Hodgkin's disease); *allergic disorders* (asthma, hay fever, urticaria, drug reactions); *infections* (scarlet fever, erythema multiforme); *parasitic infestations* (trichinosis, ecchynococcosis); *genital* (ovarian tumors); *miscellaneous* (polyarteritis nodosa, sarcoidosis); *irradiation; poisons* (phosphorus, black widow spider bite).

Decreased Concentration (eosinopenia): Bone marrow failure, hypoadrenalism.

—**basophil counts.** *Normal Concentration:* 0–150/μL (or mm^3) (0%–1.8% of WBC).

Increased Concentration (basophilia): *Thyroid* (myxedema); *spleen* (postsplenectomy); *kidneys* (nephrosis); *infections* (varicella, variola); *blood* (chronic myelocytic leukemia, polycythemia vera, myeloid metaplasia, Hodgkin's disease, chronic hemolytic anemias).

Decreased Concentration: Thyroid (hyperthyroidism); *genital* (pregnancy); *irradiation; blood* (bone marrow failure); *drugs* (chemotherapy, glucocorticoids).

lymphocyte counts. *Normal Concentration:* 1500–4000/μL (or mm^3) (19%–52% of WBC).

Increased Concentration (lymphocytosis): *Lungs* (tuberculosis, viral pneumonia); *liver* (infectious hepatitis); *bowel* (cholera); *blood* (infectious lymphocytosis, infectious mononucleosis, lymphocytic leukemia, malignant lymphoma); *general infections* (rubella, brucellosis, systemic syphilis, toxoplasmosis, pertussis).

Decreased Concentration (lymphopenia): *Acute infections* (viral, HIV); *neoplasm* (carcinoma, lymphoma); *irradiation; drugs* (corticosteroids, cancer chemotherapy); *idiopathic.*

monocyte counts. *Normal Concentration:* 200–950/μL (or mm^3) (2.4%–11.8% of WBC).

Increased Concentration (monocytosis): *Bowel* (ulcerative colitis, regional enteritis); *blood* (monocytic leukemia, myeloid metaplasia, recovery from agranulocytosis); *congenital* (Gaucher's disease); *neoplasm; infections; protozoal* (malaria, kala-azar, trypanosomiasis); *rickettsial* (Rocky Mountain spotted fever, typhus); *bacterial* (subacute bacterial endocarditis, tuberculosis, brucellosis); *miscellaneous and multiple system* (systemic lupus erythmatosus, sarcoidosis, syphilis).

platelet counts (thrombocytes). *Normal Concentration:* 150,000–400,000/μL (or mm^3).

Increased Concentration (thrombocytosis or thrombocythemia). *Bone* (rheumatoid arthritis); *muscles* (exercise, bleeding, burns); *heart* (acute heart disease); *liver* (cirrhosis); *spleen* (postplenectomy); *pancreas* (pancreatitis); *blood* (myeloproliferative diseases [polycythemia vera, myelocytic leukemia], iron-deficiency anemia); *malignancy, acute infections, collagen disorders.*

Decreased Concentration (thrombocytopenia): *Spleen* (hypersplenism [congestive splenomegaly, splenectomy, sarcoidosis, splenomegaly, Felty's syndrome]); *blood* (anemias [aplastic, myelophthisic, pernicious anemia, acquired hemolytic anemia, folate deficiency, contact with foreign substances in heart-lung machine during cardiac surgery], polycythemia vera, myelocytic leukemia, thrombocytopenic purpura, primary hemorrhagic thrombocytopenia, massive blood transfusions, May-Hegglin anomaly, surgical operation in general); *infections* (subacute bacterial endocarditis, sepsis, AIDS, typhus); *congenital* (Gaucher's disease, Kasabach-Merrit syndrome); *irradiation; drugs* (marrow suppressants, nitrogen mustard, cancer chemotherapy, chloramphenicol, tranquilizers, antipyretics, heavy metals); *chemical imbalance* (azotemia, heatstroke); *poisons* (benzol, insect bites).

all cellular elements of the blood (erythrocytes, leukocytes, platelets). *Increased Concentration* (pancytosis): Dehydration, polycythemia vera, the myeloproliferative syndromes. *Decreased Concentration* (pancytopenia): *Bones* (marrow failure, multiple myeloma, carcinomatous invasion); *bacterial infections* (tuberculosis); *viral infections* (hepatitis); *blood* (multiple myeloma, lymphoma, pernicious anemia or folate deficiency, myeloblastic leukemia, paroxysmal hemoglobinuria, myelofibrosis); *collagen disease* (systemic lupus erythematosus); *irradiation; drugs* (cancer chemotherapy, chloramphenicol); *poisons* (benzene).

coagulation factors

Prothrombin time (PT). Normal: 11–15 s. *Prolonged Time:* Deficiencies in any of clotting factors I, II, V, VII, or X; liver disease; disseminated intravascular coagulation; vitamin K deficiency; steatorrhea; idiopathic; Goumadin administration; greatly decreased or abnormal fibrinogen.

Partial Thromboplastin Time (PTT). Normal: 22–39 s (activated). *Prolonged time:* Deficiency of *any of* clotting factors I, II, V, VIII, IX, X XI, XII; disseminated intravascular coagulation; therapeutic doses of heparin; *drugs,* lupus erythematosus, and other antibody-mediated inhibitors of clotting factor activity.

Fibrinogen. Normal: 150–350 mg/dL. *Increased Concentration:* During menstruation; pregnancy, infections; hyperthyroidism. *Decreased Concentration:* Congenital afibrinogenemia; disseminated intravascular coagulation; circulating anticoagulants; fibrinolysis.

URINALYSIS

So much information about the patient's health can be rapidly obtained from examination of the urine that many physicians insist on personally performing this simple analysis in the small laboratories of an outclinic, hospital nursing unit, or office. Optimally, urine is collected as a midstream specimen from the first voiding in the morning and examined within one-half hour. This practice tests renal concentrating ability and permits identification of casts before they disintegrate.

color. *Pathophysiology:* Either clear or cloudy (from precipitated normally excreted urates, phosphates, or sulfates), the urine is usually yellow to amber from urochrome pigments. Other colors provide clues to the presence of abnormal substances for which chemical tests should be applied: *dark yellow to green* (bile or bilirubin); *red to black* (erythrocytes, hemoglobin, myoglobin, homogentistic acid [plus sodium hydroxide]); *purple to brown* (on standing in the sunlight from porphyrins).

acidity. Normal range of pH is from 4.6 to 8.0. Monitoring urinary pH helps physicians attempting to alkalinize or acidify the urine to enhance the solubility and excretion of certain substances and drugs.

specific gravity. *Pathophysiology:* An index of weight per unit volume, the specific gravity measures the kidney's ability to dilute or concentrate urine in response to the secretion of antidiuretic hormone (ADH). Fasting during 8 h of sleep should produce a first morning specimen with a specific gravity exceeding 1.018.

Normal Range: 1.003–1.030 achieved with forced water drinking and fasting, respectively.

Increased Specific Gravity: Fasting and dehydration, glycosuria, proteinuria, radiographic contrast media.

Decreased Specific Gravity: Compulsive water drinking, diabetes insipidus.

Fixed Specific Gravity (isosthenuria = 1.010): Severe renal parenchymal damage from many causes (gout, prolonged potassium deficiency, hypercalcemia, myeloma kidney, sickle cell disease).

proteinuria. *Pathophysiology:* Normally an adult excretes undetectable concentrations of protein (5–15 mg/dL). Tubular and glomerular disease may produce measureable proteinuria.

Low Concentrations: Pyelonephritis, fever, benign orthostatic proteinuria, idiopathic focal glomerulonephritis.

High Concentrations: Glomerulonephritis, diabetes mellitus, systemic lupus erythematosis, renal vein thrombosis, amyloidosis, and other causes of the nephrotic syndrome.

glucose. *Pathophysiology:* A function of the plasma glucose concentration, the glomerular filtration and tubular reabsorption of glucose, normal levels of glucose in randomly collected fresh urine specimens are undetectable at less than 25 mg/dL, less than 100 mg/dL during a glucose tolerance test. Dip sticks, impregnated with glucose oxidase and an indicator color, provide a convenient, rapid, and semiquantitative estimate for the patient and physician. Progressively diminished glucose utilization in a patient with uncontrolled diabetes mellitus leads to lypolysis with increasing plasma and urinary concentrations of acetoacetic acid, beta-hydroxybutyric acid, and ketones, which should be sought with other tests.

Normal Range: 3–25 mg/dL.

Increased Concentrations: Hyperglycemia in diabetes mellitus; infrequently with renal abnormalities, including acute tubular damage, hereditary renal glycosuria, and proximal tubular dysfunction as in the Fanconi syndromes.

urinary sediment. *Pathophysiology:* Normally excreted erythrocytes, leukocytes, hyalin casts, and crystals (urate, phosphate, oxalate) are found in the sediment of a fresh specimen collected after a night's fast. Centrifuge 10 mL of urine in a conical tube for 5 min, decant the supernatant, flick the tube to disperse formed elements in the remaining drop, and place it on a slide under a coverslip to examine with the high-power objective of a microscope (hpf). Abnormal numbers of cells and casts or any bacteria reveal the presence of disease.

Erythrocytes: Normally, 0–5 RBC/hpf can be observed in concentrated specimens. *Microscopic hematuria* may occur with fever and exercise and many lesions of the urinary tract from glomerulus to urethra. Cases of *gross hematuria* include coagulation defects, renal papillary necrosis, renal infarction, sickle cell disease, glomerulonephritis, Goodpasture's syndrome, stone or carcinoma of the kidney, hemorrhagic cystitis, stone or carcinoma of the bladder, and prostatitis.

Leukocytes: Normally, 0–10 WBC/hpf can be seen in concentrated specimens. In addition to neutrophils excreted into the urine from the same anatomic sites as erythrocytes, leukocytes from vaginal exudates frequently contaminate routine specimens collected from women. When pyuria exceeding 10 WBC/hpf is present in an uncontaminated specimen, a site of infection in the urinary tract should be sought.

Casts: Occasional *hyalin casts,* arising from the normal renal tubular secretion of mucoproteins, are seen in fresh concenrated specimens. Finding many broad, fine, or coarse *granular casts* (composed of serum proteins like albumin, IgG, transferrin, haptoglobin) in urine containing excessive protein, however, indicates renal parenchymal disease, especially when accompanied by red cell casts. The urine of patients with the nephrotic syndrome, who exhibit glomerular proteinuria and hyperlipoproteinuria, contains *fatty casts,* casts with *doubly refractile fat bodies,* and *maltese crosses* when examined in polarized light. *Red cell casts,* containing 10 to 50 distinct erythrocytes and doubly refractile fat bodies, indicate glomerular disease (glomerulonephritis). *White cell casts* are found in the urinary sediment of patients with pyelonephritis, polyarteritis, exudative glomerulonephritis, and renal infarction. *Bacteria* accompanying white cell casts indicate urinary tract infection. Broad orange or brown *hematin casts* occur in acute tubular injury and chronic renal failure.

(From: DeGowin RL: DeGowin's Diagnostic Examination, 6th ed, New York, McGraw-Hill, Inc., 1995.)

Appendix D

Units of Measurement and Terminology for the Description of Exercise and Sport Performance (Publications Advisory Subcommittee, IOC Medical Commission)

UNITS FOR QUANTIFYING HUMAN EXERCISE

Mass: kilogram (kg)

Distance: meter (m)

Time: second (s)

Force: newton (N)

Work: joule (J)

Power: watt (W)

Velocity: meters per second ($m \cdot s^{-1}$)

Torque: newton-meter ($N \cdot m$)

Acceleration: meters per second^2 ($m \cdot s^{-2}$)

Angle: radian (rad)

Angular Velocity: radians per second ($rad \cdot s^{-1}$)

Amount of Substance: mole (mol)

Volume: liter (L)

TERMINOLOGY

Concentric Action: One in which the ends of the muscle are drawn closer together.

Eccentric Action: One in which a force external to the muscle overcomes the muscle force and the ends of the muscle are drawn further apart.

Endurance: The time limit of a person's ability to maintain either an isometric force or a power level involving combinations of concentric or eccentric muscle actions. (SI unit: second)

Energy: The capability of producing force, performing work, or generating heat. (SI unit: joule)

Exercise: Any and all activity involving generation of force by the activated muscle(s). Exercise can be quantified mechanically as force, torque, work, power, or velocity of progression.

Exercise Intensity: A specific level of muscular activity that can be quantified in terms of power (energy expenditure or work performed per unit of time), the opposing force (e.g., by free weight of weight stack), isometric force sustained, or velocity of progression.

Force: That which changes or tends to change the state of rest or motion in matter. (SI unit: newton) A muscle generates force in a muscle action.

Free Weight: An object of known mass, not attached to a supporting or guiding structure, which is used for physical conditioning and competitive lifting.

Isometric Action: One in which the ends of the muscle are prevented from drawing closer together, with no change in length.

Mass: The quantity of matter of an object that is reflected in its inertia. (SI unit: kilogram)

Muscle Action: The state of activity of muscle.

Power: The rate of performing work; the product of force and velocity. The rate of transformation of metabolic potential energy to work or heat. (SI unit: watt; note $1 \text{ joule} \cdot s^{-1} = 1 \text{ watt}$)

Strength: The maximal force or torque a muscle or muscle group can generate at a specified or determined velocity.

Torque: The effectiveness of a force to overcome the rotational inertia of an object. The product of force and the perpendicular distance from the line of action of the force to the axis of rotation. (SI unit: newton-meter)

Weight: The force exerted by gravity on an object. (SI unit: newton; traditional unit: kilogram of weight.) (*Note:* mass = weight/acceleration resulting from gravity)

Work: Force expressed through a displacement but with no limitation on time. (SI unit: joule) (*Note:* 1 newton ×1 meter = 1 joule)

From *Jrnl Strength Cond Res* 1994;8(2):126.

Appendix E
Fracture Eponyms

Aviator's astragalus. Implies a variety of fractures of the talus; described after World War I as "rudder bar is driven into foot during plane crash."

Barton's fracture. Displaced articular lip fracture of the distal radius; may be associated with carpal subluxation. Fracture configuration may be in a dorsal or volar direction.

Bennett's fracture. Oblique fracture of the first metacarpal base separating a small triangular fragment of the volar lip from the proximally displaced metacarpal shaft.

Bosworth fracture. Fracture of the distal fibula with fixed displacement of the proximal fragment posteriorly behind the posterolateral tibial ridge.

Boxer's fracture. Fracture of the fifth metacarpal neck with volar displacement of the metacarpal head.

Burst fracture. Fracture of the vertebral body from axial load, usually with outward displacement of the fragments. May occur in the cervical, thoracic, or lumbar spine.

Chance fracture. Distraction fracture of the thoracolumbar vertebral body with horizontal disruption of the spinous process, neural arch, and vertebral body.

Chauffeur's fracture (Hutchinson's fracture). Oblique fracture of the radial styloid initially attributed to the starting crank of an engine being forcibly reversed by a backfire.

Chopart's fracture and dislocation. Fracture or dislocation involving Chopart's joints (talonavicular and calcaneocuboid) of the foot.

Clay-shoveler's (coal-shoveler's) fracture. Spinous process fracture of the lower cervical or upper thoracic vertebrae. Injury initially attributed to workers attempting to throw a full shovel of clay upward, but the clay, adhering to the shovel, caused a sudden flexion force opposite to the neck musculature.

Colles' fracture. General term for fractures of the distal radius with dorsal displacement, with or without an ulnar styloid fracture.

Cotton's fractures. Trimalleolar ankle fracture with fractures of both malleoli and the posterior lip of the tibia.

Die-punch fracture. Intraarticular fracture of the distal radius with impaction of the dorsal aspect of the lunate fossa.

Dupuytren's fracture. Fracture of the distal fibula with rupture of the distal tibiofibular ligaments and lateral displacement of the talus.

Duverney's fracture. Fracture of the iliac wing without disruption of the pelvic ring.

Essex-Lopresti's fracture. Fracture of the radial head with associated dislocation of the distal radioulnar joint.

Galeazzi's fracture. Fracture of the radius in the distal third associated with subluxation of the distal ulna.

Greenstick fracture. Incompletely fractured bone in a child, with a portion of the cortex and periosteum remaining intact on the compression side of the fracture.

Hangman's fracture. Fracture through the neural arch of the second cervical vertebra (axis).

Hill-Sachs fracture. Posterolateral humeral head compression fracture caused by anterior glenohumeral dislocation and impaction of the humeral head against the anterior glenoid rim.

Holstein-Lewis fracture. Fracture of the distal third of the humerus with entrapment of the radial nerve.

Hutchinson's fracture. See *Chauffeur's fracture.*

Jefferson's fracture. Comminuted fracture of the ring of the atlas caused by axial compressive forces. Fractures usually occur anterior and posterior to the lateral facet joints.

Jones fracture. Diaphyseal fracture of the base of the fifth metatarsal.

Lisfranc's fracture dislocation. Fracture and/or dislocation involving Lisfranc's (tarsometatarsal) joint of the foot. Lisfranc was one of Napoleon's surgeons. He described traumatic foot amputation through the level of the tarsometatarsal joint.

Maisonneuve's fracture. Fracture of the proximal fibula with syndesmosis rupture and associated fracture of the medial malleolus or rupture of the deltoid ligament.

Malgaigne's fracture. Unstable pelvic fracture with vertical fractures anterior and posterior to the hip joint.

Mallet finger. Flexion deformity of the distal interphalangeal joint caused by separation of the extensor tendon from the distal phalanx. The deformity may be secondary to direct injury of the extensor tendon or an avulsion fracture from the dorsum of the distal phalanx, where the tendon inserts.

Monteggia's fracture. Fracture of the proximal third of the ulna with associated dislocation of the radial head.

Nightstick fracture. Isolated fracture of the ulna secondary to direct trauma.

Posadas's fracture. Transcondylar humeral fracture with displacement of the distal fragment anteriorly and dislocation of the radius and ulna from the bicondylar fragment.

Pott's fracture. Fracture of the fibula 2 to 3 inches above the lateral malleolus with rupture of the deltoid ligament and lateral subluxation of the talus.

Rolando's fracture. Y-shaped intraarticular fracture of the thumb metacarpal.

Segond's fracture. Avulsion fracture of the lateral tibial condyle from the bony insertion of the iliotibial band.

Shepherd's fracture. Fracture of the lateral tubercle of the posterior talar process.

Smith's fracture. Fracture of the distal radius with palmar displacement of the distal fragment. Also referred to as a reverse Colles' fracture.

Stieda's fracture. Avulsion fracture of the medial femoral condyle at the origin of the medial collateral ligament.

Straddle fracture. Bilateral fractures of the superior and inferior public rami.

Teardrop fracture. Flexion fracture or dislocation of the cervical spine with associated triangular anterior fragment of the involved vertebrae. Injury complex is unstable, with posterior ligamentous disruption.

Tillaux's fracture. Fracture of the lateral half of the distal tibial physis during differential closure of the physis. The medial part of the tibial physis has already fused.

Torus fracture. Impaction fracture of childhood as the bone buckles instead of fracturing completely.

Walther's fracture. Ischioacetabular fracture that passes through the pubic rami and extends toward the sacroiliac joint. The medial wall of the acetabulum is displaced inward.

Hart RG, Rittenberry TJ, Uehara DT: Handbook of Orthopaedic Emergencies. Philadelphia, Lippincott-Raven, 1999.

Appendix F
Major Movements of the Body and the Muscles Acting on the Joints Causing the Movement

The Muscles Acting at the Joints That Cause the Movement

Joint Movement	Description	Muscles
Inversion (supination) of the *ankle*	Sole of foot turns inward	Tibialis anterior Tibialis posterior Flexor digitorum longus Flexor hallucis longus
Eversion (pronation) of the *ankle*	Sole of foot turns outward	Peroneus longus Peroneus brevis Peroneus tertius Extensor digitorum longus
Dorsiflexion of the *ankle*	Toes move toward shin	Tibialis anterior Extensor digitorum longus Peroneus tertius Extensor hallucis longus
Plantar flexion of the *ankle*	Toes move away from the shin	Gastrocnemius Soleus Plantaris Peroneus longus Peroneus brevis Tibialis posterior Flexor digitorum longus Flexor hallucis longus
Knee flexion	Bend at the knee, making the angle smaller	Biceps femoris Semitendinosus Semimembranosus Sartorius Gracilis Popliteus Gastrocnemius
Knee extension	Straighten the knee, making the angle larger	Rectus femoris Vastus lateralis Vastus intermedius Vastus medialis
Medial (internal) rotation of the *knee*	Knee turns inward (knee must be bent)	Semitendinosus Semimembranosus Sartorius Gracilis
Lateral (external) rotation of the *knee*	Knee turns outward (knee must be bent)	Biceps femoris

The Muscles Acting at the Joints That Cause the Movement—cont'd

Joint Movement	Description	Muscles
Hip flexion	Bend at the hip, which reduces the angle	Iliopsoas Pectineus Rectus femoris Sartorius Gluteus maximus
Hip extension	Straighten at the hip, which increases the angle	Biceps femoris Semitendinosus Semimembranosus
Hip abduction	Leg moves away from the body at the hip	Gluteus medius Gluteus minimus
Hip adduction	Leg moves toward the body at the hip	Gracilis Pectineus Adductor magnus Adductor longus Adductor brevis
Medial (internal) rotation of the *hip*	Leg rotates inward at the hip	Gluteus minimus Gluteus medius Gluteus maximus Semitendinosus Semimembranosus Pectineus Gracilis Tensor fasciae latae
Lateral (external) rotation of the *hip*	Leg rotates outward at the hip	Iliopsoas Sartorius Biceps femoris Adductor brevis Adductor magnus Piriformis Obturator Internus/externus Quadratus femoris Gemelli superior/inferior
Transverse *pelvic girdle* rotation	Twisting movement at the hip and waist	External oblique Internal oblique Erector spinae (sacrospinalis)
Anterior *pelvic girdle* rotation	Pelvic tilt or "suck and tuck"	External oblique Internal oblique Rectus abdominis
Lumbar flexion	With hips locked, bend forward at the lumbar vertebrae	External oblique Internal oblique Rectus abdominis
Lumbar extension	With hips locked, bend backward at the lumbar vertebrae	Erector spinae (sacrospinalis)
Cervical flexion	Chin moves toward the chest	Sternocleidomastoid Rectus capitis anterior Longus capitis

Continued

The Muscles Acting at the Joints That Cause the Movement—cont'd

Joint Movement	Description	Muscles
Cervical extension	Chin moves away from the chest	Rectus capitis lateralis Rectus capitis posterior Obliquus capitis superior Semispinalis capitis
Cervical rotation	Head rotates from side to side	Sternocleidomastoid Obliquus capitis inferior Semispinalis capitis
Lateral bending (flexion) of the *cervical spine*	Ear moves toward the shoulder	Levator scapulae Rectus capitis lateralis Obliquus capitis superior
Lateral bending (flexion) of the *trunk*	Trunk moves side to side (no movement at the hip)	External oblique Internal oblique Erector spinae (sacrospinalis)
Shoulder elevation	Shoulder shrug	Levator scapulae Trapezius Rhomboids
Shoulder depression	Shoulders move downward	Pectoralis minor Trapezius
Scapular abduction (protraction)	Scapulas move further apart	Pectoralis minor Serratus anterior Rhomboids
Scapular adduction (retraction)	Scapulas move closer together	Levator scapulae Trapezius
Upward rotation of the *scapula*	Left (from rear) scapula rotates clockwise and right scapula counterclockwise	Serratus anterior Trapezius
Downward rotation of the *scapula*	Right (from rear) scapula rotates clockwise and left scapula counterclockwise	Rhomboids Pectoralis minor Levator scapulae
Shoulder adduction	Arms move sideways inward toward the body	Latissimus dorsi Teres major Pectoralis
Shoulder abduction	Arms move sideways away from the body	Deltoid (middle) Supraspinatus
Shoulder flexion	Arms straight up in front of the body	Deltoid (anterior) Pectoralis (clavicular)
Shoulder extension	Arms move from straight up in front of body to the anatomic position	Deltoid (posterior) Pectoralis (sternal) Latissimus dorsi Teres major
Shoulder hyperextension	Arms move from anatomic position to behind the body	Deltoid (posterior)
Medial rotation of the *shoulder*	Humerus rotates inward at the shoulder	Latissimus dorsi Teres major Pectoralis major
Lateral rotation of the *shoulder*	Humerus rotates outward at the shoulder	Infraspinatus Teres minor
Horizontal *shoulder* adduction	With arm straight at shoulder height to the side, move arm toward the midline	Pectoralis Deltoid (anterior)

The Muscles Acting at the Joints That Cause the Movement—cont'd

Joint Movement	Description	Muscles
Horizontal *shoulder* abduction	With arm straight at shoulder height at the midline, move arm toward the side of the body	Deltoid (middle and posterior) Infraspinatus Teres minor Biceps brachii
Elbow flexion	Bend elbow, making the angle smaller	Brachialis Brachioradialis
Elbow extension	Straighten elbow, making the angle larger	Triceps brachii (long, lateral, and medial)
Supination of *radio-ulnar joint*	Palm is turned upward	Biceps brachii Supinator
Pronation of *radio-ulnar joint*	Palm is turned downward	Pronator teres
Wrist flexion	Wrist bends down, making angle smaller	Flexor carpi radialis Flexor carpi ulnaris
Wrist extension	Wrist bends up, making angle larger	Extensor carpi radialis Extensor carpi ulnaris

ANALYSIS OF BASIC WEIGHT TRAINING EXERCISES*

Chin-Up

Exercise description: Using a horizontal bar suspended above the head, grasp the bar with the palms toward the body. Pull the body vertically upward until the chin passes the bar, and then return downward in a controlled manner to the initial hanging position.

Joint Movement	Primary Muscles Involved	Phase of Isotonic Contraction
UPWARD MOTION		
Elbow flexion	Biceps brachii Brachialis Brachioradialis	Concentric
Shoulder extension	Latissimus dorsi Teres major Deltoid (posterior) Pectoralis	Concentric
Scapula adduction	Trapezius Rhomboids Levator scapulae	Concentric
Shoulder depression	Trapezius Pectoralis	Concentric

*A more detailed description of the proper lifting technique for these basic weight training exercises can be found in most weight training textbooks (e.g., Sandler D: Weight Training Fundamentals. Champaign, IL, Human Kinetics, 2003). Further information on structural kinesiology and the analysis of other weight training exercises can be found in Thompson CW, Floyd RT: Manual of Structural Kinesiology, 14th ed. Boston, McGraw-Hill, 2001.

Continued

Chin-Up—cont'd

Joint Movement	Primary Muscles Involved	Phase of Isotonic Contraction
DOWNWARD MOTION		
Elbow extension	Biceps brachii	Eccentric
	Brachialis	
	Brachioradialis	
Shoulder flexion	Latissimus dorsi	Eccentric
	Teres major	
	Deltoid (posterior)	
	Pectoralis	
Scapula abduction	Trapezius	Eccentric
	Rhomboids	
	Levator scapulae	
Shoulder elevation	Trapezius	Eccentric
	Pectoralis	

Latissimus Pull-Down

Exercise description: Gasp the bar suspended over the head with palms facing away from the body. Pull the bar downward until the bar touches the shoulders behind the head, and then return upward in a controlled manner to the initial position.

Joint Movement	Primary Muscles Involved	Phase of Isotonic Contraction
DOWNWARD MOTION		
Elbow flexion	Biceps brachii	Concentric
	Brachialis	
	Brachioradialis	
Shoulder adduction	Latissimus dorsi	Concentric
	Teres major	
	Pectoralis	
Scapula adduction	Trapezius	Concentric
	Rhomboids	
	Levator scapulae	
Shoulder depression	Trapezius	Concentric
	Pectoralis	
UPWARD MOTION		
Elbow extension	Biceps brachii	Eccentric
	Brachialis	
	Brachioradialis	
Shoulder abduction	Latissimus dorsi	Eccentric
	Teres major	
	Pectoralis	
Scapula abduction	Trapezius	Eccentric
	Rhomboids	
	Levator scapulae	
Shoulder elevation	Trapezius	Eccentric
	Pectoralis	

Bent Knee Sit-Up

Exercise description: While lying on your back with knees bent, arms across the chest, and feet on the floor, curl upward until the elbows touch the thighs, and then return downward in a controlled manner to the initial supine position.

Joint Movement	Primary Muscles Involved	Phase of Isotonic Contraction
UPWARD MOTION Lumbar flexion	Rectus abdominis External oblique Internal oblique	Concentric
DOWNWARD MOTION Lumbar extension	Rectus abdominis External oblique Internal oblique	Eccentric

Squat

Exercise description: With a bar across the shoulders behind the head, bend at the knees and waist moving downward to a position where the thighs are parallel with the floor, and then return upward in a controlled manner to the standing position.

Joint Movement	Primary Muscles Involved	Phase of Isotonic Contraction
DOWNWARD MOTION Hip flexion	Gluteus maximus Biceps femoris Semitendinosus Semimembranosus	Eccentric
Knee flexion	Rectus femoris Vastus lateralis Vastus medialis Vastus intermedius	Eccentric
Ankle dorsiflexion	Gastrocnemius Soleus	Eccentric
UPWARD MOTION Hip extension	Gluteus maximus Biceps femoris Semitendinosus Semimembranosus	Concentric
Knee extension	Rectus femoris Vastus lateralis Vastus medialis Vastus intermedius	Concentric
Ankle plantar flexion	Gastrocnemius Soleus	Concentric

Leg Press

Exercise description: Using a leg press machine, position the feet about shoulder width apart. Push the foot pad forward until the knees are extended, and then return backward in a controlled manner to the initial position.

Joint Movement	Primary Muscles Involved	Phase of Isotonic Contraction
FORWARD MOTION		
Hip extension	Gluteus maximus	Concentric
	Biceps femoris	
	Semitendinosus	
	Semimembranosus	
Knee extension	Rectus femoris	Concentric
	Vastus lateralis	
	Vastus medialis	
	Vastus intermedius	
BACKWARD MOTION		
Hip flexion	Gluteus maximus	Eccentric
	Biceps femoris	
	Semitendinosus	
	Semimembranosus	
Knee flexion	Rectus femoris	Eccentric
	Vastus lateralis	
	Vastus medialis	
	Vastus intermedius	

Bench Press

Exercise description: While lying on your back, grasp the bar with hands shoulder width apart and palms facing toward the feet. Lower the bar in a controlled manner to a position across the chest, and then push the bar upward to the initial position.

Joint Movement	Primary Muscles Involved	Phase of Isotonic Contraction
DOWNWARD MOTION		
Elbow flexion	Triceps brachii	Eccentric
Shoulder extension	Pectoralis	Eccentric
	Deltoid (anterior)	
Scapula adduction	Serratus anterior	Eccentric
	Pectoralis	
UPWARD MOTION		
Elbow extension	Triceps brachii	Concentric
Shoulder flexion	Pectoralis	Concentric
	Deltoid (anterior)	
Scapula abduction	Serratus anterior	Concentric
	Pectoralis	

Shoulder Press

Exercise description: Grasp the bar with hands shoulder width apart and palms facing forward. Push the bar upward until the elbows are extended, and then lower the bar in a controlled manner to the initial position.

Joint Movement	Primary Muscles Involved	Phase of Isotonic Contraction
UPWARD MOTION		
Elbow extension	Triceps brachii	Concentric
Shoulder flexion	Pectoralis	Concentric
	Deltoid (anterior)	
Shoulder elevation	Trapezius	Concentric
	Rhomboids	
	Levator scapulae	
DOWNWARD MOTION		
Elbow flexion	Triceps brachii	Eccentric
Shoulder extension	Pectoralis	Eccentric
	Deltoid (anterior)	
Shoulder depression	Trapezius	Eccentric
	Rhomboids	
	Levator scapulae	

Arm Curl

Exercise description: While standing holding the bar with palms facing forward, curl the bar upward while bending at the elbow until the bar reaches shoulder height, and then lower the bar in a controlled manner to the initial position.

Joint Movement	Primary Muscles Involved	Phase of Isotonic Contraction
UPWARD MOTION		
Elbow flexion	Biceps brachii	Concentric
	Brachialis	
	Brachioradialis	
DOWNWARD MOTION		
Elbow extension	Biceps brachii	Eccentric
	Brachialis	
	Brachioradialis	

Triceps Push-Down

Exercise description: While standing holding the bar at chin level with palms facing down, push the bar downward until the elbows are extended, and then raise the bar in a controlled manner to the initial position.

Joint Movement	Primary Muscles Involved	Phase of Isotonic Contraction
DOWNWARD MOTION		
Elbow extension	Triceps brachii	Concentric
UPWARD MOTION		
Elbow flexion	Triceps brachii	Eccentric

Leg Curl

Exercise description: While lying prone on the bench with your heels hooked under the pad, curl the weight forward until the pad reaches the buttocks, and then lower the weight backward in a controlled manner to the initial position.

Joint Movement	Primary Muscles Involved	Phase of Isotonic Contraction
FORWARD MOTION Knee flexion	Biceps femoris Semitendinosus Semimembranosus	Concentric
BACKWARD MOTION Knee extension	Biceps femoris Semitendinosus Semimembranosus	Eccentric

Knee Extension

Exercise description: While sitting on the bench with your feet hooked under the pad, extend the weight upward until the knees are extended, and then lower the weight in a controlled manner to the initial position.

Joint Movement	Primary Muscles Involved	Phase of Isotonic Contraction
UPWARD MOTION Knee extension	Rectus femoris Vastus lateralis Vastus medialis Vastus intermedius	Concentric
DOWNWARD MOTION Knee flexion	Rectus femoris Vastus lateralis Vastus medialis Vastus intermedius	Eccentric

Heel Raise

Exercise description: While standing with a bar supported on your shoulders, raise your body upward until you are standing on your toes, and then lower your body in a controlled manner to the initial position.

Joint Movement	Primary Muscles Involved	Phase of Isotonic Contraction
UPWARD MOTION Plantar flexion	Gastrocnemius Soleus	Concentric
DOWNWARD MOTION Dorsiflexion	Gastrocnemius Soleus	Eccentric

Glossary

Abductor "lurch" Gluteus medius gait resulting from weak or nonfunctioning hip abductor muscles. The patient lurches toward the weak side to place the center of gravity over the hip.

Abiotrophy A degeneration or failure of microscopic or macroscopic structure of a body tissue or part.

Accessory movements Joint movements that are necessary for a full range of motion, but that are not under direct voluntary control of the individual.

Accountability Being accountable or responsible for the moral and legal requirements of proper patient care. Systematic, reliable, and appropriate investigative questioning, listening, and active participation at all levels of patient care.

A-C joint Acromioclavicular joint.

Actin A protein found in muscle fibers that acts with myosin to bring about contraction and relaxation. Also called actinin.

Active transport Transmission of topical medications into tissues via acoustic energy of ultrasound as a result of increased cell membrane permeability.

Adhesions Tissue structures normally separated that adhere together because of injury.

Aerobic capacity Degree of aerobic fitness. Also referred to as cardiovascular endurance, cardiovascular fitness, or cardiorespiratory fitness.

Afferent neural input Nerves and sensory organs that carry or transmit information from the periphery to the central nervous system (*see also* mechanoreceptor system).

Afferent receptors Five classes: mechanoreceptors, thermoreceptors, nociceptors, chemoreceptors, and electromagnetic receptors.

Age-related drug effects Liver metabolic activity declines with increasing age. The drug dose may have to be reduced in elderly patients.

Age-adjusted maximum heart rate (AAMHR) Expressed as 220 − age = MHR.

Allograft Transplant tissue used from cadavers. Commonly the ACL can be reconstructed with an allograft.

Amplitude Width or breadth of range or extent, such as amplitude of accommodation or amplitude of convergence.

Annulus Any ring-shaped structure, such as the outer edge of an intervertebral disk.

Antalgic gait Because of pain in the stance phase (while walking through on the foot), the time spent on the affected side is shortened compared with that on the normal side.

Anterior cruciate ligament (ACL) Deep ligament within the knee that crosses anteriorly to the posterior cruciate ligament.

AO classification of fracture fixation devices Also referred to as ASIF (the Association for the Study of International Fixation). A group of general and orthopedic surgeons was founded in 1956 by Maurice E. Müller to develop a series of screws, plates, and other internal fixation devices. In addition, the AO group (Arbeitsgemeinschaft für Osteosynthesefragen) established a system of fracture classification and management.

Arthrokinematics Study of motion within the joints. Description of joint typography.

Arthroplasty Surgery to reconstruct joints.

Arthroscopy Examination of a joint interior using an arthroscope.

Articular cartilage Thin layer of hyaline cartilage on joint surfaces. Concentration of collagen, proteoglycans, and water influences tensile forces, compression, shear, and permeability.

Articular cartilage biomechanical function Acts to increase load distribution and provides a wear-resistant surface that reduces wear.

Articular cartilage composition Chondrocytes, matrix, type II collagen, proteoglycans, and noncollagenous proteins.

Articular cartilage injury and repair Intrinsic repair depends on the nature and extent of the injury. Trauma that penetrates cartilage but not subchondral bone leaves a defect that does not heal. Penetration of subchondral bone stimulates intense vascular response that allows weak fibrous tissue to fill the defect.

Atraumatic multidirectional bilateral instability (AMBRI) Atraumatic multidirectional bilateral instability that responds to rehabilitation, but occasionally requires an inferior capsular shift surgical procedure.

Atrophy Reduction in size of an anatomic structure; frequently related to disuse or decreased blood supply.

Autograft A tissue or organ removed from one site and placed in another within the same individual.

Avascular necrosis (AVN) Tissue death from a lack of blood supply.

"Back school" Education model to inform individuals about spine anatomy, injury, self-care, fitness, activities of daily living, and ergonomic modifications.

"Bag of bones technique"   Sling and swath procedure used to help stabilize severe comminuted intercondylar fractures of the elbow in elderly people with poor bone quality.

Balance   The ability to maintain equilibrium with gravity, both statically and dynamically.

Ballistic stretching   Method of dynamic stretching involving rapid bouncing.

Bankart lesion   Seen surgically as a detachment of the glenoid labrum and sometimes a bone fragment from the glenoid.

Base of support   The distance between a person's feet while standing and during ambulation. The area over which the center of gravity widens or narrows in response to maintain balance in relation to the center of gravity.

Behaviors   *Dominance:* exercising control or influence. *Submission:* passive and quick to comply. *Hostility:* unresponsive and insensitive. *Warmth:* responsive and sensitive.

Bennett's fracture   Fracture: subluxation of proximal first metacarpal.

Bioavailability   The percentage of the drug that reaches the systemic circulation. Intravenous (IV) drugs have 100% bioavailability.

Biomechanical ankle platform system (BAPS)   A commercial or hand-made disk used to challenge a patient's balance.

Biotribology   The division of tribology that focuses on understanding the friction, lubrication, and wear of diarthrodial joints.

Bladder technique   The therapeutic technique of ultrasound transmission applied over a water-filled small balloon placed directly over the injured area that serves as a coupling medium.

Blood pressure adaptations   Resistance exercise leads to decreased heart rate, reduced blood pressure, and decreased double product.

Bone to bone end-feel   A sudden, hard, nonyielding sensation that is felt at the end range of motion. An example is terminal elbow extension.

Bone callus   Subsequent scarring of bone following a fracture.

Bone injury and repair: inflammation   Fracture site hematoma. Granulation tissue forms around fracture site. Osteoblasts and fibroblasts proliferate.

Bone matrix   Organic components: 40% dry weight of bone, collagen, proteoglycans, glycoproteins, and phospholipids.

Bone types   Normal bone is lamellar. Immature or pathologic bone is woven, not stress oriented. Mature lamellar bone is cortical or cancellous.

Borg scale   A scale of measurement of relative perceived exertion.

Boutonnière deformity   A fixed deformity of the finger consisting of flexion of the proximal interphalangeal joint and extension of the distal interphalangeal joint. A result of rheumatoid destruction of the extensor tendon mechanism at the proximal interphalangeal joint and also secondary to trauma without arthritis.

Boxer's fracture   Volarly displaced impacted fracture of the neck of the fifth or fourth metacarpal, caused by striking a closed-fist hand on a hard object.

Bursitis   Inflammation of a bursa.

Cadence   Number of steps or strides taken per unit of time.

Calcaneal gait   Weakness of gastroc-soleus muscle groups that results in reduced foot propulsion during the toe-off period of the stance phase of gait.

Cancellous bone   Spongy, porous, lattice-like tissue within midshaft of long bone.

Capsular and noncapsular pattern   Every synovial joint under muscular control possesses a characteristic pattern of limitation. An example of a capsular pattern is described by Barak, Rosen, and Sofer. The capsular pattern of the shoulder "involves external rotation as the most limited movement, abduction as less limited, internal rotation still less limited, and flexion as the least limited movement." If a lesion exists that does not correspond to a characteristic, predetermined capsular pattern, it is called a noncapsular pattern. (From Barak T, Rosen ER, Sofer R: Basic concepts of orthopaedic manual therapy. In Gould JA, ed. Orthopaedic and Sports Physical Therapy, 2nd ed. St Louis, Mosby, 1990.)

Capsular end-feel   An abnormal feel encountered during the performance of mobilization techniques. An elastic resistance is encountered prior to the normal range of motion. Usually, this end-feel is related to a specific capsular restriction.

Capsular pattern   Limitation of movement or a pattern of pain at a joint that occurs in a predictable pattern.

Capsulitis   Inflammation of the capsule.

Cardiovascular endurance   The capacity of the aerobic energy system to perform work. Also referred to as cardiovascular fitness, aerobic capacity, and cardiorespiratory fitness.

Carpal tunnel syndrome   A compression entrapment neuropathy of the median nerve within the wrist, commonly caused by repetitive motions of the wrist.

Carrying angle   Viewing the upper extremity in the anterior-posterior (AP) frontal plane, the angle observed at the axis of the elbow between the upper arm and lower arm.

Center of gravity   Point in a body where the body mass is centered. Anterior to the second sacral vertebra. However, the center of gravity is not constant, but varies in location with reference to changes in movement and position.

Cervical spondylosis   Chronic degenerative disk disease of the cervical spine. Occurs most often in the fourth and fifth decades of life and characteristically affects men more often than women. Commonly affects the C5-C6 and C6-C7 segments.

Chondrocytes   Cartilage cells.

Circuit training   A method of physical exercise in which activities are arranged in sets so that the participant moves quickly from one activity to another with minimum rest between sets.

Claw toe   Dorsiflexion of the metatarsophalangeal joints associated with hammer toe deformities and often with a clavus foot.

Clearance of drugs   Measurement of how fast substances are removed from the blood and excreted in the urine.

Closed-ended questions   Technique that requires a "yes" or "no" answer. This method effectively directs specific responses aimed at details of the patient's condition.

Closed kinetic chain exercise (CKC)   Any exercise where the distal or terminal exercising segment is weight bearing or "fixed." Functional exercises that use concentric and eccentric muscle contractions in a synchronous fashion to produce functional movement in which motion at one joint produces motion at all of the other joints in the kinetic chain in a predictable manner.

Close-packed   The most congruent position of a joint. The joint surfaces are aligned, and the capsule and ligaments are taut.

Codman's pendulum exercises   Exercises for a stiff shoulder in which the patient is bent over at the waist (90 degrees) and the hand hangs like a pendulum toward the floor. A weight may be placed in the hand, and the arm is then moved through various arcs to increase the range of motion in that shoulder.

Collagen   Fibrous protein of connective tissue, ligament, cartilage, bone, and skin.

Collagen in ligaments   Collagen represents 70% to 80% of the dry weight of ligament. Ninety percent of collagen in ligament is type I; about 10% is type III.

Colles' fracture   Fracture of the distal end of the radius with the lower fragment displaced posteriorly.

Communication   Any process in which a message containing information is transferred, especially from one person to another, via any of a number of media.

Compact bone   The thick outer portion of bone that surrounds the medullary (marrow) cavity. Also called cortical bone.

Compression   Occurs when two forces or loads are applied toward each other.

Compression fracture   Crumbling or smashing of cancellous bone by forces acting parallel to the long axis of the bone (applied particularly to vertebral body fractures).

Compression neuropathy   Loss of motor or sensory nerve function (acute or chronic) because of extrinsic compression. Entrapment can occur within tight fibroosseous tunnels or as a result of tumor, hemorrhage, or metabolic changes, causing swelling of soft tissues around the nerve.

Concentric contraction   A shortening contraction of muscle produced by tension that results in the approximation of the origin and insertion of the contracting muscle.

Constrained   A type of total joint implant (TKR) that sacrifices the cruciates (ACL, PCL, or both). Also referred to as a conforming implant.

Continuous passive motion (CPM)   A technique for maintaining or increasing the amount of movement in a joint with the use of a mechanical device that applies force to bring about motion in a joint without normal muscle function.

Contracture   Shortening of muscle tissue, joint capsule, ligament, tendon, and other soft tissues resulting from paralysis, spasm, or fibrosis of tissue around the joint.

Controlled-protected motion   Therapeutic technique that calls for gentle, specific motion that does not place unwanted force or stress on injured or healing tissues. The joint or joints affected can be protected with a cast-brace or range-limiting hinge brace.

Contusion   Bruise of any tissue but without disruption.

Convex-concave rule   "When the concave surface is stationary and the convex surface is moving, the gliding movement in the joint occurs in a direction opposite to the bone movement." If the convex surface is mobile, the gliding motion occurs in the same direction as the bone movement. (From Barak T, Rosen ER, Sofer R: Basic concepts of orthopaedic manual therapy. In Gould JA, ed. Orthopaedic and Sports Physical Therapy, 2nd ed. St Louis, Mosby, 1990.)

Coordination   The production of volitional accurate, smooth, purposeful, controlled, dynamic movements.

Cortical bone   The thick outer portion of bone that surrounds the medullary (marrow) cavity. Also called compact bone. Eighty percent of adult skeleton.

Creep   A viscoelastic property in which there is a change in the shape (deformation) of tissue without actual loss of continuity. A constant force increases deformation of a material over time as long as the force is maintained.

Criteria for ligament healing   Torn ligament fibers must be in continuity and confined in well-vascularized soft tissue bed, with controlled stress to stimulate healing. Continuous protection against inappropriate stress.

Cryokinetics   Application of cold alternated with therapeutic exercise to induce the physiologic effects of cold and stimulate the effects of exercise to propagate function.

Cumulative trauma disorder   A soft-tissue injury that is characteristically caused by overuse or repetitive motion.

Deep zone   Largest part of the articular cartilage. Contains the largest collagen fibrils and has the highest proteoglycan content and lowest water content.

Deformations   Temporary deformations display transient elastic properties. Permanent deformations display plastic properties. Change in loads results in change in deformations.

De Quervain's tenosynovitis   Repetitive motion injury that affects the tendons of the abductor pollicis longus and extensor pollicis brevis as they pass within the first dorsal compartment of the wrist.

Deceleration   A decrease in the speed or velocity of an object or reaction.

Degenerative joint disease (DJD)   Also called osteoarthritis.

Delayed onset muscle soreness (DOMS)   Muscle weakness, restricted range of motion, and diffuse tenderness that occur 24 to 48 hours after intense or prolonged muscle activity.

Delayed union   The speed of callus formation (fracture healing) is slower than anticipated, but this does not imply expectancy of total healing or a nonunion.

Dinner fork deformity   Resultant characteristic angular deformity of the radius following a Colles' fracture.

Direct muscle injury   Lacerations, surgical incisions, contusions, or blunt trauma.

Disk   An avascular and aneural (except that the outer fibers are innervated) structure comprised of the annulus (fibroelastic cartilage) and nucleus (mucopolysaccharide gel) that provides stability and movement between the vertebral bodies within each segment.

Dislocation   Complete displacement of a bone from its normal position at the joint surface, disrupting the articulation of two or three bones at that junction and altering the alignment.

Distribution of drugs   The transfer of drugs from one compartment of the body to another.

Double product   Refers to heart rate × systolic blood pressure. Elevation of double product indicates an increase in myocardial oxygen consumption.

Double support   The point within the gait cycle in which both feet are in contact with the ground and weight transfer occurs from one foot to the other.

Drug half-life   The time it takes for 50% of the dose of the drug to be cleared from the body.

Dupuytren's contracture   Disease affecting the palmar fascia of the hand, causing the ring and little finger to contract toward the palm.

Eccentric contraction   A muscle contraction in which tension is produced but lengthening of the muscle occurs. The origin and insertion of the contracting (lengthening) muscle moves further apart during the contraction. Also referred to as a negative contraction or negative work.

Elastic deformation   The viscoelastic property of soft tissues to "deform" under slow rates of stress then return to normal resting length and tension.

Electric stimulation for fracture repair   Generally used for treatment of nonunion fractures. Constant direct or pulsed electromagnetic fields externally applied stimulation enhances production of insulin-like growth factor (IGF) in osteoblast cells.

Electrically evoked muscle stimulation   Reeducation of asynchronous muscle contraction. Elicits muscle vasodilation, reduces muscle atrophy, stimulates muscle strength, and improves joint range of motion. *Caution:* Electrically evoked muscle contractions may create greater fatigue via synchronous muscle firing.

Empty end-feel   An abnormal end-feel encountered during the performance of mobilization techniques. Motion that is very limited by significant pain without muscle spasm. This end-feel is not characterized by any mechanical block or restriction.

End-feel terms   Firm, hard, soft or spongy, loose, capsular, bony bloc, springy bloc, and empty.

Endomysium   A fibrous sheath of connective tissue that enfolds striated muscle fiber within a fasciculus.

Epicondylitis   Inflammation of the common wrist extensor origin or inflammation of the common flexor tendon and pronator teres at the medial epicondyle or lateral epicondyle of the elbow.

Epimysium   A fibrous sheath that enfolds a muscle and extends between the bundles of muscle fibers, such as the perimysium. It is sturdy in some areas but more delicate in others, such as those areas where the muscle moves freely under a strong sheet of fascia. The epimysium also may fuse with fascia that attaches a muscle to a bone.

Ergonomics   A scientific discipline devoted to the study and analysis of human work, especially as it is affected by individual anatomy, psychology, and other human factors.

Extruded disk   An injury to the intervertebral disk in which the nucleus extends through the annulus but the nuclear material remains confined by the posterior longitudinal ligament.

Fasciculus   Small bundle or cluster (referring to muscle, tendon, or nerve fibers).

Fast twitch (type II-white glycolytic) muscle fiber   Muscle fiber type with high levels of myosin-ATPase. These muscle fibers are recruited for activities that require speed, strength, and power.

Fibroelastic cartilage   A type of cartilage that is composed of water, four types of collagen (of which type I represents approximately 90%), proteoglycans, and elastin. The menisci of the knee are an example of fibroelastic cartilage.

Fibrotic adhesions   Chronic inflammation leading to fibrous adhesions in the joint capsule, ligaments, fascia, and tendon.

Fighter's fracture   A fracture to the neck of the second, third, fourth, or fifth metacarpal. Also referred to as a boxer's fracture.

Foot-flat   The point in the gait cycle when the entire foot is in contact with the floor. Shock absorption is a primary action during the foot-flat period.

Force couple   Force couple occurs when a moment is created by equal, noncolinear, parallel but opposite directed forces. The moment created is called a couple.

Four-point gait pattern   Using crutches as an example, the patient advances the crutch opposite the involved limb first, followed by the involved limb, then advances the crutch toward the uninvolved limb, and finally advances the uninvolved limb.

Free nerve endings   A receptor nerve ending that is not enclosed in a capsule. A typically free nerve ending consists of a bare axon that may be myelinated or unmyelinated. They are often found in fibrous capsules, ligaments, or synovial spaces and may be sensitive to mechanical or biochemical stimuli.

Full weight bearing (FWB)   Weight bearing status that allows no restrictions.

Functional capacity evaluations   Specific functional testing procedure designed to identify and quantify physical limitations, restrictions, and risk factors associated with specific job tasks.

Gait   Walking pattern.

Gamekeeper's thumb   A traumatic rupture of the ulnar collateral ligament of the metacarpophalangeal joint of the thumb, usually a hyperabduction injury. Also called skier's thumb.

Glide   An accessory joint motion.

Golgi tendon organs (GTO)   Inhibitory sensory receptors located within the myotendinous junction.

Grades of movement

Grade I: Small-amplitude motions at the beginning of joint range of motion.

Grade II: Large-amplitude motions that do not affect the limits of available range of motion.

Grade III: Large-amplitude motions that affect the full limits of available range of motion.

Grade IV: Small-amplitude motions at the end range of available joint motion.

Gross dissection of ligament   Ligament surrounded by loose connective tissue or synovium if the ligament is intraarticular.

Hallux valgus   The big toe bends toward the other toes.

Hammer toe   Descriptive of a variety of deformities of the second to fifth toes; increased flexion of the distal toe, causing prominence of the bones of the dorsal aspect of the proximal interphalangeal joint.

Hard or springy tissue stretch   A normal end-feel encountered during the performance of mobilization techniques. The most common normal end-feel at the end range of motion of joints. Examples are terminal knee extension and wrist flexion where elastic resistance and a springy stretch are felt at the end range of motion.

Heel-off   When the heel of the weight bearing limb initially raises from the floor. At this point, weight is unloaded from the weight bearing limb and is shifted or transferred to the opposite limb.

Heel-strike   The instant foot contact is made with the ground. Ideally the heel should initiate contact.

Hemiarthroplasty   Partial reconstructive surgery of a joint. The hip is an example of when the femoral head is replaced and not the acetabulum. A total hip replacement is when both the femoral head and the acetabulum are replaced.

Herniated nucleus pulposus (HNP)   A broad term referring to more specific nomenclature concerning various stages of disk injury. Three general categories of HNP include disk protrusion, extruded disk, and sequestrated disk.

Hill-Sachs lesion   Seen radiographically as an indentation of the posteromedial humeral head, which occurs at the time of the dislocation. Also called hatchet head deformity.

Histochemical changes with exercise   Increase in motoneuron metabolism and efficient activation with endurance training, pronounced increase in oxidative enzymes, and improved supply of adenosine triphosphate.

Hooke's law   Stress is proportional to strain up to a limit, which is called the proportional limit.

Hyaline cartilage   Flexible, glassy, translucent cartilage (see articular cartilage).

Hypermobility grades   Grade 3 is considered normal. Grade 4 represents slightly increased motion. Grade 5 represents significant increased instability. Grade 6 represents total instability.

Hypertrophy   Increase in diameter of structure.

Hypomobility grades   0 = ankylosis; grade 1 represents greatly decreased range of motion; grade 2 represents minimal decreased range of motion.

Immobilization   Method of stabilizing a structure, limb, or joint by internal fixation, casting, bracing, splinting, traction, or any means to limit motion and protect healing tissues.

Impingement   Pressure transmitted from one tissue to the next, such as subacromial rotator cuff impingement.

Indirect muscle injury   An injury where the muscle or musculotendinous junction becomes injured by sudden stretch or concentric or eccentric muscle contraction.

Inflammation (phase I of healing)   Localized increase in blood supply, resulting in small vessel dilation or migration of white blood cells into the tissue. Inflammation is the normal response of living tissue to an injury with tissue alteration. The inflammatory process mobilizes the body's defense mechanism to initiate the healing process and react against any microbes that may be introduced at the site of the injury with resultant heat, pain, swelling, and loss of function.

Intercondylar fractures of the humerus   Fractures that extend between the condyles of the humerus and involve the articular surfaces of the elbow joint.

Intrathoracic pressure   Tendency to increase with resistance exercise; intrathoracic pressure limits venous return.

Intrinsic material properties   Deformational properties of an object that does not depend on size or shape.

Iontophoresis   The use of electric current to transmit ions of specific medications into tissues for analgesic and anti-inflammatory effects.

Isometric contraction   A type of muscle contraction where tension is developed but no joint motion takes place.

Joint congruency   Articular position regarding concave and convex joint surfaces. A joint is in congruence when both articulating surfaces are in contact throughout the total surface area of the joint.

Joint involvement of fractures   If the fracture involves a joint, bone union may be delayed secondary to dilution of fracture hematoma from synovial fluid.

Joint motions   Nonaxial-facets, coaxial-knee, biaxial-wrist, and triaxial-subtalar joint

"Joint play"   The application of accessory joint motion (e.g., glide, roll, slide, and spin) "as a response to an outside force but not as a result of voluntary movement." (From Barak T, Rosen ER, Sofer R: Basic concepts of orthopaedic manual therapy. In Gould JA, ed. Orthopaedic and Sports Physical Therapy, 2nd ed. St Louis, Mosby, 1990.)

Joint stability   Two general factors: close- and loose-packed position.

Joint surface motions   Rotation, rolling, and gliding.

Karvönen method   An equation used to establish a training heart rate. The training intensity range for the Karvönen method is 50% to 85% of the VO_2max. The Karvönen method uses the difference between the maximal heart rate (HR max) and the resting heart rate (HR rest), which is known as the maximum heart rate reserve (HR max reserve).

Kinesthesia   The recollection of movement, weight, resistance, and position of the body or parts of the body.

Kyphosis   Round shoulder deformity; humpback; dorsal kyphotic curvature; may refer to any forward-bending area or deformity in the spine.

Lamellar bone: biomechanical function   Lamellar bone increases stiffness and strength of bone with a corresponding increase in brittleness.

Lauge-Hansen classification   Based on five possible positions of the foot at the time of injury: supination-adduction, supination-eversion, pronation-eversion, pronation-abduction, and pronation-dorsiflexion.

Legg-Calvé-Perthes disease   Aseptic epiphyseal ischemic necrosis of the capital femoral epiphysis in children.

Ligament   Bands of strong fibrous connective tissue that bind together the articular ends of bones and cartilage at the joints, to facilitate or limit motion.

Ligament gross morphology   Dense, white, hypovascular, or homogenous appearance.

Ligament maturation of healing   This level of healing takes 12 months or longer. Increased ligament contraction and increased tensile strength. Maturation is not achieved before 12 months. After 1 year, ligament tensile strength is between 50% and 70% of normal.

Linear elastic material   Three fundamental stress-strain characteristics: stress and strain are directly proportional; strain is totally recovered when stress is removed; material is not sensitive to the rate of loading.

Listening   An effective communication tool. Demonstrates interest and concern for the patient and his or her individual needs.

Loads   The force sustained by the body. Types of loads include compression, tension, shear, and torsion.

Loose end-feel   An abnormal end-feel felt during the performance of joint mobilization techniques. Primarily, this end-feel is characterized by joint hyper mobility. Typically no resistance is felt at the end range of motion, signifying extraordinary joint looseness.

Loose-packed   Also referred to as the joint resting position. In a loose-packed position, the joint capsule and supporting ligaments are not stressed. For example, when the knee joint is flexed 30 degrees, the intracapsular space is increased and supporting ligaments become more relaxed. The joint loose-packed position is ideal for applying joint mobilization techniques.

Low-load prolonged stretch   Therapeutic technique used to enhance tissue extensibility by preheating the affected area, applying an external load (0.5% of body weight) to the area to stretch soft-tissue contractures, and maintaining a passive, pain-free stretch for 20 to 60 minutes.

Mallet finger Acute rupture of the terminal end of the distal extensor tendon. This may be intratendinous or bony. This arises as a result of a direct axial blow to the digit. This digit is left with an inability to extend the distal interphalangeal joint (extensor lag). There is usually full passive movement of the digit.

Mallet toe Flexion of the distal joint of the second to fifth toes, such that the toenails are pointing into the ground when walking.

Malunion Bone heals in abnormal position or alignment.

Manipulation Passive intervention motion of high velocity at end ranges of available joint motion.

Matrix and cellular proliferation phases of healing Phase III: Neovascular granulation tissue visible at torn ends of ligament at 2 weeks postinjury. Fibroblasts are the predominant cell type. Ligament scar is very cellular. There is an increase in collagen content.

Mechanical instabilities of the ankle Chronic laxity of the ankle ligaments. A functional instability defines a subjective "giving way" of the ankle, but does not demonstrate instability or laxity of the supporting ligaments.

Mechanisms of Heat Transmission Conduction: direct contact with heat or cold; convection: transmission of air or water over the skin's surface; radiation: transmission of heat source to a cooler area.

Mechanoreceptors Mechanical deformation stimulates free nerve endings, Ruffini endings, pacinian corpuscles, muscle spindles, and Golgi tendon organs.

Mechanoreceptor system Joint receptors that provide information concerning joint displacement, velocity and amplitude of joint movement, pressure, stretch, and pain. The mechanoreceptor system includes Ruffini mechanoreceptors, pacinian mechanoreceptors, type III mechanoreceptors, and free nerve endings. This afferent neural input system is important in regulating adaptive changes in joint movement and body position.

Medial collateral ligament Strong fibrous ligament on the medial side of the knee connecting the femur with the tibia.

Meniscal repair Surgical technique that attempts to suture and approximate torn portions of the meniscus. If a tear is present in a vascularized portion of the meniscus, the repair technique is favored over subtotal meniscectomy in order to maintain as much viable meniscus tissue as possible.

Meniscectomy Excision of the medial or lateral meniscus. There are other menisci in the body, but meniscectomies usually are done on the knee.

Meniscus A crescent-shaped fibrocartilaginous disk between two joint surfaces.

Meniscus gross anatomy Extension of the tibia peripheral border is thick, convex, and attached to the capsule; the opposite border tapers to a thin free edge. Medial meniscus is semicircular; lateral meniscus is nearly circular. Tibial portion of capsular attachment of medial meniscus is referred to as the coronary ligament.

Meniscus neuroanatomy Horns of the meniscus are innervated; there is less innervation of the bodies of the meniscus. The central third of the meniscus is aneural. The sensory afferent arc may provide proprioception information concerning joint position.

Meniscus vascular anatomy Blood supply from the lateral and medial genicular arteries. Vessels penetrate 10% to 30% of the periphery of the medial meniscus and 10% to 25% of the lateral meniscus.

Metabolism of drugs Chemical change or modification of drugs in the body. Typically metabolism takes place in the liver; however, metabolism also takes place in the kidney, lungs, and circulation.

Midstance The period during stance where the body is directly over the weight bearing leg. This action serves to "rollover" the foot into single-limb support during stance.

Midswing The action where the non–weight bearing limb is advanced to where the limb passes directly beneath the body.

Miserable malalignment syndrome An anatomic malalignment of the lower extremity, which is characterized by femoral anteversion (internal femoral rotation), "squinting" patella (patellae face toward each other), proximal external tibial rotation, and foot pronation. This malalignment syndrome commonly is seen with extensor mechanism disorders of the knee.

Mobility Complex volitional, high-level gross motor and sophisticated fine-motor activity.

Mobility at fracture site Excessive mobility interferes with vascularization of fractures and hematoma, and it disrupts bridging callus.

Mobilization An attempt to restore joint motion or mobility or decrease pain associated with joint structures via manual selective grades of passive accessory joint movement. Passive intervention motion within and at end range of joint motion with varying degrees of speed and amplitude.

Muscle fatigue Failure to maintain a required or expected repetitive force.

Muscle fiber changes with fatigue Declined force production; reduced relaxation of fatigued muscle. Reduced impulse conduction, decreased electromyographic activity, increased sodium (Na^+), decreased potassium (K^+), and reduced phosphocreatine (PCR).

Muscle spasm Sudden contraction of muscle, usually in reflexive response to stimulus from an external source.

Muscle spindle A specialized proprioceptive sensory organ composed of a bundle of fine striated intrafusal muscle fibers innervated by gamma nerve fibers. Their nuclei are gathered together near the center of each fiber to form a nuclear sac, which is surrounded in turn by sensory, annulospiral nerve endings, all enclosed in a fibrous sheath.

Myofibrils Individual muscle fibers are composed of myofibrils, which lie parallel to each other and the muscle fiber itself.

Myosin A cardiac and skeletal muscle protein that makes up close to one half of the proteins that occur in muscle tissue. The interaction of myosin and actin is essential for muscle contraction.

Nerve entrapment Compression of nerve tissue related to bony overgrowth, inflammation, disk bulge, muscular hypertrophy, and repetitive motion.

Neuroma Benign tumor of the nerve.

Neuromuscular fatigue Acetylcholine is reduced with repetitive activation of motor neuron terminals. May be a contributory factor in local muscle fatigue.

Neuromuscular response to stretch Golgi tendon organs (GTOs) are stimulated by the presence of muscular tension. GTOs act to inhibit tension development in muscle, promoting muscle relaxation. Muscle spindles respond to stretch via stretch reflex and reciprocal inhibition.

Nonconstrained A type of implant used for joint reconstruction (TKR). This type of implant retains the cruciate ligaments (cruciate sparing implant).

Nonunion Failure of progression of healing with expectation of no further healing.

Non–weight bearing (NWB) Weight bearing status that does not allow contact or loading of the involved limb.

Nucleus pulposus A mucopolysaccharide gel contained within the concentrically arranged rings of fibroelastic cartilage called the annulus fibrosus of the intervertebral disk.

Olecranon Curved process of the ulna at the elbow.

Open-ended questions Allows patients the opportunity to provide substantial information concerning their care. A technique to facilitate rapport and let the patient see that the PTA is effectively listening.

Open reduction and internal fixation (ORIF) A surgical technique where a fracture is visualized by surgical exposure (open), manually realigned into anatomic apposition (reduction), then stabilized with an internal fixation device.

Osteoarthritis Degenerative joint disease affecting articular cartilages and the synovial membranes.

Osteoblasts Bone-forming cells. Increased endoplasmic reticulum, increased Golgi apparatus, and increased mitochondria.

Osteoclasts Remodeling cells of bone, resorb bone. Bone resorption generally is more rapid than bone formation.

Osteocytes Bone cells. Ninety percent of mature skeleton. Former osteoblasts that serve to maintain bone.

Osteokinematics Study of movement of bone segments around a joint axis.

Osteomalacia Softening of bones.

Osteoporosis Abnormal loss of bone density.

Osteotomy Excision of all or part of a bone.

Overload A system of progressive, incremental demand in order to stimulate growth and strength.

Oxygen consumption and circuit training Circuit exercise training may increase peak oxygen consumption 4% in men and 8% in women.

Pacinian mechanoreceptors Encapsulated afferent nerve tissue that responds to changes in joint position and pressure. Type II mechanoreceptors.

Partial weight bearing (PWB) Weight bearing status assigned to a patient that is frequently graded in a percentage of the patient's body weight.

Patella: biomechanical function Acts to distribute forces across the distal femur. Lengthens the lever arm of the quadriceps extensor mechanism.

Pathologic fractures A group or classification of fractures caused by tumors (malignant or primary bone disease), osteoporosis (most common), microtrauma from repetitive overload (stress fractures), or metastatic bone disease (second most common).

Pelvic "list" Rotation of the pelvis within the frontal plane of the body during gait.

Perimysium Noncontractile connective tissue that surrounds the fasciculus.

Pharmacokinetics Four separate areas represent pharmacokinetics: absorption, distribution, metabolism, and excretion.

Physiologic effects of cold Reduced localized tissue temperature, reduced localized cell metabolism, decreased blood flow via vasoconstriction, reduced nerve conduction velocity, and analgesia.

Physiologic effects of heat Increase in localized superficial temperature, increase in localized and superficial cell metabolism, vasodilation and increased blood flow, superficial increase in capillary permeability, increased elasticity of dense connective tissue, reduced muscle spasms, and analgesia.

Physiologic movement Movement that occurs as a result of active or passive joint range of motion. This type of joint motion can be visualized and measured by goniometric assessment.

Piccolo traction Manually applied traction used to minimize joint compressive forces during mobilization. Piccolo traction is used to describe a stage I traction technique. The force used to deliver a grade I traction is not enough to actually separate the joint surfaces, but only to neutralize joint pressure.

Piezoelectric effect A negative electric charge toward the concave or compression side of a force applied to a bone. An electropositive charge is seen on the tension or convex side of the bone. The negative-charge side responds by stimulating osteoblasts, whereas the positive-charge side (tension side) responds by increasing osteoclast activity.

Pilon fracture Distal tibia compression fracture where a vertical or axial load compresses the tibia into the talus.

Plantar fasciitis A chronic inflammatory reaction of the plantar aponeuroses (fascia) at the insertion into the calcaneus. Also referred to as heel spur syndrome because of the occasional development of a calcaneal exostosis (spur).

Plyometrics A system of physical exercise that is based on the neurophysiologic responses from the Golgi tendon organs (GTO) and muscle spindles that involve ballistic, high-velocity movement to develop power and speed of movement.

Posterior cruciate ligament A deep ligament within the knee that crosses posteriorly to the anterior cruciate ligament.

Proactive supervision The patient avoids being placed in a reactive position by using probing questions and appropriate communications skills, accountability, listening, and responsibility.

Probing questions Techniques of questioning patients leading to insightful, rewarding, and responsive care.

Progressive resistance exercise (PRE) A system or program of resistance exercise that systematically and incrementally prescribes progressive amounts of externally applied stress or resistance to stimulate adaptive physiologic responses to enhance strength. Examples are the DeLorme PRE program, the Oxford technique, and the daily adjustable progressive resistance exercise (DAPRE) technique.

Proprioception Sensibility to position, whether conscious or unconscious. Afferent information sense of anatomic location or position. Either static (proprioception) or dynamic (kinesthesia).

Proprioceptive neuromuscular facilitation (PNF) Stretching and facilitation technique that uses the neurophysiologic organs (GTO) and muscle spindles to enhance muscle contraction and joint motion and to inhibit resistance to increased muscle flexibility.

Protected motion Therapeutic principle and technique where specific motion limitations are allowed but unwanted motions are avoided or eliminated in order to protect healing tissues.

Protrusion Displaced nuclear material causes a discrete bulge in the annulus, but no material escapes through the annular fibers (protrusion of disk).

Proximal femoral intertrochanteric osteotomy A specific surgical procedure used to reduce pain and improve function of the hip related to advanced osteoarthritis by surgically changing the femoral neck-shaft angle in order to expose healthy articular cartilage, thereby improving joint surface congruity.

Purpose of communication To gather information relevant to the patient's problem; to establish rapport and to provide confidence. To facilitate understanding of the patient's problem to assist in comprehensive patient management.

Q-angle Made by intersection of lines drawn from antero-superior iliac spine (ASIS) to midpatella and from mid-patella to anterior tibial tuberosity.

Radicular signs Neurologic signs of radiating pain and paresthesias (numbness and tingling).

Range of motion (ROM) Extent of movement within a given joint.

Red-on-red A zone classification concerning location of a tear within the meniscus. Red-on-red refers to the tear being vascular on both sides of the tear. Zone I.

Red-on-white A zone classification concerning location of a tear within the meniscus. Red-on-white refers to the tear being vascular on one side (red) and avascular (white) on the other side. Zone II.

Reduced muscle fatigue Partly caused by relative increase in mitochondria, as well as capillary neovascularization from specific high-volume training.

Reducing acute cardiovascular responses to resistance exercise Minimize Valsalva maneuver; reduce or minimize large muscle group exercise; use submaximal repetitions. Avoid near-maximum or maximum resistance.

Reflex sympathetic dystrophy (RSD) Usually posttraumatic (major or minor) pain dysfunction syndrome. Thought to result from abnormal modulation of afferent pain signals with possible short circuiting of somatic and autonomic nerve fibers. Attendant autonomic nervous system hyper-activity produces abnormal peripheral small vessel response to cold and heat stimulus. Symptoms include hyperpathia (increased pain at rest), allodynia (painful response to a nonpainful stimulus), erythema brawny edema, joint stiff-ness, and loss of skin elasticity. Osteoporosis and complete loss of dexterity result. Also referred to as complex regional pain syndrome (CRPS).

Remodeling of bone The process of tissue restructuring in response to stress. Occurs long after the fracture has clinically healed. Woven bone formed during the repair phase is replaced with lamellar bone. Bone remodeling is affected by mechanical function according to Wolff's law. Removal of external stress can lead to significant bone loss. Bone remodels in response to stress and responds to piezoelectric charges.

Remodeling (phase II) of healing tissue A process that alters the structure of connective tissue in response to stress.

Remodeling (phase III) of healing tissue Decreasing fibroblasts and macrophages. Markedly decreased vascularity and increased density of collagen, with improved alignment.

Remodeling and maturation (phases III and IV) of heal-ing tissue Decreased cellularity; water content declines toward normal; collagen concentration and proportion of type III to type I declines toward normal.

Repair phase of fractures (phase II of healing) Primary callus forms in about 2 weeks. Soft callus involving enchon-dral ossification occurs if fracture is not in continuity. Amount of callus is indirectly proportional to the degree of immobili-zation. Primary cortical healing occurs with immobilization and near-anatomic reduction.

Responsibility A component of active involvement of all areas of patient care.

Roll An accessory joint motion.

Ruffini mechanoreceptors Type I mechanoreceptors that respond slowly to static joint position.

SAID principle Specific adaptations to imposed demands. A fundamental exercise principle that states that tissues respond and adapt specifically to the type of stress or demand placed on the tissue. For example, high-intensity exercise of short duration yields specific physiologic adaptations specific to this type of stress.

Salter-Harris fracture Epiphyseal fracture in children involving epiphyseal growth plate, the seriousness of which could arrest growth or cause deformity.

Scaphoid fracture A fracture of the scaphoid bone of the carpals. Recognized as the most common fracture to the carpal bones. Fractures of the scaphoid are related to a high incidence of avascular necrosis and nonunion caused by the vascular anatomy of the proximal pole of the scaphoid.

Scar tissue The healing or union of torn or injured tissue with connective tissue.

Scoliosis Abnormal lateral curvature of the spine.

Sequestrated disk Injury to the intervertebral disk in which the nucleus is free within the canal.

Shear Two parallel forces or loads that slide past each other.

Short wave diathermy *Advantages:* Treats larger areas com-pared with ultrasound; delivers uniform thermal energy effects; applies therapeutic stretching techniques for a longer duration posttreatment compared with ultrasound; requires less dedicated clinician treatment time compared with ultrasound.

Single-support The time during the stance phase when only one foot is in contact with the ground.

Skier's thumb A traumatic rupture of the ulnar collateral ligament of the metacarpophalangeal joint of the thumb, usually a hyperabduction injury. Also called gamekeeper's thumb.

Slide An accessory joint motion.

Slow twitch (type I-red oxidative) muscle fiber Muscle fiber type that possesses more mitochondria, triglycerides, and enzymes. These fatigue-resistant fibers are recruited for muscular endurance activities.

Smith's fracture Reverse Colles' fracture. Distal fragment displaced volarly.

Snuffbox The anatomic "snuffbox" is an area on the dorsum of the thumb formed by extension of the thumb.

Soft-tissue approximation A normal joint end-range feel. This type of joint end-range feel is characterized by a yielding compression of muscular tissue compression during joint flexion.

Specificity   Specific and predictable physiologic adaptations a muscle goes through in response to a specific training stimulus.

Spin   An accessory joint motion.

Spinal stenosis   Narrowing of the spinal canal, constricting and compressing nerve roots that give rise to symptoms of neurogenic or spinal claudication. This condition is most commonly acquired from degenerative arthritic changes that encroach on the diameter of the canal, producing symptoms of nerve root compression.

Spondylolisthesis   Not a true dislocation because it rarely occurs as a result of trauma or muscle imbalance; rather a forward displacement of one vertebral body over another, usually occurs as the result of a defect in the pars interarticularis.

Spondylolysis   Disruption of the pars interarticularis (a portion of bone between each of the joints of the back), allowing one vertebral body to slide forward on the next. May be referred to as pars interarticularis defect, acute (traumatic) dissociation of pars interarticularis, or posterior elements (lamina) with or without spondylolisthesis.

Spongy bone   Spongy bone is less dense and is more elastic than compact or cortical bone. Approximately 20% of the adult skeleton is spongy or cancellous bone.

Sprain   Stretching or tearing of ligaments (fibrous bands that bind bones together at a joint), varying in degree from being partially torn (stretched) to being completely torn (ruptured). After a sprain, the fibrous capsule that encloses the joint may become inflamed, swollen, discolored, and painful. Involuntary muscle spasm and sometimes a fracture avulsion may occur.

Springy block   An abnormal end-feel in which full motion is limited by a soft or springy sensation occasionally accompanied by pain.

Stability   Bodies that have a wide base of support and a center of gravity that is relatively caudal and close to the base of support demonstrate the greatest stability. Equilibrium is a form of stability.

Steady state   When the rate of drug administration becomes equal to the rate of drug clearance. This maintains the plasma concentration at a constant level.

Step length   Linear distance between two consecutive contralateral contacts of the lower extremities.

Steppage gait   Muscular weakness of the ankle dorsi flexors that is characterized by extreme hip flexion and knee flexion during swing through to prevent dragging the toes on the ground.

Strain   1. Stretching or tearing of a muscle or its tendon (fibrous cord that attaches the muscle to the bone it moves) that may result in bleeding into the damaged muscle area, which causes pain, swelling, stiffness, and muscle spasm, followed by a bruise. 2. The relative measure of the deformation of a body as a result of loading. Strain equals the change in length or original length of a tissue.

Strength   The maximal load that a structure can withstand before functional failure occurs (load strength) or the maximal energy that a structure can withstand before functional failure occurs (energy strength).

Stress   The force per unit area of a structure and a measurement of the intensity of the force. Units of measure are newtons per square meter or pound force per square foot. The amount of tension or load placed on tissues. Intensity of internal force. Stress equals force divided by area. It can be compressive, tensile, or shear. 3. A force required to maintain the deformation of viscoelastic material diminishes with time until equilibrium is reached.

Structure and function (of articular cartilage)   Proteoglycans and water provide stiffness to compression; proteoglycans contribute resiliency and durability. Articular cartilage is a nonhomogeneous tissue. Elaborate organization of cells and matrix that varies considerably in depth.

Subacromial rotator cuff impingement   The tendons of the rotator cuff are crowded, buttressed, or compressed under the coracoacromial arch, resulting in mechanical wear, stress, and friction.

Subchondral bone   Bone directly under any cartilaginous surface.

Subluxation   Incomplete or partial dislocation in that one bone forming a joint is displaced only partially from its normal position.

Subluxing peroneal tendon   Either an acute or chronic subluxation of the peroneal tendons resulting from a loose retinaculum or a shallow peroneal groove, which results in instability.

Subtotal meniscectomy   Surgical removal of part of a torn meniscus.

Summary of ligament biochemistry   Dense, regular connective tissue, cells, water, collagen, proteoglycans, fibronectin, and elastin.

Summary-type statements   Techniques that validate understanding of the patient's needs. Help to clarify and specify patient's awareness and place emphasis on listening and responding appropriately.

Supracondylar fractures   A fracture of the distal third of the humerus.

Swing phase   The time in which one limb is entirely non-weight bearing throughout the gait cycle. The swing phase occupies approximately 40% of the gait cycle.

Systemic effects of orthopedic implant material   Allergic reactions and toxicity are two common systemic effects of implants. Cobalt chrome and nickel are reported to be associated with allergic reactions.

Tachyphylaxis   Rapid reduction or loss of a drug's effect after administration.

Tendinitis   Inflammation of a tendon.

Tennis elbow   Inflammation of the wrist and finger extensor muscles at the lateral epicondyle.

Tenocytes   Tendon cells.

Tenosynovitis   Inflammation of the tendon sheath. Causes are multifactorial. Repetitive and nonspecific overuse are implicated.

Thoracic outlet (inlet) syndrome   Mechanical problem related to the exit of arteries and nerves at the base of the neck leading down the arm; can also involve the vein bringing blood back from the arm (inlet).

Three-point gait pattern   The advancing of both crutches and the involved limb. The uninvolved limb is advanced; then the sequence is repeated.

Tibial plateau fractures   Various fracture patterns related to the proximal tibia. Generally classified as nondisplaced or displaced.

Tibial stem and tray: biomechanical function In a total knee arthroplasty, the tibial stem effectively reduces shear forces at the bone–implant interface and distributes loads across the maximal tibia.

Toe-off The instant where the knee of the weight bearing limb flexes and preparation occurs for the swing phase. Also referred to as preswing.

Toe-touch weight bearing (TTWB) Minimal contact of the involved limb with the ground during gait. Also referred to as touch-down weight bearing.

Tolerance Responsiveness or effect of drugs may be reduced with continued use.

Total hip precautions Postoperative precautions following total hip replacement that involve patient education on avoiding hip flexion greater than 90 degrees, hip and leg adduction past midline, and internal hip rotation.

Total hip replacement (THR) Surgical procedure that replaces the proximal femoral component, as well as the acetabulum.

Traction Pull on a limb or part thereof. Skin traction (indirect traction) is applied by using a bandage to pull on the skin and fascia where light traction is required; however, skeletal traction (direct traction) uses pins or wires inserted through bone and is attached to weights, pulleys, and ropes.

Transition zone of articular cartilage Several times the volume of the superficial zone. Contains large collagen fibrils.

Traumatic unidirectional injury with a Bankart lesion (TUBS) Frequently requires surgery.

Trendelenburg gait Weakness of the gluteus medius is characterized by the pelvis dropping toward the unaffected limb during the single-limb support period of the stance phase.

Tribology The science that deals with friction lubrication and wear of interacting joint surfaces in motion.

Two-point gait pattern The patient characteristically uses each crutch with opposing leg.

Ultimate strength Maximum strength obtained by a material.

Ultrasound for fracture healing Clinical studies demonstrate that low-intensity pulsed ultrasound stimulates bone growth and fracture repair healing in nonunions.

Valgus overload Medial valgus stress overload occurs to the capsuloligamentous structures as a result of repetitive valgus stress to the elbow.

Vascular access channel A surgical incision created to provide blood flow (vascular access) to a part of the meniscus that is avascular.

Vascular changes with local muscle fatigue Local and diffuse ischemia creates a decrease in force production, which may prolong fatigue.

Vascular zone I "Red-on-red." The location of the tear is vascular on both sides. Reparable, intrinsic healing is possible.

Vascular zone II "Red-on-white." The location of the tear is vascular on one side. Reparable, intrinsic healing is possible.

Vascular zone III "White-on-white." The tear is avascular on both sides. Not repairable, no blood supply to support the healing process.

Velocity Displacement divided by the time taken for that displacement (cm/sec). A change of position with respect to time. Velocity is also a vector, possessing both speed and direction.

Viscoelastic Stress and strain behavior is time and rate dependent.

VO$_2$max Maximum oxygen uptake.

Volkmann's ischemic contracture Contracture of the fingers, and sometimes the wrists, with loss of muscle power caused by vascular blockage.

Weight bearing as tolerated (WBAT) Status assigned to patients for whom pain tolerance is the predominant limiting factor.

White-on-white A zone classification of an injury to the meniscus. White-on-white indicates that the injury is avascular on both sides. Zone III.

Wolff's law The scientific law that states that bone forms and remodels in the direction of forces acting on it.

Work The product of force multiplied by the displacement through which the force moves.

Young's modulus of elasticity A measure of the stiffness of a material or its ability to resist deformation. Elasticity equals stress divided by strain.

Zone of calcified cartilage Separates cartilage from subchondral bone. Forms anchor for hyaline cartilage to attach to bone.

Zones of articular cartilage Superficial zone is the thinnest zone. Gliding surface of joint is covered with a thin, clear liquid that is almost entirely frictionless.

Index

A

A-band of sarcomere, *77, 177*
Abdominal exercises
    for lumbar sprains and strains, 366-367, *368*
    for spondylolisthesis, 375
Abduction
    hip, *243*
        for groin pulls, *349*
        for Legg-Calvé-Perthes disease, 345-346
        post-fracture, *339, 340*
    humeral-ulnar, 432
    measurement of, *5b*
    shoulder, *242*
        glenohumeral instability and, 399, *400, 401,* 403-404
        impingement during, *393, 394, 395*
        multiangle isometric, *86*
Abductor "lurch," 223, *224t*
Abiotrophy, 253
Abrasion, cartilage repair by, *167, 168,* 315
Absorption, drug, 208
Acceleration
    in gait cycle, *220, 222, 223t*
    linear and angular, 245
    movement and, 244
    Newton's law of, 248-249
    running and changes in, *244*
Accessory joint motions
    assessment of, 32
    convex-concave rule for, *230, 231*
    grades of, 231-232
    types of, 230
Accountability for patient care, 5-6, 10
Acetabulum
    fractures of, 350-353
    surgical replacement of, 343
Acetylcholine (ACH), 77, 178
Achilles tendon
    ruptures of, 187, 269, *270*
        healing of, 188-189
        management and rehabilitation for, 189, 270-271, *272*
        Thompson test for, 269, *271*
    tendinitis of, 268-269
ACL injuries. *See* Anterior cruciate ligament (ACL) injuries.
Acoustic streaming in ultrasound, 41-42
Acromioclavicular sprains and dislocations, 405-408

Actin, 76-77, 177
Active recovery, 102
Active transport of topical medications, 53
Activities of daily living (ADLs), modifying
    for carpal tunnel syndrome, 438
    after meniscectomy, 308
    for rotator cuff impingement, 394
Adaptable scar, 65
Adduction
    ankle sprain from, *260*
    hip, *243*
        for groin pull, *348, 349*
        for MCL sprain, 142, *143*
        for patellofemoral conditions, *312, 313*
        post-fracture, *339, 340*
        after total arthroplasty, 343, *344*
    humeral-ulnar, 432-433
    shoulder, *242*
Adenosine triphosphate (ATP)
    aerobic exercise and, 100
    formation of, 178
    muscle contraction and, 77, 94
Adhesion, platelet, 125
Adhesions
    fibrotic, description of, 72
    after flexor tendon injuries of hand, 447
    formation of, 65, *66*
    joint stability and, 67
    noncapsular motion and, 233
Adhesive capsulitis of shoulder, 404-405
Adjunctive interventions, physical agents as, 38
Adolescents, strength training for, 91-92
Aerobic capacity, 100
Aerobic exercise
    activities for, 101-102
    Borg Scale of perceived exertion during, *101b*
    measuring and prescribing, 100-101
    muscle fibers and, 77
    orthopedic considerations during, 102-103, *104*
    physiologic changes with, 100
    prescription recommendations for, *100b*
    rehabilitation with
        for Achilles tendon injuries, 268-269, *270*
        after ACL reconstruction, 297, *298, 299*
        for ankle sprains, 264

Note: Page numbers in *italics* indicate figures; page numbers followed by *t* indicate tables and *b,* boxes.

Aerobic exercise—cont'd
    after fasciotomy of lower leg, 272
    after foot/ankle stress fractures, 276
    for glenohumeral stabilization, 400, *402*
    after hip arthroplasty, 344
    for hip soft-tissue injuries, 346-347
    after lumbar discectomy, 373
    after lumbar fractures, 376
    for lumbar strains, 366
    after peroneal tendon repair, 268
    for plantar fasciitis, 278
    after proximal femoral osteotomy, 342
    strength training with, 104-105
Aerobic metabolism, 100, 178
Afferent neural input, 108
Afferent receptors, 115
Age-adjusted maximum heart rate (AAMHR), 100
Aggregation, platelet, 125
Aging
    articular cartilage changes with, 165*t*
    drug metabolism and, 214
    tendon changes with, 190
Air-stirrup brace for ankle, *143*
Allografts
    for ACL reconstruction, 294
    for fracture repair, 158
    for PCL reconstruction, 302
Alpha-motor neurons, 178
AMBRI shoulder instability pattern, 400, 415
American College of Sports Medicine guidelines, 100, 101
American Heart Association guidelines, 28
American Physical Therapy Association (APTA) guidelines, 14-15, 21, 38, 49
Aminoglycosides, 209
Amortization phase in plyometrics, 87
Amplitude of movement
    joint mobilization and, 231-232
    mechanoreceptors for, 108
Anabolic energy metabolism, 178
Anaerobic exercise, muscle fibers and, 77
Anaerobic metabolism, 100, 178
Anatomic position, *240*
Anatomic "snuffbox," 443, 449
Angiogenesis in tissue healing, 125
    fractures and, 154
    muscle injuries and, 179, 180
    tendon injuries and, 189
Angiogenic growth factors, 125, 132, 180
Angle of application of force, 245-246
Angular motion, biomechanics of, 244-245, 246
Ankle
    Achilles injuries of, 187, 188, 190, 268-271, *272*
    edema measurement in, 20*b*
    fractures of, 273-274, 276
    gait and rotation of, 221, *222*
    mobilization techniques for, 281-283
    movement patterns for, *243*
    range of motion in, 5*b*
    sprains of
        aerobic activities for, 103, *104*
        chronic instability after, 265-266, *267*
        lateral, 260-265
        medial, 265
        remobilization and exercise for, 142, *143*
    subluxing peroneal tendons of, 266-268
Ankle weights, 92

Annulus
    nuclear herniation through, 369
    structure and function of, 360, *361*
Anoxia, nerve compression and, 195
Antalgic gait
    description of, 223, 226
    after total hip replacement, 343
Anterior, definition of, 240*b*
Anterior compartment of lower leg, 272
Anterior cruciate ligament (ACL) injuries, 290-300
    additional features for, 325
    history and physical examination for, 290, *291-292*
    MCL injuries with, 304
    mechanism of, *291*
    meniscal injury with, 309
    rehabilitation for, 142, 295-300
    stability tests for, 292-294
    surgical repair and healing of, 139, 294-295
Anterior drawer test
    of ankle, *261*
    of knee, *71*
        for ACL injuries, 293
        for PCL injuries, 300, *301*
Anterior-posterior mobilization of hip, 353, *354*
Anteroposterior plane
    description of, 240, *241*
    movements in, 241, *242*, *243*
Antibiotic beads for open fractures, 210
Antibiotics, 205
    action of, 208
    prophylaxis and treatment with, 209-211
    types of, 208-209
Anticoagulants, 201
Antiinflammatory agents, 205
    action of, 130, *131*, *211*, *213*
    nonsteroidal, 212
    steroidal, 211-212, 372
AO/ASIF classification system for fractures, 152, 157*b*
    of ankle, *273*
    of supracondylar femur, *317*
Apex stretch, side-lying, *382*
Apley's compression and distraction test, 306-307
Apophyseal injury, weight lifting and, 92
Apoptosis, cellular, 133, 134
Arachidonic acid
    inflammatory metabolites of, 130, *131*, 211-212
    inhibition of, *211*, 212, *213*
Arch deformities, 278-279
Armchair push-ups, *339*
Arms
    aerobic activities for, 103
    balance training for, 113, *114*
    elevation of, for rotator cuff impingement, *394*, 395
Arterial pressure index (API), 200
Arteries
    anatomy of, 179, 198
    bone nutrient, 150, *151*
    injuries to, 199, 201
Arteriography, percutaneous, 200
Arthritis, hip, 354. *See also* Osteoarthritis.
Arthrocentesis for knee effusion, 290
Arthrofibrosis of elbow, mobilization for, 432
Arthrokinematics
    accessory movements in, 32, 230
    description of, 234
Arthrometers, knee ligament, 293-294

Arthroplasty
  hip
    partial, 342
    prosthesis fixation for, 343
    total, 343-345, 354
  patellofemoral, 315
  total joint, infections in, 209, 211
  total knee, 320-322, 326
  total shoulder, 413
Arthroscopy
  for ACL reconstruction, 294-295
  for articular cartilage repair, 166
  for glenohumeral stabilization, 402
  for meniscal repair, 171
  for osteochondral autografting, 167-168
  for patellofemoral chondromalacia, 315
  for PCL reconstruction, *302*
Articular cartilage
  additional features for, 172
  biochemical changes in, 165*t*
  composition of, 163-164
  function of, 164, 253
  healing and repair of, 165-166
    alternative surgeries for, 167-169
    depth of injury and, *167*
    glucosamine/chondroitin supplements for, 169-170
    hyaluronic acid injection for, 170
    immobilization and, 164-165
    rehabilitation and, 163
    techniques for stimulating, 166-167
  injury and degeneration of, 165, *166*
  layers in, *163*, 163*t*
Assessment. *See also* Physical assessment.
  definition of, 14
  SOAP documentation for, 34
Assistive devices
  assessing need for, 33
  gait pattern instruction for, 224, *225*
  negotiating stairs with, 225-226
  selection of, 226
  stretching exercises using, 69, *70*
  weight bearing status and, 224-225
Association for the Study of Internal Fixation (ASIF/AO), fracture
    classification by, 152, 157*b*, *273*, 317
ATP. *See* Adenosine triphosphate (ATP).
Atrophy
  articular cartilage, 164-165
  ligament, 139-140
  muscle
    assessment of, 30
    electrical stimulation for, 50-51, 52
    exercise and, 81
    immobilization and, 185
Autogenic inhibition in muscle contraction, 63
Autografts
  for ACL reconstruction, 294-295, 325
  arthroscopic osteochondral, 167-168
  for fracture repair, 158
  for PCL reconstruction, 302
  for peripheral nerve repair, 198
  vascular, 200
Autologous chondrocyte transplantation, 168-169
Autolysis, cellular, 133
Autolytic wound débridement, 117-118
Autonomic nervous system, pain mediation by, *26*
Avascular necrosis (AVN)
  ACL autografts and, 295

Avascular necrosis (AVN)—cont'd
  hip fractures and, 335-336
  patellar fractures and, 315
  proximal humerus fractures and, 411
  scaphoid fractures and, 442, 443
Avulsion fractures, 151-152
  calcaneal, *274*
  mallet finger with, 446
  pelvic, *350*
Axial extension of cervical spine, 384, *385*
Axonotmesis, 194-195, 201
Axons, nerve, *195*

B

Back. *See also* Lumbar spine; Thoracic spine.
  injuries to, aerobic activities for, 102
  low
    flexibility tests for, *71, 72*
    movement patterns for, *243*
    torque effects on, *246*
  low, dysfunction of
    pain related to, 369
    prevention and education for, 376, 377*b*
    treatment options for, 360, *361*
  strength measurement for, 363-364
Back school model, 376, 377*b*
Bacterial adherence to implants, 210
Bactericidal and bacteriostatic drugs, 208
"Bag of bones technique" for intercondylar fractures, 429
Balance
  additional features for, 115
  assessment of, 33
  description of, 108, 115
  exercises for
    after ACL reconstruction, 297, *299*
    for ankle sprains or instability, 263, *264, 266, 267*
    progressive, 110-113
    proprioceptive, 113, *114*
    after total hip replacement, 345
  functional training for, 110
  improving, principles for, 252-253
  mechanoreceptors for, 108
  tests for, 108-110
Balance board. *See* Wobble board, balance training on.
Ballistic movements in plyometrics, 88
Ballistic stretching, 59, 61-62, *63*
Bankart lesion
  description of, 397, *398*, 415
  surgical repair of, 400, 402
Barbells, 93
Base of support
  definition of, 115
  gait and, *220*
  lifting and, 363
  stability and, 253
Basement membrane, muscle, 176
Basic dimensional model of behavior, 6, 8, *9*
"Bayonet" sign in miserable malalignment syndrome, *311*
Beam nonuniformity ratio (BNR) in ultrasound, 42
Behavior
  basic dimensional model of, 6, 8, *9*
  categories of, 6
  description of, 10
  pain and, 25-26
Bending, effects of, 250, *251*
Bennett's fracture, 444, *445*
Beta-motor neurons, 178

Bicycle ergometers
  after ACL reconstruction, 297
  after hip fractures, 338
  for lumbar strains, 366
  recumbent, *102*
  seated, *101*, *104*
  single-leg, *103*
Bioavailability, drug, 208, 214
Biofeedback, step-ups with, *298*, *313*
Biofilm, bacterial, 210
Biomechanical ankle platform system (BAPS). *See also* Wobble
      board, balance training on.
  for ankle sprains, *264*
  balance training with, 111, *112*, *113*
Biomechanics
  additional features for, 253
  body movements in, *242-243*
  cardinal planes in, *241*
  concepts in, 241, 244
  definition and application of, 237, 240
  directional terms in, *240b*
  energy in, 252
  equilibrium in, 252-253
  kinematics in, 244-245
  kinetics in, 245-250
  lumbar spinal, 360-361, *362*
  mechanical loading in, 250-252
  reference terminology for, 240-241
Biotribology, 253
Bipolar hip prosthesis, 342, 354
Bladder technique in ultrasound, 53
Blood flow, exercise and, 94. *See also* Vascular supply.
Blood pressure
  assessment of, *5b*, 27
  exercise and, 28, 105
Blood vessels, anatomy of, 179, 198
Blunt trauma, severe, 190. *See also* Contusions.
Body parts
  cardinal planes dividing, *241*
  directional terms for, *240b*
  major movements of, *242-243*
Bone. *See also* Fractures.
  assessment of, 31-32
  collagen in, *150*
  healing of
    additional features for, 159
    complications of, 155
    components of, 153
    factors influencing, 157-158
    fixation devices for, 155-157
    objectives for, 148
    phases and process of, 154
    primary vs. secondary, 153
    rehabilitation techniques during, 159
    stimulation of, 158
  heterotopic, formation of, 181, 190
  lamellar, biomechanical function of, 253
  loss of
    aging and, 153
    immobilization and, 139, 140, 153, 154-155
  remodeling of, 149-150, 276
  structure and function of, 148-149
  types of, 148, *149*, 159
  vascular supply to, 150, *151*
Bone callus, formation of, 154, 156
Bone cells, types of, 148

Bone cement, polymethylmethacrylate
  antibiotic-impregnated, 210, 211
  for hip prosthesis, 343
  for knee prosthesis, 321
Bone grafts for fracture repair, 158, 443
Bone plates
  for fracture fixation, 155, 156t, 157, 158t
  for hip fracture, *337*
  for intercondylar humerus fracture, 428, *429*
Bone to bone end-feel, 29, 232
Bone-patellar tendon-bone autografts
  for ACL reconstruction, 294-295, 325
  for PCL reconstruction, *302*
Borg Scale of relative perceived exertion, 101b
"Bounce home" test for meniscal injury, 307
Boutonnière deformity, 447
Bow-leg deformity, tibial osteotomy for, 322-323
Boxer's fracture, 444-445
Braces
  for ankle sprains, *143*, 263, 264
  counterforce, for "tennis elbow," 423, *424*
  for fracture fixation, 157
  for Legg-Calvé-Perthes disease, 345-346
  limited range of motion
    after ACL reconstruction, 295, 297
    example of, *140*
    for ligament healing, 140, 142
    for muscle healing, 186
    after PCL injury or repair, 302
  for MCL sprains, 305
  for scoliosis, 380
Brachial plexus, compression of, 385, *386*
Bradykinin, 117
Brawny edema, 20-21
Breaking point, 72
Breath-holding
  blood pressure and, 27
  lifting and, 363
Brief assertion, *7*
Bristow procedure for glenohumeral stabilization, 402, *404*
Bucket-handle tear of meniscus, *306*
Bunionectomy, 280
Bursae, assessment of, 32
Bursitis, trochanteric, 346-347
"Butterfly" stretch for groin pull, 348

C

Cable column systems
  cam-based, resistive torque in, 248
  for hip strengthening, 338, *341*
  for shoulder strengthening, 400
  for strength training, 93
Cable tensiometry for strength measurement, 79, *80*
Cadence, gait and, 220
Calcaneal gait, 224
Calcaneus
  anterior glide of, 282
  fractures of, *274*, *275*, 283
Calcification, fibrocartilage, 154
Calcified zone of articular cartilage, 163t, 172
Calcium
  deficiency of, osteomalacia and, 153
  muscle contraction and, 77, 176, 178
Calf raises for Achilles tendon, 271, *272*
Calf stretches, static, *62*
Callus formation, bone, 154, 156
Cam-based pulley systems, 248

Cancellous bone, 148-149, 153, 159
Cancer, physical agent use and, 43, 44, 52
Canes
    negotiating stairs with, 225-226
    stretching exercises with, 69, *70*
    types of, 226
Capacitive plates in diathermy, 44-45
Capillaries, *121*
Capsular end-feel, 29, 32, 233
Capsular pattern of joint movement, 233, 234
Capsular shift for glenohumeral stabilization, 402, *404*
Capsulitis, adhesive shoulder, 404-405
Capsulorrhaphy for glenohumeral stabilization, 402
Cardinal planes
    illustration of, *241*
    movements in, 240-241, *242-243*
Cardiorespiratory fatigue, 28
Cardiovascular endurance, 100
Carpal bones
    fractures of, 442-444
    instability of, sprains and, 440, *441*
    mobilization of, *448*, 449
Carpal tunnel syndrome, 438-439
"Carrying angle" of elbow, 429-430
Cartilage
    additional features for, 172
    articular
        biochemical changes in, 165*t*
        composition of, 163-164
        degeneration of, *166*
        function of, 164, 253
        healing and repair of, 165-170
        immobilization and, 164-165
        injury to, 165
        layers in, *163*, 163*t*
    in bone healing, 154
    calcification of, fracture repair and, 154
    fibroelastic (*See also* Meniscus)
        injury and healing of, 171-172
        structure and function of, 170-171
    healing of, rehabilitation and, 163
Casts
    for Achilles tendon injuries, 269, 270
    for ankle fractures, 274
    for ankle sprains, 263, 265
    for foot/ankle stress fractures, 276
    for fracture healing, 156*t*, 157
    for metacarpal fractures, 445
    for scaphoid fractures, 443
    for skier's thumb, 444
    for subluxing peroneal tendons, 267
    for wrist sprains, 440
Catabolic energy metabolism, 178
Catching balls for balance testing, 109
Cavitation in ultrasound, 41
Cell body, nerve, *195*
Cells
    bone, 148
    of inflammation and repair, *119*, 128, 130, *134*
    injury and repair of, 133
    regeneration of, 134
    structure of, 128
Center of gravity (mass)
    description of, 115, 240, 244
    gait and, 220
    lifting and, 363
    stability and, 253

Centers for Disease Control and Prevention guidelines, 17
Central canal stenosis, 387
Centralization of pain
    assessment of, 24
    definition of, 23
    in lumbar disc herniation, 370
Cephalosporins, 209
Ceramic bone grafts, 158
Cerclage wiring for patellar fractures, 315, *317*
Cervical retraction exercises, 384, *385*
Cervical spine
    compression and distraction tests for, 387
    disc injuries of, 384-385
    mobilization of, 386-387
    scoliosis of, 380-382, *383*
    spondylolysis of, 385
    sprains and strains of, 382-384, *385*
    thoracic outlet syndrome and, 385-386
Charcot's neuropathy, 283
Chest press for glenohumeral stabilization, 399, *400*
Children
    Legg-Calvé-Perthes disease in, 345-346
    strength training for, 91-92
Chondrocytes
    in articular cartilage, 163
    autologous transplantation of, 168-169
    calcification of, 154
Chondroitin sulfate
    endogenous, function of, 124
    oral administration of, 169-170
Chondromalacia, 315
Chondroplasty
    for articular cartilage repair, 167, *168*
    patellofemoral, 313, 315
Chrisman-Snook procedure for ankle stabilization, 265, *266*
Circuit training, 104
    oxygen consumption and, 105
    weight training in, 86, 87*t*
Circumferential measurement of edema, 20
Claudication
    neurogenic, 373-374, 387
    vascular, 24, 387
"Claudication time," 24
Clavicular fractures, 409-410
Claw toes, 280-281
Clearance, drug, 214
Clinical Performance Instrument (CPI), 14, 33-34
Closed fractures, 152
Closed kinetic chain (CKC) exercise. *See also* Strength training.
    after ACL reconstruction, 297-300
    balance training with, 110-113, *114*
    description of, 88-89, 94
    for glenohumeral stabilization, 399, 400, *401*, *402*, *403*, 404
    after hip fractures, 338
    after MCL injuries, 305
    after meniscal surgeries, 308, 309
    for patellofemoral conditions, 313, 314, 315
    after PCL injury or repair, 302, 303
    after proximal humerus fractures, 412
    after total hip replacement, 344, *345*
Closed-ended questions, 6, 7, 8, 10
Close-packed joint position, 230-231
Coagulation
    thromboembolic disease and, 200, 201
    tissue healing and, 117, 125, *126*, *127*

Codman's pendulum exercises
for adhesive capsulitis, 405
for glenohumeral stabilization, 398
after rotator cuff repair, 396, 397
after shoulder arthroplasty, 413
techniques for, 69, *70*, 71
Coefficient of friction, 249*b*
Cold agents. *See also* Ice.
application of, 45-47
physiologic effects of, 39, 45, 54
Cold ischemia, 201
Collagen
in articular cartilage, 163-164, 166, 167
in bone, 148, *150*
in connective tissue, 58, 124
function of, *121*
in ligaments, 138, 144
in meniscal tissue, 170
in muscle, 176, 179
overview of, *129*
in tendons, 187, 188, 447
tissue healing by, 118, 122*b*, *127*
coagulation and, *126*
fibroplasia and, 130
inflammatory phase and, *119*
remodeling phase and, *120*, 125, 128
types of, 164*t*
Collagen bundles, *58*, *121*
Collagenases, interstitial, 179
"Collar and cuff" sling for elbow fracture, 429
Colles's fractures, 441-442, *443*
Comminuted fractures, 151
distal radial, 441, *442*
intercondylar humeral, 428-429
olecranon, 430, 431
patellar, *317*
radial head, 430
Communication
with patient, 5-6
purpose of, 10
with rehabilitation team, 4-5
skills for, 6, *7*
Compact bone, 148-149, 153, 159
Compartment syndromes
of lower leg, 272
signs and symptoms of, 21
thoracolumbar, 362
Complete fractures, 151
Complete muscle tears, 179
Compound fractures
definition of, 152
infection after, 209-210
Compression
cervical cord, surgeries for, 385
cervical spine, test using, 387
cold application with, 46-47
description of, 234
intermittent pneumatic, 201
intraneural tissue, *196*
joint
assessment using, 32
resistance exercise and, 84, 90, *91*
knee, Apley's test using, 306-307
lateral patellar
causes of, 310-311
nonoperative rehabilitation for, 312-313
postoperative rehabilitation for, 313-315

Compression—cont'd
neurovascular, thoracic outlet syndrome and, 385-386
physiologic effects of, 250, *251*
in RICE program, 262-263 (*See also* RICE)
after total knee replacement, 321
Compression fractures, 151
distal tibial, 274-275
humeral head, 397-398, 415
lumbar spinal, 375-376
proximal tibial, *319*
Compression neuropathy, 195-197
of median nerve, 438-439
spinal, tests for, 362
Concave-convex rule of joint motion, *230*, 231
Concentric exercises, 80-81, 82*b*
for lateral epicondylitis, 423
modification of, 9
during muscle healing, 186
Concentric muscle contractions
description of, 77, *78*
gait cycle and, 222-223
tension and energy produced by, 80-81
Conduction, heat transmission by, 39, 53
Congestive heart failure, edema in, 21
Congruence, joint, 230-231
Connective tissue
additional features for, 134-135
collagen in, *129*
composition and functions of, *121*, 124
healing of
cell injury and repair in, 133
cells and mediators for, 128, 130, *131*, 131*t*-133*t*
mechanisms of, 122*b*
necrotic process in, *134*
phases of, 117-118, *119-120*, 124-128
repair vs. regeneration in, 134
in muscle, 76, 94, 176
in peripheral nerves, 194, *195*, 201
properties of, 58-59, *60*
in tendon, 187
vascular, 198
Consolidation in tissue healing, 122*b*
Constrained knee implants, 320
Contact force, 249
Continuous aerobic activities, 101-102
Continuous diathermy, 44
Continuous passive motion (CPM)
after ACL reconstruction, 295-296
during bone healing, 159
during cartilage healing, 166-167
during ligament healing, 141-142
machine for, *141*
after total knee replacement, 321
Continuous ultrasound, effects of, 41, 42
Contractile proteins, 76-77, 177
Contractile tissue. *See also* Muscles; Tendons.
assessment of, 29-31
properties of, 29
proteins in, 94, 177
structure of, *76*, 77
Contractility, 29
Contraction in tissue healing, *120*, 122*b*. *See also* Muscle contractions.
Contract-relax in PNF stretching, 63, *64*
Contractures
definition of, 65
distal interphalangeal, 446-447

Contractures—cont'd
  Dupuytren's, 445-446
  elbow flexion, 432
  formation of, *120*
  stretching, 65-71
  Volkmann's ischemic, *427*
Contrast bath, 47
Controlled motion, tendon healing and, 190
Controlled substances, classes of, 208
Contusions
  hip or pelvic, 349-350
  muscle
    description of, 176, 190
    healing of, 179
    heterotopic bone formation and, 181
    therapeutic interventions for, 186*b*
  thoracic spinal, 378
Convex-concave rule of joint motion, *230*, *231*
Coordination. *See also* Balance.
  definition of, 108, 115
  mechanoreceptors for, 108
  tests for, 5*b*, 108-110
Coracoclavicular ligament tears, 405-406, *407*
Coracoid transfer for glenohumeral stabilization, 402, *404*
Coronal plane
  description of, 240, *241*
  movements in, 240-241, *242*, *243*
Cortical bone, 148-149, 153, 159
Corticosteroids, 205
  antiinflammatory action of, 130, *131*, 211, *213*
  epidural, for lumbar disc herniation, 372
  intraarticular/paraarticular injection of, 211-212
Counterforce brace for "tennis elbow," 423, *424*
Coupling media in ultrasound, 42
COX-2 inhibitors, 212
Coxa plana, 345-346
CPM. *See* Continuous passive motion (CPM).
Creep
  description of, 72, 253
  mechanical stress and, 58
  nerve tissue and, 194
Creeping substitution in fracture healing, 155
Crepitus, joint, 32
Criterion-based rehabilitation programs, 257
Critical mapping, 257
Cross-country ski machines, 103
Crush injury, physeal, *152*
Crutches
  features of, 226
  gait pattern instruction for, 224, *225*
  negotiating stairs with, 225-226
Cryokinetics, 46, 53
Cryostretch, 46
Cryotherapy. *See also* Ice.
  application of, 45-47
  physiologic effects of, 39, 45, 54
Cubital tunnel syndrome, 433
Cueing, prompting vs., 8
Cuff weights, 92
Cumulative trauma disorders of wrist and hand, 438-439. *See also* Overuse injuries.
Cyclooxygenase, inhibition of, *211*, 212
Cytokines and growth factors
  inflammatory response and, 125, 212, 214
  in muscle healing, 180
  tissue regeneration and, 134
  types and functions of, 130, 131*t*-133*t*

D
Daily adjustable progressive resistance exercise (DAPRE) program, 85
Data collection skills, 14, 15
Davies model of exercise progression, 81*b*
De Quervain's tenosynovitis, 439
Débridement
  articular cartilage, 167
  autolytic wound, 117-118
Deceleration
  in gait cycle, *220*, *222*, 223*t*
  movement and, 244
Deep, definition of, 240*b*
Deep posterior compartment of lower leg, 272
Deep tendon reflexes, grading scale for, 5*b*
Deep vein thrombosis (DVT), 19, 200-201
Deep zone of articular cartilage, 172
Deformation
  description of, 72
  elastic and plastic, 58, *59*, *60*
  load and limits for, 250, *252*
Degenerative joint disease (DJD), 341. *See also* Osteoarthritis.
Degradative enzymes, healing and, 179-180
Delayed onset muscle soreness (DOMS), 83-84
  cryotherapy for, 46
  definition of, 176
  treatment techniques for, 84*t*
Delayed union of fracture, 155
DeLorme PRE protocol, 85
Deltoid ligament sprains, 265
Demolition, 134
Dendrites, *195*
Denervation
  description of, 201
  muscle, electrical stimulation for, 50-51
Density, definition of, 244
Depth jump, plyometric, *87*
Diathermy, 44-45, 54
Dimensional model of behavior, 6, 8, 9
Dinner fork deformity of wrist, *442*
Direct current, 159
Direct muscle injury
  definition of, 176
  therapeutic interventions for, 186*b*
Disc, intervertebral
  displacement of, 387
  herniation of
    cervical, 384-385
    lumbar, 368-373
    signs of, 362
    thoracic, 378
  structure and mechanics of, 360-361, *362*
Disc protrusion, 369
Discectomy for lumbar herniation, 372, *373*
Discontinuous aerobic activities, 102
Dislocations
  acromioclavicular joint, 405-408
  arterial injuries with, 200*t*, 201
  elbow, fractures with, 430, 431-432
  glenohumeral, 397-404, 415
  hip, 336, *338*
    complications of, 354
    post-arthroplasty, 343
Displacement, movement and, 244
Distal, definition of, 240*b*
Distal fractures, *115*
  radial and ulnar, 441-442, *443*
  tibia compression, 274-275

Distal interphalangeal (DIP) joint deformities, 446-447
Distal realignment of patella, 314-315
Distraction
  cervical spine, 387
  elbow, *432*
  hip, 353
  humeral head, 414
  joint, assessment using, 32
  knee, Apley's test of, 306-307
  metacarpal phalangeal, 449
  proximal interphalangeal, *283*
  scapular, *414*
  talar, 282
  wrist, *448*, 449
Distribution, drug, 208, 214
DJD. *See* Osteoarthritis.
Documentation
  of assessment data, 33-34
  for edema, 20*b*
  for pain, 21-23
  for physical agent interventions, 53
  SOAP format for, 34*b*
  for strength testing, 29*b*
Dominance
  description of, 6, 10
  dimensions of, *8, 9*
DOMS. *See* Delayed onset muscle soreness (DOMS).
Doppler flow detection of vascular occlusion, 200
Dorsiflexion
  exercises for
    for Achilles tendon injuries, 269, 270-271, *272*
    after ankle fractures, 274
    for ankle sprains or instability, 263, 265-266
    after calcaneal fractures, 275
    after peroneal tendon repair, 268
  gait and, 221, *222*
  illustration of, *243*
  measurement of, 5*b*
Double crush syndrome, 197
Double product, description of, 105
Double support in gait cycle, 220
Double varus, tibiofemoral, 325
Double-leg stance test (DLST), 108-109
Double-leg static balance training, 110, 111*b*
Drilling, cartilage repair by, 167, *168*
Drug Enforcement Agency (DEA), U.S. Federal, 208
Drugs. *See* Medications.
Dumbbells, 93
Duplex ultrasonography for vascular injury, 200, 201
Dupuytren's contracture, 445-446
Duration of training
  for aerobic exercise, 100*b*, 101
  for strength programs, 82*b*
Duty cycle in ultrasound, 42
DVT. *See* Deep vein thrombosis (DVT).
Dynamic, definition of, 240
Dynamic balance
  definition of, 108
  progressive exercises for, 110, 111-113, *114*
  tests for, 109, 110
Dynamic stretching, 59, 61-62, *63*
Dynamometry for strength measurement, 79-80
Dynasplint appliance for stretching, 69, *70*
Dyspnea
  fatigue and, 28
  pulmonary embolism and, 201

E

Eccentric exercises, 80-81, 82*b*
  after glenohumeral stabilization, 404
  for lateral epicondylitis, 423, *424*
  modification of, 9
  for muscle healing, 186
  for tendon healing, 189
Eccentric muscle contractions
  description of, 77, *78*
  gait cycle and, 222-223
  tension and energy produced by, 80-81
Edema
  after ACL reconstruction, 295
  in deep vein thrombosis, 201
  documenting, 20*b*
  electrical stimulation for, 50
  inflammation and, 16, 117, *119*, 212, *213*
  measurement of, 5*b*, 19-21
  pitting, scale for rating, 21*b*
  in reflex sympathetic dystrophy, 448
  RICE for, 262-263
  treatment modifications for, 8, 9
Education, normative model of PTA, 15
Effective radiating area (ERA) in ultrasound, 42
Effusion, knee, 8, 290
Ehlers-Danlos syndrome, 134
Elastic bands and cords, exercises with
  for Achilles tendinitis, 269
  for ankle strengthening, 263, 267
  for knee sprains, *300*
  for patellofemoral conditions, *313*
  for strength training, 92
  after total hip replacement, *344, 345*
Elastic deformation
  description of, 58, *59*
  limit point for, 250, *252*
Elastica externa/interna, 199
Elasticity, Young's modulus of, 72
Elastin
  in ligaments, 138
  structure and function of, 58, *121*, 124
  in tendons, 187
Elbow
  additional features for, 433
  epicondylitis of
    lateral, 422-424
    medial, 424-425
  fractures of, 427-432
  lever action of, *247, 248*
  mobilization of, 432-433
  movement patterns for, *242*
  range of motion in, 5*b*
  valgus stress overload of, 425-427
Elderly
  osteoporosis in (*See* Osteoporosis)
  strength training for, 90-91
Electrical stimulation, 47-48
  for edema, 50
  for fracture repair, 53, 158
  impedance and, 48
  for knee rehabilitation, *298*
  medication delivery with, 53
  for muscle denervation and atrophy, 50-51, 159
  for muscle healing, 186, 186*b*
  for nerve healing, 198
  for pain, 48-50
  precautions and contraindications for, 52-53

Electrical stimulation—cont'd
    for reflex sympathetic dystrophy, 448
    for scaphoid graft healing, 443
    techniques for application of, 51-52
Electrically evoked muscle stimulation, 53
Electrodes, placement of, 50
Electromagnetic resonance in diathermy, 44
Elevation in RICE program, 262-263. *See also* RICE.
Elmslie-Trillat procedure for patellar realignment, *314*
Embolism, pulmonary, 200, 201
Empiric evidence for physical agent efficacy, 38
Empty end-feel, 29, 232-233
End-feel, joint
    capsular, 32
    MCL sprain and, 304
    "muscle spasm," 30
    types of, 29, 232-233, 234
Endomysium, 76, 125, 176
Endoneurium, 194, *195*
Endoplasmic reticulum, 128
Endotenon, 187
Endothelium, vascular, 198
Endurance
    additional features for, 105
    aerobic exercise for (*See also* Aerobic exercise)
        measuring and prescribing, 100-101
        methods of, 101-102
        orthopedic considerations during, 102-103, *104*
        physiologic changes with, 100
    cardiovascular, 100
    local muscular, circuit training for, 103-104
    muscle fiber types and, 77
    strength and, 79, 104-105
Energy, categories of, 252
Enoxaparin. *See* Low-molecular-weight heparin.
Enzymes
    degradative, healing and, 179-180
    oxidative, exercise and, 104
Epicondylitis
    lateral, 422-424
    medial, 424-425
Epidermal growth factor (EGF), 180
Epimysium, 76, 125
Epineurial neurorrhaphy, *197*
Epineurium, 194, *195*
Epiphyseal fractures, 152
Epitenon, 187
Epithelialization, *120*
Equilibrium, maintenance of, 252-253
Equipment, exercise. *See* Exercise equipment.
Ergonomics, 376-378
Erythema
    assessment of, 18-19
    inflammation and, 16, 117, *119*, 212
E-stim. *See* Electrical stimulation.
Evaluation, definition of, 14
Evaporation, cooling by, 47
Eversion, ankle, 5*b*, *243*
Evidence for physical agent efficacy, 38
Examination, definition of, 14
Excision
    olecranon, 431
    radial head, 430, 432
Exercise. *See also* Aerobic exercise; Range of motion (ROM);
        Strength training; Stretching.
    abnormal responses to, 28*t*
    blood pressure and, 27, 105

Exercise—cont'd
    bone healing and, 159
    cartilage healing and, 166-167, 171-172
    compartment syndrome from, 272
    cryotherapy with, 46
    design variables for, 82*b*, 94
    fatigue during, 28
    fever and, 17
    heart rate during, 26, 100-101
    inflammatory reactions after, 16, 17
    intramuscular temperature and, 59
    ligament healing and, 140-141
    modifications for, 9, 94
    muscle response to, 76, 81-83
    orthopedic disorders and, 108
    oxygen saturation and, 28
    progressive hip, *338-340*
    soreness after, 46, 83-84, 176
    tendon healing and, 189-190
    vascular response to, 94
    vital signs and, 28
Exercise equipment
    aerobic, 101-103, *104*
    balance training, 111, *112*, 113, *114*
    biomechanics of, 248
    continuous passive motion, 141-142
    strength testing/training, 80, *81*, 82*b*, 92-94,
        363-364
    stretching with, 67-68, *69*, *70*
Exertion
    perceived, scales for rating, 28, 101*b*
    strength and, 79
Exertional compartment syndrome, 272
Extension
    cervical, 383, 384, *385*
    elbow
        humeral-ulnar abduction for, 432
        olecranon fracture and, 431
    hip
        for iliopsoas muscle strain, 349
        post-fracture, *340*, *341*
        after total arthroplasty, 344, *345*
    illustrations of, *242*, *243*
    knee
        after ACL reconstruction, 295, 296, *297*, *299*, *300*
        after hip fractures, *339*, *340*
        for MCL injuries, 305
        modifications for, 9*b*
        for PCL injuries, 302, 303
        stretches for, 68, *69*
        after total hip replacement, *345*
    lumbar
        nucleus pulposus movement during, 361, *362*,
            370
        spondylolisthesis and, 375
    lumbar and thoracic
        for kyphosis, 380
        for lumbar disc injuries, *370*, *371*, *372*, *373*
        for lumbar sprains or strains, 365, *366*, *367*, 368
        for thoracic muscle injuries, 378, *379*
    measurement of, 5*b*
    wrist, for lateral epicondylitis, *423*
Extension lag in distal interphalangeal joint, 446
External fixation devices
    for Colles's fracture, 441, *442*
    fracture healing and, 156*t*
    types of, 157

External rotation
  hip
    test for, 71, *72*
    total arthroplasty and, 344
  measurement of, *5b*
  shoulder, *242*
    glenohumeral instability and, 399, 403-404
    for scapular stabilization, *395*
Extracellular matrix
  components and functions of, 124
  healing and formation of, *118*, 125, 138, 145
Extruded disc, 369

F

Fasciculi, muscle, 76, 176
Fasciectomy for Dupuytren's contracture, 445, *446*
Fasciitis, plantar, 277-278
Fasciotomy
  for compartment syndromes of lower leg, 272
  for plantar fasciitis, 278
Fast twitch (FT) muscle fibers
  description of, 77, 94
  exercise and adaptation of, 83, 181, 184-185
  immobilization effects on, 185
  types of, 177-178
Fat, subcutaneous
  function of, *121*
  heat conduction by, 40
  impedance of, 48
Fatigue, assessment of, 28. *See also* Muscle fatigue.
Feet. *See* Foot.
Femoral head
  replacement of, 342, 343-345
  vascular supply to, 335, *336*, 354
Femoral neck fracture, 335, *336*
Femoral nerve tension sign, 362
Femur
  anatomy of, patellofemoral pathology and, 325
  fractures of, *151*
    malunion of, *155*
    supracondylar, 317-318, 325
  patellar posture relative to, *310*
  proximal osteotomy of, 341-342
Fever, precautions for, 17-18
Fibrin clot in fracture repair, 154
Fibroblast growth factor (FGF), 125, 132, 180
Fibroblasts
  function of, *121*, 124
  in tendon, 187, 189
  in tissue healing, *120*, 125, 130
Fibrodysplasia, palmar, 445-446
Fibroelastic cartilage, 170. *See also* Meniscus.
Fibromyalgia, 30
Fibronectin, 124, 130
Fibroplasia in tissue healing, *120*, *122b*, 125, 130
Fibrotic adhesions, 72
Fibulocalcaneal ligament tears, *261*, 264
Fighter's fracture, 444-445
Figure-of-eight bandage for clavicular fracture, *409*
Figure-of-eight edema measurement technique, *20b*
Fingers
  Boutonnière deformity of, 447
  Dupuytren's contracture of, 445-446
  flexor tendon injuries of, 447-448
  mallet, 446-447
First-class lever, 247
"First-pass effect" of drugs, 208

"Five Ls" of lifting, 362-363
Fixation, fracture. *See also* Open reduction with internal fixation
    (ORIF).
  biomechanics of, 155-156
  devices for, 156-157
  external, 156
  healing responses to, 153, *156t*
  objectives for, 148
Fixed-load circuit, 104
Flatfoot, 278-279
Flexibility. *See also* Range of motion (ROM); Stretching.
  additional features for, 72
  assessment of, 30-31
  connective tissue properties and, 58-59, *60*
  definition of, 58
  measuring, 71, *71-72*
  stretching exercises for
    ballistic, 61-62, *63*
    low load, prolonged, 65-71
    proprioceptive neuromuscular facilitation, 62-63, *64-65*
    static, 59-61, *62*
Flexion
  cervical
    for disc injuries, 384
    for sprains and strains, 383, *384*, *385*
  elbow
    humeral-ulnar adduction for, 432-433
    olecranon fracture and, 431
  hip
    for iliopsoas muscle strain, 349
    post-fracture, *339*, *341*
    after total arthroplasty, 343, 344
  illustrations of, *242*, *243*
  knee
    after ACL reconstruction, 295, 296
    gait and, 221, *222*, 226
    after hip fractures, *340*
    for MCL injuries, 305
    after patellar fractures, 315, 317, 318
    after PCL reconstruction, 303
    stretches for, 67-68
    after tibial osteotomy, 323
    after total arthroplasty, *321*
  lumbar
    exercises for, 360, *361*
    fractures and, 376
    nucleus pulposus movement during, 361, *362*, 366, 370
    for spinal stenosis, 374
  measurement of, *5b*
  wrist, for lateral epicondylitis, *423*
Flexor tendon injuries of hand, 447-448
Fluoroquinolones, 209
Foam padding, balancing exercises on, *111b*
Foam test, 109
Food and Drug Administration (FDA), 208
Foot
  arch deformities of, 278-279
  fractures of
    calcaneal, *274*, *275*, 283
    stress, 276
    talar, 275
  gait and motion of, 221, *222*
  mobilization techniques for, 281-283
  Morton's neuroma of, 279-280
  plantar fasciitis of, 277-278
  toe deformities of, 280-281
Foot flat in gait cycle, *220*, *222*, *223t*

Footwear
    coefficient of friction for, 249*b*
    toe deformities from, 280, 281
Foraminal stenosis, 387
Force couple, description of, 246, 253
Force(s)
    aspects of, 245-246
    definition of, 79, 244
    effects of, *246, 249, 250*
    equilibrium and, 252-253
    levers and, 247-248
    mechanical loading, 250-252
    muscle contraction and, 94
    "overload," counterforce brace for, 423, *424*
    types of, 249-250
Forearm exercises for lateral epicondylitis, 423, *424*
Forward bend of trunk, *339*
Forward-bending test for disc herniation, 370
Four-point gait pattern, 224
Fractures
    additional features for, 159
    ankle, 273-274
    ankle sprains and, 262, 265
    arterial injuries with, 200*t*, 201
    calcaneal, *274, 275,* 283
    classifications of, 151-153
    clavicular, 409-410
    femoral head, hemiarthroplasty for, 342
    femur, supracondylar, 317-318, 325
    finger avulsion, 446
    fixation of
        biomechanics of, 155-156
        devices for, 156-157
    foot and ankle stress, 276
    Galeazzi's, 433
    healing of
        complications of, 155
        electrical stimulation for, 53
        factors influencing, 157-158
        immobilization and, 153, 154-155
        phases and process for, 154
        primary vs. secondary, 153
        rehabilitation techniques during, 159
        stabilization type and, 156*t*
        stimulation of, 158
        ultrasound for, 54
    hip
        classification and fixation of, 335-337
        rehabilitation after, 338-340, *341*
        subtrochanteric, problems with, 354
    humeral
        distal, *426,* 427-428
        intercondylar, 428-429
        proximal, 410-412
    humeral head impaction, 397-398, 415
    infection after, 209-210
    Lisfranc's, 283
    lumbar, *374,* 375-376
    metacarpal, 444-445
    Monteggia's, 433
    objectives for managing, 148
    olecranon, 430-432
    pars interarticularis, lumbar, *374, 375*
    patellar
        treatment of, 315, 317, 326
        types of, *317,* 325
    pelvic and acetabular, 350-353

Fractures—cont'd
    radial and ulnar, distal, 441-442, *443*
    radial head, 429-430
    scaphoid, 442-444
    scapular, 408-409
    signs and symptoms of, 31-32
    talar, 275
    tibial
        distal compression, 274-275
        medial stress, 277
        proximal, 318-320
Free nerve endings, 108
Freiberg's infraction, 283
Frequency of training
    aerobic exercise and, 100*b*, 101
    strength training and, 82*b*, 89, *90, 91*
Friction, 249
    applied force and, *250*
    coefficient of, 249*b*
    pulling force and, *249*
    stability and, 252-253
Frontal axis, movement around, 241
Frontal plane
    description of, 240, *241*
    movements in, 240-241, *242, 243*
"Frozen shoulder," 404-405
Fulcrum, lever, 247
Full weight bearing (FWB), 225
Functional balance training, 110
Functional capacity evaluations (FCEs), 376-378
Functional electrical stimulation (FES), 52
Functional instability, ankle, 266
Functional measurement of flexibility, 31

G
Gait, 217
    abnormalities of, 223-224
    additional features for, 226
    assessment of, 33
    assistive devices for
        negotiating stairs with, 225-226
        patient instruction for, 224, *225*
        selection of, 226
        weight bearing status and, 224-225
    definition of, 220
    knee flexion and ankle rotation in, *222*
    muscle function during, 223*t*
    muscle weakness and, 224*t*
    pelvic list in, *221*
    pes planus and, 279
    phases of, *220,* 222-223
    rehabilitation of
        after bunionectomy, 280
        after hip fractures, 338
        for lumbar strains, 366
        for spinal stenosis, 374
        after total hip replacement, 345
    terms and concepts for, 220-221
Gait cycle, *220,* 226
Galeazzi's fracture, 433
Gamekeeper's thumb, 444
Gamma-motor neurons, 178
Gastrocnemius/soleus complex
    exercises for
        for Achilles tendon injuries, *269, 271, 272*
        after calcaneal fractures, *275*
        for medial tibial stress, 277

Gastrocnemius/soleus complex—cont'd
  stretching, *62*
  gait mechanics and, *223t, 224t*
Gastrointestinal tract, NSAIDs and, 212
"Gate" system of pain control, 49
Gelatinases, 179
General adaptation syndrome, 94
Glenohumeral joint
  description of, 415
  instability and dislocation of, 397-404, 415
    nonoperative management of, 398-400, *401, 402, 403*
    operative management and rehabilitation for, 402-404
    pathophysiology of, 397-398
    shoulder impingement and, 393
  mobilization of
    proximal humerus fractures and, 410, 412
    techniques for, 413, 414, *415*
Glenoid fractures, 408-409
Glenoid labrum
  anatomy of, *398*
  avulsion of, *397, 398*
Glides
  ankle, 282
  distal metatarsal, 282, *283*
  glenohumeral, 414, *415*
  hip, 354
  joint motion via, 230, *231*
  metacarpal phalangeal, 449
  patellar, 323-324
  proximal interphalangeal, 283
  scapular, 413-414
  tibiofemoral, *324*
  traction vs., *232*
  wrist, *448, 449*
Gliding zone of articular cartilage, *163t*
Glucosamine sulfate, 169-170
Glucose metabolism, 178
Gluteus maximus/medius, gait mechanics and, *223t, 224t*
Glycocalyx "slime," 210
Glycogenolysis and glycolysis, 178
Glycoproteins, 124, 128
Glycosaminoglycans (GAGs)
  in articular cartilage, 163, 164
  oral administration of, 169-170
  tissue healing and, 128
  types of, 124, 134-135
Godfrey posterior tibial sag test, 301, *302*
"Golfer's elbow," 424-425
Golgi apparatus, 128
Golgi tendon organs (GTOs), 62, *63*
Goniometric measurements
  of flexibility, 31, 71
  standard, *5b*
Grades of injury, ligament, 139
Grafts
  for ACL reconstruction, 294-295, 325
  arthroscopic osteochondral, 167-168
  for fracture repair, 158, 443
  for PCL reconstruction, 302
  for peripheral nerve repair, 198
  vascular, 200
Granulation tissue
  description of, 135
  formation of, *118, 120*
Granulocyte-macrophage colony-stimulating factor (GM-CSF), *133t*
Granulomatosis, 15
Gravitation, law of, 250. *See also* Center of gravity (mass).

Greater trochanteric bursitis, 346-347
Greenstick fractures, 151
Grip strength, measurement of, *80*
Groin pull, 348-349
Gross dissection of ligament, 144
Ground reaction forces, 249
Ground substance, 124, 135
Group fascicular neurorrhaphy, *197*
Growth factors. *See* Cytokines and growth factors.
Guarding, reflex muscle, 52, *66*
Guide to Physical Therapist Practice (APTA), 14, 49
"Gunstock deformity" of elbow, 430
Guyon's canal, 449

H
Half-life, drug, 214
Hallux valgus, 280
Hammer, forearm exercises with, 423, *424*
Hammer toes, 280-281
Hamstrings
  flexibility tests for, *71, 72*
  gait mechanics and, *223t*
  strains of, 347-348
  strengthening
    after ACL reconstruction, 296, 299
    after PCL injury or repair, 302, 303
    after tibial osteotomy, 323
    after total hip replacement, *344*
  stretches for
    knee extension with, 68, *69*
    for patellofemoral disorders, 312
    static, *60, 61*
  tightness of, patellofemoral compression and, *311*
Hand
  Boutonnière deformity of, 447
  Dupuytren's contracture of, 445-446
  flexor tendon injuries of, 447-448
  mallet finger of, 446-447
  metacarpal fractures of, 444
  mobilization of, 448-449
  thumb sprains of, 444
Handwashing, 17
Hard callus, formation of, 154, 156
"Hard" signs of arterial injury, 199, 201
Hard-tissue stretch end-feel, 232
Harness for acromioclavicular injuries, 406
Haversian bone, 148
H-band of sarcomere, *77*
Healing, tissue. *See* Tissue healing.
Heart attack, pain patterns in, 24, *25*
Heart rate
  age-adjusted maximum and target, 100-101
  assessment of, *5b*, 26
  exercise and abnormal, *28t*
Heat
  application of
    contrast bath for, 47
    diathermy for, 44-45
    hot packs for, 39-40
    paraffin for, 40-41
    skin assessment during, *40b*
    stretching exercises and, 59, 66, 67, *68*
    ultrasound for, 41-44
  inflammation and, 16, 117, *119*, 212
  physiologic effects of, 39, 54
  transmission of, 53-54
Heel off in gait cycle, *220, 222, 223t*

Heel orthosis
    for Achilles tendon injuries, 269, 270
    for plantar fasciitis, 278
Heel raises after Achilles tendon rupture, 270-271, *272*
Heel slides after hip fracture, *340*
Heel spur syndrome, 277-278
Heel strike in gait cycle, *220, 222, 223t*
Hemarthrosis
    of knee, 8, 290
    signs of, 33
Hemiarthroplasty
    hip, 342
    shoulder, 413
Hemi-walkers, 226
Heparin, 201
Herniated nucleus pulposus (HNP)
    cervical, 384-385
    classification of, 387
    lumbar
        classification of, 368-369
        invasive management of, 372-373
        nonsurgical rehabilitation for, 369-372
        tests for, 362
    pain assessment for, 23-24, 370
    thoracic, 378
Heterolysis, cellular, 133
Heterotopic bone formation
    muscle trauma and, 181, 190
    olecranon fracture-dislocation and, 431, 432
High tibial osteotomy, 322-323, *323*, 325
Hill-Sachs lesion, 397-398, 415
Hip
    additional features for, 354
    dislocation of, 337, *338*
    external rotation test for, 71, *72*
    fractures of
        classification and management of, 335-337
        rehabilitation after, 338-340, *341*
    hemiarthroplasty of, 342
    Legg-Calvé-Perthes disease of, 345-346
    mobilization techniques for, 353-355
    movement patterns for, *243*
    progressive exercises for, *339-340*
    prosthetic, fixation of, 343
    proximal femoral osteotomy for, 341-342
    range of motion in, *5b*
    soft-tissue injuries of, 346-350
    total replacement of, 343-345
Hip abductors, gait mechanics and, *223t*
Hip adductors
    gait mechanics and, *223t*
    strains of, 348-349
Hip flexors
    gait mechanics and, 223
    "pull" of, 349
    stretching, *340*
Hip pointer, 349-350
Histamine, tissue injury and, 117, 212, *213*
Histochemical changes in endurance training, 105
HNP. *See* Herniated nucleus pulposus (HNP).
Hold-relax in PNF stretching, 63, *65*
Homan's sign, reliability of, 19, 201
Hooke's law, 72
Hopping, 87, 111
Horizontal plane
    description of, *241*
    movements in, 240, *242, 243*

Hostility
    description of, 6, 10
    dimensions of, *8, 9*
Hot packs, application of, 39-40. *See also* Heat.
Hueter-Volkmann law, 150
Hughston jerk test for ACL stability, 293
Humeral head
    distraction of, 414
    impaction fracture of, 397-398, 415
Humeral-ulnar abduction and adduction, 432-433
Humerus
    anatomy of, *410*
    fractures of
        intercondylar, 428-429
        proximal, 410-412
        supracondylar, *426*, 427-428
    proximal, prosthesis for, *413*
Hunting effect, 46
Hyaline cartilage, 163. *See also* Articular cartilage.
Hyaluronic acid, intraarticular injection of, 170
Hydroxyproline in collagen, 164
Hyperemia, reactive, 94
Hyperextension
    cervical injuries from, 382, 383
    thumb sprain from, *444*
    wrist injuries from, 439, *440*, 443
Hyperflexion, cervical injuries from, 382
Hypermobility, joint, 234
Hyperplasia
    intimal, 199
    muscle, strength training and, 83
Hypersensitivity to cold, 46, 47
Hypertrophy
    cellular, injury and, 133
    ligament, exercise and, 140-141
    muscular
        assessment for, 30
        children and, 92
        elderly and, 90-91
        strength training and, 81, 83
Hypomobility, joint, 234
Hypotension, orthostatic, 27

I
I-bands of sarcomere, 177
Ice
    for Achilles tendon injuries, 268, 269, 270
    application of, 45-46
    after glenohumeral stabilization, 402
    for hip soft-tissue injuries, 346, 347
    after low-load, prolonged stretch, 67
    for medial tibial stress syndrome, 277
    in RICE program, 262 263 (*See also* RICE)
Ice massage, 45, 46
Iliopectineal bursitis, 347
Iliopsoas muscle
    gait mechanics and, *223t*
    strain of, 349
Iliotibial band stretches
    for patellar tracking disorders, *312*, 313
    for trochanteric bursitis, 346
Ilium
    contusions of, 349-350
    fractures of, 350, *351*
Immobilization
    effects of
        articular cartilage and, 164-165

Immobilization—cont'd
    bone and, 153, 154-155
    ligaments and, 139-140, 141
    muscle and, 183-184, 188
    tendons and, 188
    techniques and rehabilitation for
        for Achilles tendon injuries, 269, 270
        after ACL reconstruction, 295, 297
        for acromioclavicular sprain/dislocation, 406, 407
        for adhesive capsulitis, 404-405
        for ankle sprains, 263-265
        after ankle stabilization surgery, 265, 266
        for carpal tunnel syndrome, 438-439
        for clavicular fractures, 409
        for De Quervain's tenosynovitis, 439
        after flexor tendon repair of hand, 447
        for glenohumeral instability/dislocation, 398, 402
        after high tibial osteotomy, 323
        for humeral fractures, 410-411, 427, 428, 429
        for knee fractures, 315, 317, 318
        for MCL sprains, 305
        after meniscal repair, 309
        for metacarpal fractures, 444-445
        for muscle injuries, 185, 186b
        for olecranon fracture-dislocation, 430-431
        after patellar realignment, 314
        after PCL injury or repair, 302, 303
        for pelvic/acetabular fractures, 351
        after peroneal tendon repair, 267-268
        for radial head fractures, 430
        after rotator cuff repair, 396, 397
        for scaphoid fractures, 443-444
        for scapular fractures, 408, 409
        after shoulder arthroplasty, 413
        for skier's thumb, 444
        after total knee replacement, 321
        for wrist sprains, 439-440
Impacted fractures
    description of, 151
    of humeral head, 397-398, 415
Impedance, electrical stimulation and, 48
Implants. *See* Grafts; Internal fixation devices; Prostheses.
Impulse, definition of, 244
Impulse inertial exercise apparatus, 94
Incomplete fractures, 151
Incomplete muscle tears, 179
Indirect muscle injury
    definition of, 176
    therapeutic interventions for, 186b
Inductive coil applicators in diathermy, 44-45
Inductive coupling in electrical stimulation, 159
Induration, thrombophlebitis and, 19
Inertia
    definition of, 244
    Newton's law of, 248
Inertial training, 94b
Infection control
    fever and, 17
    paraffin use and, 41
Infections
    antibiotics for, 205, 208-209
    bone healing and, 158
    prevention and treatment of, 209-211
    skin color and, 18
    temperature and, 17
    tissue healing and, 127
Inferential current (IFC) units, 49
Inferior, definition of, 240b

Inflammation
    acute vs. chronic, 16-17, 212-214
    antiinflammatory agents for, 205, 211-212, 213
    cardinal signs of, 16, 117, 119, 212
    contraindications and precautions for, 16
    description of, 15-16
    RICE for, 262-263
    skin color and, 18-19
    systemic, 135
    temperature and, 17
    tissue healing and
        bone, 154, 159
        cartilage, 165-166
        cells and mediators for, 128, 130, 131, 131t-133t
        ligament, 138, 144
        muscle, 178-179
        processes during, 117-118, 119, 125, 127
        tendon, 187
Insulin-like growth factor (IGF), 125, 130
Intensity of training
    aerobic exercise and, 100-101
    strength training and, 82b, 89, 90, 91
Intercondylar fractures of humerus, 428-429
Interferon γ, 133t
Interleukins
    inflammation and, 212, 214
    tissue healing and, 125, 130, 131t-132t
Intermittent claudication, 24
Intermittent pneumatic compression, 201
Internal fixation devices. *See also* Open reduction with internal
        fixation (ORIF).
    for acromioclavicular stabilization, 407, 408
    for ankle fractures, 274
    fracture healing and, 155, 156t
    for hip fractures, 337
    infection related to, 209-210
    for intercondylar humerus fractures, 428, 429
    for patellar fractures, 315, 317
    for proximal humerus fractures, 410
    for supracondylar femur fractures, 317, 318
    for tibial plateau fractures, 320
    types of, 157, 158t
Internal rotation
    hip
        illustration of, 243
        after joint replacement, 343, 344
    measurement of, 5b
    shoulder, 242, 395
Intertrochanteric hip fractures, 335, 336, 337
Intertrochanteric osteotomy of femur, 341-342
Interval training, 102
Intervertebral disc. *See* Disc, intervertebral.
Intimal hyperplasia, 199
Intraarticular fractures, 152
Intrathoracic pressure, exercise and, 105
Intrinsic material properties, 253
Inversion, ankle, 5b, 243
Inversion ankle sprains
    chronic instability after, 265-266, 267
    clinical examination of, 261-262
    mechanisms and classification of, 260-261
    rehabilitation for, 262-265
Iontophoresis, 53
Irritability, contractile tissue, 29
Ischemia
    cold, description of, 201
    nerve compression and, 195
    supracondylar humerus fractures and, 427

Ischial bursitis, 347
Ischial tuberosity, avulsion fractures of, *350*
Isoinertial back strength testing, 363, 364
Isoinertial contractions, 79
Isokinetic exercise
    ACL stability testing with, 299
    isotonic vs., 82*b*
    muscle contractions in, 77, 79
    strength testing with, 80, 363, 364
    systems and protocols for, 93
    velocity spectrum training in, 84-85
Isometric exercise. *See also* Strength training.
    back strength testing with, 363-364
    during bone healing, 159
    modification of, 9
    multiple-angle, *86*
    during muscle healing, 185-186
    progressive training with, 80-81, 82*b*
    rule of tens for, 86
Isometric muscle contractions, 77, 80-81
Isostation B-200, back strength testing with, 364
Isotonic exercise. *See also* Strength training.
    equipment and systems for, 93
    isokinetic vs., 82*b*
    knee extension with, 9*b*, 67-68
    muscle contraction velocity in, 84, 85
    muscle contractions in, 77, 79
    plyometric vs., 88
    progressive training with, 80-81, 82*b*
    strength testing with, 80, *81*
Isthmic spondylolisthesis, lumbar, 374, 375

J

Jogging. *See* Running.
"Joint play," 230
Joints. *See also* Arthroplasty; Cartilage; Mobilization, joint.
    accessory motions of, 32, 230, *231*, 253
    assessment of, 32-33
    compressive loads on, 84, 90, *91*
    congruency of, 230-231
    contractures of, stretching, 65-71
    convex-concave rule for, *230*, 231
    corticosteroid injections into, 211-212
    end-feel in, 29, 30, 32, 232-233, 234
    fractures involving, 159
    hyaluronic acid injections into, 170
    hypermobility/hypomobility of, 234
    immobilization and, 139-140
    major movements of, *242-243*
    mechanoreceptors in, 108
    range of motion in (*See also* Range of motion (ROM))
        capsular/noncapsular patterns of, 233, 234
        definition of, 58
        grades for, 231-232, 234
        measuring, 5*b*, 31, 71
    of shoulder complex, 415
    stability of, 71, 234
Judgments, making, 14, 15
Jumps, plyometric, 87

K

Karvonen formula for target heart rate, 100-101
Keratan sulfate, 124
Kienböck's disease, 449
Kinematics
    concepts in, 244-245
    definition of, 240
Kinesthesia, 108

Kinesthetic ability training device (KAT), *112*, 113
Kinetic energy, 252
Kinetics
    definition of, 240, 245
    forces in
        aspects of, 245-246
        coefficient of friction for, 249*b*
        effects of, *246*, 249
        types of, 249-250
    levers in, 246-248
    Newton's laws of motion in, 248-249
Kirschner wires, 428, *429*
Knee
    additional features for, 325-326
    anterior drawer test of, *71*
    contractures of, stretching, *66*, 67-69
    fractures of, 315-320
    gait and flexion of, 221, *222*, 226
    high tibial osteotomy for, 322-323
    ligament injuries of
        anterior cruciate, 290-300
        degrees of, 290
        healing of, 138-139
        medial collateral, 303-305
        posterior cruciate, 300-303
        remobilization and exercise for, 141-144
    meniscus of
        composition and functions of, 170-171, 305, *306*
        injury and repair of, 171-172, 305-309
    mobilization techniques for, 323-325
    movement patterns for, *243*
    osteoarthritis of, strength training and, 90, *91*
    patellofemoral conditions of, 309-315
    range of motion in, 5*b*
    reconstruction of, 320-322
    rehabilitation of
        isokinetic systems for, 93*b*
        treatment modifications during, 8-9
Knee extension machines, 67-68
Knee-to-chest exercises
    for hip rehabilitation, *340*
    for low back problems, *361*
    for spinal stenosis, 374
Knight's DAPRE program, 85
Knock-knees, tibial osteotomy for, 322-323
Korotkoff sounds, 27
Krebs cycle, 178
KT1000/KT2000 knee ligament arthrometers, 293*b*, 294
Kyphosis, 378-380, 386

L

Labile cells, 134
Lachman examination for ACL stability, 293
Lactate/lactic acid, 178
Lamellar bone, 148, 253
Lamina, vascular, 179, 198
Laminectomy, decompression, 375
Laminin, 124
Laminotomy with decompression discectomy, 372, *373*
Lat bar pull-down for thoracic muscle injuries, *379*
Lateral, definition of, 240*b*
Lateral ankle sprains
    chronic instabilities after, 265-266, *267*
    clinical examination of, 261-262
    mechanisms and classification of, 260-261
    rehabilitation for, 262-265
Lateral collateral ligament, injuries of, 300
Lateral compartment of lower leg, 272

Lateral epicondylitis of elbow, 422-424
Lateral meniscus of knee, *306*
Lateral retinacular release of patella, 314
Lateral trunk exercises for scoliosis, *381, 382, 383*
Lauge-Hansen classification of ankle fractures, *273*
Leading questions, *7*
Leg curls after ACL reconstruction, 296
Leg press
    after ACL reconstruction, *297*
    for patellofemoral conditions, *313*
    after PCL injuries, 302
Leg raises
    after ACL reconstruction, *142*
    after hip fractures, 338, *341*
    for lumbar strains, 365
Legend drugs, regulation of, 208
Legg-Calvé-Perthes (LCP) disease, 345-346
Legs
    aerobic activities for, *102*, 103, *104*
    balance training for, 110-113
    in lifting mechanics, 363
Letornel classification of acetabular fractures, 351, *352*
Leukocytes
    function of, *121*
    in inflammatory response, 213, 214
    in ligament healing, 138
    in tissue healing, *119*, 125, 128, 130
Leukotrienes
    inhibition of, *211*, 212, *213*
    synthesis of, 130, *131*, 213
Levers
    classification of, 246-248
    in lifting mechanics, 362-363
Lifting
    after lumbar disc injuries, 371, 372
    mechanics of, 362-363
    torque during, *246*
Ligament-augmentation devices (LAD), 294
Ligaments
    adhesions of, joint motion and, 233
    anatomy of, 138, 144, 145, *188*
    ankle, chronic instabilities of, 265-266, *267*
    assessment of, 32-33
    elbow, stability of, 433
    healing of
        ACL autografts and, 295
        additional features for, 144-145
        exercise and, 140-141
        immobilization and, 139-140
        nonsurgical vs. surgical repair and, 139
        phases of, 138-139
        remobilization and exercise for, 141-144
        therapeutic considerations during, 144*t*
    injuries of
        acromioclavicular, 405-408
        ankle, 260-265
        cervical spinal, 382-384, *385*
        grades of, 139
        knee, 290-305, 325
        lumbar spinal, 367-368
        ulnar collateral of thumb, 444
        ulnar medial collateral, 425-427
        wrist, 439-440, *441*, 441*b*
    mechanical properties of, 138
    stability tests for
        ACL, 292-294, 299
        ankle, 261, *262*, 262*b*

Ligaments—cont'd
    MCL, 304
    PCL, 300-301
    ulnar MCL, *425*
    triangular fibrocartilage complex, 449
Lincosamide antibiotics, 209
Line of application of force, 245, *246*
Line of gravity, stability and, 253
Linear elastic material, 253
Linear force, 79
Linear motion, biomechanics of, 244-245
Lipids in extracellular matrix, 124
Lipoxygenase, inhibition of, *211*, 212
Lisfranc's fracture, 283
Listening, 5, 10
Load-deformation curve, 250, *252*
Loading, mechanical, 250-252
Load(s)
    definition of, 250
    in lifting mechanics, 362
    types of, 72, 250, *251*
Local muscular endurance, 103-104
Long-axis distraction
    of hip, 353
    metacarpal phalangeal, 449
    proximal interphalangeal, *283*
    of talus, 282
    of wrist, *448*, 449
Longitudinal axis, movement around, 240
Longitudinal tear of meniscus, *306*
Loose end-feel, 233
Loose-packed joint position, 230-231
Lordosis
    in lifting mechanics, 363
    maintaining/enhancing
        lumbar disc injuries and, *370*, 371-372
        lumbar sprains and, 368
Low back. *See* Back; Lumbar spine.
Low-load, prolonged stretch
    Codman's pendulum exercises for, 69, *70*, 71
    commercial tools for, 69, *70*
    technique and application of, 66-69
Low-molecular-weight heparin, 201
Lumbar spine
    additional features for, 387
    disc herniation of
        classification of, 368-369
        invasive management of, 372-373
        nonsurgical rehabilitation for, 369-372
    ergonomics and functional capacity evaluations for, 376-378
    fractures of, 375-376
    injuries of
        back school model for, 376, 377*b*
        epidemiology of, 360
        treatment of, 360, *361*
    lifting fundamentals for, 362-363
    ligament sprains of, 367-368
    measuring strength of, 363-364
    mechanical stress on, 250
    mobilization of, 386-387
    muscle strains of, 364-367
    scoliosis of, 380-382, *383*
    spondylolysis and spondylolisthesis of, 374-375
    stenosis of, 373-374
    structure and mechanics of, 360-362
"Lungs" in lifting mechanics, 363

Lymph nodes, fever and, 17-18
Lymph nodes and vessels, *18*
Lymphocytes
  in inflammatory response, 213, 214
  in tissue healing, 125, 138
Lysosomes, 128

M

MacConaill's classification of accessory joint movements, 230, *231*
Macrocycle, periodization program, 89, 90
Macrolide antibiotics, 209
Macrophages
  in chronic inflammation, 214
  function of, *121*
  in tissue healing, *119*, 125, 128, 130
Magnusen-Stack procedure for glenohumeral stabilization, 402
Malleolar fractures of ankle, 273-274
Mallet finger, 446-447
Mallet toes, 280-281
Malnutrition, bone healing and, 158
Malunion, fracture
  description of, 155
  subtrochanteric hip, 336
Manipulation, joint, 234
Manual muscle testing
  description of, 79
  format for recording, 29*b*
  scales for, *5b, 79b*
  techniques for, 29-30
Mass. *See also* Center of gravity (mass).
  definition of, 244
  kinetic energy and, 252
  stability and, 252, 253*b*
Massage
  for carpal tunnel syndrome, 439
  ice, 45, 46
  after palmar fasciectomy, 445
  for reflex sympathetic dystrophy, 448
Mast cells
  function of, *121*
  histamine release from, 212, *213*
Matrix
  bone, components of, 148, 159
  extracellular
    components and functions of, 124
    healing and formation of, *118*, 125, 138, 145
Matrix metalloproteinases (MMPs), 179-180
Maturation
  in ligament healing, 138, 144, 145
  in tissue healing, 122*b*, 125, *127*, 128, 135
Maximal oxygen uptake (VO$_2$ max), 100
Maximal volitional isometric contraction (MVIC), 51
Maximum heart rate (MHR), age-adjusted, 100
Maximum heart rate reserve (MHR reserve), 100-101
Maximum static friction, 249, *250*
McGill-Melzack Pain Questionnaire, *22*
MCL. *See* Medial collateral ligament (MCL).
McMurray test for meniscal injury, 307
Measurement
  of aerobic intensity, 100-101
  of arch varus and valgus, 278
  of back strength, 363-364
  of edema, 19, 20, 21*b*
  of flexibility, 31, 71, *71-72*
  of knee ligament stability, 293-294
  of muscle strength, 29-30, 79-80
  of pain, 21-22, *23*

Measurement—cont'd
  of quadriceps angle, *311*
  scales for, 4, *5b*
  of vital signs, 17, 26-28
Mechanical advantage (MA), 247
Mechanical instability, ankle, repair of, 265, *266*, *267*
Mechanical loading, 250-252
Mechanical Research Council Grading System for nerve recovery, 198
Mechanical strain or stress, 250, *251*
Mechanoreceptors
  in anterior cruciate ligament, 325
  description of, 115
  loss of, hip arthroplasty and, 345
  in meniscus of knee, 170
  in tendon, 187
  types of, 108
Medial, definition of, 240*b*
Medial ankle sprains, 265
Medial collateral ligament (MCL)
  knee, injuries of, 303-305, 325
    ACL injuries with, 300
    healing of, 138-139
    intraarticular effusion and, 290
    mechanisms of, 303-304
    mobilization and exercise for, 142, *143*, 144
    rehabilitation for, 304-305
    surgical vs. nonsurgical repair of, 139
    tests for, 304
  ulnar
    rupture of, *426*
    stability test for, *425*
    valgus stress overload of, 425-427
Medial epicondylitis of elbow, 424-425
Medial meniscus of knee, *304*, *306*
Medial tibial stress syndrome, 276-277
Medial valgus stress overload of elbow, 425-427
Median nerve, compression neuropathy of, 438-439
Medications
  additional features for, 214
  antibiotic, 208-211
  anticoagulant, 201
  antiinflammatory
    action of, 130, *131*, *211*, *213*
    nonsteroidal, 212
    steroidal, 211-212, 372
  classification of, 208
  common orthopedic, 205
  pharmacokinetics/pharmacodynamics of, 208
  topical, delivery of
    iontophoresis for, 53
    phonophoresis for, 43
Meniscectomy, 171-172, 308
Meniscus
  composition and function of, 170-171, 172, 305, *306*
  injuries of
    ACL injuries with, 300
    additional features for, 172, 325, 326
    clinical examination of, 306-307
    healing after, 171
    management of, 307-308
    mechanisms of, 306
    medial, MCL injuries and, *304*
    rehabilitation after, 163, 171-172, 308-309
    types of, 305-306
  surgical repair of, 171, 308
Meralgia paresthetica, 195
Mesocycle, periodization program, 89, 90

Metabolism
  aerobic vs. anaerobic, 100
  drug, 208, 214
  muscle tissue, 178
Metacarpal fractures, 444-445
Metacarpal phalangeal joint, mobilization of, 449
Metal implants
  bacterial adherence to, *210*
  diathermy and, 45
  electrical stimulation and, 53
Metaphyseal fractures, *152*
Metatarsals
  mobilization of, 282, *283*
  stress fractures of, 276
Microcycle, periodization program, 89-90
Microfracture, cartilage repair by, 167, *168*
Microtrauma, muscle or tendon, 176. *See also* Overuse injuries.
Midstance and midswing in gait cycle, *220*, 222, 223*t*
Milwaukee brace for scoliosis, 380
Minitrampoline, balance training on, 111, 113, *114*
  after ACL reconstruction, *299*
  for ankle sprains, *264*
Miserable malalignment syndrome, 310
Mitochondria
  aerobic metabolism in, 100, 178
  functions of, 128
Mobile WAD of Henry, 433
Mobility
  description of, 115
  at fracture site, 32, 159
Mobilization, joint, 217
  additional features for, 234
  ankle, foot and toe, 281-283
  articular surfaces and, *230*
  capsular and noncapsular patterns in, 233
  clinical application of, 233-234
  convex-concave rule for, *230*, 231
  definition of, 230, 234
  elbow, 432-433
  end-feel during, 29, 30, 32, 232-233
  grades of, 231-232, 234
  hip, 353-355
  indications and contraindications for, 233
  knee, 323-325
  ligament healing and, 141-144
  principles of, 230-231
  shoulder, 413-414, *415*
    for adhesive capsulitis, 405
    after proximal humerus fractures, 410, 412
  spinal, 386-387
  tendon healing and, 187-188
  traction and glide in, *232*
  wrist and hand, 448-449
Mode of activity, definition of, 101
Modifications, treatment, 8-9
Moment arm of force, 246, 247
Moment arm of resistance, 247-248
Moment of force, 246
Momentum, 244
Monocytes
  in inflammatory response, 213, 214
  in tissue healing, *119*, 125, 128, 130
Monteggia's fracture, 433
Morton's neuroma, 279-280
Motion, Newton's laws of, 248-249
Motor end plates, 178
Motor nerves
  assessing recovery of, 198
  injury to, 194

Motor nerves—cont'd
  regeneration of, 180
  types of, 178
Motor units
  components of, 178
  "size principle" in recruitment of, 181, 184
Movement, biomechanics of. *See* Biomechanics.
Multiple-angle isometrics, 86
Mumford procedure, 415
Muscle contractions
  comparison of, 80-81, 82*b*
  during gait cycle, 222-223
  physiology of, 76-77, 94, 176, 178
  types of, 77-79, 94
  velocity of, 84-85
Muscle fatigue
  assessment of, 28
  electrical stimulation and, 51, 52
  local muscular endurance and, 103-104
  physiological changes with, 105
Muscle fibers
  contractile unit of, 77, 177
  exercise and adaptation of, 83, 182-183
  fatigue and changes in, 105
  immobilization and, 184-185
  organization of, *76*, 125, 176
  types of, 77, 94, 177-178
Muscle spasm, 30, 52, 232
Muscle spindles, stretch reflex and, 62-63, *64*
Muscles
  assessment of, 29-31
  bioenergetics of, 178
  biology of, 76-79, 176-178
  delayed onset soreness of, 46, 83-84, 176
  electrical stimulation for, 50-52
  exercise effects on, 76, 81-83, 94
  flexibility of, 30-31
  gait and function of, 223-224
  healing of
    processes during, 178-180
    rehabilitation techniques during, 185-186
  immobilization and, 139, 140, 185-186, 189
  injuries of
    blunt, 190
    classification of, 180-181
    overuse, 31
    types of, 176
    weight lifting and, 92
  palpation of, 30
  posterior thigh, *348*
  resistance exercise and adaptation of, 181, 184, *182-184*
  smooth vascular, 198
  strain of (*See* Strain)
  strength testing for, 5*b*, 29-30, 79-80 (*See also* Strength)
  stretching
    active exercises for, 59-63, *64-65*
    contractures and, 65-71
    evaluating pain while, 30
    responses to, 59
  tears of, 179
  viscoelastic properties of, 59, 125
Musculoskeletal structures, assessment of, 29-33
Musculotendinous junction, 187
Myelin sheath, *195*
Myocardial infarction, pain patterns in, 24, *25*
Myofibers. *See* Muscle fibers.
Myofibrils
  contractile proteins in, 94, 177
  structure of, 76, 77

Myosin, 76-77, 177
Myositis ossificans
 muscle trauma and, 181, 190
 olecranon fracture-dislocation and, 431, 432

N

National Osteoporosis Foundation, 32
Neck, movement patterns for, *242*
Necrosis, tissue or cellular. *See also* Avascular necrosis (AVN).
 description of, 134
 processes in, *127, 133, 134*
Neer's stages of rotator cuff impingement, 393, 415
Nerve blocks, sympathetic, 448
Nerve entrapment in carpal tunnel syndrome, 438, 439
Nerves, peripheral. *See also* Mechanoreceptors.
 additional features for, 201
 architecture of, *195*
 connective tissue of, *121*, 201
 disorders of, electrical stimulation for, 50-51
 injury to
  causes and classification of, 194-195, 201
  compression or traction and, 195-197
  hip dislocation and, 354
  recovery after, 197-198
  regeneration after, 180
  surgical repair of, 197, 201
 mechanical behavior of, 194
 resistance exercise and, 182-183
 vascular supply to, 194, *196*, 201
 visceral pain transmission by, 25, *26*
Neurapraxia, 194, 197
Neurogenic claudication, 373-374, 387
Neurogenic low back pain, 369
Neuroma, plantar interdigital, 279-280
Neuromuscular electrical stimulation (NMES), 49, 51. *See also* Electrical stimulation.
Neuromuscular fatigue, 103-104, 105
Neuromuscular junction, 178
Neuropathy
 Charcot's, 283
 compression and traction, 195-197, 362
 median nerve, 438-439
Neurorrhaphy, 197, 201
Neurotmesis
 description of, 195, 201
 surgical repair of, 197
Neutral phrase or question, 7
Neutrophils, *119*, 128, 138
Newton's laws of motion, 248-249
NMES. *See* Neuromuscular electrical stimulation (NMES).
Node of Ranvier, *195*
Noncapsular pattern of joint movement, 233
Nonconstrained knee implants, 320-321
Noncontact force, 249, 250
Noncontractile muscle tissue
 functions of, 125, 176
 types of, 76, 94
Nonsteroidal antiinflammatory drugs (NSAIDs), 205
 action of, 130, *131, 211, 212, 213*
 adverse reactions to, 212
Nonunion, fracture
 description of, 155
 scaphoid, 442, 443
 subtrochanteric hip, 336
Non-weight bearing (NWB) status, 224-225
Normal reaction force, 249
Normative Model of Physical Therapist Assistant Education (APTA), 15, 21, 38
Nucleus, muscle fiber, *76*

Nucleus pulposus. *See also* Herniated nucleus pulposus (HNP).
 fluid mechanics of, 361, *362*, 366, 370
 structure and function of, 360, *361*

O

Objective data
 examples of, 9
 SOAP documentation of, 34
Oblique fractures, 151
Olecranon
 fractures of, 430-432
 valgus stress overload and, 425
One-arm cycling, *103*
Open fractures
 definition of, 152
 infection after, 209-210
Open kinetic chain (OKC) exercise, 88-89. *See also* Strength training.
 after ACL reconstruction, 296
 example of, *89*
 after PCL injury, 302
Open reduction with internal fixation (ORIF)
 for ankle fractures, *274*
 for Colles's fractures, 441, 442
 description of, 157
 for hip fractures, 336
 infection after, preventing and treating, 209-210
 for intercondylar humerus fractures, 428, *429*
 for lumbar spine fractures, 376
 for metacarpal fractures, 445
 for olecranon fractures, 431
 for patellar fractures, 315, *316, 317*
 for pelvic/acetabular fractures, 350, 351
 for proximal humerus fractures, 410-411
 for radial head fractures, 430
 for scaphoid fractures, 443
 for skier's thumb, 444
 for supracondylar femur fractures, 317, *318*
 for tibial plateau fractures, 318, *320*
 for wrist sprains, 440
Open-ended questions, 6, *7*, 8, 10
"Opiate" system of pain control, 49
Organelles, cell, 128
Orthopedic management. *See* Physical therapy (PT); Rehabilitation.
Orthosis
 for Achilles tendon injuries, 269, 270
 for hallux valgus, 280
 hip abduction, 345-346
 for lumbar spondylolisthesis, 375
 for pes planus or cavus, 279
 for plantar fasciitis, 278
 for toe deformities, 281
Orthostatic hypotension, 27
Os trigonum, 283
Oscillations in joint mobilization, 231-232, 233
Osteoarthritis. *See also* Degenerative joint disease (DJD).
 aerobic activities for, 103
 cartilage changes in, 165*t*
 causes and stages of, 165, *166*
 glucosamine/chondroitin supplements for, 169-170
 of hip
  arthroplasty for, 343
  intertrochanteric osteotomy for, 341-342
 hyaluronic acid injections for, 170
 of knee
  arthroplasty for, 320
  tibial osteotomy for, 322-323
  valgus and varus deformity in, *322*
 rehabilitation and, 163

Osteoarthritis—cont'd
  shoulder arthroplasty for, 413
  strength training and, 90, *91*
Osteoblasts, 148, 153, 159
Osteochondral autograft transplantation system (OATS), 167-168
Osteoclasts and osteocytes, 148, 153, 159
Osteoinduction, 158
Osteokinematics, 234
Osteomalacia, 153
Osteon, 148
Osteonecrosis of hip
  arthroplasty for, 342, 343
  description of, 354
  fractures and, 335
Osteoporosis, 152-153
  fractures associated with
    intercondylar humeral, *429*
    lumbar, 375
    physical assessment and, 31-32
  kyphosis and, 379
Osteotendinous junction, 187
Osteotomy
  high tibial, 322-323, 325
  for medial valgus stress overload, 426
  proximal femoral, 341-342
"Overload forces," counterforce brace for, 423, *424*
Overload principle, 83
Over-the-counter drugs, regulation of, 208
Overuse injuries
  of Achilles tendon, 268-269
  assessment of, 31
  classification of, 134
  definition of, 176
  of elbow, 422-427
  of medial tibia, 276-277
  treatment strategy for, 135
  of wrist and hand, 438-439
Oxford exercise program, 85
Oxidative enzymes, 104
Oxidative phosphorylation, 100, 178
Oxygen consumption
  aerobic exercise and, 100
  circuit training and, 105
Oxygen saturation, measurement of, 27-28

P

Pacinian mechanoreceptors, 108
Pain
  anterior knee
    causes of, 310-311
    nonoperative rehabilitation for, 311-313
    postoperative rehabilitation for, 313-315
  assessment of, 21-26
  in deep vein thrombosis, 200
  delayed onset muscle, 46, 83-84, 176
  fracture-associated, 31-32
  in heart attack, *25*
  inflammation and, 16, 17, 117, *119*, 212, *213*
  intermittent claudication, 24
  low back
    categories of, 369
    evaluation of, 362, 370
    prevalence of, 360
    prevention and education for, 376, *377b*
    strains or sprains with, 364
  management of
    cryotherapy for, 46

Pain—cont'd
    electrical stimulation for, 48-50, 52
    hot packs for, 39
    joint mobilization and, 233
    for Morton's neuroma, 279
    for reflex sympathetic dystrophy, 448
    RICE for, 262-263
    treatment modifications for, 8, 9
  measurement of, *5b*, 21-23
  mechanoreceptors for, 108
  in medial tibial stress syndrome, 276
  neurogenic claudication, 374
  on palpation or stretching, 30
  patient behavior and, 25-26
  pleuritic, pulmonary embolism and, 201
  "red flag" patterns for, 24, *25*
  referred, 24
  during strength testing, 30
  after total hip replacement, 343
  trigger points for, 25, 30, 47
  visceral, 24-25, *26*, 369
Pallor, assessment of, 19
Palmar fascia, Dupuytren's contracture of, 445-446
Palpation
  ankle, *262b*
  pain or tenderness on, 30
  of pain trigger points, 25
  of plantar fascia, 277
Paraffin, 40-41
Paratenon, 187
Parrot-beak tear of meniscus, *306*
Pars interarticularis, fractures and defects of, 374-375
Partial weight bearing (PWB), 225
Passive osteoconduction, 158
Patella
  biomechanical function of, 253
  fractures of
    treatment of, 315, 317, 326
    types of, *317*, 325
  lateral compression and tracking disorders of
    description of, 310-311
    nonoperative rehabilitation for, 311-313
    postoperative rehabilitation for, 313-315
  mobilization of
    glides for, 323-324
    after total knee replacement, 322
  postures of, 310, 325
  resurfacing, 320-321
  stretching
    after ACL reconstruction, 295, *296*, 299
    after tibial osteotomy, 322
    for tracking disorders, *312*
Patellofemoral joint
  cartilage defects at, exercises for, 166
  compression of, resistance exercise and, *84*
  mobilization of, 323-324
  pathologies of, 309-315
    additional features for, 325, 326
    compression and tracking, 310-311
    rehabilitation for, 312-315
Pathologic fractures, 152-153
Patient supervision
  additional features for, 10
  basic skills for, 6-8
  components of, 4
  by rehabilitation team, 4-6
  treatment modifications during, 8-9

Pause, description of, 7
PCL injuries. *See* Posterior cruciate ligament (PCL) injuries.
Pectorals, stretching
    for kyphosis, 380
    for thoracic outlet syndrome, *386*
Pelvic "list" in gait mechanics, 221
Pelvic tilt
    for low back problems, *361*
    after lumbar discectomy, 373
    for spinal stenosis, 374
Pelvis
    contusions of, 349-350
    fractures of, 350-353
    gait and rotation of, 221
Penicillins, 208-209
Peptic ulcers, NSAIDs and, 212
Perimysium, 76, 125, 176
Perineurium, 194, *195*
Periodization of strength training, 89-90, *91*, 94
Peripheral arterial disease (PAD), 24
Peripheral nervous system (PNS), injury to, 194-198.
        See also Nerves, peripheral.
Peripheralization of pain
    assessment of, 24
    definition of, 23
    in lumbar disc herniation, 370
Peroneal tendons, subluxing, 262, 266-268
Peroneus brevis muscle, rerouting, 265, *266*
Peroxisomes, 128
Pes planus and cavus, 278-279
Pharmacodynamics, 208
Pharmacokinetics, 208, 214
Pharmacology, definitions in, 208, 214. *See also*
    Medications.
Phonophoresis
    for Achilles tendinitis, 269
    description of, 43
Phospholipids
    in extracellular matrix, 124
    inflammatory mediators from, 130, *131, 211*
Physeal plates
    fractures of, *152*
    injury to, weight lifting and, 92
Physical agents
    additional features for, 53-54
    APTA guidelines for, 38
    documentation for, 53
    electrical, 47-53
    evidence for efficacy of, 38
    inflammation and use of, 15
    thermal, 39
        cold, 45-47
        combination, 47
        hot, 39-45
Physical assessment
    APTA guiding documents for, 14-15
    documentation of, 33-34
    of edema, 19-21
    of fatigue, 28
    of inflammation, 15-17
    of musculoskeletal structures, 29-33
    of pain, 21-26
    of redness and skin color changes, 18-19
    scales of measurement for, 4, *5b*
    of temperature, 17-18
    of vital signs, 26-28
Physical capacity assessments (PCAs), 376-378

Physical therapy (PT). *See also* Rehabilitation.
    APTA guiding documents for, 14-15
    criterion-based programs in, 257
    pain control in, 49
    philosophical differences in, 10
    physical agent use in, 38
    PTA's role in, 4, 14
    therapist-assistant relationship in, 15, *16*
Physioball
    balance training on, *112*, 113, *114*
    for glenohumeral stabilization, 400, *403*
    for lumbar spinal strengthening, *366*, 367
Physiologic joint motions, 230, 231-232
Piccolo traction, 232, 233
Piezoelectric effect
    bone remodeling and, 150, 153, 158
    description of, 159
Pigmentation, skin, 19
Pilon fractures, 274-275
Pins
    for acromioclavicular stabilization, *407*
    for wrist sprains, 440, *441*
Pitting edema, 20, 21
Pivot shift test for ACL stability, 293
Plan, SOAP documentation for, 34
Planes, cardinal
    illustration of, *241*
    movements in, 240-241, *242-243*
Plantar fasciitis, 277-278
Plantar flexion
    for Achilles tendon injuries, 269, 270-271
    after ankle fractures, 274
    for ankle instabilities, 265-266
    after calcaneal fractures, 275
    gait and, 221, *222*
    illustration of, *243*
    for lateral ankle sprains, 103, *104, 260, 263*
    measurement of, *5b*
    after peroneal tendon repair, 268
Plantar interdigital neuroma, 279-280
Plasma cells, *121*
Plastic deformation
    description of, 58, *60*
    failure point for, 250, *252*
Platelet plug, formation of, 117, 125, *126, 127*
Platelet-derived growth factors (PDGF)
    in muscle healing, 180
    in tissue healing, 125, 130, 132
Pleuritic pain, 201
Plyoball. *See* Physioball.
Plyometrics
    description of, 87-88
    impulse inertial system for, 94
    after peroneal tendon repair, 268
Pneumatic compression, intermittent, 201
PNF. *See* Proprioceptive neuromuscular facilitation (PNF).
Point of application of force, 245, *246*
Polar fractures of patella, *316*
Polymethylmethacrylate (PMMA) cement
    antibiotic-impregnated, 210, 211
    for hip prosthesis, 343
    for knee prosthesis, 321
Polymorphism, muscle fiber, 184-185
Polymorphonuclear (PMN) leukocytes, *119*, 128, 138
Polysaccharide glycocalyx, *210*
Position, potential energy and, 252
Position sense, 108

Positive talar tilt, 283
Posterior, definition of, 240*b*
Posterior compartments of lower leg, 272
Posterior cruciate ligament (PCL) injuries
    ACL injuries with, 300
    clinical examination of, 300-301, *302*
    management and rehabilitation for, 301-303
    mechanisms of, 300, *301*
    repair and healing of, 139
Posterior tibial artery, 283
Postural extension, "all fours," 372
Postural kyphosis, 379-380
Postural stress test (PST), 109
Posture
    enhancement of
        for cervical sprains and strains, 383-384
        for kyphosis, 380
        for spinal stenosis, 374
        for thoracic outlet syndrome, 386
    maintaining lordotic
        lifting and, 363
        lumbar disc injuries and, *370*, 371-372
        lumbar sprains and, 368
Potential energy, 252
Power, definition of, 79, 244. *See also* Strength.
PRE. *See* Progressive resistive exercise (PRE).
Pregnancy, physical agent use during, 40, 44, 52
Press-ups for rotator cuff impingement, *395*
Pressure
    definition of, 244
    force and, 250
    intrathoracic, exercise and, 105
    lumbar intradiscal, 360-361
    mechanoreceptors for, 108
Primary cortical healing, 153, 154
Primary varus, tibiofemoral, 325
Proactive supervision, 6, 10
Probing questions, 6, *7*, 10
Pro-glide appliance for stretching, 69, *70*
Progressive balance training, 110-113, *114*
Progressive resistive exercise (PRE)
    Davies model for, 81*b*
    muscle contractions types in, 80-81
    protocols for, 85-87
    therapeutic parameters for, 82*b*
Prolapsed disc, 369, 378
Proline in collagen, 164
Prompting, cueing vs., 8
Pronation exercise for lateral epicondylitis, 423, *424*
Pronation-abduction/lateral rotation injuries of ankle, *273*
Pronator syndrome, 433
Prone extension exercises
    for kyphosis, 380
    for lumbar disc injuries, *370*, 371
    for lumbar sprains or strains, 365, *366*, 367, 368
    for thoracic muscle injuries, 378, *379*
Prophylaxis, preoperative antibiotic, 209
Proprioception
    description of, 108, 115
    exercises for
        after Achilles tendon rupture, 270, *271*
        after ACL reconstruction, 297, *299*
        for adhesive capsulitis of shoulder, 405
        for ankle sprains or instability, 263, *264*, 266, *267*
        for glenohumeral stabilization, 400, *402*, *403*, 404
        after knee fractures, 318, 320-321
        after peroneal tendon repair, 268

Proprioception—cont'd
        after subtotal meniscectomy, 308
        after total hip replacement, 345
        for upper extremity, 113, *114*
    functional training for, 110
Proprioceptive closed-chain neuromuscular training, 94
Proprioceptive neuromuscular facilitation (PNF), 59, 62-63, *64-65*
Prostaglandins
    inflammation and, 117, 130, 212
    inhibition of, *211*, 212, *213*
    synthesis of, *131*
Prostheses
    for ACL reconstruction, 294
    hip
        fixation of, 343
        types of, 342, 343, 354
    infection prevention for, 210-211
    knee, 320-321
    metal
        bacterial adherence to, *210*
        diathermy and, 45
        electrical stimulation and, 53
    proximal humeral, *413*
    total shoulder, 412-413
Protected motion
    for ligament healing, 142, *143*, 144
    for tendon healing, 189
Proteoglycans
    in articular cartilage, 163, 164
    in connective tissue, 124, 128
    oral administration of, 169-170
Protocols, rehabilitation, 257, 295
Protrusion, disc, 369, 378
Proximal, definition of, 240*b*
Proximal femoral osteotomy, 341-342
Proximal fractures, *115*
    of humerus, 410-412
    of tibia, 318-320
Proximal interphalangeal (PIP) joint
    flexion deformity of, 447
    mobilization of, 283
Proximal realignment of patella, 314
Psychogenic low back pain, 369
Pubic rami fractures, 350, *351*
Pulling, friction and, *249*
Pulmonary embolism (PE), 200, 201
Pulse, assessment of, 5*b*, 26. *See also* Heart rate.
Pulse oximetry, 27-28
Pulsed short wave diathermy (PSWD), 44
Pulsed ultrasound, effects of, 41, 42
Push-ups
    armchair, *339*
    standing wall, 400, *403*

Q
Q4 behavioral model, 6, 8, *9*
Quad canes, 226
Quadriceps
    eccentric contraction of, 77, *78*
    gait mechanics and, 223*t*, 224*t*
    strengthening
        after ACL reconstruction, 296, 297, *298*, 299
        after knee fractures, 315, 317, 318
        after MCL injury, 305
        for patellofemoral conditions, 312-313, 314, 315
        after PCL injury or repair, 301-302, 303
        after tibial osteotomy, 323

Quadriceps angle (Q angle), 310, *311*
Quadriceps "set"
    isometric contraction in, 77
    knee extension stretch with, 68, *69*
Quinolones, 209

R

Radial acceleration, 245
Radial deviation, *242*
Radial head fractures, 429-430, *431*, 432
Radial zone of articular cartilage, 163*t*
Radiation, heat transmission by, 44, 54
Radical surgeries for patellar realignment, 314-315
Radicular signs
    in lumbar disc herniation, 362, 370, 371, 372
    in lumbar strains, 366
Radius, distal fractures of, 441-442, *443*
Range of motion (ROM). *See also* Mobilization, joint; Stretching.
    ankle, testing, 262*b*
    capsular/noncapsular patterns of, 233, 234
    definition of, 58
    end-feel during, 29, 30, 32, 232-233, 234
    exercises for
        after ACL reconstruction, 295-296, 297, 299
        for adhesive capsulitis of shoulder, 405
        for ankle sprains, 263
        after ankle stabilization surgery, 265-266
        after articular cartilage repair, 166-167
        for carpal tunnel syndrome, 438-439
        for cervical sprains and strains, 383
        after clavicular fractures, 409-410
        for De Quervain's tenosynovitis, 439
        after flexor tendon repair of hand, 447-448
        for glenohumeral instability/dislocation, 398-399, 403-404
        after high tibial osteotomy, 323
        after hip fractures, 338, *339-340*
        for hip soft-tissue injuries, 346-347, 348, 349
        after intercondylar humerus fractures, 429
        after knee arthroplasty, *321*
        after lumbar discectomy, 373
        for medial valgus stress overload, 426
        after meniscal surgeries, 171-172, 308, 309
        for Morton's neuroma, 279-280
        during muscle healing, 186, 186*b*
        after olecranon fracture-dislocation, 431
        after palmar fasciectomy, 445, 446
        after patellar realignment, 314
        after PCL injury or repair, 302, 303
        after pelvic fractures, 351
        after peripheral nerve repair, 197-198
        after radial head fractures, 430
        after rotator cuff repair, 396, 397
        after shoulder arthroplasty, 413
        after supracondylar humerus fractures, 427
        for wrist sprains, 440, 441*b*
    grades for, 231-232, 234
    measurement of, 5*b*, 31, 71
    movement patterns for, *242-243*
    physiologic vs. accessory motion during, 230
    after total hip arthroplasty, 345, 354
Rating of Perceived Exertion (RPE), 28
Reach test, 109
Reaction, Newton's law of, 249
Reactive hyperemia, 94
Reciprocal inhibition in PNF stretching, 63
Recognition of patient status changes, 9
Record keeping. *See* Documentation.

Recovery. *See also* Rest.
    active, 102
    connective tissue, property of, 58
Redness, skin
    assessment of, 18-19
    inflammation and, 16, 117, *119*, 212
"Red-on red" and "red-on-white" zones, meniscal tears in, 171, 172, 307
Referred pain, 24
Reflective statement, *7*
Reflex, stretch
    measurement of, 5*b*
    sensory receptors involved in, 62, *63, 64,* 72
Reflex muscle guarding, 52, *66*
Reflex sympathetic dystrophy (RSD), 448
Regeneration
    peripheral nerve, 180
    tissue, process of, *120, 127,* 134, 135
Rehabilitation
    ankle/foot
        for Achilles rupture, 270-271, *272*
        for Achilles tendinitis, 268-269
        for plantar fasciitis, 278
        for sprains, 262-265
        after stabilization surgery, 265-266
        for subluxing peroneal tendons, 267-268
        for toe deformities, 280, 281
    during bone healing, 148, 159
    during cartilage healing, 163, 166-167
    for compartment syndromes of lower leg, 272
    criterion-based programs for, 257
    exercise in, 108
        aerobic, 101-105
        balance training, 110-113, *114*
        strength training, 81*b,* 82*b,* 85-90, 92-94
        stretching, 59-71, *72*
    hip
        post-fracture, 338-340, *341*
        after proximal femoral osteotomy, 342
        after total arthroplasty, 344-345
    joint mobilization techniques in, 233-234
    knee
        after ACL reconstruction, 295-300
        isokinetic protocol for, 93*b*
        isotonic modifications for, 9*b*
        for MCL injuries, 304-305
        after meniscal injury/repair, 163, 171-172, 308-309
        for patellofemoral conditions, 311-315
        for PCL injuries, 301-303
        after total arthroplasty, 321-322
    during ligament healing, 141-144
    for lumbar disc herniation, 369-373
    modifications during, 8-9
    during muscle healing, 185-186
    after peripheral nerve injury, 198, 201
    shoulder
        for glenohumeral instability/dislocation, 398-400, *401,* 402-404
        for rotator cuff impingement/tears, 393-394, 396-397
    during tendon healing, 188
    for wrist sprains, 440, 441*b*
Rehabilitation team
    patient supervision by, 4-6
    philosophical differences in, 10
Remodeling
    bone
        fracture healing and, 154, 158, 159

Remodeling—cont'd
    immobilization and, 154-155
    mechanical stress and, 149-150, 153, 276
    connective tissue
        adhesions or contractures in, 65
        description of, 72, 135
        duration of, *118*
        processes during, 118, *120*, 125, *127*, 128
    in ligament healing, 138, 145
    in tendon healing, 187
Repetitions, exercise
    periodization program for, 89-90, *91*
    rule of tens for, 86
    therapeutic parameters for, 82*b*
Repetitive motion injuries of wrist and hand, 438-439. *See also*
        Overuse injuries.
Resistance
    levers and, 247-248
    low-load, prolonged stretch with, *66*, *68*
    therapeutic parameters for, 82*b*
Resistance training. *See* Strength training.
Resistive torque, 247-248
Respirations, assessment of, 5*b*, 26-27
Responsibility for patient care, 4, 10
Rest
    in interval training, 102
    in periodization program, 89, *90*
    in RICE program, 262-263 (*See also* RICE)
    rule of tens for, 86
    therapeutic parameters for, 82*b*
Resting heart rate (RHR), 100-101
Resurfacing, patellar, 320-321
"Reverse Colles's fracture," 441-442, *443*
Reversibility of training, 61-62, 83
Rheumatoid arthritis, joint replacement for, 320, 343, 413
RICE
    after ACL reconstruction, 295
    for ankle sprains, 262-263, 265
    for MCL sprains, 305
    for muscle healing, 186
    after PCL injury, 302
    for tendon healing, 187
Rigid internal fixation. *See* Internal fixation devices; Open
        reduction with internal fixation (ORIF).
Rods, intramedullary
    for fracture fixation, 155, 158*t*
    for hip fractures, *337*
Roll, joint motion via, 230, *231*
ROM. *See* Range of motion (ROM).
Rotary force, 79
Rotation
    ankle and pelvic, gait and, 221, *222*
    biomechanics of, 244-245, *246*
    hip
        post-fracture, *339*
        test for external, 71, *72*
        after total arthroplasty, 343, 344
    illustrations of, *242*, *243*
    joint, measurement of, 5*b*
    shoulder
        glenohumeral instability and, 399, 403-404
        for rotator cuff impingement, *395*
Rotator cuff
    impingement or tears of, 393-394
        Neer's stages for, 393, 415
        rehabilitation for, 394-395
        surgical management of, 396-397, 413

Rotator cuff—cont'd
    "SITS" muscles of, 415
    strengthening, for glenohumeral stabilization, 399
Rough endoplasmic reticulum, 128
Rowing machines
    aerobic training on, 103
    scapular strengthening on, *379*, 380
RSD. *See* Reflex sympathetic dystrophy (RSD).
Rubber band traction of hand, *447*
Ruffini mechanoreceptors, 108
Rule of tens in isometric exercise, 86
Running
    after ACL reconstruction, 299, 300
    after peroneal tendon repair, 268
    velocity and acceleration changes during, *244*
Russian stimulation, 51-52

S
Sagittal axis, movement around, 240-241
Sagittal plane
    description of, 240, *241*
    movements in, 241, *242*, *243*
SAID principle for strength training, 81-82, 94
Salter-Harris fractures, 152
Sarcolemma, *76*, 176
Sarcomeres
    definition of, 76
    immobilization effects on, 185
    structure of, *77*, 177
Sarcoplasmic reticulum, 176
Satellite cells in muscle healing, 180
Scalene stretch for thoracic outlet syndrome, *386*
Scaphoid fractures, 442-444
Scapholunate advanced collapse, 449
Scaption for rotator cuff impingement, *395*
Scapular fractures, 408-409
Scapular muscles, strengthening
    for kyphosis, 380
    for thoracic spinal muscle injuries, 378, *379*
Scapular stabilization exercises
    for adhesive capsulitis, 405
    for glenohumeral instability/dislocation, 399, 404
    for proximal humerus fractures, 410
    for rotator cuff impingement, 394, 395, 397
    after shoulder arthroplasty, 413
Scapulothoracic joint, mobilization of, 414
Scar tissue
    formation and maturation of, 122*b*
    massage of, 446
    in muscle healing, 179
    remodeling of, *127*, 128
    stretching contractures from, 65, *66*
    in tendon healing, 188
    tissue repair by, 134
Sciatica
    lumbar disc herniation with, 362, 370, 371, 372
    lumbar strains with, 366
Scoliosis, 380-382, *383*
"Scooping" of tibiofemoral joint, 325
Screws
    for acromioclavicular stabilization, *408*
    for ankle fracture, *274*
    for fracture fixation, 155, 157, 158*t*
    for hip fracture, *337*
    for intercondylar humerus fractures, 428, *429*
Secondary fracture healing, 153, 154
Second-class lever, 247

Sensory nerves
    assessing recovery of, 198
    injury to, 194
    regeneration of, 180
Sequestrated disc, 369
Serotonin, tissue injury and, 117
Sesamoiditis, 283
Sets
    in isometric contractions, 77
    periodization program for, 89-90, *91*
    therapeutic parameters for, *82b*
Shear
    description of, 234
    effects of, 250, *251*
"Shin splints," 276
Shoes
    coefficient of friction for, *249b*
    toe deformities from, 280, *281*
Short wave diathermy, 44-45, 54
Shoulder
    acromioclavicular sprains/dislocations of,
        405-408
    additional features for, 415
    adhesive capsulitis of, 404-405
    fractures of
        clavicular, 409-410
        proximal humeral, 410-413
        scapular, 408-409
    glenohumeral instability/dislocation of, 397-404
    mobilization of, 405, 413-414, *415*
    movement patterns for, *242*
    multiangle isometric abduction of, *86*
    range of motion in, *5b*
    rotator cuff impingement of, 393-397
    stabilization of, cervical stretch and, 383
    stretching exercises for, 69, *70*, *71*, 380
    total arthroplasty of, 412-413
Shoulder press for glenohumeral stabilization,
    399, *400*
Simple fractures, 152
Single support in gait cycle, 220
Single-leg stance test (SLST), 109
Single-leg static balance training
    for ankle sprains/instability, *264*, *267*
    description of, 110, *111b*
Sit and reach test, *71*
Sitting, lumbar disc injuries and, 371, *372*, *373*
Sit-ups
    partial, for lumbar spine, *361*, 366, *367*, 374
    physioball, balance training with, *112*, 113
    side-lying, for scoliosis, 382, *383*
"Size principle" in motor unit recruitment, 181, 184
Skeletal muscles. *See* Muscles.
Skier's thumb, 444
Skin
    assessment of, heat application and, 39, *40b*, 45
    preparation of, electrical stimulation and, 48
Skin color
    assessing changes in, 18-19
    inflammation and, 16, 117, *119*, 212
    reflex sympathetic dystrophy and, 448
Slack, joint, 232
SLAP lesion of glenoid labrum, 415
Slide, joint motion via, 230
Slide board
    hip abduction/adduction on, *349*
    shoulder exercises on, *401*

Slings
    for acromioclavicular injuries, 406
    for intercondylar humerus fracture, 429
    for proximal humerus fractures, 410
    for scapular fractures, 408, 409
Slipped capital femoral epiphysis (SCFE), 354
"Slipped disc." *See* Herniated nucleus pulposus (HNP).
Slow twitch (ST) muscle fibers
    description of, 77, 94
    exercise and adaptation of, 83, 181, 185
    immobilization effects on, 185
    types of, 177-178
Slow-reversal-hold in PNF stretching, 63, *65*
Smith's fracture, 441-442, *443*
Smoking, bone healing and, 158
Smooth endoplasmic reticulum, 128
Smooth muscle, vascular, 198
"Snuffbox," anatomic, 443, 449
SOAP documentation format, 34
Soft callus, formation of, 154, 156
"Soft" signs of arterial injury, 199, 201
Soft-tissue approximation end-feel, 29, 232
Soleus. *See* Gastrocnemius/soleus complex.
Somatosensory system, balance control by, 33
Soreness, delayed onset muscle, 46, 83-84, 176
Sound head, ultrasound, 42
Spasms, muscle, 30, 52, 232
Specificity of training, 61-62, 83
Speed of limb movement, muscle contraction velocity
    and, 84
Spin, joint motion via, 230, *231*
Spinal fusion
    for scoliosis, 382
    for thoracic disc injuries, 378
Spinal nerve root compression, 195, 362
Spinal stenosis, 373-374, 387
Spine. *See* Cervical spine; Lumbar spine; Thoracic spine.
Spine stabilization
    cervical, 383, *384*, *385*
    lumbar, 368, 376
Spiral fractures, 151
Splints
    for ankle fractures, 274
    for carpal tunnel syndrome, 438
    for flexor tendon injuries of hand, *447*
    for fracture stabilization, 157
    for lateral epicondylitis, 422
    after palmar fasciectomy, 445
    physiologic, pain and, 52
    for plantar fasciitis, 278
    for radial head fractures, 430
    for reflex sympathetic dystrophy, 448
    for rotator cuff repair, 397
    after shoulder arthroplasty, 413
    for wrist sprains, 440
Spondylogenic pain, 369
Spondylolisthesis, lumbar, 374-375
Spondylolysis
    cervical, 385
    lumbar, 374-375
Spongy bone, 148-149, 153, 159
Sprains
    acromioclavicular, 405-408
    ankle
        instability after, 265-266, *267*
        lateral, 260-265
        medial, 265

Sprains—cont'd
  cervical spinal, 382-384, *385*
  knee, 290
    anterior cruciate, 290-300, 325
    medial collateral, 303-305, 325
    posterior cruciate, 300-303
  ligament
    assessment of, 32-33
    healing of, 138-139
    remobilization and exercise for, 141-144
    surgical repair of, 139
  lumbar spinal, 367-368
  strains vs., 176
  ulnar collateral, 444
  wrist, 439-440, *441*, 441*b*
"Spray and stretch," 47
Springy block, 232
Springy-tissue stretch end-feel, 232
"Squinting" patellae, 310
Stability
  ankle, tests for, 261, *262*, 262*b*
  description of, 115
  elbow ligament, 433
  fracture fragment, 32
  joint
    factors for, 234
    measuring, 71
  knee, tests for
    ACL, 292-294, 299
    MCL, 304
    PCL, 300-301
  maintaining, principles for, 252-253
  ulnar MCL, test for, *425*
Stabilization, fracture. *See* Fixation, fracture; Open reduction
  with internal fixation (ORIF).
Stair steppers
  aerobic training on, 103
  exercises on
    for glenohumeral stabilization, 400, *401*
    after hip fractures, 338
    for knee sprains, *297, 298, 299, 302*
Stairs, negotiating
  assistive devices for, 225-226
  patellofemoral conditions and, 311-312
Stance phase of gait
  definition of, 220
  divisions of, *220, 222,* 223*t,* 226
  knee flexion in, 221, *222*
Standing hamstring stretch, *60*
Standing toe-touch flexibility test, 71, *72*
Staple capsulorrhaphy for glenohumeral stabilization, 402
Static, definition of, 240
Static balance
  definition of, 108
  progressive exercises for, 110-113, *114*
  tests for, 108-109
Static stretching exercises, 59, *60,* 61, *62*
Steady state, drug, 214
Steinman pin for acromioclavicular stabilization, *407*
Stellate fractures of patella, *316*
Stener's lesion, 449
Step length, gait and, 220
Steppage gait, 223, 224*t*
Step-ups, short-arc
  after ACL reconstruction, 297, *298*
  for patellofemoral conditions, *313*
  after PCL injuries, 302

Steroids. *See* Corticosteroids.
Stiffness, knee, after supracondylar fractures, 325
Straight-leg test for nerve root compression, 362
Strain
  definition of, 58, 72
  hip, musculotendinous, 347-349
  mechanical, 250, *251*
  muscle
    causes of, 179
    cervical, 382-384, *385*
    definition of, 176
    delayed onset soreness vs., 83
    lumbar, 364-367
    therapeutic interventions for, 186*b*
    thoracic spinal, 378
  tendon, healing of, 188
Strength
  additional features for, 94
  definition of, 79
  determinants of, 76
  measurement of
    for ankle, 262*b*
    for back, 363-364
    format for recording, 29*b*
    manual muscle testing for, 5*b*, 79*b*
    methods for, 29-30, 79-80
  muscle fiber types and, 77
  ultimate, description of, 72
Strength training
  additional features for, 94
  closed/open kinetic chain exercise for, 88-89
  delayed onset soreness after, 83-84
  electrical stimulation with, 51-52
  endurance training with, 104-105
  equipment for, 92-94
  isotonics vs. isokinetics for, 82*b*
  muscle contraction types in, 77-79, 80-81
  muscle contraction velocity in, 84-85
  during muscle healing, 185-186
  muscular adaptation to, 81-83, 181-183, *185*
  neural adaptation to, 182-183
  for older populations, 90-91
  periodization programs for, 89-90
  plyometrics for, 87-88
  progressive
    Davies model for, 81*b*
    muscle contraction types in, 80-81
    protocols for, 85-87
    therapeutic parameters for, 82*b*
  reducing cardiovascular responses to, 105
  rehabilitation with
    for Achilles tendon injuries, 269, 270-271, *272*
    after ACL reconstruction, 296-300
    for acromioclavicular sprain/dislocation, 407, 408
    for adhesive capsulitis of shoulder, 405
    for ankle sprains or instabilities, 263, 266, *267*
    after calcaneal fractures, 275
    for carpal tunnel syndrome, 438, 439
    for cervical sprains and strains, 383, 384, *385*
    for epicondylitis, 423, *424*
    after fasciotomy of lower leg, 272
    after flexor tendon repair of hand, 447-448
    after foot/ankle stress fractures, 276
    for glenohumeral instability/dislocation, 398, 399-400,
      401, 402, 403, 404
    after high tibial osteotomy, 322
    after hip arthroplasty, 344, *345*

Strength training—cont'd
    after hip fractures, 338, *341*
    for hip soft-tissue injuries, 346, 347, 348-349
    after intercondylar humerus fracture, 429
    after knee fractures, 315, 317, 318, 319-320
    for kyphosis, 379-380
    after lumbar discectomy, 372-373
    after lumbar fractures, 376
    for lumbar spondylolisthesis, 375
    for lumbar sprains or strains, 365-367, 368
    after MCL injuries, 305
    for medial valgus stress overload, 426-427
    after meniscal surgeries, 172, 308, 309
    after metacarpal fractures, 445
    for Morton's neuroma, 280
    after olecranon fracture-dislocation, 431, 432
    for patellofemoral disorders, 312-313, 314, 315
    after PCL injury or repair, 301-302, 303
    after pelvic fractures, 350, 351
    after peroneal tendon repair, 268
    for plantar fasciitis, 278
    after proximal femoral osteotomy, 342
    after proximal humerus fractures, 410, 412
    after radial head fractures, 430
    for rotator cuff impingement, 395
    after rotator cuff repair, 396-397
    for scoliosis, 380-381, 382, *383*
    after shoulder arthroplasty, 413
    for skier's thumb, 444
    after supracondylar humerus fractures, 427-428
    for thoracic muscle injuries, 378, *379*
    for thoracic outlet syndrome, 386
    for wrist sprains, 440, 441*b*
  weight lifting vs., 91-92
  for younger populations, 91-92
Stress
  applying, effects of, 58, *59*, 60
  bone remodeling and, 149-150, 153, 276
  definition of, 58, 72, 253
  mechanical, 250, *251*
Stress fractures
  foot and ankle, 276
  lumbar spinal, 374, 375
  medial tibial, 277
Stress relaxation, nerve tissue and, 194
Stretch reflex
  measurement of, 5*b*
  sensory receptors involved in, 62, *63*, *64*, 72
Stretching
  ballistic, 61-62, *63*
  cold application with, 46, 47
  connective tissue response to, 58-59, *60*
  heat application with, 39
  mechanoreceptors for, 108
  during muscle healing, 186, 186*b*
  muscle hypertrophy and, 83
  neuromuscular response to, 62, *63*, *64*, 72
  pain or tenderness during, 30
  PNF techniques for, 62-63, *64-65*
  rehabilitation with
    for Achilles tendon injuries, 269, 270-271, *272*
    after ACL reconstruction, 295, 296, *297*, 299
    for ankle sprains, 263, *264*
    for cervical sprains and strains, 383, 384, *385*
    for epicondylitis, 422-423, *424*
    after high tibial osteotomy, 322
    after hip fractures, *340*

Stretching—cont'd
    for hip soft-tissue injuries, 346, 347-348, *349*
    for kyphosis, 380
    for lumbar sprains or strains, 365, 368
    for medial tibial stress syndrome, 277
    for medial valgus stress overload, 425
    after palmar fasciectomy, 445
    for patellofemoral conditions, *312*, 313, 315
    for plantar fasciitis, 278
    for rotator cuff impingement/tears, 394-395, 396, 397
    for scoliosis, 380-382
    for thoracic outlet syndrome, 386
  of soft-tissue contractures, 65-71
  static, 59, *60*, 61, *62*
  ultrasound with, 43
Stride length, gait and, 220
Stroke volume, 105
Stromelysins, 179
Subacromial decompression, 396
Subacromial rotator cuff impingement, 393-397, 415
Subchondral bone, cartilage healing and, 166
Subclavian artery/vein, compression of, 385, *386*
Subcutaneous fat
  function of, *121*
  heat conduction by, 40
  impedance of, 48
Subjective data, SOAP documentation for, 34
Subluxation
  glenohumeral, 397-404
  patellofemoral, 325
Subluxing peroneal tendons, 262, 266-268
Submission
  description of, 6, 10
  dimensions of, *8*, *9*
Subtotal meniscectomy, 171, 308
Subtrochanteric hip fractures
  complications of, 336, 354
  types of, 335, *337*
Summary statements, 6, 7, 10
Superficial, definition of, 240*b*
Superficial posterior compartment of lower leg, *272*
Superior, definition of, 240*b*
Supervision, patient. *See* Patient supervision.
Supination exercise for lateral epicondylitis, 423
Supracondylar fractures
  of femur, 317-318, 325
  of humerus, *426*, 427-428
Supraspinatus tendon, rotator cuff impingement and, 393, 394
Surface changes for balance training, 111*b*
Surgical procedures. *See also* Open reduction with internal fixation (ORIF).
  ankle/foot
    for Achilles tendon rupture, 270
    for ankle sprains, 264, 265
    for ankle stabilization, 265, *266*, *267*
    for hallux valgus, 280
    for Morton's neuroma, 279
    for plantar fasciitis, 278
    for subluxing peroneal tendons, 267
    for toe deformities, 281
  antibiotic prophylaxis for, 209
  arterial injuries associated with, 199*t*
  for articular cartilage repair, 166, 167-169
  for compartment syndromes of lower leg, 272
  elbow
    for medial valgus stress overload, 426

Surgical procedures—cont'd
    for olecranon fracture-dislocation, 431, 432
    for radial head fractures, 430
  for fracture fixation and repair, 155, 157, 158
  hip
    for partial joint replacement, 342
    prosthesis fixation in, 343
    proximal femoral, 341-342
    for total joint replacement, 343-345
  knee
    for ACL reconstruction, 294-295
    for meniscal injuries, 171, 308, 309, 325
    for patellofemoral disorders, 313-315
    for PCL reconstruction, 302
    for total joint replacement, 320-322, 326
    for valgus/varus deformities, 322-323
  for ligament repair, 139
  for nerve repair, 197-198, 201
  shoulder
    for acromioclavicular dislocation, 407, *408*
    for glenohumeral stabilization, 400, 402-404
    for rotator cuff impingement/tears, 396-397
    for total joint replacement, 412-413
  spinal
    for cervical cord compression, 385
    for lumbar disc herniation, 372, *373*
    for lumbar spondylolisthesis, 375
    for scoliosis, 382
    for thoracic disc injuries, 378
  for tendon repair, 188
  for vascular repair, 200
  wrist/hand
    for carpal tunnel syndrome, 438-439
    for De Quervain's tenosynovitis, 439
    for Dupuytren's contracture, 445, *446*
    for flexor tendon injuries, 447
    for scaphoid fractures, 443
Sutures, acromioclavicular stabilization with, *408*
Swelling. *See* Edema.
Swing phase of gait
  definition of, 220
  divisions of, *220, 222,* 223*t*
Syndesmosis, 283
Synovial fluid, 164
Systemic inflammation, 135

T

"T" fractures
  intercondylar humeral, 428-429
  supracondylar femur, *317, 318*
Tachyphylaxis, drug, 214
Tachypnea, pulmonary embolism and, 201
Talar fractures, 275
Talar tilt test for ankle stability, 261, *262,* 283
Talofibular ligament tears, *260, 261*
  surgical repair of, 265, *267*
  test for, 261
Talus
  anatomy of, 283
  posterior glide and distraction of, 282
Tandem walking test, 109
Tangential acceleration, 245
Tanner stages of development, 91
Taping ankle sprains, 263, 264
Target circuit, 104
Target heart rate (THR), 100-101
Tarsal tunnel syndrome, 283

Temperature
  assessment of, 17-18
  tissue extensibility and, 58-59, 61
Tenderness, muscle, 30
Tendinitis, 187
  Achilles, 268-269
  elbow, 422-425
  healing of, 187
  rehabilitation techniques for, 188
  rotator cuff, 393-395
  signs of, 31
Tendons
  additional features for, 190
  anatomy of, 187-189
  flexibility of, 30-31
  healing of
    mobilization vs. immobilization and, 189-190
    phases of, 187-189
    rehabilitation techniques during, 189
  injuries of
    in hand or finger, 446-448
    overuse, 31
    types of, 176, 187
  stretching and palpating, 30
  subluxing peroneal, 262, 266-268
"Tennis elbow," 422-424
Tenoblasts and tenocytes, 187, 188
Tenosynovitis, De Quervain's, 439
TENS. *See* Transcutaneous electrical nerve stimulation (TENS).
Tens, rule of, in isometric exercise, 86
Tension
  description of, 234
  mechanical, effects of, 250, *251*
  muscle contraction, 79, 80
Tension-band wires
  for fracture fixation, 157, 158*t*
  for patellar fractures, 315, *317*
Tetracyclines, 209
Thera-band. *See* Elastic bands and cords, exercises with.
Therapists, different philosophies of, 10
Thermal agents, 39. *See also* Ice; RICE.
  application of
    for adhesive capsulitis of shoulder, 405
    for cervical sprains and strains, 383
    for joint mobilization, 281, 353, 449
    for lumbar muscle strains, 364
    for Morton's neuroma, 279
    for stretching exercises, 59, 66, 67, *68*
  cold, 45-47, 53
  combination, 47
  hot, 39-45, 54
"Thermometer" pain rating scale, *23*
Thermotherapy, 39
Third-class lever, 247, *248*
Thompson test for Achilles tendon rupture, 269, *271*
Thoracic outlet syndrome, 385-386
Thoracic spine
  disc injuries of, 378
  kyphosis of, 378-380
  mechanical stress on, 250
  mobilization of, 386-387
  muscle injuries of, 378
  prone extension exercises for, 365, *366, 367*
  scoliosis of, 380-382, *383*
Three-point gait pattern, 224, *225*
Thromboembolic disease, 200-201
  assessment for, 19
  hip surgeries and, 338, 343

Thrombophlebitis, 19
Thromboxanes
    in inflammatory response, 212
    inhibition of, *211*
    synthesis of, 130, *131*
Thumb
    De Quervain's tenosynovitis of, 439
    skier's, 444
Tibia
    anatomy of, 325
    fractures of
        distal compression, 274-275
        proximal, 318-320
    high osteotomy of, 322-323, 325
    medial stress syndrome of, 276-277
Tibial nerve, 283
Tibial plateau fractures, 318-320
Tibial stem and tray, 253
Tibialis anterior, gait mechanics and, 223*t*, 224*t*
Tibialis posterior tendon, rupture of, 283
Tibiofemoral joint
    mobilization of, 324-325
    surgical realignment of, 322-323
Tidemark in articular cartilage, 163*t*
Tilt table for pelvic fractures, 351
Time, movement and, 244
Tissue healing. *See also under* Connective tissue.
    bone, 153-159
    cartilage, 164-172
    inflammation during, 15
    joint mobilization and, 233
    ligament, 138-146
    muscle, 178-180, 185-186
    nerve, 180, 197-198
    review of, 117-118, *119-121,* 122*b*
    RICE program for, 262-263
    tendon, 187-189
    vascular, 198
Tissue inhibitors of metalloproteinases (TIMPS), 179-180
Toe curls
    for Morton's neuroma, 280
    for plantar fasciitis, 278
Toe off in gait cycle, *220,* 222, 223*t*
Toe touch weight bearing (TTWB), 225
Toes
    deformities of, 280-281
    mobilization techniques for, 281-283
    Morton's neuroma of, 279-280
Tolerance, drug, 214
Tone, muscle, 30
Torque
    application of, 246
    definition of, 79, 244
    lifting and, *246*
    resistive, 247, *248*
Torsion, effects of, 250, *251*
Total hip precautions, 343-344
Total joint arthroplasty
    of hip, 343-345, 354
    infections in, 209, 211
    of knee, 320-322, 326
    of shoulder, 413
Touch down weight bearing (TDWB), 225
Towel stretch
    for ankle sprains, *264*
    for knee extension, 68, *69*
Trabecular bone, 148-149, 153, 159

Tracking disorders, patellar
    causes of, 310-311
    nonoperative rehabilitation for, 312-313
    postoperative rehabilitation for, 313-315
Traction. *See also* Distraction.
    for acetabular fractures, 351
    for cervical spondylosis, 385
    for flexor tendon injuries of hand, *447*
    for fracture immobilization, 157
    for hip fractures and dislocations, 336
    in joint mobilization, 232, 233
    for lumbar disc injuries, 371
Traction neuropathy, 195-197
Training heart rate (THR), 100-101
Transcutaneous electrical nerve stimulation (TENS). *See also* Electrical stimulation.
    for edema, 50
    neuromuscular stimulation vs., 51
    for pain, 49-50
Transducer, ultrasound, 42
Transfer training
    after lumbar discectomy, 372
    after total hip replacement, 344
Transforming growth factor β (TGF-β)
    in muscle healing, 180
    in tissue healing, 125, 130, 133*t*
Transition zone of articular cartilage, 163*t*, 172
Translatory motion, biomechanics of, 244-245
Transverse fractures, 151
    patellar, 315, *316*
    physeal, *152*
    supracondylar, *318*
Transverse plane
    description of, 240, *241*
    movements in, *242, 243*
Treadmills
    aerobic training on, 101, *102*
        for glenohumeral stabilization, 400, *401*
        for lumbar strains, 366
        after proximal femoral osteotomy, 342
    standard, *101*
    underwater, *102*
Treatment modifications, 8-9
Trendelenburg gait, 33, 223
Triangular fibrocartilage complex, 449
Tribology, 253
Tricarboxylic acid cycle, 178
Trigger points
    applying cold agents to, 47
    palpation of, 25, 30
Triple varus, tibiofemoral, 326
Tripod gait pattern, 224
Trochanteric bursitis, 346-347
Trochanteric hip fractures, 335, *336,* 337
Tropocollagen, *150*
Troponin and tropomyosin, 77, 177
Trunk, exercises for
    balancing, *112,* 113
    forward bend, *339*
    for lumbar sprains and strains, 365-367, *368*
    for scoliosis, 381-382, *383*
TUBS shoulder instability pattern, 400, 415
Tumor growth, ultrasound and, 43, 44
Tumor necrosis factor (TNF)
    in inflammation, 212, 213
    in tissue healing, 125, 130, 133*t*
Tunica adventitia/media/intima, 179, 198

Two-point gait pattern, 224, *225*
Type I/type II muscle fibers. *See* Fast twitch (FT) muscle fibers; Slow twitch (ST) muscle fibers.

U

Ulna, distal fractures of, 442
Ulnar collateral ligament sprain, 444
Ulnar deviation, *242*
Ulnar tunnel syndrome, 449
Ultimate strength, description of, 72
Ultrasound, 41-44
   application of
      for Achilles tendon injuries, 269, 270
      guidelines for, 43, *44b*
      techniques for, 42-43, 53
   diathermy vs., 45
   duplex, for assessing vascular injury, 200, 201
   effects of, 41, 42
   for fracture healing, 54, 158
   indications for, 41-42
   medication delivery via, 43
   passive stretching with, *43*, 67
   precautions and contraindications for, 43-44
Unadaptable scar, 65
Unipolar femoral prosthesis, 342
Upper body ergometer (UBE), *102, 103*

V

Valgus, hindfoot, 278
Valgus deformity
   hallux, 280
   knee, tibial osteotomy for, 322-323
   after radial head fracture, 430
Valgus stress
   for elbow extension, 432
   thumb sprain from, *444*
   ulnar MCL rupture from, *426*
Valgus stress overload, medial elbow, 425-427
Valgus stress test
   for knee sprains, 304
   for ulnar sprains, *425*
Valsalva maneuver
   blood pressure and, 27
   lifting and, 363
Vapocoolant sprays, 47
Varus, forefoot, 278
Varus deformity
   knee, tibial osteotomy for, 322-323
   after radial head fracture, 430
   tibiofemoral, forms of, 325, *326*
Varus force for elbow flexion, 432-433
"Vascular access channel" for meniscal repair, 171
Vascular claudication, 24, 369, 387
Vascular endothelial growth factor (VEGF), 132, 180
Vascular injury, 198-200
Vascular low back pain, 369
Vascular supply
   of articular cartilage, 164
   of bone, 150, *151*
   of femoral head and neck, 335, *336*, 354
   of intervertebral disc, 368
   of meniscus, 171, 172, 307, *308*
   muscle healing and, 179
   of peripheral nerves, 194, *196*, 201
   of scaphoid, 442, *443*
   of supraspinatus tendon, 393
   of tendon, 185, 187

Vasodilation, tissue healing and, *119*
Vasomotor reflexes, abnormal, 448
Vastus medialis oblique
   strengthening, patellar tracking and, 312-313
   surgical advancement of, 314
Veins
   anatomy of, 198-199
   thrombosis of, 19, 200-201
Velocity
   definition of, 79, 253
   in joint mobilization, 231
   joint motion, mechanoreceptors for, 108
   kinetic energy and, 252
   linear and angular, 245
   movement and, 244
   muscle contraction, 84-85
   running and changes in, *244*
Velocity spectrum training, 84-85
Vertebrae. *See also* Cervical spine; Lumbar spine; Thoracic spine.
   compression and tension stresses on, 250, *251*
   compression fractures of
      lumbar, 375-376
      pain with, 31-32
Vestibular system, balance control by, 33
Virchow's triad, 200, 202
Visceral pain
   assessment of, 24-25
   low back dysfunction and, 369
   transmission of, *26*
Viscoelastic properties
   of connective tissue, 58-59, *60*, 125
   description of, 72
   of peripheral nerves, 194
Vision, balance and, 33, 110
Visual analog scales for pain, *23*
Vital signs
   assessment of, 17, 26-28
   exercise and, 28, 105
   monitoring, pelvic fractures and, 351
Volkmann's ischemic contracture, *427*
Volume, definition of, 244
Volumetrics, edema measurement using, 19, 20

W

Walkers, 226
Walking. *See also* Gait.
   assessing gait during, 33
   for lumbar strains, 366
Wall pulleys, 93, 400
Wall slides
   after ACL reconstruction, 297, *298*
   for knee flexion, *67*
   after total knee replacement, *322*
Wands, stretching exercises with, 69, *70*
Warfarin, 201
Warmth (behavioral)
   description of, 6, 10
   dimensions of, *8, 9*
Warm-up, pre-exercise, 59, 61, 62
"Watershed zone" of supraspinatus tendon, 393
Weakness, muscle
   gait abnormalities and, 223-224, *224t*
   lumbar nerves and, 387
Weight, mass vs., 244
Weight bearing, 224-225
   after ACL reconstruction, 296, 297
   after articular cartilage injury, 166, 167

Weight bearing—cont'd
    after hip arthroplasty, 343, 344
    after hip fractures and dislocations, 336, 338
    after meniscal surgeries, 172, 308, 309
    after PCL injury or repair, 302, 303
    after pelvic fractures, 350, 351
    after pilon fractures, 274-275
    after proximal femoral osteotomy, 342
Weight bearing as tolerated (WBAT), 225
Weight lifting. *See also* Strength training.
    injuries from, 92
    lumbar spondylolisthesis and, 375
    strength training vs., 91-92
Weight-pulley system for balance testing, 109
Weights
    knee extension stretch with, *66, 68*
    types of, 92, 93
"Whiplash," 382
Whirlpool therapy
    for elbow fractures, 429, 430
    after palmar fasciectomy, 445
"White-on-white" zone, meniscal tears in, 171, 172, 307, *308*
Williams flexion exercises for back, *361*, 374
Wobble board, balance training on, 111, *112, 113*
    after Achilles tendon rupture, *271*
    after ACL reconstruction, *299*
    for ankle sprains, *264*
    for glenohumeral stabilization, 400, *402*
Wolff's law, 149-150, 153
Work, definition of, 79, 244

Work:rest ratio in interval training, 102
Woven bone, 148
Wrist
    carpal tunnel syndrome of, 438-439
    De Quervain's tenosynovitis of, 439
    ligament injuries of, 439-440, *441*, 441*b*
    mobilization of, 448-449
    movement patterns for, *242*
    scaphoid fractures of, 442-444
    strengthening exercises for, 423, *424*
Wrist cock-up splints
    for carpal tunnel syndrome, 438
    for lateral epicondylitis, 422
Wrist extensors
    common origin of, 433
    overuse injury of, 422-424
Wrist flexors, overuse injury of, 424-425

Y

"Y" fractures
    intercondylar humeral, 428-429
    supracondylar femur, *317, 318*
Young's modulus of elasticity, 72

Z

Z-line of sarcomere, *77*, 177
Zones
    articular cartilage, 163, 172
    meniscus vascular, 171, 172, 307, *308*